Elbow Ulnar Collateral Ligament Injury

Joshua S. Dines
Christopher L. Camp • David W. Altchek
Editors

Elbow Ulnar Collateral Ligament Injury

A Guide to Diagnosis and Treatment

Second Edition

Springer

Editors
Joshua S. Dines
Department of Orthopedic Surgery
Hospital for Special Surgery
New York, NY
USA

Christopher L. Camp
Department of Orthopedic Surgery
Mayo Clinic
Rochester, MN
USA

David W. Altchek
Department of Orthopedic Surgery
Hospital for Special Surgery
New York, NY
USA

ISBN 978-3-030-69566-8 ISBN 978-3-030-69567-5 (eBook)
https://doi.org/10.1007/978-3-030-69567-5

This Springer imprint is published by the registered company Springer Nature Switzerland AG
The registered company address is: Gewerbestrasse 11, 6330 Cham, Switzerland

Foreword

I can think of few textbooks more timely in the field of sports medicine than the following on elbow ulnar collateral ligament injuries. The first edition was written in 2014 and it was prior to the 2014 season during which two of the forefathers of baseball medicine passed away: Dr. Frank Jobe and Dr. Lewis Yocum. Now, in 2020, the topic of UCL injuries is no less relevant.

I can think of no better tribute to these men than this book which features chapters written by many of their former students, fellows, and colleagues. David and Josh, the editors, have assembled all of the current thought leaders in the field to address the topic of ulnar collateral ligament (UCL) injury in a more thorough way than has been done before. Not only does the monograph cover the basics like exam and imaging of the elbow in a thorough and readable way but it also tackles complicated topics such as revision UCL reconstruction and UCL reconstruction in high school athletes. Furthermore, there is an outstanding section on nonoperative treatment as well as postoperative rehabilitation, which will surely be of interest to surgeons and non-surgeons alike.

As UCL injuries continue to be more common, I am confident that this book will find its way on to the shelves of all doctors, therapists, and trainers who treat these injuries.

Neal S. ElAttrache,
Kerlan-Jobe Orthopaedic Clinic
Los Angeles, CA, USA

Preface

Since the initial description of elbow ulnar collateral ligament reconstruction by Dr. Frank Jobe, the use of the procedure to save the careers of baseball players (and other athletes) at all levels of play has increased exponentially. Our initial edition focused on helping doctors, therapists, and trainers learn more about the diagnosis and treatment of injuries of the UCL. To that end, we assembled a world-class group of authors to review the biomechanics and pathophysiology of throwing injuries. Keys to performing a physical exam in this unique group of patients were highlighted in the text as were pearls to interpreting imaging studies. Ample coverage was given to the variety of techniques that have been used to reconstruct the UCL since Dr. Jobe's initial description of the technique that he used to reconstruct pitcher Tommy John's ligament.

For this second edition of the book, many of the original contributor groups are back with additional chapters on the use of novel repair techniques, the use of biologics to prevent surgery, and advanced thoughts on injury prevention and recovery. We hope that this book helps readers gain a better understanding of UCL injuries with the goal of not only improving outcomes after UCL reconstruction but also preventing these injuries.

New York, NY, USA — Joshua S. Dines
Rochester, MN, USA — Christopher L. Camp
New York, NY, USA — David W. Altchek

Contents

Contributors

Christopher S. Ahmad, MD New York Yankees, Center for Shoulder, Elbow, and Sports Medicine, Columbia University Irving Medical Center, New York, NY, USA

Frank J. Alexander, MS, ATC Center for Shoulder, Elbow, and Sports Medicine, Columbia University Irving Medical Center, New York, NY, USA

David W. Altchek, MD Sports Medicine and Shoulder Service, Hospital for Special Surgery, New York, NY, USA

Department of Orthopedic Surgery, Sports Medicine and Shoulder Service, Sports Medicine Institute, Hospital for Special Surgery, New York, NY, USA

Alex J. Anatone, MD Hospital for Special Surgery, New York, NY, USA

Michael E. Angeline, MD Mercy Health System, Janesville, WI, USA

John M. Apostolakos, MD, MPH Department of Orthopedic Surgery, Sports Medicine and Shoulder Service, Sports Medicine Institute, Hospital for Special Surgery, New York, NY, USA

Abigail Bacharach, MS Orthopaedics Department, Hospital for Special Surgery, New York, NY, USA

Asheesh Bedi, MD Department of Orthopaedic Surgery, University of Michigan, Ann Arbor, MI, USA

Alexandra D. Berger, BA University of Miami, Jupiter, FL, USA

Alexander M. Brown, MD American Sports Medicine Institute, Andrews Sports Medicine and Orthopaedic Center, Birmingham, AL, USA

Curtis Bush, MD Texas Orthopedic Associates, Fort Worth, TX, USA

E. Lyle Cain, MD American Sports Medicine Institute, Andrews Sports Medicine and Orthopaedic Center, Birmingham, AL, USA

Christopher L. Camp, MD Department of Orthopedic Surgery, Mayo Clinic, Rochester, MN, USA

James B. Carr II, MD Sports Medicine Institute, Hospital for Special Surgery, West Palm Beach, FL, USA

Peter N. Chalmers, MD Department of Orthopaedic Surgery, University of Utah, Salt Lake City, UT, USA

Christopher Chin, BS Sports Medicine and Shoulder Service, Hospital for Special Surgery, New York, NY, USA

Joseph H. Choi, MD Orthopaedic Surgery, Seton Hall Orthopedics, Paterson, NJ, USA

Alexander Christ, MD Hospital for Special Surgery, New York, NY, USA

Garrett V. Christensen, BS Department of Othopaedic Surgery, University of Utah, Salt Lake City, UT, USA

Michael C. Ciccotti, MD Orthopaedics Sports Medicine Fellow, The Steadman Clinic and Steadman Philippon Research Institute, Vail, CO, USA

Michael G. Ciccotti, MD The Everett J. and Marian Gordon Professor of Orthopaedic Surgery, Division of Sports Medicine, The Rothman Institute, Thomas Jefferon University, Philadelphia, PA, USA

Stan A. Conte, PT, DPT, ATC Conte Sport Performance Therapy, Scottsdale, AZ, USA

John E. Conway, MD TCU Baseball, Texas Orthopedic Associates, LLP, Fort Worth, TX, USA

John V. Crues III, MD, MS RadNet, Inc., Los Angeles, CA, USA

Terrence S. Daley-Lindo, MD Department of Orthopedics, Orlando Health, Orlando, FL, USA

Elizabeth R. Dennis, MD Department of Orthopaedic Surgery, Hospital for Special Surgery, New York, NY, USA

David M. Dines, MD Orthopaedic Surgery, Sports Medicine and Shoulder Service, Hospital for Special Surgery, New York, NY, USA

Joshua S. Dines, MD Department of Orthopedic Surgery, Sports Medicine and Shoulder Service, Sports Medicine Institute, Hospital for Special Surgery, New York, NY, USA

Christopher C. Dodson, MD Rothman Institute, Philadelphia, PA, USA

Brittany Dowling, MS Sports Performance Center, Midwest Orthopaedics at Rush, Chicago, IL, USA

Jeffrey R. Dugas, MD Andrews Sports Medicine and Orthopaedic Center, Birmingham, AL, USA

L. T. C. Josef K. Eichinger, MD Shoulder and Elbow Surgery, Department of Orthopaedics, Medical University of South Carolina, Charleston, SC, USA

Neal S. ElAttrache, MD Kerlan-Jobe Orthopaedic Clinic, Los Angeles, CA, USA

Todd S. Ellenbecker, DPT, MS, SCS, OCS, CSCS Medical Services ATP Tour, Rehab Plus Sports Therapy Scottsdale, Scottsdale, AZ, USA

Brandon J. Erickson, MD Department of Sports Medicine, Rothman Orthopaedic Institute, New York, NY, USA

Rachel Faber, MD Department of Orthopaedics, Orlando Regional Medical Center, Orlando, FL, USA

Lauren M. Fabian, MD Orthopaedic Specialty Group, Fairfield, CT, USA

Larry D. Field, MD Upper Extremity Service and Sports Medicine Program, Mississippi Sports Medicine and Orthopaedic Center, Jackson, MS, USA

Michael A. Flaherty, MD The Bone and Joint Center, Capital Region Orthopaedics Group, Albany, NY, USA

Salvatore J. Frangiamore, MD, MS Cleveland Clinic Sports Medicine, Cleveland Clinic Foundation, Garfield Heights, OH, USA

Jan Fritz, MD Radiology and Imaging, MRI Division, Hospital for Special Surgery, New York, NY, USA

Elizabeth C. Gardner, MD Department of Orthopaedic Surgery, Yale University, New Haven, CT, USA

Christopher Garrett, MD Department of Orthopaedics, Orlando Health, Orlando, FL, USA

Albert O. Gee, MD Orthopaedics and Sports Medicine, University of Washington Medical Center, Seattle, WA, USA

David C. Gerhardt, MD Andrews Sports Medicine and Orthopaedic Center, Birmingham, AL, USA

Brian Grawe, MD Department of Orthopaedics and Sports Medicine, University of Cincinnati Academic Health Center, Cincinnati, OH, USA

Timothy B. Griffith, MD Peachtree Orthopedics, Atlanta Braves, Atlanta, GA, USA

Eric W. Guo, BS Department of Orthopedic Surgery, Henry Ford Hospital, Detroit, MI, USA

Sheref E. Hassan, MD Orthopedic Surgery and Sports Medicine, Landa Spine and Orthopedic Center, Old Bridge, NJ, USA

Andrew R. Jensen, MD, MBE Department of Orthopaedic Surgery, University of California, Los Angeles, Santa Monica, CA, USA

Matthew D. LaPrade, BS Department of Orthopedic Surgery, Mayo Clinic, Rochester, MN, USA

Xinning Li, MD Sports Medicine and Shoulder Surgery, Department of Orthopaedics, Boston University School of Medicine, Boston, MA, USA

Orr Limpisvasti, MD Kerlan-Jobe Orthopaedic Clinic, Los Angeles, CA, USA

Vincent A. Lizzio, MD Department of Orthopedic Surgery, Henry Ford Hospital, Detroit, MI, USA

Gary M. Lourie, MD The Hand and Upper Extremity Center of Georgia, Atlanta Braves, Atlanta, GA, USA

Brett Lurie, MD Radiology and Imaging, MRI Division, Hospital for Special Surgery, New York, NY, USA

Travis G. Maak, MD Department of Orthopaedic Surgery, University of Utah, Salt Lake City, UT, USA

Leonard C. Macrina, MSPT, SCS, CSCS Champion Physical Therapy, Waltham, MA, USA

Lenny Macrina Co-Founder and Director of Physical Therapy, Champion PT & Performance, Waltham, MA, USA

Eric C. Makhni, MD MBA Department of Orthopedic Surgery, Henry Ford Hospital, Detroit, MI, USA

Joe Manzi, MS Sports Medicine Institute, Hospital for Special Surgery, New York, NY, USA

Kathryn McElheny, MD Sports Medicine Institute, Hospital for Special Surgery, New York, NY, USA

Susie Muir, MD, PhD RadNet, Inc., Los Angeles, CA, USA

Anand M. Murthi, MD Shoulder and Elbow Surgery, MedStar Union Memorial Hospital/Georgetown University School of Medicine, Baltimore, MD, USA

Naveen S. Murthy, MD Department of Radiology, Mayo Clinic, Rochester, MN, USA

Levon N. Nazarian, MD The William E. Conrady, MD Professor of Radiology, Sidney Kimmel Medical College of Thomas Jefferson University, Philadelphia, PA, USA

Fiona E. Nugent, FNP-BC Center for Shoulder, Elbow, and Sports Medicine, Columbia University Irving Medical Center, New York, NY, USA

Michael J. O'Brien, MD Department of Orthopaedics, Tulane University Medical Center, New Orleans, LA, USA

Robert S. O'Connell, MD Department of Orthopaedic Surgery, Virginia Commonwealth University, Richmond, VA, USA

Thomas O'Hagan, MD, MED Rothman Institute, Philadelphia, PA, USA

Daryl C. Osbahr, MD Orlando Health Orthopedic Institute, Orlando, FL, USA

Miguel Pelton, MD Cleveland Clinic Sports Medicine, Cleveland Clinic Foundation, Garfield Heights, OH, USA

William Piwnica-Worms, MS Orthopaedics Department, Hospital for Special Surgery, New York, NY, USA

Hollis G. Potter, MD Radiology and Imaging, MRI Division, Hospital for Special Surgery, New York, NY, USA

Andrew J. Rosenbaum, MD Orthopaedic Surgery, The Bone and Joint Center, Albany Medical Center, Albany, NY, USA

Marcus A. Rothermich, MD Department of Orthopaedic Surgery, Andrews Sports Medicine and Orthopaedic Center, Birmingham, AL, USA

Felix H. Savoie III, MD Department of Orthopaedics, Tulane University School of Medicine, New Orleans, LA, USA

Mark S. Schickendantz, MD Cleveland Clinic Sports Medicine, Cleveland Clinic Foundation, Garfield Heights, OH, USA

Brian M. Schulz, MD Los Angeles Angels and Anaheim Ducks, Cedars-Sinai Kerlan-Jobe Institute, Anaheim, CA, USA

Ryan S. Selley, MD Department of Orthopaedic Surgery, Hospital for Special Surgery, New York, NY, USA

Benjamin C. Service, MD Orlando Health Orthopedic Institute, Orlando, FL, USA

Brandon A. Simonetta, MD Department of Orthopedic Surgery, Orlando Health Orthopedic Institute, Orlando, FL, USA

Spencer M. Stein, MD Sports Medicine, Orthopedic Surgery, Kerlan-Jobe Institute, Los Angeles, CA, USA

Charlton Stucken, MD Rothman Institute, Philadelphia, PA, USA

Robert Z. Tashjian, MD Department of Orthopaedic Surgery, University of Utah, Salt Lake City, UT, USA

Ryan R. Thacher, MD Department of Orthopedic Surgery, Hospital for Special Surgery, New York, NY, USA

Christin A. Tiegs-Heiden, MD Department of Radiology, Mayo Clinic, Rochester, MN, USA

Evan E. Vellios, MD Southern California Orthopedic Institute, Van Nuys, CA, USA

James E. Voos, MD Department of Orthopaedic Surgery, University Hospitals Cleveland, Cleveland, OH, USA

Tony Wanich, MD High Mountain Orthopedics, Wayne, NJ, USA

Kenneth Durham Weeks III, MD OrthoCarolina, Charlotte, NC, USA

Alex E. White, MD Department of Orthopedic Surgery, Hospital for Special Surgery, New York, NY, USA

Kevin E. Wilk, MD Associate Clinical Director, Champion Sports Medicine, A Select Medical Facility, Birmingham, AL, USA

Vice President of Clinical Education & Research, Select Medical, Birmingham, AL, USA

Director Rehabilitative Research, American Sports Medicine Institute, Birmingham, AL, USA

Eric N. Windsor, BA, MS Department of Orthopaedic Surgery, Hospital for Special Surgery, New York, NY, USA

Melissa A. Wright, MD Department of Orthopaedics, MedStar Union Memorial Hospital, Baltimore, MD, USA

Joshua Wright-Chisem, MD Department of Orthopedic Surgery, Sports Medicine and Shoulder Service, Sports Medicine Institute, Hospital for Special Surgery, New York, NY, USA

Lewis A. Yocum, MD Kerlan-Jobe Orthopaedic Clinic, Los Angeles, CA, USA

Jonathan S. Yu, BS Hospital for Special Surgery, New York, NY, USA

John M. Zajac, PT New York Mets Baseball Club, Flushing, NY, USA

Anatomy and Biomechanics of the Medial Ulnar Collateral Ligament

1

Miguel Pelton, Salvatore J. Frangiamore, and Mark S. Schickendantz

Introduction

The medial ulnar collateral ligament (MUCL) has three distinct components. These include the anterior bundle, posterior bundle, and transverse or oblique ligament. The anterior bundle of the UCL complex is the primary static stabilizer to valgus stress on the medial elbow. It primarily acts to resist valgus and extension stress from 70 to 120° of elbow flexion. The anterior bundle of the UCL is composed of an anterior and a posterior band. The anterior band is more isometric, but generally tight in extension, whereas the posterior band is tight in flexion. The posterior bundle is a fan-like structure that originates from the medial epicondyle and inserts into the medial posterior aspect of the olecranon. Lastly, the transverse bundle is often indistinguishable from the capsule and has both its origin and insertion on the proximal ulna at the olecranon and sublime tubercle, respectively.

The mean length and width of the anterior bundle of the UCL is 31.9 mm (range 21.1–53.9 mm) and 5.95 mm (range 4.5 mm–7.6 mm), respectively [1–8]. The anterior bundle originates at the medial epicondyle of the humerus at approximately 8.5 mm distal and 7.8 mm anterior to the center of medial epicondyle of the humerus with a surface area of 17–45 mm [1]. The anterior position relative to the medial epicondyle is important to conceptualize during UCL reconstruction, as posterior tunnel position is a common error. This can decrease graft isometry and result in a graft which is overly tight in flexion [9] (Figs. 1.1 and 1.2).

The exact distal insertion site of the anterior bundle has been a topic of controversy [1, 4, 10]. It was once described at the apex of the sublime tubercle, at a site 5.5 mm distal to the articular surface. Now, more recent literature suggests a more elongated, tapered footprint measuring 66.4–187.6 mm^2, and an average of 5.3 mm (1.5 mm–7.6 mm) distal to the center of the sublime tubercle along the ulnar UCL ridge [1–3, 5–7, 10–13] (Fig. 1.3). Those authors suggest that the wide variability of distal attachments may be due to the inclusion of the underlying joint capsule in addition to the tendinous structure of the AB of the anterior bundle. It remains to be seen if changes to distal tunnels should be made to better reconstruct native anatomy [14–17]. Camp and colleagues recently assessed an alteration to the distal tunnel insertion using cadaveric reconstructions with palmaris autograft

M. Pelton · S. J. Frangiamore (✉)
M. S. Schickendantz
Cleveland Clinic Sports Medicine, Cleveland Clinic Foundation, Garfield Heights, OH, USA

J. S. Dines et al. (eds.), *Elbow Ulnar Collateral Ligament Injury*,
https://doi.org/10.1007/978-3-030-69567-5_1

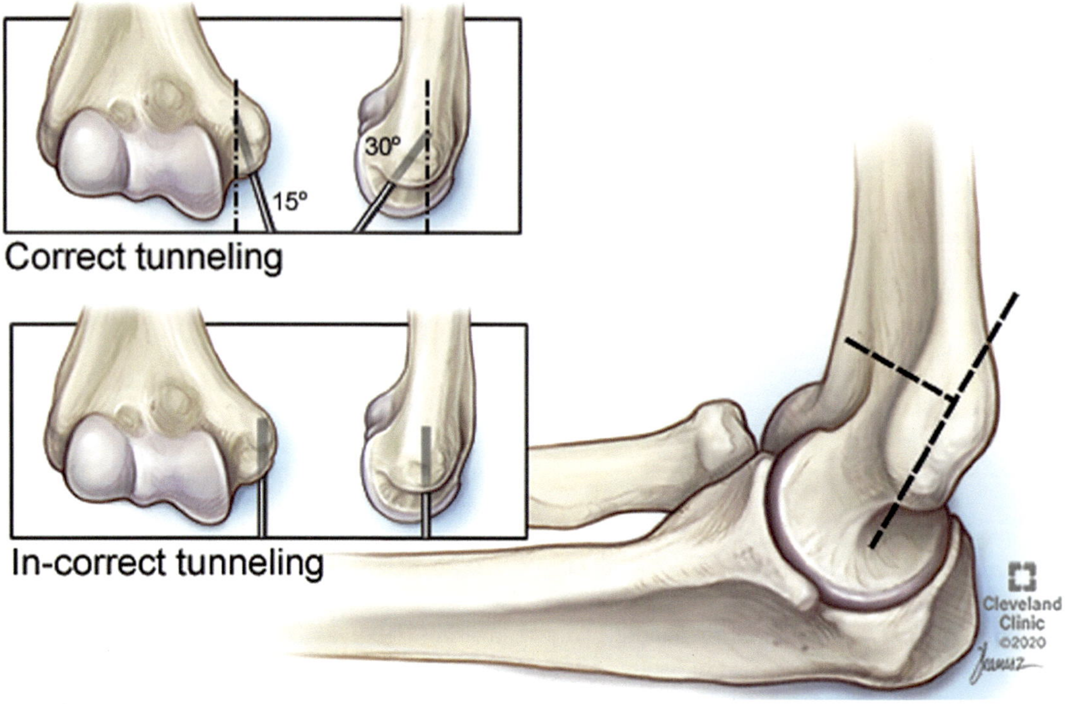

Fig. 1.1 Correct and incorrect tunnel reconstruction in both sagittal and coronal planes

Fig. 1.2 Illustration demonstrating Docking technique with correct tunnel trajectories and allograft reconstruction in place

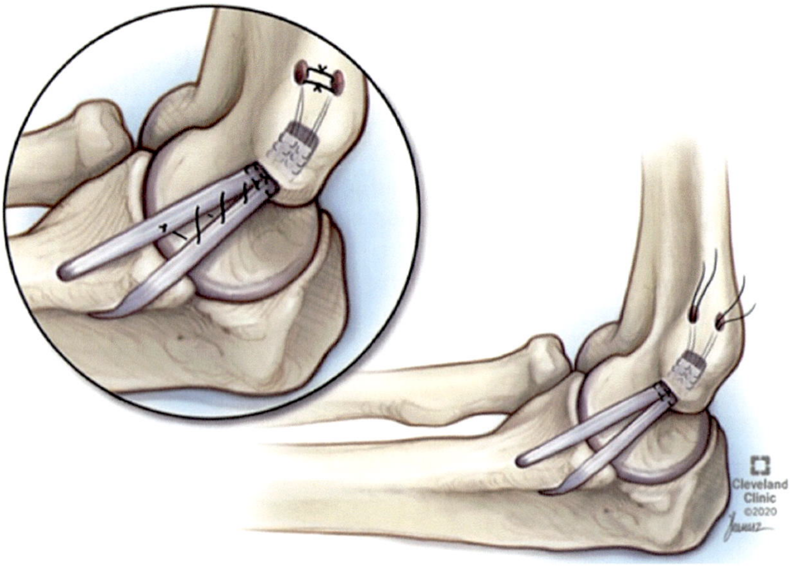

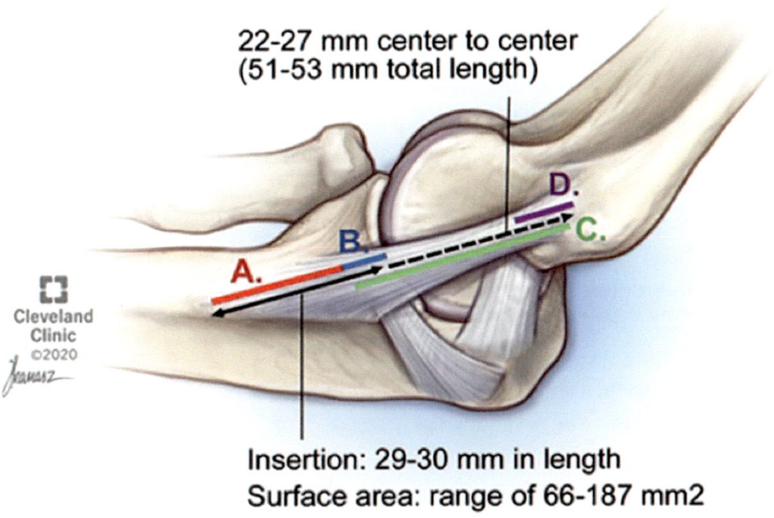

Fig. 1.3 Medial side of the elbow demonstrating the expanded ulnar footprint of the anterior bundle of the ulnar collateral ligament. (**a**) insertion length, (**b**) articular surface to proximal ulnar footprint 5.5 mm, (**c**) center of humeral footprint to the center of ulnar footprint, (**d**) length of distal humeral origin surface area 17–45 mm^2 (center of origin 8.5 mm distal and 7.8 mm lateral to medial epicondyle)

versus the traditional docking technique [18]. They demonstrated a higher mean ultimate load to failure with anatomical reconstruction over the traditional docking technique [18].

Biomechanics of Medial Ulnar Collateral Ligament Complex

Anterior Bundle (Anterior Band, Posterior Band, and Central Band)

The primary biomechanical role of the mUCL is to provide valgus stability of the elbow, especially in overhead throwing athletes. Morrey et al. demonstrated that with an intact radial head, the mUCL provides 31% and 54% of valgus stability of 0° and 90° of elbow flexion, respectively [6, 19]. Moreover, the authors noted that an intact mUCL allowed for only 3° of valgus opening in full extension and 2° of valgus opening in full flexion.

Similar findings have been reported in several other studies, which have demonstrated 2° to 8° of valgus laxity with an intact mUCL [2, 20, 21]. To quantify when the mUCL has the most laxity with a loaded elbow, Safran et al. analyzed 12 cadaveric specimens with 2 Nm load applied to the elbow in 30° of flexion and reported 10.7° of valgus laxity with the forearm in neutral rotation [8]. Callaway et al. expanded on these findings by loading the elbow with 2 Nm at 30° and 90° of flexion and reported a valgus laxity of 3.6° [22]. The former of these two studies did not quantify the amount of inherent valgus laxity specimens had prior to testing, which makes direct comparison of the two studies challenging. However, it is thought the amount of mUCL valgus laxity is greatest at 30° of flexion [8].

The anterior bundle has been shown to impart the greatest resistance to valgus loads. It is not an isometric stabilizer but changes length throughout progressive elbow flexion [23–25]. Studies have demonstrated a change of 2.8–4.8 mm as the elbow progresses from extension to full flexion [20, 26]. One cadaveric sectioning study sought to define the contribution to valgus stability of three distinct sections of the anterior bundle insertion [27]. They describe the proximal, middle, and distal third segments of insertional footprint at the sublime tubercle. A 5 Nm valgus load was applied at 30°, 60°, 90°, and 120° of flexion. Ulnohumeral joint gapping showed no significant difference between the intact state and sectioning of both the middle and distal insertion segments. However, there was a significant difference in joint gapping when the proximal segment was sectioned. One reason for this may be the relative thinning of the AB as it inserts distally on the sublime tubercle. In 16 cadaveric specimens, Frangiamore et al. found the posterior distal portion of the AB contributed the most to overall valgus elbow rotational stability and stiffness [28]. This was most apparent at 90° and 120° of elbow flexion. Those authors also found that the anterior insertions contributed most to elbow stability at lower flexion angles [28]. Thus, reconstruction techniques may take all these properties into account as more investigations are performed.

Some literature suggest that the presence of the middle or central band acts as an adjunct to impart some valgus stability [23, 28, 29]. Unlike the anterior and posterior bands, this central band was originally thought to be relatively static and taut throughout elbow motion [28]. One recent biomechanical cadaveric study sought to understand the load distribution between the anterior and posterior bands of the AB during the range of motion through the transition point of the central band [30]. The three bands were sequentially transected and then load tested in varying angles with valgus stress. The lesser flexion angles, 0° and 30°, saw the highest slack in the posterior band and the highest structural stiffness in the anterior band. The authors concluded that at higher flexion angles of 60–90°, the anterior band saw the highest slack and the middle band demonstrated the greatest stiffness. Further in vitro research is needed to further elucidate the role of the proposed central or middle band of the anterior bundle MUCL with pertinent clinical applications.

Posterior Bundle

Several studies have sought to define the contribution of the posterior bundle of the mUCL to valgus stability by sectioning the mUCL and measuring valgus angles during elbow range of motion [22, 31–34]. The posterior bundle (PB) of the UCL is a broader and thinner part of the UCL complex, originating from the humeral epicondyle and broadly inserting on the medial ulna. The PB provides valgus stability at flexion angles >120° [21]. Rahman et al. built a computational elbow joint model simulating varying levels of MUCL deficiencies [35]. When either the anterior or posterior bundle was transected, there was more valgus instability. However, there was less instability in the posterior bundle deficient condition. Additionally, less contact pressure at the cartilage surface was noted only in the anterior bundle deficient and entire mUCL deficient conditions. In agreement with other literature, these data indicate a smaller role of the posterior bundle in imparting medial elbow joint stability [36–40].

Transverse Ligament

The transverse ligament of the MUCL was thought not to impart any inherent stability as it does not cross the ulnohumeral joint, is not consistently present, or is poorly developed [19, 22, 23]. Others suggest that it is the confluence of collagen fibers from the transverse bundle with the anterior bundle that can contribute to valgus stability [10, 38]. Kimata and colleagues recently describe this connection in 42 cadaveric specimens [39]. The transverse bundle contributed to the distal half of the anterior bundle insertion in 73% of the elbows (Type I). In the remaining 27% of specimens, the transverse bundle contributed to the entire anterior bundle insertion (Type II). Female cadavers were more likely to show Type II anatomy at the medial elbow. These fibers were all represented in a perpendicular fashion to the anterior bundle fibers. Future biomechanical studies will further elucidate what role, if any, the transverse ligament contributes to elbow stability.

Anatomy of the Medial Elbow Complex Dynamic Stabilizers

The dynamic stabilizers of the elbow are made up of the flexor–pronator muscle complex that cross the elbow joint. Specifically, the flexor digitorum superficialis (FDS), flexor carpi ulnaris (FCU), pronator teres (PT), and brachialis (BR) make up

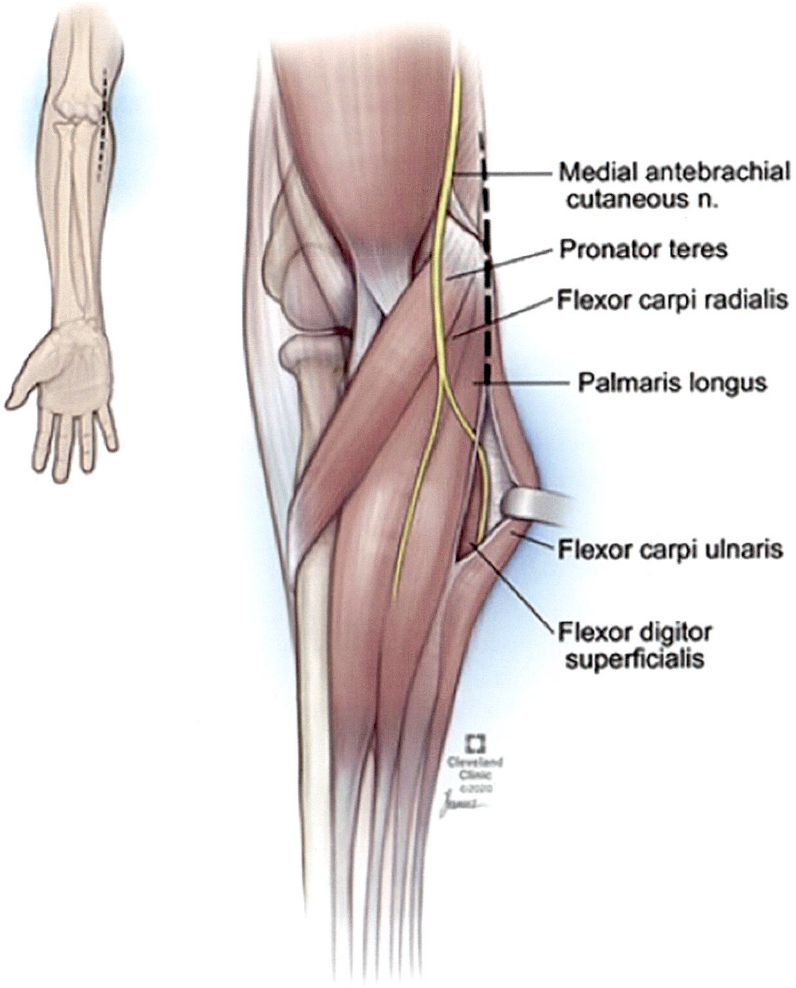

Fig. 1.4 Illustration demonstrating the contents and relationships of the flexor–pronator mass. (**a**) Dashed line indicates incision for MUCL reconstruction

what is often referred to as the flexor–pronator mass. They play an integral role in valgus stability during the throwing motion and studies have demonstrated an increased risk of UCL injury when these are deficient [32]. The medial antebrachial cutaneous nerve arises from the medial cord of the brachial plexus. This nerve must be observed and retracted in any proposed reconstruction incision (Fig. 1.4). The forearm flexors primarily insert proximally on the humerus as part of the common flexor insertion, 4.4 mm posterior to the medial epicondyle [1]. The common flexor insertion has been reported to have a surface area of 127.9 mm^2 (range, 89.5–166.3 mm^2) [1, 10]. The FDS and FCU also have demonstrated secondary ulnar insertions near the attachment of the AB of thc UCL [33]. The FDS ulnar tendinous insertion has been reported to be overlapped with the AB for 46% of its length, until inserting 6.8 mm distal to the sublime tubercle of the ulna [1]. The FCU ulnar insertion has been reported to be 1.9 mm posterior and 1.3 mm proximal to the sublime tubercle and overlaps 21% with the AB during its proximal to the distal course (Fig. 1.5).

The pronator teres (PT) inserts just proximal to the common flexor humeral insertion, 9.4 mm

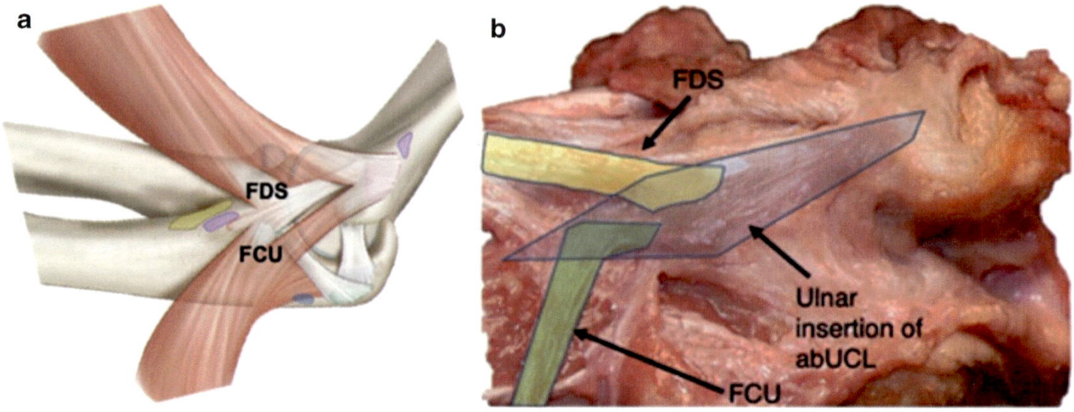

Fig. 1.5 (**a**) Illustration and (**b**) cadaveric view of relationship of ulnar insertion of the anterior bundle of the UCL and the ulnar footprints of the FCU and FDS

proximal from the medial epicondyle. The footprint of this humeral insertion has been reported to be 40.1 mm^2 (range, 33–47 mm^2) [1]. The PT then courses distally to insert 14.5 mm distal to the sublime tubercle, which is 24.5 mm distal to the joint line. It should be highlighted that the PT ulnar insertion is a thin tendinous structure that runs between the brachialis muscle and the anterior bundle of the UCL.

Microanatomy and Biomechanical Properties

The microstructural organization of the mUCL as it relates to biomechanical properties has recently been investigated [36, 37, 40]. Smith and colleagues performed a cadaveric study using tensile forces to measure real-time microstructural collagen changes in 34 specimens [36]. Through the use of a polarization camera, the characteristics stress–strain curve could be obtained for both the anterior and posterior bundles. The AB was found over the PB to have a larger elastic modulus in both the toe region (2.73 MPa [interquartile range, 1.1–5.6 MPa] vs 0.65 MPa [0.44–1.5 MPa respectively) and the linear region (13.77 MPa [4.8–40.7 MPa] vs 1.96 MPa [0.58–9.3 MPa] respectively). Additionally, the AB demonstrated larger stress values, stronger collagen alignment, and more uniform collagen organization during stress-relaxation. The posterior bundle collagen fibers showed more disorganized fibers in zero, transitional and linear regions of the stress–strain curve. However, under loading, the magnitude of change of the collagen fibers was minimal. These authors opine that the data provide a basis to describe the relatively static nature of the mUCL bundles which is not well suited to large tensile forces. In comparison to the other ligaments, such as the ACL and PCL, microstructural properties of the UCL change less under load. The overall alignment is weaker and more dispersed before the application of load. These data may explain why mUCL is less compliant and more vulnerable to injury with the high valgus loads that may be seen during throwing.

Conclusion

The anterior bundle of the medial ulnar collateral ligament is responsible for the primary valgus stability of the elbow. Proximally, it inserts in an anterior and distal position relative to the center of the epicondyle and distally at the sublime tubercle with an elongated tapered insertion. Distally, the UCL is intimately associated with ulnar attachment of the forearm flexors and must be taken into consideration during dissection. With an increased understanding of the anatomy and biomechanics of the UCL and its anatomic relationships, reconstruction approaches and techniques can be further refined to reflect these changes.

References

1. Frangiamore SJ, Moatshe G, Kruckeberg BM, et al. Qualitative and quantitative analyses of the dynamic and static stabilizers of the medial elbow: an anatomic study. Am J Sports Med. 2018;46:687–94.
2. Alcid JG, Ahmad CS, Lee TQ. Elbow anatomy and structural biomechanics. Clin Sports Med. 2004;23(4):503–17, vii.
3. Beckett KS, McConnell P, Lagopoulos M, Newman RJ. Variations in the normal anatomy of the collateral ligaments of the human elbow joint. J Anat 197 Pt. 2000;3:507–11.
4. Dugas JR, Ostrander RV, Cain EL, Kingsley D, Andrews JR. Anatomy of the anterior bundle of the ulnar collateral ligament. J Shoulder Elb Surg. 2007;16:657–60.
5. Eygendaal D, Valstar ER, Söjbjerg JO, Rozing PM. Biomechanical evaluation of the elbow using roentgen stereophotogrammetric analysis. Clin Orthop Relat Res. 2002:100–5.
6. Morrey BF, An KN. Articular and ligamentous contributions to the stability of the elbow joint. Am J Sports Med. 1983;11(5):315–9.
7. Regan WD, Korinek SL, Morrey BF, An KN. Biomechanical study of ligaments around the elbow joint. Clin Orthop Relat Res. 1991:170–9.
8. Safran M, Ahmad CS, Elattrache NS. Ulnar collateral ligament of the elbow. Arthroscopy. 2005;21(11):1381–95.
9. Lall AC, Beason DP, Dugas JR, Cain ELJ. The effect of humeral and ulnar bone tunnel placement on achieving UCL graft isometry: a cadaveric study. Arthroscopy. 2019.
10. Camp CL, Jahandar H, Sinatro AM, Imhauser CW, Altchek DW, Dines JS. Quantitative anatomic analysis of the medial ulnar collateral ligament complex of the elbow with implications for reconstructive surgery. J Shoulder Elb Surg. 2018;e127:27.
11. Farrow LD, Mahoney AP, Sheppard JE, Schickendantz MS, Taljanovic MS. Sonographic assessment of the medial ulnar collateral ligament distal ulnar attachment. J Ultrasound Med. 2014;33:1485–90.
12. Farrow LD, Mahoney AJ, Stefancin JJ, Taljanovic MS, Sheppard JE, Schickendantz MS. Quantitative analysis of the medial ulnar collateral ligament ulnar footprint and its relationship to the ulnar sublime tubercle. Am J Sports Med. 2011;39:1936–41.
13. Hoshika S, Nimura A, Yamaguchi R, Nasu H, Yamaguchi K, Sugaya H, Akita K. Medial elbow anatomy: a paradigm shift for UCL injury prevention and management. Clin Anat. 2019;32:379–89.
14. Andrews JR, Jost PW, Cain EL. The ulnar collateral ligament procedure revisited: the procedure we use. Sports Health. 2012;4:438–41.
15. Dines JS, ElAttrache NS, Conway JE, Smith W, Ahmad CS. Clinical outcomes of the DANE TJ technique to treat ulnar collateral ligament insufficiency of the elbow. Am J Sports Med. 2007;35:2039–44.
16. Erickson BJ, Chalmers PN, Bush-Joseph CA, Verma NN, Romeo AA. Ulnar collateral ligament reconstruction of the elbow: a systematic review of the literature. Orthop J Sports Med. 2015;2325967115618914:3.
17. Marshall TJ, Frangiomore S, Schickendantz M. Medial ulnar collateral ligament reconstruction: restoring the ulnar footprint. Tech Should Elbow Surg. 2017;18:62.
18. Camp CL, Bernard C, Benavitz B, Konicek J, Altchek DW, Dines JS. Reconstruction of the medial ulnar collateral ligament of the elbow: biomechanical comparison of a novel anatomic technique to the docking technique. Orthop J Sports Med. 2019;7:2325967119857592.
19. Morrey BF, An KN. Functional anatomy of the ligaments of the elbow. Clin Orthop Relat Res. 1985;201:84–90.
20. Bryce CD, Armstrong AD. Anatomy and biomechanics of the elbow. Orthop Clin North Am. 2008;39:141–54, v.
21. Floris S, Olsen BS, Dalstra M, Søjbjerg JO, Sneppen O. The medial collateral ligament of the elbow joint: anatomy and kinematics. J Shoulder Elb Surg. 1998;7:345–51.
22. Callaway GH, Field LD, Deng XH, Torzilli PA, O'Brien SJ, Altchek DW, Warren RF. Biomechanical evaluation of the medial collateral ligament of the elbow. J Bone Joint Surg Am. 1997;79:1223–31.
23. Fuss FK. The ulnar collateral ligament of the human elbow joint. Anatomy, function and biomechanics. J Anat. 1991;175:203–12.
24. Hotchkiss RN, Weiland AJ. Valgus stability of the elbow. J Orthop Res. 1987;5:372–7.
25. Mullen DJ, Goradia VK, Parks BG, Matthews LS. A biomechanical study of stability of the elbow to valgus stress before and after reconstruction of the medial collateral ligament. J Shoulder Elb Surg. 2002;11:259–64.
26. Armstrong AD, Ferreira LM, Dunning CE, Johnson JA, King GJW. The medial collateral ligament of the elbow is not isometric: an in vitro biomechanical study. Am J Sports Med. 2004;32:85–90.
27. Erickson BJ, Fu M, Meyers K, Camp CL, Altchek DW, Coleman SH, Dines JS. The middle and distal aspects of the ulnar footprint of the medial ulnar collateral ligament of the elbow do not provide significant resistance to valgus stress: a biomechanical study. Orthop J Sports Med. 2019;2325967118825294:7.
28. Kaufmann RA, Wilps T, Musahl V, Debski RE. Elbow biomechanics: soft tissue stabilizers. J Hand Surg Am. 2020;45(2):140–47.
29. Kholinne E, Zulkarnain RF, Lee H-J, Adikrishna A, Jeon I-H. Functional classification of the medial ulnar collateral ligament: an in vivo kinematic study with computer-aided design. Orthop J Sports Med. 2018;2325967118762750:6.
30. Jordan D, Schimoler P, Kharlamov A, DeMeo PJ, Miller MC. Correlation of force to deformation of the anterior bundle of the medial collateral ligament

through consideration of band laxity. J Orthop Res. 2019;37:2027–34.
31. Armstrong AD, Dunning CE, Faber KJ, Duck TR, Johnson JA, King GJ. Rehabilitation of the medial collateral ligament-deficient elbow: an in vitro biomechanical study. J Hand Surg Am. 2000;25:1051–7.
32. Lin F, et al. Muscle contribution to elbow joint valgus stability. J Shoulder Elb Surg. 2007;16:795–802.
33. Cinque ME, Schickendantz M, Frangiamore S. Review of anatomy of the medial ulnar collateral ligament complex of the elbow. Curr Rev Musculoskelet Med. 2020;13:96–102.
34. Alolabi B, Gray A, Ferreira LM, Johnson JA, Athwal GS, King GJW. Rehabilitation of the medial- and lateral collateral ligament-deficient elbow: an in vitro biomechanical study. J Hand Ther. 2012;25:363–73.
35. Rahman M, Cil A, Stylianou AP. Medial collateral ligament deficiency of the elbow joint: a computational approach. Bioengineering (Basel). 2018;5(4):84.
36. Smith MV, Castile RM, Brophy RH, Dewan A, Bernholt D, Lake SP. Mechanical properties and microstructural collagen alignment of the ulnar collateral ligament during dynamic loading. Am J Sports Med. 2019;47:151–7.
37. Paletta GAJ, Klepps SJ, Difelice GS, Allen T, Brodt MD, Burns ME, Silva MJ, Wright RW. Biomechanical evaluation of 2 techniques for ulnar collateral ligament reconstruction of the elbow. Am J Sports Med. 2006;34:1599–603.
38. Berg EE, DeHoll D. Radiography of the medial elbow ligaments. J Shoulder Elb Surg. 1997;6:528–33.
39. Kimata K, Yasui M, Yokota H, Hirai S, Naito M, Nakano T. Transverse ligament of the elbow joint: an anatomic study of cadavers. J Shoulder Elb Surg. 2019;28:2253–8.
40. York T, Kahan L, Lake SP, Gruev V. Real-time high-resolution measurement of collagen alignment in dynamically loaded soft tissue. J Biomed Opt. 2014;066011:19.

Clinically Relevant Elbow Anatomy and Surgical Approaches

2

Xinning Li and L. T. C. Josef K. Eichinger

Pertinent Anatomy of the Thrower's Elbow

Osseous Anatomy

The elbow is primarily a ginglymus or hinge joint, but in reality consists of three bony articulations including ulnohumeral, radiocapitellar, and radioulnar joint. The primary arc of motion during throwing motions is flexion and extension through the ulnohumeral articulation; however, some pronation–supination does occur through the ulnohumeral and radioulnar joints. In full extension, the elbow has a normal valgus-carrying angle of 11–16°. Morrey and An determined the osseous anatomy's contribution to resistance to valgus stress remains fairly constant throughout elbow motion [1]. In full extension, roughly one-third of valgus force was resisted by the ulnar collateral ligament (UCL) (31%), one-third by the anterior capsule (38%), and one-third by the bony architecture (31%). At 90° of flexion, the UCL increased its relative contribution to 54%, whereas the anterior capsule provided only 10% to valgus stability, and the bony anatomy contribution remained relatively unchanged at 36%.

X. Li (✉)
Sports Medicine and Shoulder Surgery, Department of Orthopaedics, Boston University School of Medicine, Boston, MA, USA

L. T. C. J. K. Eichinger
Shoulder and Elbow Surgery, Department of Orthopaedics, Medical University of South Carolina, Charleston, SC, USA

Muscular Anatomy

Flexor–Pronator Mass

The flexor–pronator mass is a collection of muscles that form a common origin from the medial epicondyle. These muscles can be viewed and organized into superficial and deep layers or groups. Pronator teres, flexor carpi radilais (FCR), flexor carpi ulnaris (FCU), flexor digitorum superficialis (FDS), and palmaris longus (PL) muscle are found in the superficial layer. In the deep layer, three muscles are found and composed of flexor digitorum profundus (FDP), flexor pollicus longus (FPL), and pronator quadratus (PQ) muscles (Fig. 2.1). The combined function is to perform wrist flexion and forearm pronation. An analysis of the primary muscles of the flexor–pronator group (pronator teres, FDS, FCU, and flexor carpi radialis) indicates that their dynamic action applies a varus moment and therefore resisting valgus force across the elbow [2]. In relation to throwing mechanics; however, electromyogram (EMG) studies indicate that the

J. S. Dines et al. (eds.), *Elbow Ulnar Collateral Ligament Injury*,
https://doi.org/10.1007/978-3-030-69567-5_2

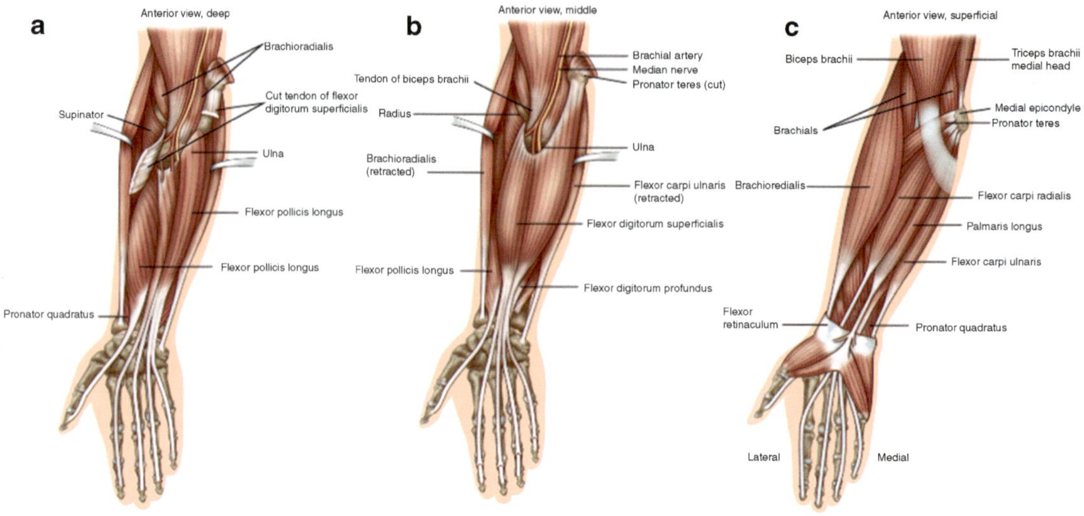

Fig. 2.1 Anterior view of the superficial and deep components of the elbow flexor–pronator mass

flexor muscles do not reflect a compensatory increase in activity in throwers with valgus instability. Furthermore, both flexor carpi radialis and pronator teres show a paradoxical decrease in activity in throwers with valgus instability after medial ulnar collateral ligament (MUCL) rupture [2, 3]. It is unclear whether the decrease in EMG activity is a cause or effect of MUCL injuries. Despite these EMG findings, ruptures of the flexor–pronator mass and medial epicondylitis can occur in the clinical setting of MUCL injuries of throwers indicating some level of contribution of the muscles to function and likely stability [4, 5]. An anatomic analysis revealed that the FCU muscle is the predominant musculotendinous unit overlying the UCL essentially independent of elbow flexion and forearm rotation [6]. The only other muscle with less frequent contribution to coverage was the FDS. Several authors have reported FCU as the biggest contributor to valgus stability in MUCL deficient elbows [7, 8]. In contrast, despite suboptimal muscle coverage, Udall et al. [9] showed FDS as the greatest contributor to valgus stability of the elbow due to its bulk (increased cross-sectional area). Furthermore, Hoshika et al. reported that contraction of the FDS of the index and middle fingers contributes the most to stabilization of the elbow against valgus stress [10].

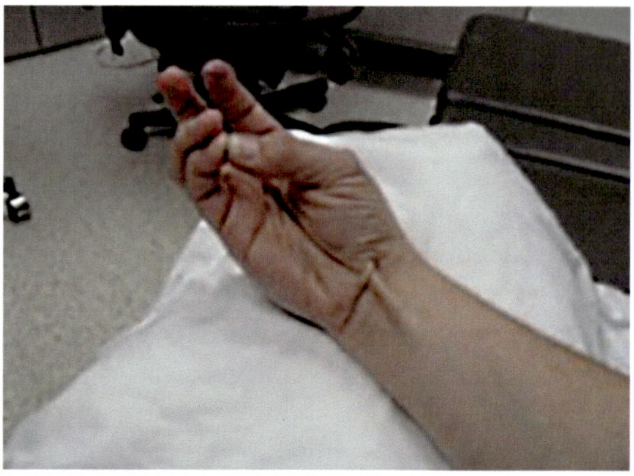

Fig. 2.2 The presence of the palmaris longus can be verified preoperatively by opposing the thumb and small finger together, which creates a characteristic appearance over the volar surface of the wrist

Palmaris Longus Tendon

The PL tendon is an ideal source of graft for MUCL reconstruction; however, it is clinically absent in 15% of the population with incidences varying widely depending on ethnicity [2]. Clinically, the presence of the PL can be verified by opposing the thumb and small finger together, which creates a characteristic appearance over the volar surface of the wrist (Fig. 2.2). The PL tendon is located between the flexor carpi radialis tendon and the FDS tendons at the level of the wrist.

Nerve Anatomy

Medial Antebrachial Cutaneous Nerve

The medial antebrachial cutaneous nerve arises from the medial cord of the brachial plexus. In the distal brachium, the nerve travels medial to the brachial artery. The nerve then courses down the ulnar aspect of the forearm and enters the deep fascia with the basilica vein. It is responsible for sensation over the medial aspect of the elbow. Branches pass 3–60 mm distal to the medial epicondyle and are at risk with the typical longitudinal incision used in UCL reconstructive surgery [11]. Identification and protection of these nerve branches protect from iatrogenic injury and prevent the development of painful, symptomatic neuromas or superficial sensory derangement. The nerves are encountered immediately after skin incision (Fig. 2.3) and are variable in their size, appearance, and distribution [12].

Ulnar Nerve

The surgical approach to the UCL demands a clear understanding of the location of the neurovascular structures. The ulnar nerve is the most thought of neurologic structure in regard to UCL

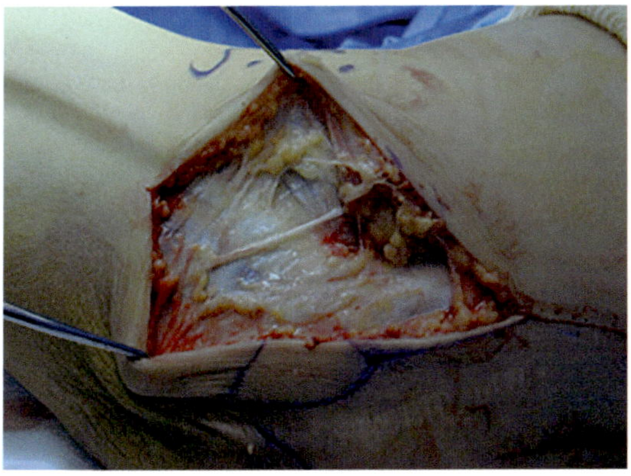

Fig. 2.3 The medial antebrachial sensory nerve is encountered immediately after the skin incision during the approach for the UCL reconstruction. Care is taken to identify and protect this nerve throughout the procedure to prevent injury

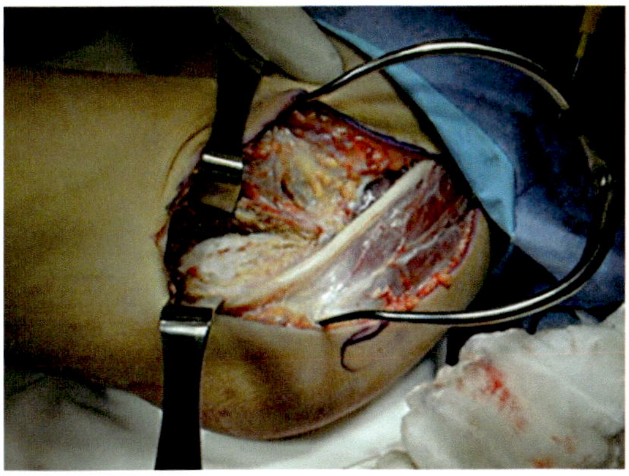

Fig. 2.4 The ulnar nerve descends along the posteromedial aspect of the humerus and then enters the cubital tunnel posterior to the medial epicondyle

reconstructive surgery. The ulnar nerve descends along the posteromedial aspect of the humerus and then enters the cubital tunnel posterior to the medial epicondyle (Fig. 2.4). After exiting the cubital tunnel, the ulnar nerve gives off an articular sensory innervation branch and then enters the flexor compartment of the forearm. It is positioned under the FCU adjacent to the ulna. The nerve innervates the FCU and the medial half of flexor digitorum profundus.

The ulnar nerve courses with the ulnar artery and distally in the hand it is responsible for sensory innervation of the ulnar 1.5 digits and intrinsic hand motor function as well. A muscle-splitting approach for UCL reconstruction can be performed without detachment of the flexor–pronator mass of the forearm [11, 13]. Exposure for this technique is performed either through a naturally occurring raphe that delineates the separation between the FCU and the remaining flexor muscle mass or simply in-line between the medial epicondyle and sublime tubercle (Fig. 2.5). This region is a natural watershed area between motor innervation of the ulnar nerve and median nerve as verified through cadaveric analysis. This approach, therefore, avoids iatrogenic denervation to these muscles [11, 13]. It is essential that during the muscle splitting approach that a sharp retractor is never used posterior medially to prevent injury to the ulnar nerve (Fig. 2.6).

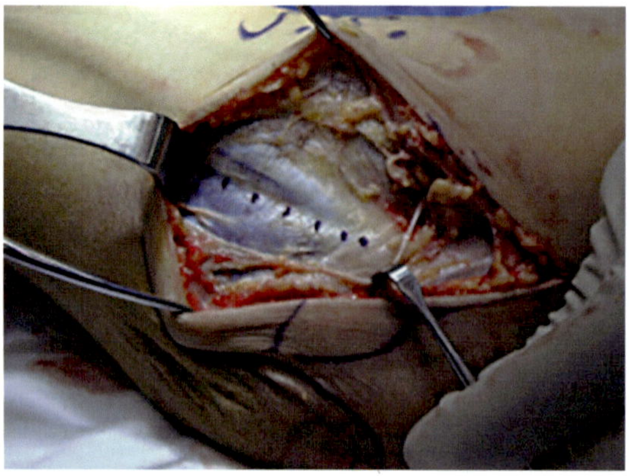

Fig. 2.5 Exposure for the muscle-splitting approach is performed through a naturally occurring raphe that delineates the separation between the flexor carpi ulnaris and the remaining flexor muscle mass (*blue dots*) or simply in-line between the medial epicondyle and sublime tubercle

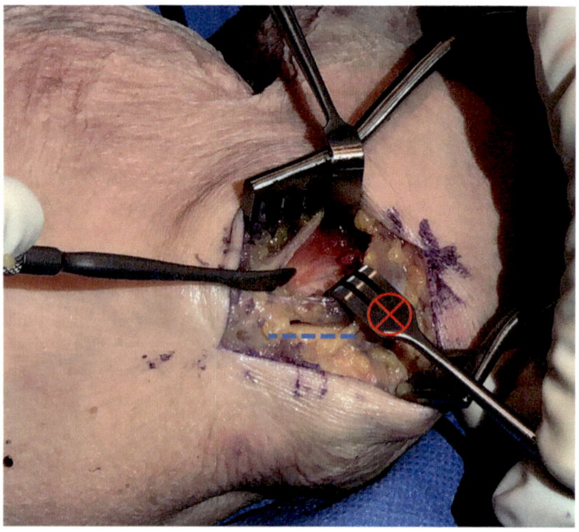

Fig. 2.6 Muscle-splitting approach is performed with the ulnar nerve in the cubital tunnel (*blue dots*). Sharp retractors should never be used in the posterior and medial direction to prevent iaotrogenic injury to the ulnar nerve

Ligamentous Anatomy

Medial Ulnar Collateral Ligament

The medial ulnar collateral ligament (MUCL) of the elbow is composed of three bundles, including the anterior, posterior, and transverse bundles [1, 14]. The transverse bundle has also been described as the oblique bundle [13]. The anterior bundle is composed of two different histological layers and two different functional bands. The deep layer is confluent with the joint capsule, while the superficial layer is a more distinct structure above the capsule with thick parallel fibers with a mean width of 4–5 mm [15]. An anatomic and biomechanical evaluation of the MUCL revealed that the anterior bundle can be further delineated into two distinct functional sub-units, the anterior and posterior bands [16]. The anterior and posterior bands of the anterior bundle of the MUCL perform reciprocal functions with the anterior band functioning as the primary restraint to valgus rotation at 30°, 60°, and 90° of flexion. The anterior and posterior bands are equal functioning restraints at 120° of flexion while the posterior band acts as a secondary restraint at 30° and 90° of flexion (Fig. 2.7) [16].

The anterior bundle arises from the inferior aspect of the medial epicondyle [17] and inserts immediately adjacent to the joint surface on the ulna near the sublimis tubercle. The anterior bundle widens slightly from proximal to distal and can be subdivided into anterior and posterior bands of equal width. The bands tighten in a reciprocal fashion as the elbow is flexed and extended (bottom frame), and they are separated by easily identifiable isometric fibers (arrows). The posterior bundle arises from the medial epicondyle slightly posterior to its most inferior portion. It inserts broadly on the olecranon process. The posterior bundle appears to be a thickened joint capsule when the elbow is extended. As the elbow is flexed, the ligament tightens and fans out to form a sharp edge that is perpendicular to the long axis of the ulna. Furthermore, the anterior bundle originates from the anteroinferior edge of the medial humeral epicondyle with an origin measuring 45.5 ± 9.3 mm^2 in diameter and inserts onto the sublime tubercle on the ulna in an area measuring 127 ± 35.7 mm^2 in diameter [18].

The anterior bundle of the MUCL is the primary restraint to valgus stress from 20° to 120° of flexion and is the critical structure requiring reconstruction after injury in throwers. Because its origin is slightly posterior to the axis of the

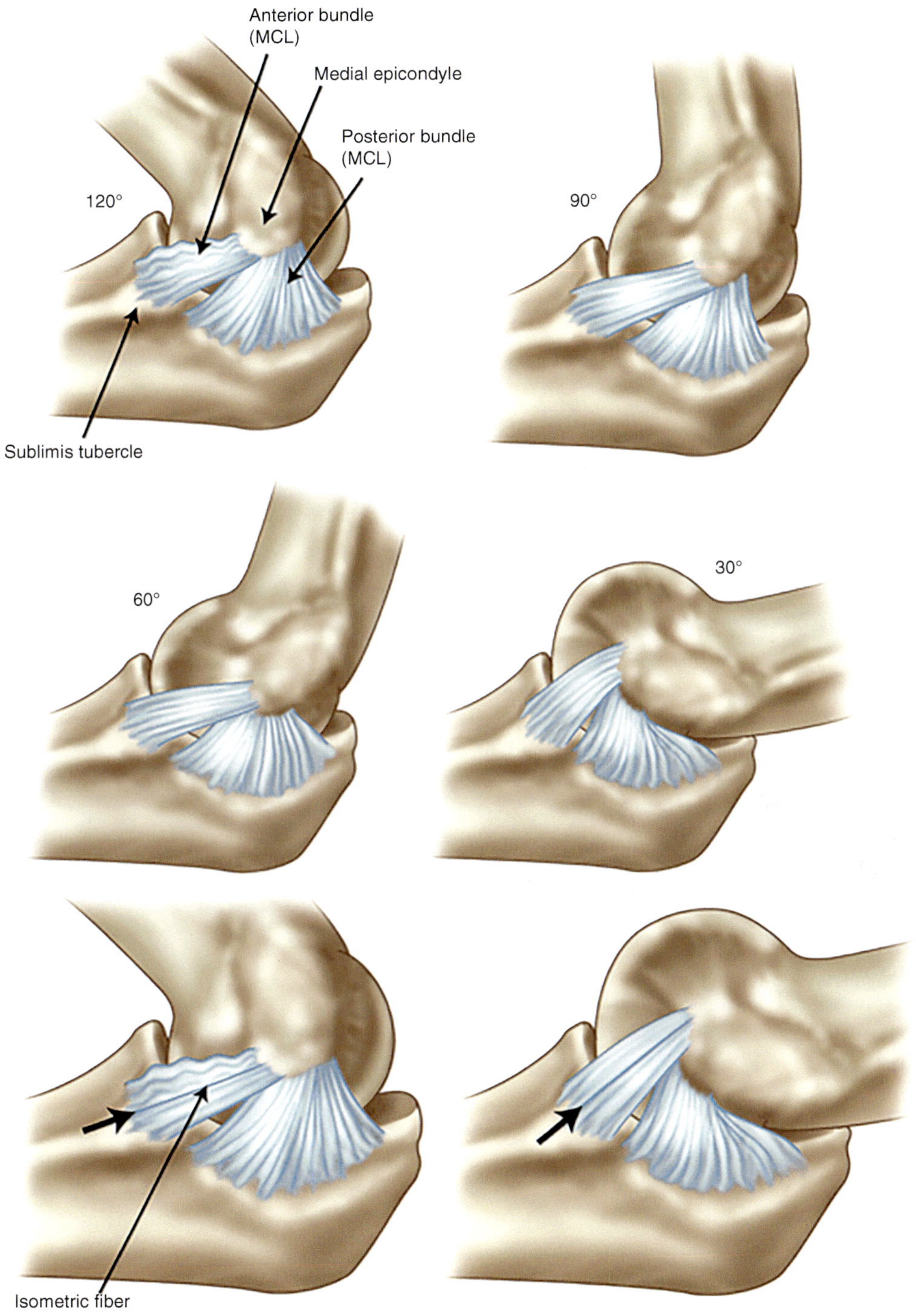

Fig. 2.7 Illustrations of the anatomy of the medial collateral ligament (*MCL*) of the elbow at 30°, 60°, 90°, and 120° of flexion. The anterior bundle arises from the inferior aspect of the medial epicondyle (ME) and inserts immediately adjacent to the joint surface on the ulna near the sublimis tubercle. The anterior bundle widens slightly from proximal to distal and can be subdivided into anterior and posterior bands of equal width. The bands tighten in a reciprocal fashion as the elbow is flexed and extended (*bottom frame*), and they are separated by easily identifiable isometric fibers (*arrows*). The posterior bundle arises from the ME slightly posterior to its most inferior portion. It inserts broadly on the olecranon process. The posterior bundle appears to be thickened joint capsule when the elbow is extended. As the elbow is flexed, the ligament tightens and fans out to form a sharp edge that is perpendicular to the long axis of the ulna

elbow, there is a cam effect created so that the ligament tension increases with increasing flexion. The anterior bundle of the MUCL is the strongest of the different components with a mean load to failure of 260 N [19]. The posterior bundle is not a significant contributor to valgus stability unless the remaining structures of the MUCL are sectioned. The posterior bundle of the MUCL is thinner and weaker than the anterior bundle, originates from the medial epicondyle and inserts onto the medial margin of the semilunar notch and acts only as a secondary stabilizer of the elbow beyond 90° of flexion [20]. Lastly, the oblique bundle or transverse ligament does not span the ulnohumeral joint but instead acts to increase the greater sigmoid notch as a thickening of the joint capsule [21].

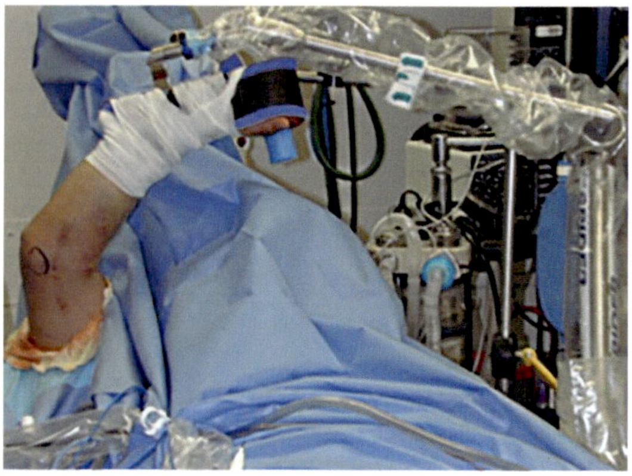

Fig. 2.8 Arthroscopic elbow evaluation is performed with the operative extremity in an arm holder and positioned across the patient's chest utilizing the Spider Limb Positioner. (Smith & Nephew, Tenet Medical Engineering, Memphis, TN)

Relevant Surgical Approaches

Positioning

UCL reconstruction is performed with the patient under either regional block or general anesthesia in the supine position with the extremity outstretched onto an arm board. A pneumatic tourniquet is placed on the upper arm and inflated to 200–250 mmHG during the graft harvest and critical portions of the procedure. Routine sterile prep and drape of the extremity is done under sterile conditions. Diagnostic elbow arthroscopy is performed before graft harvest and UCL reconstruction.

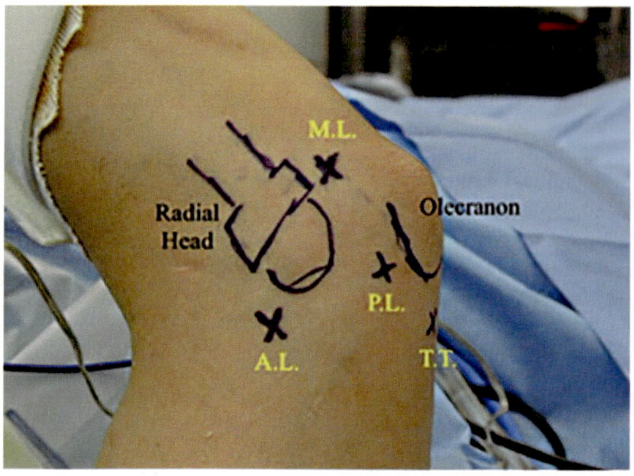

Fig. 2.9 Commonly utilized elbow arthroscopy portals for evaluation prior to the UCL reconstruction procedure. Midlateral (*M.L.*), Anterolateral (*A.L.*), Posterolateral (*P.L.*), and Trans-triceps (*T.T.*) portal sites

Elbow Arthroscopy

Arthroscopic evaluation is performed with the operative extremity in an arm holder and positioned across the patient's chest utilizing the Spider Limb Positioner (Smith & Nephew, Tenet Medical Engineering, Memphis, TN) (Fig. 2.8). An 18-gauge spinal needle is used to enter the joint via the "soft spot" or "direct lateral portal" that is located in the middle of a triangle formed by the lateral epicondyle, radial head, and olecranon. Forty to 50 ml of normal saline is injected to distend the elbow joint before trocar insertion to prevent articular cartilage damage. Distension of the joint will move the soft tissue along with the neurovascular structures away from the capsule, thus minimizing the risk of injury. The direct or mid-lateral (ML) portal (Fig. 2.9) is excellent for viewing and evaluations of the posterior compartment, specifically, the radioulnar joint, inferior surfaces of the capitellum, and radial head. It is relatively safe, passes between the plane between the anconeus and triceps muscle and within 7 mm of the lateral antebrachial cutaneous nerve [22, 23].

An anterolateral (AL) portal (Fig. 2.9) is the first portal established in the elbow arthroscopy sequence before the UCL reconstruction to examine the anterior and medial elbow compartment. More importantly, we perform an arthroscopic stress test on every patient to confirm valgus instability. This is done (viewing from the AL portal) with the forearm in full pronation and the elbow in 70° of flexion, an opening of 2 mm between the humerus and ulna with valgus stress is considered a positive sign of valgus instability. The AL portal is preferred for examination and viewing of the anterior and medial side of the elbow joint. Andrews and Carson [24] originally described this portal position as 3 cm distal and 1 cm anterior to the lateral epicondyle. Recent anatomic cadaver studies have shown that the 3 cm distal location places the trochar in very close proximity to the radio nerve, which significantly increases the risk of injury [17, 25]. Thus, several authors have moved this portal more anterior and less distal. Plancher et al. [23] advocate an AL portal placed in the sulcus, which is located between the radio head and the capitellum (1 cm distal and 1 cm anterior to the lateral epicondyle). Even with the newer proposed locations, the average distance of the radial nerve to the trochar in the AL portal position is between 3 and 7 mm in nondistended joints [17, 23–25], which increases to 11 mm with joint distension [17].

In order to examine the posteromedial olecranon and humeral fossa for impingement, loose bodies, and spurs, we will establish a second portal posterior and lateral to the triceps tendon (posterolateral portal). The posterolateral (PL) portal location has the largest area of safety provides excellent visualization of the posterior and posterolateral compartments. It is established approximately 3 cm proximal to the tip of the olecranon and at the lateral border of the triceps tendon. Allowing the elbow to flex (20–30°) will relax the posterior capsule and facilitate successful trochar insertion [23]. Structures at risk include the posterior antebrachial cutaneous and the lateral brachial cutaneous nerves. The scope is then advanced distally to the radiocapitellar joint to further evaluate for pathology. If debridement or removal of spurs or loose body is needed in the posteromedial gutter, then another accessory trans-triceps (TT) tendon portal (Fig. 2.9) can be created above the olecranon tip as a working portal for instrumentation. This portal is established above the tip of the olecranon through the musculotendinous junction of the triceps muscle with the elbow in a partially extended position. It is excellent for spur debridement and removing loose bodies from the posteromedial compartment. Structures at risk include the posterior antebrachial cutaneous nerve (23 mm away) and the ulnar nerve (25 mm away) when the elbow is distended [17, 23]. Once the elbow arthroscopy is finished and the graft (palmaris vs. gracillis autograft or allograft) is prepared, the medial approach to the elbow is performed to start the UCL reconstruction.

Medial Approach—Muscle Splitting

All portal sites from the elbow arthroscopy were closed with monocryl before the start of the medial exposure. The arm was then exsanguinated to the level of the tourniquet with an Esmarch bandage. An 9–10 cm incision was made with a #15 blade starting 2 cm proximal to the medial epicondyle and extending along the intermuscular septum to approximately 2 cm beyond the sublime tubercle (Figs. 2.3 and 2.5). Meticulous dissection is performed and the medial antebrachial cutaneous nerve is commonly encountered at this time (Fig. 2.3). We typically tag this nerve with a vessel loop and care is taken to avoid injury or damage. At this time, the common flexor–pronator mass is seen inserting on the medial epicondyle along with the anterior fibers of the FCU muscle. A muscle-splitting approach is performed between the raphe of the FCU and the anterior portion of the flexor–pronator mass (Fig. 2.5) which comprises of the flexor carpi radialis, PL, and the flexor digitorum superficialis. This approach is performed through a true internervous plane between the median nerve (anterior portion of the flexor–pronator mass) and the ulnar nerve (FCU muscle). It is also done within the anatomic safe zone that is defined as the region between the medial humeral epicondyle to the area that is 1 cm distal to the attachment of the anterior bundle of the MUCL on the sublime tubercle [11]. A blunt self-retainer retractor may be used to help with the exposure of the anterior bundle of the MUCL during this step of the operation. A sharp retractor should not be used with the exposure to prevent damage to the ulnar nerve (Fig. 2.6). The UCL is inspected and a longitudinal incision in line with the anterior bundle of the MUCL is made with a deep knife to expose the joint. Subsequently, the sublime tubercle is exposed with a periosteal elevator. Two small homans are placed superiorly and inferiorly to the sublime tubercle to help with the exposure. A small burr (3.0 mm) is used to create two tunnels anterior and posterior to the sublime tubercle perpendicular to each other. A small curette is used to complete the tunnels; care is taken to make sure that a 2 cm bone bridge is left between the two tunnels. At this time, the medial humeral epicondyle is exposed with periosteal elevator and a longitudinal tunnel (along the axis of the epicondyle) is created on the anterior half of the medial epicondyle/UCL footprint with a 4 mm burr (Fig. 2.10).

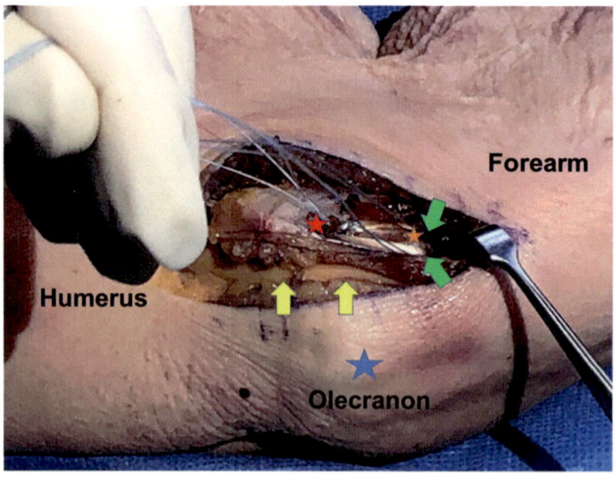

Fig. 2.10 Surgical approach to the ulnar collateral ligament (UCL) reconstruction. The osseous anatomy includes the humerus, forearm, and the Olecranon (*blue star*). The ulnar nerve (*yellow arrows*) is seen behind the medial epicondyle and a single bone tunnel is frilled with a burr into the medial epicondyle (*red star*). Two converging tunnels are drilled (*green arrows*) with the burr into the sublime tubercle (*orange star*) and the palmaris longus graft is passed through the sublime tubercle and docked into the bone tunnel in the medial epicondyle (*red star*)

Care is taken not to violate the posterior cortex of the proximal epicondyle, which would place the ulna nerve at risk and compromise graft fixation. See the pertinent chapter for more details on the tunnel position, graft shuttling, and tensioning techniques.

Medial Approach—Flexor–Pronator Mass Elevation

Alternative to the muscle-splitting technique is the flexor–pronator mass elevation or takedown described by Jobe et al. [26] as the original medial elbow approach to the UCL reconstruction procedure. A similar medial incision is made centered over the medial epicondyle and extending down past the sublime tubercle. Care is taken to protect both the medial antebrachial cutaneous nerve and the ulna nerve. First, a longitudinal split was made in the fascia and in line with the flexor muscles. At this time, the damaged MUCL is exposed and examined. Additional exposure to the UCL reconstruction procedure is provided with elevation and transection of the common flexor mass along with most of the pronator teres 1 cm distal to the medial epicondyle origin leaving a small stump of tissue for reattachment (Fig. 2.11). This approach has been shown to provide a safe and reliable method for the exposure of the anterior bundle of the MUCL and surrounding anatomy. However, detachment and

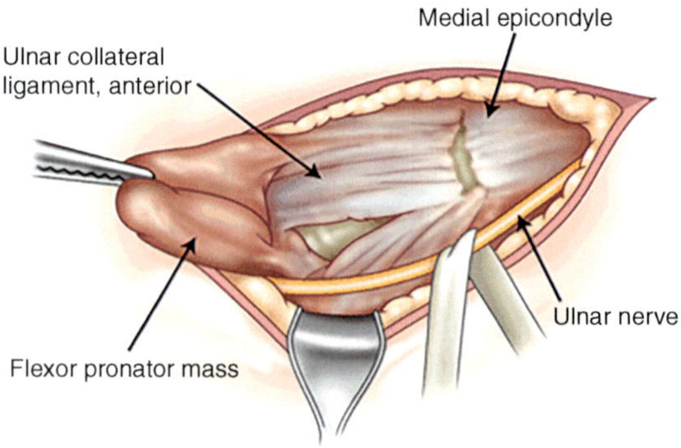

Fig. 2.11 Flexor–pronator mass is transected approximately 1 cm distal to the medial epicondyle origin and retracted to expose the damaged ulnar collateral ligament for reconstruction

reattachment of the flexor–pronator mass may create unnecessary morbidity to the patient; thus, several authors have advocated the muscle-splitting technique as a less traumatic approach to the UCL reconstruction procedure without increased risks [11, 27, 28].

References

1. Morrey BF, An KN. Functional anatomy of the ligaments of the elbow. Clin Orthop Relat Res. 1985;201:84–90.
2. An KN, Hui FC, Morrey BF, Linscheid RL, Chao EY. Muscles across the elbow joint: a biomechanical analysis. J Biomech. 1981;14(10):659–69.
3. Glousman RE, Barron J, Jobe FW, Perry J, Pink M. An electromyographic analysis of the elbow in normal and injured pitchers with medial collateral ligament insufficiency. Am J Sports Med. 1992;20(3):311–7.
4. Norwood LA, Shook JA, Andrews JR. Acute medial elbow ruptures. Am J Sports Med. 1981;9(1):16–9.
5. Safran MR. Ulnar collateral ligament injury in the overhead athlete: diagnosis and treatment. Clin Sports Med. 2004;23(4):643–63. x.
6. Davidson PA, Pink M, Perry J, Jobe FW. Functional anatomy of the flexor-pronator muscle group in relation to the medial collateral ligament of the elbow. Am J Sports Med. 1995;23(2):245–50.
7. Lin F, Kohli N, Perlmutter S, Lim D, Nuber GW, Makhsous M. Muscle contribution to elbow joint valgus stability. J Shoulder Elb Surg. 2007;16(6):795–802.
8. Park MC, Ahmad CS. Dynamic contributions of the flexor-pronator mass to elbow valgus stability. J Bone Joint Surg Am. 2004;86-A(10):2268–74.
9. Udall JH, Fitzpatrick MJ, McGarry MH, Leba TB, Lee TQ. Effects of flexor-pronator muscle loading on valgus stability of the elbow with an intact, stretched, and resected medial ulnar collateral ligament. J Shoulder Elb Surg. 2009;18(5):773–8.
10. Hoshika S, Nimura A, Takahashi N, et al. Valgus stability is enhanced by flexor digitorum superficialis muscle contraction of the index and middle fingers. J Orthop Surg Res. 2020;15:121.
11. Smith GR, Altchek DW, Pagnani MJ, Keeley JRA. muscle-splitting approach to the ulnar collateral ligament of the elbow. Neuroanatomy and operative technique. Am J Sports Med. 1996;24(5):575–80.
12. Masear VR, Meyer RD, Pichora DR. Surgical anatomy of the medial antebrachial cutaneous nerve. J Hand Surg Am. 1989;14(2 Pt 1):267–71.
13. Jones KJ, Osbahr DC, Schrumpf MA, Dines JS, Altchek DW. Ulnar collateral ligament reconstruction in throwing athletes: a review of current concepts. AAOS exhibit selection. J Bone Joint Surg Am. 2012;94(8):e49.
14. King GJ, Morrey BF, An KN. Stabilizers of the elbow. J Shoulder Elb Surg. 1993;2(3):165–74.
15. Timmerman LA, Andrews JR. Histology and arthroscopic anatomy of the ulnar collateral ligament of the elbow. Am J Sports Med. 1994;22(5):667–73.
16. Callaway GH, Field LD, Deng XH, Torzilli PA, O'Brien SJ, Altchek DW, Warren RF. Biomechanical evaluation of the medial collateral ligament of the elbow. J Bone Joint Surg Am. 1997;79(8):1223–31.
17. Lynch GJ, Meyers JF, Whipple TL, Caspari RB. Neurovascular anatomy and elbow arthroscopy: inherent risks. Arthroscopy. 1986;2(3):190–7.
18. Dugas JR, Ostrander RV, Cain EL, Kingsley D, Andrews JR. Anatomy of the anterior bundle of the ulnar collateral ligament. J Shoulder Elb Surg. 2007;16(5):657–60.
19. Regan WD, Korinek SL, Morrey BF, An KN. Biomechanical study of ligaments around the elbow joint. Clin Orthop Relat Res. 1991;Oct(271):170–9.
20. Chen FS, Rokito AS, Jobe FW. Medial elbow problems in the overhead-throwing athlete. J Am Acad Orthop Surg. 2001;9(2):99–113.
21. Ahmad CS, ElAttrache NS. Elbow valgus instability in the throwing athlete. J Am Acad Orthop Surg. 2006;14(12):693–700.
22. Adolfsson L. Arthroscopy of the elbow joint: a cadaveric study of portal placement. J Shoulder Elb Surg. 1994;3(2):53–61.
23. Plancher KD, Bishai SK. Basics of elbow arthroscopy: setup, portals, and technique. Tech in Orthop. 2006;21(4):239–49.
24. Andrews JR, Carson WG. Arthroscopy of the elbow. Arthroscopy. 1985;1(2):97–107.
25. Lindenfeld TN. Medial approach in elbow arthroscopy. Am J Sports Med. 1990;18(4):413–7.
26. Jobe FW, Stark H, Lombardo SJ. Reconstruction of the ulnar collateral ligament in athletes. J Bone Joint Surg Am. 1986;68(8):1158–63.
27. Jobe FW, El Attrache NS. In: Morrey BF, editor. Treatment of ulnar collateral ligament injuries in athletes. New York: Raven Press Limited; 1994.
28. Thompson WH, Jobe FW, Yocum LA, Pink MM. Ulnar collateral ligament reconstruction in athletes: muscle-splitting approach without transposition of the ulnar nerve. J Shoulder Elb Surg. 2001;10(2):152–7.

Ulnar Collateral Ligament: Throwing Biomechanics

3

Evan E. Vellios, Kenneth Durham Weeks III, and David M. Dines

Introduction

The overhead throwing motion is created by a complex series of coordinated movements involving different motor groups and the articulations of the upper extremity as well as the kinetic chain. The necessary kinematics of throwing place significant stresses across the joints of the upper extremity, which can lead to potential overload and injury. The shoulder and elbow are most susceptible to injury during throwing. Even though this text is centered upon ulnar collateral ligament (UCL) injury to the elbow, one must be aware of the biomechanics of the entire upper extremity in throwers in order to understand the cause and prevention of such injuries.

Recent technologic advances in motion analysis have given researchers a better understanding of the anatomic, biomechanical, and physiologic demands placed on the shoulder and elbow during throwing. Clearly, changes in kinetics and kinematics during throwing can have a significant effect upon the anatomy and lead to serious, even career-ending injury. For these reasons, it is imperative to have a comprehensive and sport-specific knowledge of muscle recruitment sequences in order to understand potential causes of anatomic failure and subsequent injury. In addition, this fundamental knowledge can lead to the development of better rehabilitation programs to prevent these injuries.

Of all overhead athletes, baseball pitchers are at the greatest risk of acute and chronic upper extremity pathology, particularly injury to the UCL and medial elbow. While some other athletes may be at risk, such as javelin throwers, tennis servers, and even football quarterbacks, pitchers carry the highest risk and have the highest incidence. Epidemiologic studies of injury patterns in baseball players have shown that there are a higher percentage of upper extremity injuries in Division I college players (58%) [1]. In fact, a study by Rothermich et al. showed that 134 (2.5%) out of 5295 Division 1 college baseball players underwent UCL surgery in 2017 alone with most being pitchers and underclassmen [2]. Moreover, a 2019 study by Leland et al. which consisted of a survey of 6135 professional baseball players (Major League, Minor League, and Dominican Summer League) showed a significant increase in the prevalence of UCL reconstruction in young (<30 years old) Minor League players (15–19%) compared to an earlier 2012 study [3]. With regard to Major League Baseball

E. E. Vellios (✉)
Southern California Orthopedic Institute, Van Nuys, CA, USA

K. D. Weeks III
OrthoCarolina, Charlotte, NC, USA

D. M. Dines
Orthopaedic Surgery, Sports Medicine and Shoulder Service, Hospital for Special Surgery, New York, NY, USA
e-mail: dinesd@hss.edu

J. S. Dines et al. (eds.), *Elbow Ulnar Collateral Ligament Injury*,
https://doi.org/10.1007/978-3-030-69567-5_3

(MLB) specifically, an early study by Conte et al. showed that approximately 30% of player days on the disabled list were the result of shoulder (and elbow) injury with pitchers comprising the majority of disability days at 48%, compared to 20% for outfielders [4]. Most of the injuries pitchers sustained were the result of repetitive overuse of the shoulder or elbow [4]. Furthermore, a recent study by Confino et al. looking at first and second round MLB draft picks from 2008 to 2016 showed that players who underwent early single-sport specialization (played only baseball from high school onwards) had a significantly higher prevalence of upper extremity injuries (primarily shoulder and elbow) and fewer total games played in the MLB than multi-sport athletes [5]. This study highlights the detrimental effects of repeated exposure of the medial elbow to the excessive forces placed upon it during throwing especially in athletes who specialize in a single sport at a young age. The purpose of this chapter is to define the biomechanics in the overhead athlete with a special emphasis upon the biomechanics of the elbow.

Biomechanics of Throwing

As a framework for the understanding of the biomechanics of the throwing shoulder, the pitching cycle is now broken down into six distinct phases, each with its own changes in muscle and joint activity at the shoulder and elbow. During this activity, the thrower must create potential energy generated from the lower extremities and transmitted upward through the pelvis to the trunk and ultimately to the smaller segments of the upper extremity, thereby creating the kinetic energy delivered to the ball in a purposeful manner. This is known as "The Kinetic Chain Theory" of throwing.

Six Phases of the Baseball Pitch

In order to understand the biomechanics of throwing, one must be aware of the six phases of pitching and the effect of the kinetic chain. The throwing motion of the overhead pitch has been divided into six segments or phases from wind-up to follow-through [6, 7].

Phase I

This initial stage is called the wind-up phase. During this phase the pitcher balances on the trailing push-off leg, while the stride leg reaches its maximum hip flexion. The arm is in slight abduction and internal rotation. The elbow is flexed and the forearm pronated.

Phase II

This stage is known as the early cocking phase, during which the ball is removed from the glove, the hands separate and the shoulder abducts and externally rotates. As this occurs, the ground reactive forces manifest in the lower body segments and these forces are then directed through the hip and pelvis of the push-off leg creating the forward movement of the body to generate the kinetic energy in the direction of the throw. As this push-off force increases so does the velocity of the throw. During this phase, there is increased activation in virtually all muscle groups of the shoulder girdle except the upper and lower trapezius with the highest degree of activation being observed in the upper trapezius (64% MVIC, multispectral visible imaging camera) and supraspinatus (51% MVIC) (Fig. 3.1; [8]). The elbow remains flexed between 80° and 90°.

Phase III

The late cocking phase is characterized by maximal shoulder abduction and external rotation. The elbow is flexed 90–120° and forearm pronation is increased to 90°. During this phase, the greatest activation is noted in the subscapularis (124% MVIC) and serratus anterior (104% MVIC) [9].

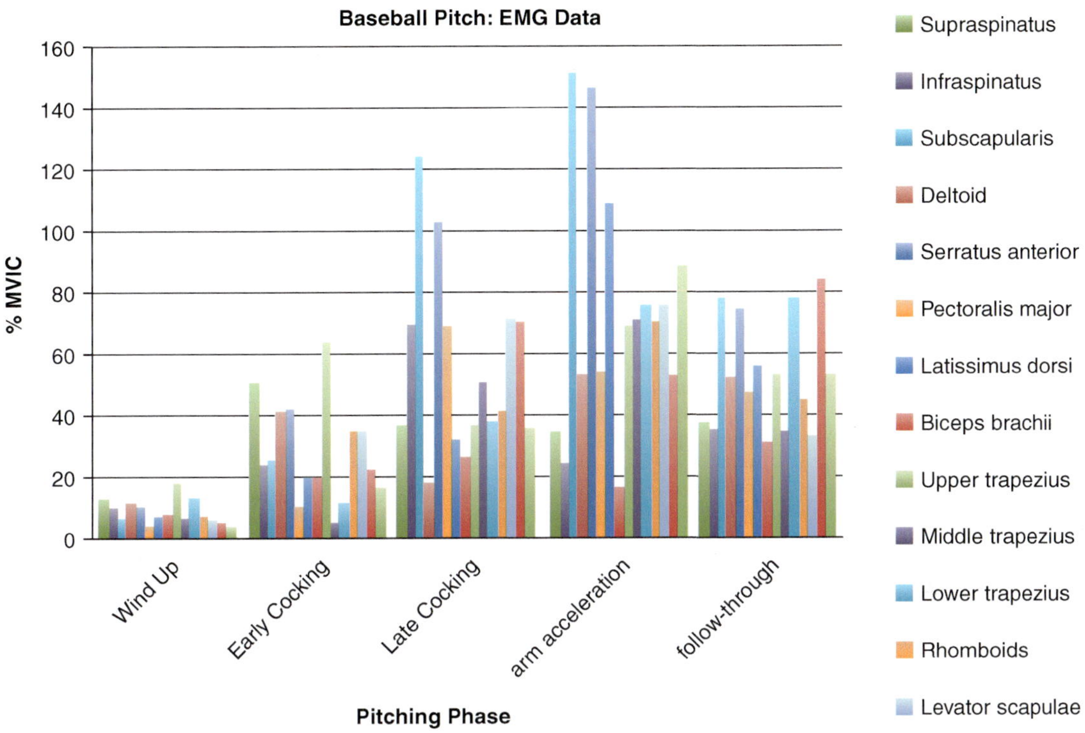

Fig. 3.1 Electromyographic analysis of the upper extremity musculature during overhead throwing. *EMG* electromyography, *MVIC* multispectral visible imaging camera

Phase IV

Acceleration is marked by the generation of a forward-directed force resulting in internal rotation and adduction of the humerus coupled with rapid elbow extension. The greatest activity is again noted in the subscapularis (152% MVIC) and serratus anterior (147% MVIC). There is also a large increase in the recruitment of the latissimus dorsi (from 32% to 110% MVIC). Stage 4 terminates with ball release and lasts 40–50 msec. During this brief amount of time, the elbow accelerates as much as 5000°/s^2 [10]. The medial elbow structures experience a tremendous valgus stress during the late cocking and early acceleration phases. Valgus forces as high as 64 N m are observed at the elbow during late cocking/early acceleration [11].

Phase V

Deceleration begins at ball release and with all muscle groups about the shoulder maximally contracting to decelerate arm rotation. Shoulder abduction is maintained at approximately 100° while the elbow reaches terminal extension at 20° short of full extension. Eccentric biceps and triceps contraction assists in slowing down elbow extension. Forceful deceleration of the upper extremity occurs at a rate of nearly 500,000°/s^2 over the short time of 50 ms [12].

Phase VI

The final stage is follow-through. This phase involves dissipation of all excess kinetic energy as the elbow reaches full extension and the throwing motion is complete.

The Kinetic Chain Theory

The kinetic chain is defined as a rapid, coordinated progression of muscle activation and force development from the legs (distal segments) to the arm during the initiation of unilateral arm throwing. Muscle activation is first seen in segments from the contralateral foot stabilizing structures and progressing through the lower legs to the pelvis and trunk and ultimately to the rapidly accelerating upper extremity. This progression captures the kinetic energy and transfers it effectively up the chain to the smaller upper extremity segments, as the shoulder is not able to generate very much force by itself. The main function of the shoulder is to harness the forces from below and to direct these forces to the arm. The forces of the kinetic chain within the upper extremity then propagate from proximal to distal resulting in a high-velocity ball release.

When looking specifically at the elbow and its interplay with the kinetic chain, two main interactions are found. First, the forearm muscle groups have been noted to assist in fine-tuning ball release. Hirashima et al. [13] analyzed pitching motions and found proximal-to-distal muscle activation, peak torque development, and force development from the trunk to the elbow. In this study of the trunk and arm muscles, the muscle activation sequencing and peak intensity proceeded from the contralateral internal and external obliques and rectus abdominis muscles to the scapular stabilizers, deltoid, and rotator cuff. Force development also proceeded in this pattern. The study showed that muscle activation around the elbow did not appear to continue in this force development sequence but rather occurred in conjunction as a way for the upper extremity to fine-tune and control the pitch. These forearm muscle activations have been called voluntary focal movements.

The second interaction between the kinetic chain and elbow is to create positions and motions that align the elbow articulation to minimize the loads dissipated to the supporting ligaments. Internal rotation of the shoulder with the elbow near full extension and forearm pronated places significantly less stress on the medial elbow. This is seen clinically as elbow injuries during pitching have been associated with mechanics in which the elbow is positioned below the shoulder during the acceleration phase.

Without adequate proximal muscle activation, the distal extremity (i.e., elbow) will experience an increased load and significant stress to generate an equivalent throwing force. Clearly, core conditioning is a critical factor in creating the appropriate timing necessary for the efficient transfer of forces up this chain, as well as in injury prevention.

Anatomy and Biomechanics of the Elbow

The medial ulnar collateral ligament (UCL) of the elbow is a frequent site of serious injury in the athlete performing overhead throwing motions, particularly the competitive baseball pitcher. The stability of the elbow stems from an intricate balance of osseous, ligamentous, and muscular forces. Injury to the UCL is rarely found in isolation and, therefore, a keen understanding of the complex anatomy and the common injuries encountered along the medial elbow is paramount.

Osseous Anatomy

The osseous anatomy of the elbow allows for flexion–extension and pronation–supination through the ulnohumeral and radiocapitellar articulations, respectively. The bony architecture of the proximal ulna and distal humerus provides approximately 50% of the overall stability of the elbow. With the elbow in 0–30° of extension, the olecranon is the primary stabilizer to varus stress. The innate resistance to varus stress of the highly congruous, interlocking ulnohumeral articulation is further increased by the normal valgus carrying angle of 11–16° with the arm fully extended. In

Table 3.1 Elbow ossification centers

Site	Age at appearance of epiphysis/apophysis	Age at closure of epiphysis/apophysis
Capitellum	18 months	14 years
Radial head	5 years	16 years
Medial epicondyle	5 years	15 years
Trochlea	8 years	14 years
Olecranon	10 years	14 years
Lateral epicondyle	12 years	16 years

contrast, the radiocapitellar joint acts as a secondary stabilizer to valgus load. The remaining stability of the elbow is afforded by the radial collateral ligament complex, the UCL complex, and the anterior joint capsule.

In the young athletic elbow, it is important to have a full understanding of the secondary ossification centers that form the distal humerus, proximal ulna, and radius. These apophyses of the elbow appear and fuse at predictable ages and are listed in Table 3.1. These growth centers do not contribute to the overall length of the arm, but are important attachment sites for muscle groups and stabilizing ligaments.

Vascular Anatomy

The vascular anatomy of the elbow consists of three arcades: posterior, lateral, and medial. The posterior arcade is formed from the medial and lateral arcades as well as the middle collateral artery. The lateral arcade is formed from the radial recurrent, interosseus recurrent, and radial and middle collateral arteries. Lastly, the medial arcade is formed by the posterior ulnar recurrent artery and inferior/superior ulnar collateral arteries. Intraosseous circulation to the elbow stems primarily from perforating branches of the previously described extra-osseus circulation [14]. Differential blood supply to portions of the UCL (proximal, midsubstance, or distal) has been hypothesized for varying success rates of nonoperative treatment for partial thickness UCL tears [15]. Recently, a cadaveric study by Buckley et al. showed a reproducibly hypovascular distal UCL insertion with a well-vascularized proximal insertion [16]. This same study showed that in the 18 cadaveric specimens roughly 49% of the length of the UCL experienced vascular penetration leaving the remaining 51% of the ligament hypoperfused. Enhanced understanding of the perfusion of the elbow and more specifically the UCL could result in more patient-specific treatment algorithms with higher rates of success.

Ligamentous Anatomy: Medial Elbow

The UCL complex consists of three ligaments: the anterior oblique (AOL), posterior oblique (POL), and the transverse ligaments. The origin of the AOL and POL is from the anteroinferior surface of the medial epicondyle.

The AOL, consisting of parallel fibers running from its origin and inserting on the sublime tubercle of the medial coronoid process, is functionally the most important due to its strength in resisting valgus stress. The AOL is 4–5 mm wide and is functionally further subdivided into anterior bands (AB) and posterior bands (PB) that provide reciprocal functions in resisting a valgus force through the range of motion. The AB is the primary restraint to valgus stress up to 90° of flexion and becomes secondary with further flexion. The PB becomes functionally more important between 60° and full flexion of the elbow. As a corollary, the PB has increased utility in the overhead athlete, as it is the primary restraint to valgus force with higher degrees of flexion. When both bands of the UCL are completely sectioned, elbow laxity is greatest at 70° of flexion.

The POL is a fan-shaped thickening of the capsule that originates from the medial epicondyle and inserts onto the medial margin of the semilunar notch. The POL is 5–8 mm wide at its midportion, is thinner than the AOL, and forms the floor of the cubital tunnel. It plays a secondary stabilizing role with the elbow in flexion beyond 90° and therefore vulnerable to valgus stress only when the anterior bundle of the AOL is completely detached.

The transverse ligament, also known as Cooper's ligament or the oblique ligament, connects the inferior medial coronoid process with the olecranon. This ligament does not cross the elbow joint and is generally believed to confer no stability against a valgus force.

Musculotendinous Anatomy

Any muscle that crosses the elbow joint does create a joint reactive force, thereby stabilizing the joint through dynamic articular compression. Morrey et al. have shown the stability conferred to the elbow by the triceps, biceps, and brachialis through an elbow model in which the medial UCL and radial head were resected [17]. In addition to these three muscles and pertinent to the overhead thrower, the flexor–pronator muscles provide further support to valgus stress across the medial elbow. Originating from the medial epicondyle, the flexor–pronator group (from proximal to distal) includes the pronator teres, flexor carpi radialis (FCR), palmaris longus, flexor digitorum superficialis, and flexor carpi ulnaris (FCU). The FCU and portions of the flexor digitorum superficialis lie directly over the anterior bundle of the medial UCL and therefore have an enhanced role in dynamic stabilization. As a corollary, electromyographic studies have shown maximal activity for the flexor–pronator muscle group during the acceleration phase of throwing.

Ulnar Nerve

The ulnar nerve has an intimate anatomic relationship with the musculotendinous and ligamentous stabilizers along the medial elbow and is thereby prone to injury during repetitive overhead throwing activities. As the nerve courses distally within the brachium, it passes through the arcade of Struthers, which is located approximately 8 cm proximal to the medial epicondyle. Descending through the midportion of the arm, the nerve then traverses the medial intermuscular septum emerging from the anterior compartment into the posterior compartment. About the elbow, the nerve rests in the cubital tunnel which is bordered anteriorly by the medial epicondyle, posteriorly by the medial head of the triceps, and superficially by Osborne's ligament. The floor of the cubital tunnel is formed by the UCL complex. Sensory fibers within the peripheral nerve are at increased risk with UCL injury given their more superficial location in relation to the motor branches. Exiting the cubital tunnel the nerve then enters the forearm between the two heads of the FCU and finally rests on the flexor digitorum profundus.

Similar to all peripheral nerves, the ulnar nerve is susceptible to injury due to elongation, compression, and inflammation. Elongation occurs during moments of arm abduction, elbow flexion, and wrist extension. A study evaluating the pressure within the ulnar nerve during various elbow and arm positions found a threefold increase in intraneural pressures with the elbow flexed at 90° and the wrist extended, which is a similar position to be seen during the late cocking and early acceleration phases of throwing [18, 19]. In addition, super physiologic elongation of the nerve may occur with a valgus stress to the elbow with an incompetent UCL causing traction neuritis. Miata et al. demonstrated in a cadaveric model that maximum ulnar nerve strain at 90° of elbow flexion nearly doubled with the UCL transected (6.8% +/− 0.7%) compared to intact (3.9% +/− 0.9%) [20]. Narrowing of the cubital tunnel occurs during elbow flexion and is one of several sources of compression. Gelberman et al. demonstrated that the diameter of the cubital tunnel decreases by nearly half during elbow flexion [21]. Compression of the nerve can also occur due to loose bodies, synovitis, thickening of Osborne's ligament, chronically inflamed and/or thickened UCL, or calcification of the UCL.

Biomechanics of Medial Elbow Injury

The significant valgus stress from overhead throwing activities creates tensile stresses that often predispose the UCL to injury. Kinematic testing has identified that the resultant valgus stress applied to the medial elbow during the acceleration phase is 64 N-m. Moreover, the static torque on the UCL during pitching has been estimated to be 32 N-m. This force approaches the known ultimate tensile strength of the UCL of 33 N-m seen in cadaveric specimens [22]. This finding provides evidence for additive dynamic musculotendinous stabilization by the flexor–pronator group as well as a cause for attenuation and eventual collateral ligament failure. In addition, during the acceleration phase, the torque produced generates approximately 500 N of compressive force at the radiocapitellar joint and an estimated 300 N of medial shear force, contributing to valgus extension overload injuries.

In addition to isolated injuries to the UCL, the combination of large valgus loads with rapid elbow extension produces three phenomena: (1) tensile stress along the other medial compartment restraints (flexor–pronator mass, medial epicondyle apophysis, and ulnar nerve), (2) shear stress in the posterior compartment (posteromedial tip of the olecranon and trochlea/olecranon fossa), and (3) compression stress in the radiocapitellar joint. These phenomena have been termed "valgus extension overload syndrome" and form the basic pathophysiologic model behind the most common elbow injuries in the throwing athlete [23]. The syndrome is signified by olecranon tip osteophytes, loose bodies in the posterior or radiocapitellar compartment, and chondromalacia along the posteromedial trochlea. Associated findings include subtle laxity of the UCL, flexor–pronator tendonitis, ulnar neuritis, and medial epicondyle apophysitis in the skeletally immature. Those physicians who treat such injuries in overhead throwing athletes must retain a high degree of suspicion for underlying UCL laxity as the cause of many of these lesions.

References

1. McFarland EG, Wasik M. Epidemiology of collegiate baseball injuries. Clin J Sport Med. 1998. https://doi.org/10.1097/00042752-199801000-00003.
2. Rothermich MA, Conte SA, Aune KT, Fleisig GS, Cain EL, Dugas JR. Incidence of elbow ulnar collateral ligament surgery in collegiate baseball players. Orthop J Sport Med. 2018. https://doi.org/10.1177/2325967118764657.
3. Leland DP, Conte S, Flynn N, et al. Prevalence of medial ulnar collateral ligament surgery in 6135 current professional baseball players: a 2018 update. Orthop J Sport Med. 2019. https://doi.org/10.1177/2325967119871442.
4. Conte S, Requa RK, Garrick JG. Disability days in major league baseball. Am J Sports Med. 2001. https://doi.org/10.1177/03635465010290040801.
5. Confino J, Irvine JN, O'Connor M, Ahmad CS, Lynch TS. Early sports specialization is associated with upper extremity injuries in throwers and fewer games played in major league baseball. Orthop J Sport Med. 2019. https://doi.org/10.1177/2325967119861101.
6. Jobe FW, Moynes DR, Tibone JE, Perry J. An EMG analysis of the shoulder in pitching: a second report. Am J Sports Med. 1984. https://doi.org/10.1177/036354658401200310.
7. Sisto DJ, Jobe FW, Moynes DR, Antonelli DJ. An electromyographic analysis of the elbow in pitching. Am J Sports Med. 1987. https://doi.org/10.1177/036354658701500314.
8. DiGiovine NM, Jobe FW, Pink M, Perry J. An electromyographic analysis of the upper extremity in pitching. J Shoulder Elb Surg. 1992. https://doi.org/10.1016/S1058-2746(09)80011-6.
9. Glousman R, Jobe F, Tibone J, Moynes D, Antonelli D, Perry J. Dynamic electromyographic analysis of the throwing shoulder with glenohumeral instability. J Bone Jt Surg – Ser A. 1988. https://doi.org/10.2106/00004623-198870020-00009.
10. Pappas AM, Zawacki RM, Sullivan TJ. Biomechanics of baseball pitching: a preliminary report. Am J Sports Med. 1985. https://doi.org/10.1177/036354658501300402.
11. Werner SL, Fleisig GS, Dillman CJ, Andrews JR. Biomechanics of the elbow during baseball pitching. J Orthop Sports Phys Ther. 1993. https://doi.org/10.2519/jospt.1993.17.6.274.
12. Fleisig GS, Andrews JR, Dillman CJ, Escamilla RF. Kinetics of baseball pitching with implications about injury mechanisms. Am J Sports Med. 1995. https://doi.org/10.1177/036354659502300218.
13. Hirashima M, Kadota H, Sakurai S, Kudo K, Ohtsuki T. Sequential muscle activity and its functional role in the upper extremity and trunk during overarm throwing. J Sports Sci. 2002. https://doi.org/10.1080/026404102753576071.

14. Yamaguchi K, Sweet FA, Bindra R, Morrey BF, Gelberman RH. The extraosseous and intraosseous arterial anatomy of the adult elbow. J Bone Jt Surg – Ser A. 1997. https://doi.org/10.2106/00004623-199711000-00007.
15. Frangiamore SJ, Lynch TS, Vaughn MD, et al. Magnetic resonance imaging predictors of failure in the nonoperative management of ulnar collateral ligament injuries in professional baseball pitchers. Am J Sports Med. 2017. https://doi.org/10.1177/0363546517699832.
16. Buckley PS, Morris ER, Robbins CM, et al. Variations in blood supply from proximal to distal in the ulnar collateral ligament of the elbow: a qualitative descriptive cadaveric study. Am J Sports Med. 2019. https://doi.org/10.1177/0363546519831693.
17. Morrey BF, An KN. Functional anatomy of the ligaments of the elbow. Clin Orthop Relat Res. 1985. https://doi.org/10.1097/00003086-198512000-00015.
18. Pechan J, Juliš I. The pressure measurement in the ulnar nerve. A contribution to the pathophysiology of the cubital tunnel syndrome. J Biomech. 1975. https://doi.org/10.1016/0021-9290(75)90045-7.
19. Apfelberg DB, Larson SJ. Dynamic anatomy of the ulnar nerve at the elbow. Plast Reconstr Surg. 1973. https://doi.org/10.1097/00006534-197301000-00014.
20. Mihata T, Akeda M, Künzler M, McGarry MH, Neo M, Lee TQ. Ulnar collateral ligament insufficiency affects cubital tunnel syndrome during throwing motion: a cadaveric biomechanical study. J Shoulder Elb Surg. 2019. https://doi.org/10.1016/j.jse.2019.02.009.
21. Gelberman RH, Yamaguchi K, Hollstien SB, et al. Changes in interstitial pressure and cross-sectional area of the cubital tunnel and of the ulnar nerve with flexion of the elbow: an experimental study in human cadavera. J Bone Jt Surg – Ser A. 1998. https://doi.org/10.2106/00004623-199804000-00005.
22. O'Holleran JD, Altchek DW. The Thrower's elbow: arthroscopic treatment of valgus extension overload syndrome. HSS J. 2006. https://doi.org/10.1007/s11420-005-5124-6.
23. Cain EL, Dugas JR, Wolf RS, Andrews JR. Elbow injuries in throwing athletes: a current concepts review. Am J Sports Med. 2003. https://doi.org/10.1177/03635465030310042601.

4 Monitoring the Throwing Motion: Current State of Wearables and Analytics

Vincent A. Lizzio, Eric W. Guo, and Eric C. Makhni

Introduction

Recently, wearable technology has emerged as a promising alternative to high-speed motion analysis for the evaluation of an athlete's throwing motion. Although this technology is relatively new, there have been several recent developments that allow for the routine collection of biomechanical data for both academic and competitive purposes. In this chapter, we review the current capabilities and limitations of wearable technology and examine how this technology might influence our approach to ulnar collateral ligament (UCL) injury risk assessment and rehabilitation.

Biomechanical Parameters of the Throwing Motion

There are several aspects of the throwing motion that have been described in the orthopedic literature. These kinetic and kinematic parameters are the primary targets for analysis and include assessments of the upper body, lower body, and trunk.

Many studies have evaluated the maximum shoulder external rotation that is achieved during the late cocking phase of the throwing motion [1–4] as well as the shoulder internal rotation during acceleration and follow-through [4–6]. Another parameter of the shoulder includes the horizontal abduction/adduction angle of the throwing shoulder which is defined as the position of the elbow when compared to the center of the torso as assessed in the sagittal plane [7, 8]. This measurement is used to quantify the anterior position (adduction) or posterior position (adduction) of the arm at the time of stride foot contact.

Several parameters of elbow motion have been evaluated as well, including elbow flexion and extension, angular velocity, and elbow valgus torque [9–13]. The throwing elbow is brought into maximum flexion during the late cocking phase and achieves maximum extension during the deceleration phase of throwing, whereas maximum elbow angular velocity occurs at ball release.

Maximum medial elbow torque occurs during the end of the late cocking phase and is a particularly intriguing biomechanical parameter due to its potential association with elbow injury risk. Although it is impossible to measure the stress placed on the UCL during the throwing motion, the calculated medial elbow torque acts as a surrogate for estimating UCL stress.

The most common forearm measurement is arm slot, which is used to describe the angle of the forearm relative to the ground at ball release and quantifies what is broadly known as over-

V. A. Lizzio · E. W. Guo · E. C. Makhni (✉)
Department of Orthopedic Surgery, Henry Ford Hospital, Detroit, MI, USA

J. S. Dines et al. (eds.), *Elbow Ulnar Collateral Ligament Injury*,
https://doi.org/10.1007/978-3-030-69567-5_4

hand, three-quarter, sidearm, or submarine throwing. In addition, arm speed can be measured using the maximum rotation of the forearm [14].

Several studies have also characterized lower body and truncal mechanics during the throwing motion. For example, researchers have investigated the impact of stride length on various biomechanical parameters, particularly for ball velocity [15–17]. Other studies have characterized forward truncal tilt at ball release and maximum upper torso rotation during the throwing motion [18–21].

Traditional Methods of Motion Capture

Traditionally, three-dimensional motion analysis has been used to quantitatively evaluate an athlete's throwing motion. This process involves an extensive setup (most commonly in a controlled laboratory setting or pitching tunnel) which includes positioning multiple cameras around the pitcher. Reflective markers are placed on specific anatomical locations on the pitcher's body. Cameras are used to triangulate the markers' positions and movements throughout the pitch. These data are processed to create a three-dimensional representation of an athlete's unique throwing motion, which is then used to calculate various kinetic and kinematic parameters.

While this method of data collection is reliable and considered the gold standard for evaluation of the throwing motion, it has several limitations that significantly inhibit its routine use for both recreational and professional baseball pitchers. First, the equipment is expensive and cumbersome. For this reason, the use of high-speed motion capture is often limited to academic institutions or professional organizations and is relatively inaccessible to the average youth or collegiate athlete. Furthermore, the elaborate setup necessary for this analysis means that data collection must occur in a controlled practice setting and cannot be performed during active competition. Thus, any data collected by this method are limited to simulation studies and cannot evaluate for changes in the throwing motion that may occur during competitive gameplay.

Motion Capture Using Wearable Technology

Recent innovations in wearable technology, particularly from the commercial sector, have been developed to overcome challenges associated with three-dimensional motion analysis. Compared to high-speed motion capture, inertial measurement units (IMUs) are significantly smaller and less expensive, making it now feasible for the average baseball player to quickly and easily evaluate their own throwing motion. Furthermore, since these devices do not require an elaborate setup, they can be used to collect data during active competition. These innovations have caused both researchers and athletes alike to consider how wearable technology can be incorporated into standard pitching practices.

One such commercially available product is the motusTHROW sensor (Motus Global, Rockville Centre, NY). Like many of the sensors used in wearable technology, this sensor contains a triaxial accelerometer and gyrometer to measure various aspects of the throwing motion throughout a pitch, including arm slot, arm speed, maximum shoulder external rotation, and medial elbow torque. The sensor is placed into an elastic athletic sleeve and positioned just distal to the medial epicondyle of the humerus (Fig. 4.1). The measurements obtained by the sensor are transmitted via Bluetooth technology to a mobile phone application (motusTHROW, v.8.6.3, Motus Global, Rockville Centre, NY) and can be evaluated in real-time or retrospectively reviewed (Fig. 4.2). This sensor has been validated against gold-standard high-speed motion analysis [14] and found to be reliable for collecting biomechanical data [22–24].

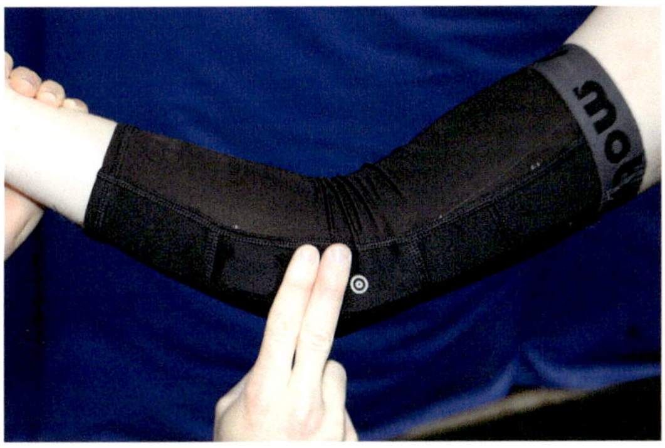

Fig. 4.1 IMU within athletic compression sleeve and positioned distal to the medial epicondyle

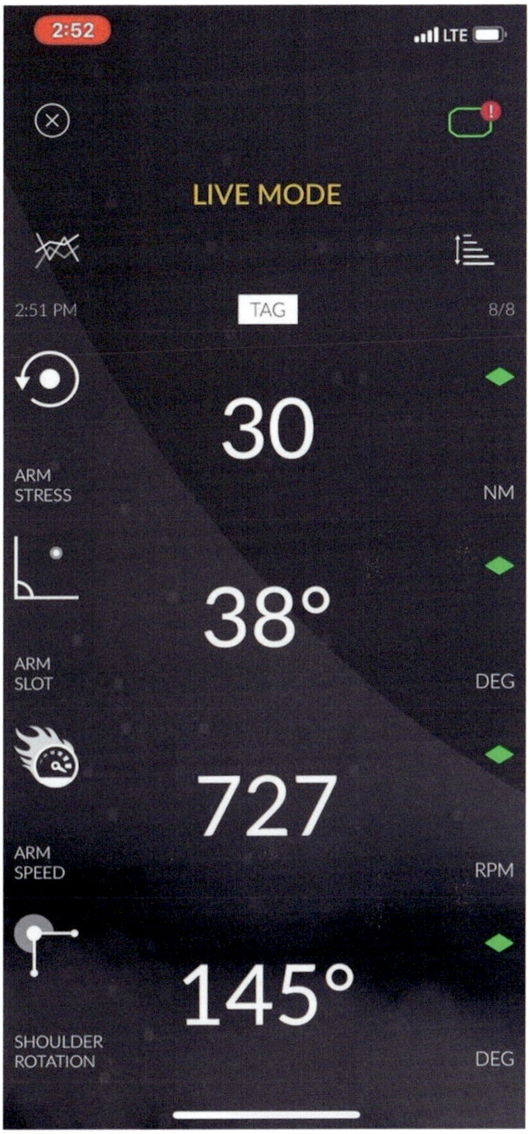

Fig. 4.2 Mobile phone application displaying biomechanical data transmitted from IMU

Evaluation of Fatigue and Workload

There are several other types of wearable technologies that do not directly measure aspects of the throwing motion, but instead evaluate other biometric data to indicate an athlete's fatigue and workload. These devices may be used in conjunction with the aforementioned motion tracking technologies to associate an athlete's physiologic fatigue with changes in their throwing motion. It has been hypothesized that physical fatigue leads to increased risk of injury due to loss of control over the dynamic stabilizers of the elbow [25–27]; therefore, monitoring an athlete's fatigue during active competition may help identify factors leading to increased UCL injury risk.

One of the most common methods of measuring fatigue is through heart rate monitoring devices [28–30]. Heart rate strongly correlates with the level of activity and overall energy expenditure, and there is evidence that post-exercise heart rate variability may correlate with short-term fatigue [31–35]. Furthermore, it is a noninvasive and relatively low-cost technique that is easily accessible to the average athlete. Although psychological factors can influence heart rate – in fact, there is some evidence that a pitcher's average heart rate may even decrease throughout the duration of a game [28] – there may be value in trending heart rate to evaluate the influence of fatigue on an athlete's throwing motion, particularly within each inning.

There are several devices available that track real-time heart rates in athletes, all of which use Bluetooth technology to transmit data in real time. The majority of these devices, including WHOOP (Whoop Inc., Boston, Massachusetts, USA), Zoom HRV (Salutron Inc., Newark, California, USA), Fitbit (Fitbit,

San Francisco, California, USA), and Apple Watch (Apple, Cupertino, California, USA) are worn on the wrist, whereas the Polar H7 (Polar Electro, Lake Success, New York, USA) and Zephyr Bioharness (Zephyr Technology Corporation, Annapolis, Maryland, USA) are worn using a chest strap and SENSE3 (Strive Tech, Bothell, Washington, USA) is worn with athletic shorts.

Analysis of Muscle Recruitment

Historically, researchers have used fine-wire electromyography (EMG) to evaluate an athlete's dynamic muscle recruitment throughout the throwing motion. Several studies have used fine-wire EMG to characterize the recruitment of specific muscles from the upper body, lower body, and even the trunk [36–41]. However, this method of data collection requires the intramuscular insertion of electrodes to measure electromyographic activity. The invasiveness of this procedure, its potential impact on an athlete's natural throwing motion, and the need to perform this study in a controlled research setting has severely limited the routine application of EMG to study the throwing motion.

Recent advancements in surface EMG has made the evaluation of muscle coordination more feasible, bypassing the need for intramuscular monitoring and instead performing these measurements non-invasively. For example, the surface EMG sensors by Delsys Trigno (Delsys, Natick, Massachusetts, USA) are positioned over targeted muscle groups using double-sided adhesive tape (Fig. 4.3). The data are then wirelessly transmitted to the associated software where the raw data are processed to reflect the timing and amount of muscle recruitment for each sensor. Other similar products include ScanVision SEMG (MyoVision, Seattle, Washington, USA), FREEEMG (BTS Bioengineering, Quincy, Massachusetts, USA), SX230 (Newport, United Kingdom), and IX-BIOx (iWorx, Dover, New Hampshire, USA).

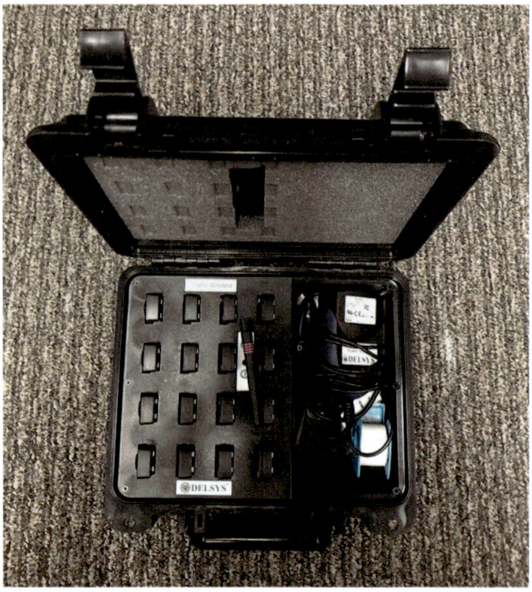

Fig. 4.3 Surface EMG sensors used to measure dynamic muscle recruitment

Wearable Technology in Orthopedic Literature

There has been a rapid increase in the application of wearable technology in the orthopedic literature. Initial studies focused on the development and validation of these IMUs, whereas subsequent studies investigated the impact of pitch type, fatigue, distance, and effort on the throwing motion.

Early IMUs were developed in an effort to more comprehensively count all throwing events performed by a pitcher during a baseball game. Murray et al. described the development of a wearable device consisting of a triaxial accelerometer and gyroscope that could tally warm-up throws and other fielding events in addition to actual pitches. They found that their IMU (Minimax S4, Catapult Innovations, Melbourne, Australia) was highly sensitive but not specific in identifying throwing events when tested with 17 youth athletes [42]. Similarly, another IMU by Rawashdeh et al. was developed and validated for detecting biomechanical differences between overhead activities (such as baseball throws and volleyball serves) and other common athletic maneuvers in 11 athletes [43]. This device was 86% accurate in counting the number of throws and hits performed by these athletes.

With advancements in wearable technology, there was a transition toward using IMUs to precisely measure various aspects of an athlete's throwing motion and find correlations among biomechanical parameters. The first study utilizing the commercially available motusThrow analyzed 82,000 throws and found that increased elbow torque was associated with greater shoulder rotation and arm speed [14]. Another study used this technology and found a strong correlation between high-speed motion capture and the wearable device, albeit with some differences in the magnitude of the measurements [44].

The reliability of this device has been evaluated in high school and collegiate pitchers, demonstrating consistent elbow torque measurements for over 96% of all fastballs, curveballs, and changeups [23]. Similar results have been found for youth and adolescent pitchers [45], but with slightly less precision for professional athletes [22].

Several studies have used this technology in the controlled laboratory setting to evaluate medial elbow stress among pitch types. These studies found that at all levels of competition, it is the fastball – not the curveball – that places the most stress on the medial elbow [22, 23, 45]. Another study evaluated the impact of fatigue on the throwing motion by having high school and collegiate pitchers undergo a simulated game consisting of 90 pitches over six innings [27]. The average medial elbow stress was found to increase over the course of the game while arm slot and ball velocity progressively decreased. Other studies have used IMUs to determine that medial elbow torque increases with increasing ball weight [24], and that elbow torque is not affected by glenohumeral internal rotation deficit [46].

The ability of these IMUs to calculate medial elbow stress has made them particularly intriguing tools for assessment during UCL reconstruction rehabilitation protocols, where the goal is to gradually increase the forces placed on the reconstructed UCL. A study by Dowling et al. used wearable technology to evaluate the throwing motion of 95 high school baseball players during a structured long-toss program that included distances ranging from 9–46 m [47]. Arm speed and shoulder external rotation increased at longer throwing distances whereas arm slot decreased at longer throwing distances. Interestingly, medial elbow torque increased up to 37 m but then plateaued at longer distances, suggesting that throwers may be achieving maximum elbow stress at shorter-than-anticipated distances of these interval throwing programs. A similar study assessed 60 healthy high school and collegiate pitchers and corroborated these findings, demonstrating no significant increase in elbow torque at distances greater than 120 feet [48]. Lastly, a study which used IMUs to evaluate partial effort pitching found that pitchers consistently underestimate their throwing effort, exhibiting 76% and 89% of maximum elbow stress at 50% and 75% of subjective maximum effort, respectively [49].

Recently, a study by Mehta et al. used IMUs to track the medial elbow torque of 18 varsity baseball pitchers for a full season in an effort to correlate elbow stress to injury risk. Over the course of the season, there were six total injuries, of which five of them occurred during throws where medial elbow torque was above the 75th percentile for all occurrences, indicating a link between particularly stressful throws and injury risk [50]. Although the sample size is limited, this is the first study to use IMUs to correlate elbow stress with injury risk for baseball pitchers.

Surface EMG analysis has been used to characterize muscular activation patterns throughout the throwing motion, particularly for lower extremity musculature such as hip adductors and abductors, quadriceps, and hamstrings [51–53]. A study by Erickson et al. demonstrated that hamstring activity is greater in the driving leg than the landing leg, which suggests that hamstring autograft harvested from the landing leg may be less disruptive to an athlete's throwing motion when undergoing UCL reconstruction [54]. A study by Oliver et al. analyzed 14 youth pitchers using surface EMG and found no significant change in muscle activation throughout a simulated game consisting of the recommended pitch limit, regardless of pitch type thrown [41].

However, another study demonstrated an increase in muscle activation for fastballs compared to curveballs when pitching from the stretch position [55].

Current Limitations of Wearable Technology

There are several limitations of wearable technology. Some of these limitations are the result of technical malfunctions and performance issues, whereas others are from difficulties with data interpretation.

Although one of the greatest advantages of wearable technology is the ability to implement data collection during the active competition, there are still barriers to performing these analyses in a reliable manner. Many IMUs have the ability to transmit data in real-time via Bluetooth technology; however, the data cannot always be transmitted to the dugout due to its relatively short range, making it unreliable for evaluating a pitcher's performance during the actual game itself. It also makes it difficult to determine if the sensors are malfunctioning or providing inconsistent measurements throughout the course of the game; if this were possible, these issues could be rectified in real-time to salvage the remaining data collection.

Retrospective review of the data also has unique challenges. IMUs indiscriminately register sudden movements of the arm as throwing events. These events could include warm-up throws, attempts to pick off a baserunner, and fielding maneuvers in addition to the full-effort pitches of interest. Thus, it becomes very difficult to retrospectively differentiate full-effort pitches from background noise in order to accurately trend biomechanical parameters throughout the course of the game.

Since the position of the IMU is vital for accuracy, it is important that these sensors are held in the correct position throughout the duration of the game. However, IMUs may shift during gameplay and compromise the reliability of data collection, especially without a researcher ensuring the accuracy of sensor placement. For example, IMUs that are positioned on the arm using athletic sleeves have a tendency to slide down the arm over time, skewing the data. While a researcher would be able to periodically check sensor placement in a controlled laboratory setting, this is not possible during active competition.

Aside from the need for more rigorous validation of IMUs [56], there are also broader concerns that calculations performed by IMUs are not necessarily representative of their intended target measurements. For example, IMUs indirectly calculate medial elbow torque using accelerometers and gyrometers but do not directly measure the force placed on the medial elbow (although it is important to note that this is a limitation for traditional high-speed motion analysis as well). Furthermore, there is concern that medial elbow torque may not be representative of UCL stress. Since it is not currently possible to directly measure UCL stress – and thus impossible to truly correlate medial elbow torque against UCL stress – it is important to keep these limitations in mind when measuring medial elbow torque using wearable technology.

Probably the greatest limitations of wearable technology at this time, technical issues aside, are those associated with the interpretation of the collected data. Since there are very little data on the impact of biomechanical parameters on injury risk, the minimal clinically significant differences of these measurements are not yet known. Again, using medial elbow torque as an example, our understanding of what constitutes high elbow torque is fairly arbitrary. Since we are still unsure how to interpret medial elbow torque in a practical sense, the measurements obtained by these IMUs are limited to relative comparisons rather than quantifiable correlations at this time.

Lastly, there is debate about whether these IMUs would actually help improve the throwing motion of young athletes. Although biomechanical parameters of the throwing motion are often described as "modifiable," many believe that an athlete's natural throwing motion is innate. For this reason, it is unlikely that pitchers would significantly alter their throwing motion based on the data collected by these wearable devices.

It is possible, however, that these athletes could alter other pitching habits (e.g., pitch counts, rest days, etc.) if they were identified as higher injury risk.

Future Outlook

There are many promising applications for wearable technology, especially for purposes of UCL injury prevention and rehabilitation. Further studies and technological advances in these IMUs will enable athletes to more routinely collect biomechanical information and make decisions using those data.

The next steps in utilizing wearable technology involve their incorporation into rehabilitation protocols for UCL reconstruction. Since these analyses occur in a controlled practice setting, it would be relatively easy to routinely analyze medial elbow stress throughout the rehabilitation process. In addition, athletes could use themselves as their own control when evaluating these measured values, assessing their own relative changes in elbow torque rather than the absolute values themselves. Given that recovering athletes often place greater-than-intended loads on the elbow during UCL rehabilitation [49] these IMUs could help guide throwing effort throughout the rehabilitation protocol.

The routine assessment of biomechanical parameters during pre-season and tracking injuries throughout the season would help researchers identify which biomechanical characteristics place athletes at greater risk for injury. Whereas this was previously impractical due to technical limitations of high-speed motion capture, wearable technology has made this type of investigation much more feasible. Further incorporation of this technology into active competition would allow researchers to analyze changes in pitching biomechanics over the course of a single game, and even throughout the duration of the competitive season. These data, when correlated with the timing of pitching-related injuries, would provide further insight into the impact of pitching mechanics on injury risk.

Ultimately, the data collected by wearable technology may even be used for in-game decision making. The most likely development may be in moving away from standardized pitch counts and toward individualized pitch limit based on an athlete's unique biomechanical data. In-game data might also be used to identify diminishing performance due to fatigue, much like ball velocity is used in today's game. Although not feasible with current IMUs, rapid innovations in wearable technology are making these developments increasingly realistic.

References

1. Miyashita K, Kobayashi H, Koshida S, Urabe Y. Glenohumeral, scapular, and thoracic angles at maximum shoulder external rotation in throwing. Am J Sports Med. 2010;38(2):363–8.
2. Miyashita K, Urabe Y, Kobayashi H, et al. Relationship between maximum shoulder external rotation angle during throwing and physical variables. J Sports Sci Med. 2008;7(1):47–53.
3. Miyashita K, Urabe Y, Kobayashi H, et al. The role of shoulder maximum external rotation during throwing for elbow injury prevention in baseball players. J Sports Sci Med. 2008;7(2):223–8.
4. Seroyer ST, Nho SJ, Bach BR, et al. The kinetic chain in overhand pitching: its potential role for performance enhancement and injury prevention. Sports Health. 2010;2(2):135–46.
5. Borsa PA, Dover GC, Wilk KE, Reinold MM. Glenohumeral range of motion and stiffness in professional baseball pitchers. Med Sci Sports Exerc. 2006;38(1):21–6.
6. Brown LP, Niehues SL, Harrah A, Yavorsky P, Hirshman HP. Upper extremity range of motion and isokinetic strength of the internal and external shoulder rotators in major league baseball players. Am J Sports Med. 1988;16(6):577–85.
7. Meyer KE, Saether EE, Soiney EK, et al. Three-dimensional scapular kinematics during the throwing motion. J Appl Biomech. 2008;24(1):24–34.
8. Takagi Y, Oi T, Tanaka H, et al. Increased horizontal shoulder abduction is associated with an increase in shoulder joint load in baseball pitching. J Shoulder Elb Surg. 2014;23(12):1757–62.
9. Aguinaldo AL, Chambers H. Correlation of throwing mechanics with elbow valgus load in adult baseball pitchers. Am J Sports Med. 2009;37(10):2043–8.
10. Anz AW, Bushnell BD, Griffin LP, et al. Correlation of torque and elbow injury in professional baseball pitchers. Am J Sports Med. 2010;38(7):1368–74.

11. Fehr S, Damrow D, Kilian C, Lyon R, Liu XC. Elbow biomechanics of pitching: does age or experience make a difference? Sports Health. 2016;8(5):444–50.
12. Fortenbaugh D, Fleisig GS, Andrews JR. Baseball pitching biomechanics in relation to injury risk and performance. Sports Health. 2009;1(4):314–20.
13. Sabick MB, Torry MR, Lawton RL, Hawkins RJ. Valgus torque in youth baseball pitchers: a biomechanical study. J Shoulder Elb Surg. 2004;13(3):349–55.
14. Camp CL, Tubbs TG, Fleisig GS, et al. The relationship of throwing arm mechanics and elbow varus torque: within-subject variation for professional baseball pitchers across 82,000 throws. Am J Sports Med. 2017;45(13):3030–5.
15. Digiovine NM, Jobe FW, Pink M, Perry J. An electromyographic analysis of the upper extremity in pitching. J Shoulder Elb Surg. 1992;1(1):15–25.
16. Ramsey DK, Crotin RL, White S. Effect of stride length on overarm throwing delivery: a linear momentum response. Hum Mov Sci. 2014;38:185–96.
17. van Trigt B, Schallig W, van der Graaff E, MJM H, Veeger D. Knee angle and stride length in association with ball speed in youth baseball pitchers. Sports (Basel). 2018;6(2):51.
18. Bullock GS, Schmitt AC, Chasse PM, et al. The relationship between trunk rotation, upper quarter dynamic stability, and pitch velocity. J Strength Cond Res. 2018;32(1):261–6.
19. Calabrese GJ. Pitching mechanics, revisited. Int J Sports Phys Ther. 2013;8(5):652–60.
20. Matsuo T, Fleisig GS. Influence of shoulder abduction and lateral trunk tilt on peak elbow varus torque for college baseball pitchers during simulated pitching. J Appl Biomech. 2006;22(2):93–102.
21. Oyama S, Yu B, Blackburn JT, et al. Effect of excessive contralateral trunk tilt on pitching biomechanics and performance in high school baseball pitchers. Am J Sports Med. 2013;41(10):2430–8.
22. Lizzio VA, Gulledge CM, Smith DG, et al. Predictors of elbow torque among professional baseball pitchers. J Shoulder Elb Surg. 2020;29(2):316–20.
23. Makhni EC, Lizzio VA, Meta F, et al. Assessment of elbow torque and other parameters during the pitching motion: comparison of fastball, curveball, and change-up. Arthroscopy. 2018;34(3):816–22.
24. Okoroha KR, Meldau JE, Jildeh TR, et al. Impact of ball weight on medial elbow torque in youth baseball pitchers. J Shoulder Elb Surg. 2019;28(8):1484–9.
25. Chalmers PN, Wimmer MA, Verma NN, et al. The relationship between pitching mechanics and injury: a review of current concepts. Sports Health. 2017;9(3):216–21.
26. Cowley JC, Gates DH. Proximal and distal muscle fatigue differentially affect movement coordination. PLoS One. 2017;12(2):e0172835.
27. Okoroha KR, Meldau JE, Lizzio VA, et al. Effect of fatigue on medial elbow torque in baseball pitchers: a simulated game analysis. Am J Sports Med. 2018;46(10):2509–13.
28. Cornell DJ, Paxson JL, Caplinger RA, et al. In-game heart rate responses among professional baseball starting pitchers. J Strength Cond Res. 2017;31(1):24–9.
29. Gillett JS, Dawes JJ, Spaniol FJ, et al. A description and comparison of cardiorespiratory fitness measures in relation to pitching performance among professional baseball pitchers. Sports (Basel). 2016;4(1):14.
30. Warren CD, Szymanski DJ, Landers MR. Effects of three recovery protocols on range of motion, heart rate, rating of perceived exertion, and blood lactate in baseball pitchers during a simulated game. J Strength Cond Res. 2015;29(11):3016–25.
31. Borresen J, Lambert MI. Autonomic control of heart rate during and after exercise: measurements and implications for monitoring training status. Sports Med (Auckland, NZ). 2008;38(8):633–46.
32. Escorihuela RM, Capdevila L, Castro JR, et al. Reduced heart rate variability predicts fatigue severity in individuals with chronic fatigue syndrome/myalgic encephalomyelitis. J Transl Med. 2020;18(1):4.
33. Mourot L, Bouhaddi M, Tordi N, Rouillon JD, Regnard J. Short- and long-term effects of a single bout of exercise on heart rate variability: comparison between constant and interval training exercises. Eur J Appl Physiol. 2004;92(4–5):508–17.
34. Schmitt L, Regnard J, Millet GP. Monitoring fatigue status with HRV measures in elite athletes: an avenue beyond RMSSD? Front Physiol. 2015;6:343.
35. Strath SJ, Swartz AM, Bassett DRJ, et al. Evaluation of heart rate as a method for assessing moderate intensity physical activity. Med Sci Sports Exerc. 2000;32(9 Suppl):S465–70.
36. Crotin RL, Kozlowski K, Horvath P, Ramsey DK. Altered stride length in response to increasing exertion among baseball pitchers. Med Sci Sports Exerc. 2014;46(3):565–71.
37. Escamilla RF, Andrews JR. Shoulder muscle recruitment patterns and related biomechanics during upper extremity sports. Sports Medicine (Auckland, NZ). 2009;39(7):569–90.
38. Glousman R, Jobe F, Tibone J, et al. Dynamic electromyographic analysis of the throwing shoulder with glenohumeral instability. J Bone Joint Surg Am. 1988;70(2):220–6.
39. Gowan ID, Jobe FW, Tibone JE, Perry J, Moynes DR. A comparative electromyographic analysis of the shoulder during pitching. Professional versus amateur pitchers. Am J Sports Med. 1987;15(6):586–90.
40. Hirashima M, Kadota H, Sakurai S, Kudo K, Ohtsuki T. Sequential muscle activity and its functional role in the upper extremity and trunk during overarm throwing. J Sports Sci. 2002;20(4):301–10.
41. Oliver GD, Plummer H, Henning L, et al. Effects of a simulated game on upper extremity pitching mechanics and muscle activations among various pitch types in youth baseball pitchers. J Pediatr Orthop. 2019;39(8):387–93.
42. Murray NB, Black GM, Whiteley RJ, et al. Automatic detection of pitching and throwing events in baseball

with inertial measurement sensors. Int J Sports Physiol Perform. 2017;12(4):533–7.
43. Rawashdeh SA, Rafeldt DA, Uhl TL. Wearable IMU for shoulder injury prevention in overhead sports. Sensors (Basel). 2016;16(11):1847.
44. Boddy KJ, Marsh JA, Caravan A, et al. Exploring wearable sensors as an alternative to marker-based motion capture in the pitching delivery. Peer J. 2019;e6365:7.
45. Okoroha KR, Lizzio VA, Meta F, et al. Predictors of elbow torque among youth and adolescent baseball pitchers. Am J Sports Med. 2018;46(9):2148–53.
46. Smith DG, Swantek AJ, Gulledge CM, et al. Relationship between glenohumeral internal rotation deficit and medial elbow torque in high school baseball pitchers. Am J Sports Med. 2019;47(12):2821–6.
47. Dowling B, McNally MP, Laughlin WA, Onate JA. Changes in throwing arm mechanics at increased throwing distances during structured long-toss. Am J Sports Med. 2018;46(12):3002–6.
48. Leafblad ND, Larson DR, Fleisig GS, et al. Variability in baseball throwing metrics during a structured long-toss program: does one size fit all or should programs be individualized? Sports Health. 2019;11(6):535–42.
49. Lizzio VA, Smith DG, Jildeh TR, et al. Importance of radar gun inclusion during return-to-throwing rehabilitation following ulnar collateral ligament reconstruction in baseball pitchers: a simulation study. J Shoulder Elb Surg. 2020;29(3):587–92.
50. Mehta S. Relationship between workload and throwing injury in varsity baseball players. Phys Ther Sport. 2019;40:66–70.
51. Campbell BM, Stodden DF, Nixon MK. Lower extremity muscle activation during baseball pitching. J Strength Cond Res. 2010;24(4):964–71.
52. Oliver GD, Keeley DW. Gluteal muscle group activation and its relationship with pelvis and torso kinematics in high-school baseball pitchers. J Strength Cond Res. 2010;24(11):3015–22.
53. Yamanouchi T. EMG analysis of the lower extremities during pitching in high-school baseball. Kurume Med J. 1998;45(1):21–5.
54. Erickson BJ, Zaferiou A, Chalmers PN, et al. Are the hamstrings from the drive leg or landing leg more active in baseball pitchers? An electromyographic study. J Shoulder Elb Surg. 2017;26(11):2010–6.
55. Smidebush M, Stewart E, Shapiro R, Chander H, Knight A. Mean muscle activation comparison between fastballs and curveballs with respect to the upper and lower extremity. J Biomech. 2019;94:187–92.
56. Driggers AR, Bingham GE, Bailey CA. The relationship of throwing arm mechanics and elbow varus torque: letter to the editor. Am J Sports Med. 2019;47(1):Np1–np5.

Medial Ulnar Collateral Ligament Injury Prevention Strategies

5

Brian M. Schulz, Spencer M. Stein, and Stan A. Conte

Introduction

Baseball is a popular sport both in the United States and worldwide and has recently seen its popularity rise [1]. More than 25 million children played baseball or softball in 2018 [1]. Unfortunately, throwing-related injuries, including injury to the medial ulnar collateral ligament (UCL), have also increased in both amateur and professional players, with one study demonstrating a 50% increase in UCL reconstructions in high school athletes between 1988 and 2003 [2]. Injury to the ulnar collateral ligament results in a significant loss of participation time. While these injuries are not completely avoidable, there are modifiable risk factors and preventative strategies to decrease their incidence. This chapter reviews the risk factors for and preventative strategies to avoid injury to the medial ulnar collateral ligament at the youth, adolescent, and adult level.

B. M. Schulz (✉)
Los Angeles Angels and Anaheim Ducks, Cedars-Sinai Kerlan-Jobe Institute, Anaheim, CA, USA

S. M. Stein
Sports Medicine, Orthopedic Surgery, Kerlan-Jobe Institute, Los Angeles, CA, USA

S. A. Conte
Conte Sport Performance Therapy, Scottsdale, AZ, USA

Youth and Adolescents

Overuse and fatigue remain a leading cause of elbow injuries among youth and adolescent baseball players. Pitching volume is the largest predictor of injury in this age group [3]. Early sports specialization has created an environment where young players are playing baseball year-round, which results in overuse. Overuse leads to arm pain, which then can lead to a more serious injury [4]. Alarmingly, when surveyed, 46% of youth baseball players stated they were encouraged at least once to keep playing despite having arm pain [5].

Early sports specialization is defined as the intensive training or competition in a single sport by children younger than 12 years old for more than 8 months per year [6]. This intense focus on a single sport prevents the athlete from participating in other sports or free play. Many athletes, parents, and coaches feel this early specialization is necessary to obtain a college scholarship or become a professional athlete. However, there is no strong evidence that this is true for baseball. Furthermore, there is evidence that early sports specialization increases the risk of injury and burnout.

In addition to overuse and fatigue, increased velocity, playing for traveling teams, early maturity, and participating in showcases increase the risk of ulnar collateral ligament injury [5, 7–9]. Pitchers that also play catcher

J. S. Dines et al. (eds.), *Elbow Ulnar Collateral Ligament Injury*,
https://doi.org/10.1007/978-3-030-69567-5_5

are at increased risk due to the large amount of throws made during the season [10]. Months played per season is another risk factor for injury. Pitchers that play more than 8 months per season are at a 5x higher likelihood of sustaining a shoulder or elbow injury that requires surgery than those who play less than 8 months per year [8]. Furthermore, the number of pitches per appearance greater than 80 pitches, fastball speed greater than 85 miles per hour, and pitching with arm fatigue were the most significant risk factors for injury requiring surgery on the shoulder or elbow [8]. Pitching for more than one team at a time and pitcher height have also been shown to be risk factors [11].

For the longest time, the curveball was blamed for throwing-related injuries leading many experts to recommend that skeletally immature players refrain from throwing these pitches. However, recent data have largely refuted that claim. Multiple studies have shown that elbow varus torque is actually lower when throwing a curveball compared to a fastball [12, 13]. Furthermore, a biomechanical study has shown no significant difference in the mechanics and arm slot for a fastball, curveball, or change up [14]. This further supports the idea that a curveball is no more dangerous than other pitches.

Despite the adoption of pitch counts and safety guidelines, overuse injuries to the elbow have continued to occur at an increased rate in this population. This can be partly attributed to a lack of awareness of the current recommendations and risk factors (Tables 5.1 and 5.2) [15]. A study of 98 baseball players between the ages of 4 and 18 showed that 62% of the participants disagreed with the statement "The more you throw, the more likely you are to get an injury" [16]. Furthermore, 57% of the respondents stated they would not seek medical attention if they experienced arm pain during a game [16]. The public perception is also flawed regarding risk factors for elbow injury and the benefits of Tommy John surgery. A questionnaire study of 189 players, 15 coaches, and 31 parents showed that 31% of coaches, 28% of players, and 25% of parents did not think the number of pitches was a risk factor [17]. Even more alarming was that 30% of coaches, 27% of parents, and 51% of players thought that Medial Ulnar Collateral Ligament Reconstruction should be performed prophylactically to improve performance.

Proper mechanics are an important aspect of injury prevention. Lower humeral internal rotation torque (HIRT), lower elbow valgus load (EVL), and higher pitching efficiency were seen in youth and adolescent pitchers that exhibited

Table 5.1 Risk factors for injury

Pitching while fatigued
Throwing too many innings over the course of the season
Not taking enough time off from baseball each year
Throwing too many innings at a single time
Inadequate rest after throwing
Pitching on consecutive days
Excessive throwing when not pitching
Playing for multiple teams at the same time
Pitching with injuries to other areas of the body
Not following proper strength and conditioning routines
Not following safe practices at Showcases
Radar gun use

Data from [15]

Table 5.2 Pitch count limits and required rest recommendations

Age	Daily max pitches (in game)	0 Days rest	1 Day rest	2 Days rest	3 Days rest	4 Days rest	5 Days rest
7–8	50	1–20	21–35	36–50	N/A	N/A	N/A
9–10	15	1–20	21–35	36–50	51–65	66+	N/A
11–12	85	1–20	21–35	36–50	51–65	66+	N/A
13–14	95	1–20	21–35	36–50	51–65	66+	N/A
15–16	95	1–30	31–45	46–60	61–75	76+	N/A
17–18	105	1–30	31–45	46–60	61–80	81+	N/A
19–22	120	1–30	31–45	46–60	61–80	81–105	106+

Data from [15]

better pitching mechanics [18]. This study looked at five basic pitching parameters that included leading with the hips, hand-on-top position, arm in the throwing position, closed shoulder position, and stride foot toward home plate. Youth pitchers were found to have lower HIRT and lower EVL when more parameters were performed correctly. In both adolescent and youth players, hand-on-top position and closed shoulder position were independently associated with lower HIRT and EVL.

Pitch Smart (www.mlb.com/pitch-smart) is a collaboration between Major League Baseball, USA Baseball, and sports medicine experts [15]. The website was designed to serve as a comprehensive resource for safe pitching practices. The goal of Pitch Smart is to provide guidelines and information players, parents, and coaches can use to avoid overuse injuries. The website serves as an excellent source of up-to-date information from experts in the field. However, studies have shown that coaches often do not adhere to pitch counts or recommendations of Pitch Smart. Knapik et al. [19] surveyed 61 coaches and found that 56% were noncompliant to age-appropriate pitch counts, and only 13% were able to identify risk factors. This shows a disconnect between preventative recommendations and what is actually occurring.

While some risk factors, including early maturity, fastball velocity, and body mass index, cannot be modified, many can. We recommend focusing on proper throwing mechanics, adhering to pitch count and rest guidelines, avoiding pitching competitively more than 8 months a year and avoiding throwing when fatigued. Young athletes should play multiple sports and avoid early specialization in baseball. Players should only play for one team at a time and should never throw with arm pain. If a player develops pain, he or she should be evaluated by a sports medicine physician and not resume throwing until symptoms have resolved. Physical therapy focusing on general conditioning and core strengthening exercises should be performed while the injured player is recovering. Furthermore, coaches should avoid the use of radar guns.

High School and College

High school and college baseball players are at risk of injury to the ulnar collateral ligament just as youth and adolescent players. These injuries, however, are often more severe and more commonly require surgery with 13% of reconstructions being performed on high school students [1]. Risk factors for these injuries mirror those of the youth and adolescent population, and most commonly are due to overuse. Similarly, the recommendations of pitch count and rest guidelines, avoiding throwing when fatigued or in pain and no competitive throwing more than 8 months a year apply to these players as well.

There has recently been an increased emphasis on pitch velocity in high school, college, and professional pitchers. This increased emphasis has led to the development of several velocity enhancement programs that have been marketed to pitchers at every level. One of the most popular programs has been the use of underweight and overweight weighted baseballs. Several studies have shown these programs are effective at increasing velocity [20–25]. While these programs have been effective, there is concern that the program or the increased velocity from the program could lead to injury. Recently, a randomized controlled trial showed that 24% of the pitchers in the weighted ball training group sustained an elbow injury either during the weighted ball training or the following season [25]. There were no players in the control group that developed an elbow injury. Driveline Baseball, based in Seattle Washington, has developed in-gym and remote training programs for pitchers looking to gain velocity [26]. The company uses a combination of motion-capture devices, barbell speed trackers, high-speed video, ball flight data, and manual tests to create a player-specific training program geared toward the goals of the individual player. Pitchers should use caution when considering these types of programs as more research is necessary to optimize the program without increasing additional risk of injury.

Dines et al. [27] showed that pathologic glenohumeral internal rotation deficit was seen more commonly in baseball players with ulnar collateral ligament insufficiency than in asymptomatic players. Furthermore, high school and college baseball players with ulnar collateral ligament injury were found to have impaired balance compared to an uninjured cohort [28]. These findings suggest that a stretching and strengthening program that focuses on improved range of motion of the shoulder, elbow and hips, strengthening of the rotator cuff, scapular stabilizers, core and lower extremities, and proprioceptive training should be integrated into the athlete's regular routine to potentially decrease injury risk.

Professional

Between 1998 and 2015, the incidence of medial ulnar collateral ligament injury and MUCL reconstruction in Major League Baseball players has increased [29]. Currently, approximately 25% of Major League Baseball players have undergone Tommy John surgery [30]. This has resulted in significant time lost for the player and monetary loss for the teams they play for. The cause of the increased incidence is likely multifactorial but previous studies have suggested that risks factors for this group of athletes include pitching mechanics and release point [31], pitching fatigue, pitch type, and pitching velocity [32]. Interestingly, in this population of athletes increased pitching volume has not been shown to be a direct risk factor [33], as it is in the youth age group. However, the importance of prevention is highlighted by Keller et al. [34] who demonstrated that revision surgery for professionals was more common in those who underwent primary surgery at a younger age and those who had less major league experience.

A recent questionnaire of Major League Baseball pitchers showed that 45% thought that injury to the ulnar collateral ligament was avoidable [35]. Fifty-five percent of the pitchers surveyed, who had a history of a UCL injury, had a history of elbow injury as an adolescent or child compared with 18% in the uninjured group. Seventy-two percent of these pitchers believed that fatigue over the season increased the risk of injury to the UCL. Furthermore, 59% of the MLB pitchers felt that a six man starting rotation in Major League Baseball would decrease the incidence of UCL injury.

The mean fastball velocity in Major League Baseball has gradually increased. Keller et al. showed that MLB pitchers who pitch a high percentage of fastballs had a higher risk of ulnar collateral ligament injury [32]. Pitching greater than 48% fastballs was a risk factor for injury to the UCL. The risk of injury increased 2% for every 1% increase in fastballs thrown. Furthermore, Chalmers et al. showed that peak velocity was an independent risk factor for ulnar collateral ligament reconstruction in MLB pitchers [36]. While increased velocity has been shown to be a risk factor, a higher velocity imparts an advantage for the pitcher. Consequently, it is unlikely that pitchers will throw at slower speeds to avoid injury.

In conclusion, UCL injury prevention, even in the professional pitcher, starts in youth baseball. Young pitchers should not pitch more than 100 innings in a single season, adhere to USA Baseball Medical/Safety Advisory Committee recommendations on pitch limits, and rest and avoid playing for more than one team at a time. Furthermore, pitchers should avoid throwing for more than 8 months in a year and avoid early baseball specialization. Players at every level of play should be discouraged from throwing with elbow pain or pitching while fatigued. Furthermore, medical professionals need to address the common misperceptions and better educate players, coaches, and parents on risk factors and current safety recommendations.

References

1. Nuckols B. Put me in, coach: youth baseball participation on the rise. USA Today. 2019;August(23):2019.
2. Petty DH, Andrews JR, Fleisig GS, Cain EL. Ulnar collateral ligament reconstruction in high school baseball players: clinical results and injury risk factors. Am J Sports Med. 2004;32(5):1158–64.
3. Fleisig GS, Andrews JR. Prevention of elbow injuries in youth baseball pitchers. Sports Health. 2012;4(5):419–24.
4. Yang J, Mann BJ, Guettler JH, Dugas JR, Irrgang JJ, Fleisig GS, et al. Risk-prone pitching activities and injuries in youth baseball: findings from a national sample. Am J Sports Med. 2014;42(6):1456–63.
5. Makhni EC, Morrow ZS, Luchetti TJ, Mishra-Kalyani PS, Gualtieri AP, Lee RW, et al. Arm pain in youth baseball players: a survey of healthy players. Am J Sports Med. 2015;43(1):41–6.

6. Popkin CA, Bayomy AF, Ahmad CS. Early sport specialization. J Am Acad Orthop Surg. 2019;27(22):e995–e1000.
7. Fleisig GS, Andrews JR, Cutter GR, Weber A, Loftice J, McMichael C, et al. Risk of serious injury for young baseball pitchers: a 10-year prospective study. Am J Sports Med. 2011;39(2):253–7.
8. Olsen SJ 2nd, Fleisig GS, Dun S, Loftice J, Andrews JR. Risk factors for shoulder and elbow injuries in adolescent baseball pitchers. Am J Sports Med. 2006;34(6):905–12.
9. Matthys SP, Vaeyens R, Coelho ESMJ, Lenoir M, Philippaerts R. The contribution of growth and maturation in the functional capacity and skill performance of male adolescent handball players. Int J Sports Med. 2012;33(7):543–9.
10. Melugin HP, Leafblad ND, Camp CL, Conte S. Injury prevention in baseball: from youth to the pros. Curr Rev Musculoskelet Med. 2018;11(1):26–34.
11. Chalmers PN, Sgroi T, Riff AJ, Lesniak M, Sayegh ET, Verma NN, et al. Correlates with history of injury in youth and adolescent pitchers. Arthroscopy. 2015;31(7):1349–57.
12. Dun S, Loftice J, Fleisig GS, Kingsley D, Andrews JR. A biomechanical comparison of youth baseball pitches: is the curveball potentially harmful? Am J Sports Med. 2008;36(4):686–92.
13. Nissen CW, Westwell M, Ounpuu S, Patel M, Solomito M, Tate J. A biomechanical comparison of the fastball and curveball in adolescent baseball pitchers. Am J Sports Med. 2009;37(8):1492–8.
14. Oliver GD, Plummer H, Henning L, Saper M, Glimer G, Brambeck A, et al. Effects of a simulated game on upper extremity pitching mechanics and muscle activations among various pitch types in youth baseball pitchers. J Pediatr Orthop. 2019;39(8):387–93.
15. https://www.mlb.com/pitch-smart. Major League Baseball; 2020.
16. Bohne C, George SZ, Zeppieri GJ. Knowledge of injury prevention and prevalence of risk factors for throwing injuries in a sample of youth baseball players. Int J Sports Phys Ther. 2015;10(4):464–75.
17. Ahmad CS, Grantham WJ, Greiwe RM. Public perceptions of Tommy John surgery. Phys Sportsmed. 2012;40(2):64–72.
18. Davis JT, Limpisvasti O, Fluhme D, Mohr KJ, Yocum LA, Elattrache NS, et al. The effect of pitching biomechanics on the upper extremity in youth and adolescent baseball pitchers. Am J Sports Med. 2009;37(8):1484–91.
19. Knapik DM, Continenza SM, Hoffman K, Gilmore A. Youth baseball coach awareness of pitch count guidelines and overuse throwing injuries remains deficient. J Pediatr Orthop. 2018;38(10):e623–e8.
20. DeRenne CBB, Hetzler RK, Ho KW. Effects of under-and-overweighted implement training on pitching velocity. J Strength Cond Res. 1994;8:247–50.
21. Derenne C, Ho KW, Murphy JC. Effects of general, special, and specific resistance training on throwing velocity in baseball: a brief review. J Strength Cond Res. 2001;15(1):148–56.
22. Derenne CSD. Effects of baseball weighted implement training: a brief review. Strength Cond J. 2009;31:30–7.
23. Escamilla RF, Speer KP, Fleisig GS, Barrentine SW, Andrews JR. Effects of throwing overweight and underweight baseballs on throwing velocity and accuracy. Sports Med. 2000;29(4):259–72.
24. Fleisig GS, Diffendaffer AZ, Aune KT, Ivey B, Laughlin WA. Biomechanical analysis of weighted-ball exercises for baseball pitchers. Sports Health. 2017;9(3):210–5.
25. Reinold MM, Macrina LC, Fleisig GS, Aune K, Andrews JR. Effect of a 6-week weighted baseball throwing program on pitch velocity, pitching arm biomechanics, passive range of motion, and injury rates. Sports Health. 2018;10(4):327–33.
26. www.drivelinebaseball.com. 2020.
27. Dines JS, Frank JB, Akerman M, Yocum LA. Glenohumeral internal rotation deficits in baseball players with ulnar collateral ligament insufficiency. Am J Sports Med. 2009;37(3):566–70.
28. Garrison JC, Arnold A, Macko MJ, Conway JE. Baseball players diagnosed with ulnar collateral ligament tears demonstrate decreased balance compared to healthy controls. J Orthop Sports Phys Ther. 2013;43(10):752–8.
29. Conte S, Camp CL, Dines JS. Injury trends in major league baseball over 18 seasons: 1998–2015. Am J Orthop (Belle Mead NJ). 2016;45(3):116–23.
30. Erickson BJ, Bach BRJ, Bush-Joseph CA, Verma NN, Romeo AA. Medial ulnar collateral ligament reconstruction of the elbow in major league baseball players: where do we stand? World J Orthop. 2016;7(6):355–60.
31. Portney DA, Buchler LT, Lazaroff JM, Gryzlo SM, Saltzman MD. Influence of pitching release location on ulnar collateral ligament reconstruction risk among major league baseball pitchers. Orthop J Sports Med. 2019;7(2):2325967119826540.
32. Keller RA, Marshall NE, Guest JM, Okoroha KR, Jung EK, Moutzouros V. Major League Baseball pitch velocity and pitch type associated with risk of ulnar collateral ligament injury. J Shoulder Elb Surg. 2016;25(4):671–5.
33. Crotin RL, Bhan S, Karakolis T, Ramsey DK. Fastball velocity trends in short-season minor league baseball. J Strength Cond Res. 2013;27(8):2206–12.
34. Keller RA, Mehran N, Marshall NE, Okoroha KR, Khalil L, Tibone JE, et al. Major League pitching workload after primary ulnar collateral ligament reconstruction and risk for revision surgery. J Shoulder Elb Surg. 2017;26(2):288–94.
35. Vance DD, Alexander FJ, Kunkle BW, Littlefield M, Ahmad CS. Professional and amateur pitchers' perspective on the ulnar collateral ligament injury risk. Orthop J Sports Med. 2019;7(6):2325967119850777.
36. Chalmers PN, Erickson BJ, Ball B, Romeo AA, Verma NN. Fastball pitch velocity helps predict ulnar collateral ligament reconstruction in major league baseball pitchers. Am J Sports Med. 2016;44(8):2130–5.

Valgus Extension Overload

6

David C. Gerhardt, Alexander M. Brown, and E. Lyle Cain

Introduction

The mechanics of baseball pitching and other high-velocity throwing sports explain the constellation of elbow injuries that occur in the overhead athlete. Valgus extension overload (VEO) syndrome is a result of repetitive high valgus moments coupled with elbow extension that lead to pathologic shear forces within the posteromedial olecranon and trochlea.

Repetitive near-tensile failure loads experienced by the anterior bundle of the ulnar collateral ligament (UCL) may eventually lead to ligament attenuation or failure. Valgus overload is then accentuated, and subtle valgus laxity may lead to stretch of the other medial structures, resulting in ulnar neuritis, flexor-pronator mass tendinopathy, or medial epicondyle apophysitis in the skeletally immature patient. Overload on the lateral side of the elbow may lead to abnormal compressive forces across the radiocapitellar articulation, resulting in chondromalacia, osteophyte formation, or osteochondral defects in younger athletes. Finally, when a valgus moment is coupled with near terminal extension, posterior shear forces may produce osteophytes at the posteromedial tip of the olecranon, with a corresponding "kissing lesion" in the olecranon fossa and posteromedial trochlea (Fig. 6.1). This is the defining lesion of VEO [1, 2].

The complex interplay between medial tensile forces, lateral compressive forces, and elbow extension are controlled by both static and dynamic stabilizers that confer varying levels of stability depending on the degree of elbow flexion. Underlying valgus laxity, resulting from injury to the UCL, must be excluded as the etiology of many of the elbow disorders in the throwing athlete, even when the presenting symptom initially appears to be unrelated [1, 2].

A recent, large epidemiologic study of elbow injuries in Major and Minor League Baseball players using injury surveillance data over a 4-year time span indicated posteromedial impingement (VEO) was the most common bone injury diagnosed during the season (67% of all bone injuries) [3]. Medial elbow injuries comprised 42.1% of all elbow injuries during the study period, with 40% of all injured players being pitchers [3]. However, posteriormedial impingement accounted for only 2.9% of all elbow injuries sustained during the season [3].

D. C. Gerhardt
Andrews Sports Medicine and Orthopaedic Center, Birmingham, AL, USA

A. M. Brown · E. L. Cain (✉)
American Sports Medicine Institute, Andrews Sports Medicine and Orthopaedic Center, Birmingham, AL, USA
e-mail: lyle.cain@andrewssm.com

J. S. Dines et al. (eds.), *Elbow Ulnar Collateral Ligament Injury*, https://doi.org/10.1007/978-3-030-69567-5_6

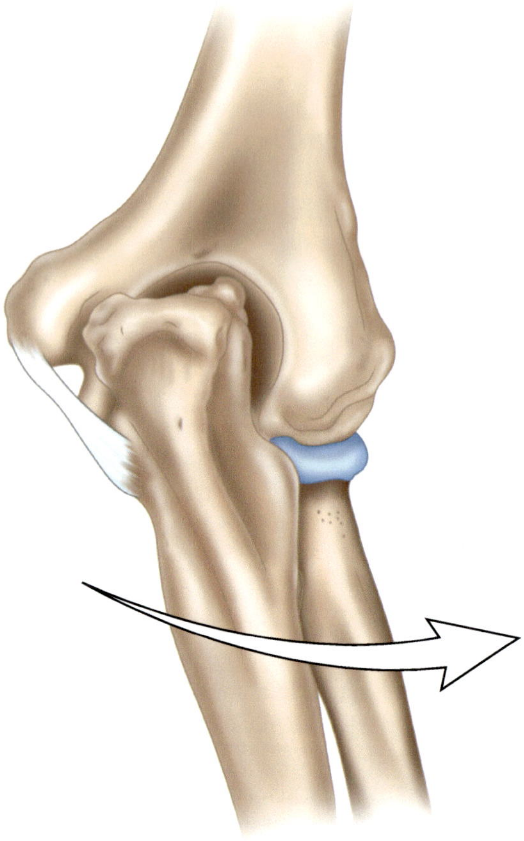

Fig. 6.1 When a valgus moment is coupled with near terminal extension, posterior shear forces produce osteophytes at the posteromedial tip of the olecranon, with a corresponding "kissing lesion" in the olecranon fossa and posteromedial trochlea. (Adapted from [66])

Anatomy and Biomechanics

The bony anatomy of the elbow consists of a modified hinge joint in which the distal humerus, radial head, and proximal ulna/olecranon articulate. Elbow stability is provided by both static and dynamic restraints. Static elbow stability results from the congruent bony articulation and ligament attachments, while dynamic stability is provided by the various muscle-tendon complexes that attach to or cross the joint. Cadaveric and biomechanical studies have helped define the relative importance of each of the individual elbow stabilizers [4–9]. A recent biomechanical study of the dynamic and static stabilizers of the medial elbow provided quantitative measurements of insertion sites relative to bony landmarks of both the anterior bundle of the ulnar collateral ligament and the muscle insertions of the common flexor muscles, adding precision to our understanding of the anatomy of the medial elbow [10].

The mechanics of high-velocity throwing can help explain elbow injuries specific to the overhead athlete [2, 11–13]. Valgus forces across the medial elbow have been estimated to reach 64 N m during the late cocking and early acceleration phases of throwing, and compressive forces of 500 N have been documented at the lateral radiocapitellar joint [2, 14]. Angular velocity has been estimated to reach 6000°/s for shoulder internal rotation and 3000–5000°/s for elbow extension during the acceleration phase of throwing [14, 15]. After early and late cocking phases, the acceleration phase initiates and the trunk rotates, the shoulder internally rotates, and the elbow extends to approximately 25° at the time of ball release. The acceleration to ball release occurs over approximately 50 ms. As the elbow extends toward ball release, forces produce a valgus and extension moment, which result in tensile forces across the medial side of the elbow, compressive forces across the lateral side of the joint, and shear forces in the posterior compartment [1, 2, 11, 15, 16]. Because the ulnohumeral joint has a greater role in stability with elbow flexion angles less than 25°, any relative valgus or microinstability during throwing as the elbow moves toward full extension at ball release, forces the posteromedial olecranon tip, olecranon fossa, and posteromedial trochlea to be exposed to higher shear forces. This phenomenon has been termed VEO syndrome and forms the basic pathophysiologic model behind the most common elbow injuries in the throwing athlete [1, 2, 16].

History and Physical Examination

A detailed history and physical examination is a crucial part of the evaluation of the overhead athlete. High-level overhead throwing athletes are often acutely aware of the phases of throwing as they impact technique and training. This depth of knowledge coupled with a detailed history of the throwing athlete can help distinguish pathologies within the elbow. In addition to the history, the superficial nature of many structures about the elbow allows the examiner to gather important information from the physical examination. When combining information from the history and the physical examination, it is important to rule out valgus instability due to UCL injury or attenuation as the primary underlying cause of associated pathologic conditions in any thrower presenting with elbow pain.

The duration and preceding timeline of the elbow pain is helpful in distinguishing VEO from other pathologies. For pitchers, any changes in accuracy, velocity, stamina, and strength are key indicators of pathology. The timing of the onset of symptoms, as well as the phase of throwing, during which pain is experienced is important [14, 17]. In athletes with medial elbow instability, nearly 85% will experience pain during the acceleration phase of throwing, whereas less than 25% will experience pain during the deceleration phase [18]. With VEO, the timing of the pain is more commonly at or just after ball release and during the deceleration phase of throwing as the elbow reaches terminal levels of extension [2, 19–21]. In the context of valgus laxity, mechanical overload of the posteromedial elbow can occur at 90° of flexion during throwing, suggesting that the process of valgus extension overloading begins higher in the flexion arc of the throwing elbow than historically suggested [22]. Approximately 60% of patients with UCL injury present after an acute episode, although many report prior medial elbow pain or treatment for flexor-pronator tendonitis or ulnar neuritis [23, 24]. VEO often presents with a slow, insidious onset of pain. Olecranon stress fractures, ulnar neuritis, flexor-pronator tendonitis, and radiocapitellar compression may have a similar pace of presentation and should be considered in the differential diagnosis. Location of the pain is helpful in further delineating the cause of the symptoms. In cases of VEO, patients typically describe pain at the posteromedial aspect of the olecranon consistent with the shearing lesion, which occurs in that location.

The physical examination of the elbow begins with inspection to evaluate the resting position of the arm. The carrying angle is the angle formed by the axis of the humerus and the axis of the forearm. A normal carrying angle is 11° of valgus in men and 13° of valgus in women [25]. In throwing athletes, carrying angles of greater than 15° can be seen due to adaptive changes from repetitive stress [26]. Further inspection of the elbow is performed systematically to evaluate bony landmarks, including the olecranon tip and the medial and lateral epicondyles, with special consideration given to the posteromedial olecranon tip.

Range of motion (ROM) should be assessed both actively and passively, as loss of motion is a common finding in VEO. Normal motion in the sagittal plane includes flexion from 0° to 140° and forearm rotation of 80–90° in both supination and pronation [27–31]. During ROM testing, crepitus, pain, or other mechanical symptoms may represent chondral irregularities, osteophyte formation, or loose bodies. The end-feel to ROM testing in extension can be an important indicator of pathology in the thrower's elbow. The endpoint in extension testing should be a firm sensation of bone engaging bone as the olecranon tip contacts the distal humerus in the olecranon fossa. Not all loss of motion in the thrower's elbow can be attributable to VEO, because anterior capsular and soft tissue contractures may play a role as well. Flexion contractures have been seen in up to 50% of professional throwers and are not always indicative of posterior olecranon pathology [26].

Palpation of the posteromedial tip of the olecranon process can help localize the pain caused by VEO. In addition to palpation, the examiner can apply a valgus stress to the flexed elbow as it is brought into extension, causing the medial aspect of the olecranon tip to impinge on the medial wall of the olecranon fossa. When this exam maneuver reproduces the patient's pain, it is considered the hallmark of VEO.

The "valgus extension overload test" is performed with the patient in a seated position and the

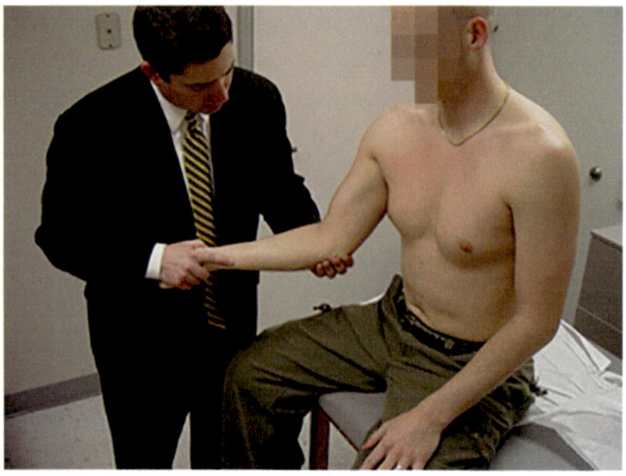

Fig. 6.2 The valgus extension overload test. The examiner repeatedly forces the slightly flexed elbow rapidly into full extension while applying a valgus stress. This maneuver reproduces pain due to impingement of the posteromedial tip of the olecranon on the medial wall of the olecranon fossa

shoulder in slight forward flexion. The examiner repeatedly forces the slightly flexed elbow rapidly into full extension while applying a valgus stress [16] (Fig. 6.2). This maneuver reproduces pain due to impingement of the posteromedial tip of the olecranon on the medial wall of the olecranon fossa. A positive finding often indicates the presence of a posteromedial olecranon osteophyte, which may occasionally be palpable at the time of physical examination [1, 2, 15, 17, 20, 21, 32].

Not all proximal olecranon pain is synonymous with VEO. Pain noted with palpation of the lateral border of the olecranon tip, rather than the medial border, should raise suspicion for an olecranon stress fracture. Additionally, while palpating the ulnar nerve proximal to the cubital tunnel, the examiner should palpate the distal medial aspect of the triceps tendon, as anomalous bands of the distal triceps insertion have been described as a cause of pain, ulnar nerve impingement, and "snapping" as they move across the medial epicondyle [33].

The diagnosis of VEO with posteromedial impingement is made only when the patient history, physical examination, and imaging studies suggest the presence of posteromedial olecranon pain with an intact, functional UCL. Underlying instability of the UCL must be excluded as the root cause of posteromedial overload .

Imaging Studies

Imaging of the elbow plays an integral role in developing an accurate diagnosis in the throwing athlete. Specialized radiographic views, computed tomography (CT), and magnetic resonance imaging (MRI) all provide pertinent information.

Standard radiographs of the elbow, including anteroposterior (AP), lateral, oblique, and axial views are often the initial imaging study. The oblique axial radiograph with the elbow in 110° of flexion helps demonstrate posteromedial olecranon osteophytes [16]. Comparison to the normal elbow may be performed if needed. Radiographs are helpful in evaluating for olecranon osteophytes but may show additional pathology such as calcification within the UCL (an indirect sign of prior injury), osteochondritis dissecans of the capitellum, or intra-articular bodies. Valgus AP stress views can be obtained if injury to the UCL is suspected; this is performed with a valgus stress radiography machine (Telos, Weiterstadt, Germany). AP views with 0, 5, 10, and 15 dN of valgus stress applied to each elbow at 25° of flexion is recommended [2]. An increase in medial joint space widening with increasing stress, compared with the uninjured side, is suggestive of medial ligamentous injury [34]. However, standard normal values are not well established, especially since uninjured baseball pitchers have been found to have increased laxity in the throwing elbow compared with the nondominant arm [24, 35].

CT is not routinely performed but may be helpful to evaluate the olecranon osteophyte size, osteophyte fragmentation, intra-articular bodies, overall elbow morphology, and olecranon stress fracture [36]. CT with intra-articular contrast may also be helpful to assist in the evaluation of the UCL [35, 37], especially in patients who are unable to undergo MRI. It is important to note that normal radiographic imaging studies do not rule out the presence of an olecranon osteophyte. Imaging of the olecranon tip and trochlea is difficult and the diagnosis of olecranon impingement is made primarily by history and physical examination, but may be confirmed with radiographs and/or CT imaging modalities.

MRI with intra-articular gadolinium contrast is the preferred imaging modality for evaluation of the UCL and may be helpful to determine the presence of olecranon osteophytes and the sequelae of VEO. MR arthrography is much more sensitive than MRI without intra-articular contrast for the detection of partial tears of the UCL [37]. MRI also identifies a reproducible pattern of pathology in throwing athletes. Marrow edema and/or chondral abnormalities within the posterior trochlea and anteromedial olecranon, synovitis in the posteromedial recess, and marginal osteophytes at the trochlea and olecranon suggest posteromedial elbow impingement [38]. MRI is also superior for identification of intra-articular bodies (both chondral and ossific), osteochondritis dessicans of the capitellum, synovial plicae, and radiographically occult stress fractures of the olecranon tip, olecranon process, posteromedial trochlea, and sublime tubercle [14, 38].

Treatment

Treatment initially consists of active rest and rehabilitation. Throwing is avoided, and the athlete is treated with rehabilitation exercises for the elbow and shoulder. Return to gradual interval throwing is allowed as symptoms resolve. In the athlete who fails to obtain symptom relief after an extended rehabilitation program, elbow arthroscopy may be considered.

Nonoperative management can be successful and has been documented in the cases of olecranon osteophyte formation in 17 world-class javelin throwers, all of whom eventually returned to competition. However, these patients were identified retrospectively, and, thus, the number of athletes with olecranon osteophytes who were unable to return to play is unknown [39]. Several authors have reported on the use of orthobiologics in the treatment of UCL insufficiency in throwers, but to date no large-scale studies have looked at this treatment option for posteromedial olecranon impingement. While the field of orthobiologics is promising, particularly for partial UCL tears in position players, an osteophyte pathology such as VEO that is recalcitrant to nonoperative treatment will likely be best treated with surgery [40–42]. Nonoperative management including rest, nonsteroidal antiinflammatories, local modalities, and strengthening exercises for the rotator cuff and flexor-pronator mass with a focus on throwing technique may allow the thrower to become asymptomatic, but will not be curative in regards to the structural pathology such as the posteromedial olecranon osteophytes and chondral lesions.

Elbow arthroscopy is indicated for the treatment of posteromedial olecranon impingement in the thrower secondary to VEO syndrome after failure of adequate conservative treatment. Elbow arthroscopy also allows for the treatment of concomitant pathology including loose body removal, osteochondral lesions (i.e., capitellum), excision of anterior osteophytes, chondromalacia of the radial head, partial synovectomy, lysis of adhesions, and evaluation of valgus instability secondary to UCL insufficiency [1, 16, 19, 21, 24, 32, 43–45].

Surgical Technique

Elbow arthroscopy has been described in lateral decubitus, prone, or supine positions [43, 46–53]. Our experience is predominantly with the patient in the supine position due to the simplicity of positioning and reproducibility with OR staff [53]. The patient is supine with the arm in 90° of abduction and the elbow in 90° of flexion suspended by an overhead arthroscopic traction device (Fig. 6.3). Elbow flexion and extension is controlled by adding or subtracting weight on a pulley system. The tourniquet is routinely set at 250 mm Hg, and a pressure-sensitive arthroscopic pump is helpful in preventing overdistension of the elbow and fluid extravasation into the soft tissues. Both a standard 4.0-mm arthroscope and 2.7-mm small joint arthroscope are routinely utilized. A 70° arthroscope is also useful for evaluation of the space along the medial and lateral gutters of the elbow capsule.

A detailed knowledge of elbow anatomy is imperative for proper portal placement and to

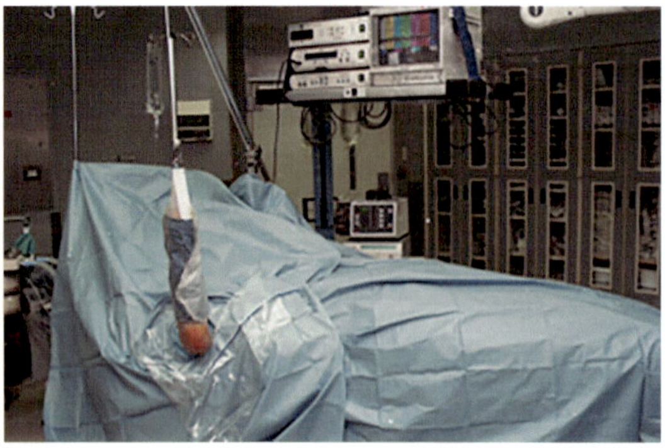

Fig. 6.3 Elbow arthroscopic positioning. The patient is supine with the arm in 90° of abduction and the elbow in 90° of flexion suspended by an overhead arthroscopic traction device

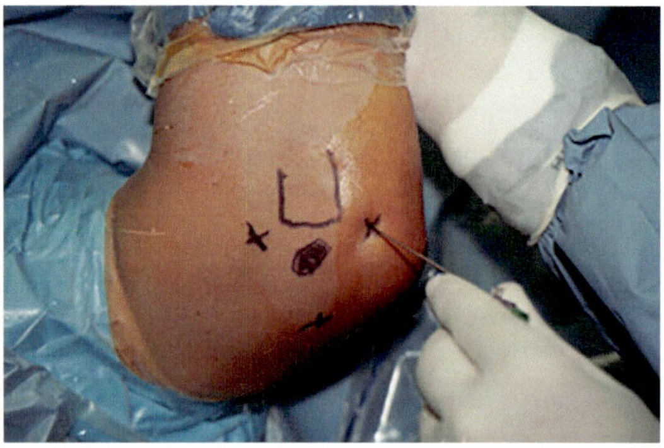

Fig. 6.4 Bony landmarks and portal locations are marked

minimize the risk of neurovascular complications. Prior to injection and incision, all bony landmarks and portal locations are marked (Fig. 6.4). The elbow joint is then distended using a saline injection into the lateral soft spot [54, 55]. The anterolateral portal is established by placement of an 18-gauge spinal needle into the anterior capsule to confirm intra-articular placement, followed by careful skin incision. A hemostat is used for blunt dissection to the anterolateral joint capsule before penetration of the capsule with a 4.0-mm blunt trocar and sheath.

The anterior compartment diagnostic arthroscopy is then begun. An anteromedial portal may be established using an 18-gauge spinal needle for portal localization. The anteromedial portal is useful as a working portal to address loose bodies, injury to the coronoid process, capitellum or radial head, or osteophyte formation within the coronoid fossa. All compartments must be thoroughly visualized in order to avoid missing critical pathology. During the evaluation of the anterior compartment, concurrent evaluation of UCL stability can be performed by placing a valgus stress on the elbow at 70° of flexion. Opening of greater than 1–2 mm suggests UCL insufficiency [56].

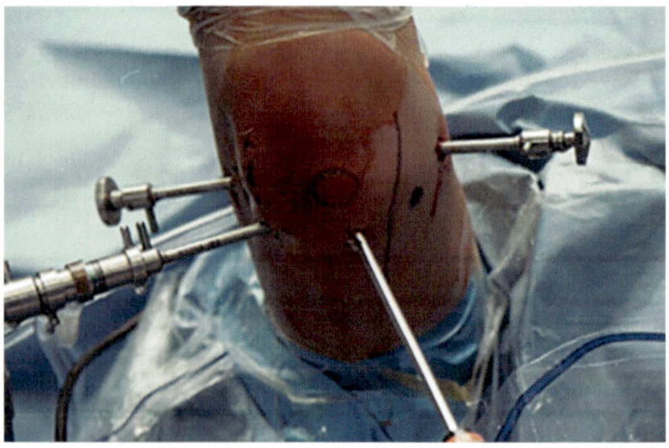

Fig. 6.5 The accessory straight posterior portal through the triceps tendon. Care is taken to avoid the ulnar nerve

A lateral soft spot portal is then established for the 2.7-mm arthroscope. A second lateral portal may be placed approximately 1 cm distal to the direct lateral portal for instrumentation of the lateral compartment. The posterior compartment is then viewed by transitioning the 2.7-mm arthroscope from the lateral portal to the posterior compartment. The elbow is extended to 30° of flexion by adding traction weight to increase the posterior working space. A posterolateral portal is established, and the 4.0 mm arthroscope is then introduced into the posterior compartment. An accessory straight posterior portal can then be established through the triceps tendon with care taken to avoid the ulnar nerve (Fig. 6.5). The posterior portals are kept as far apart as possible to allow triangulation in the posterior compartment. Viewing from the posterolateral portal, a shaver is introduced through the straight posterior portal to clear synovitis and soft tissue from the olecranon tip and olecranon fossa so that the entire bony margin of the olecranon tip can be visualized (Fig. 6.6).

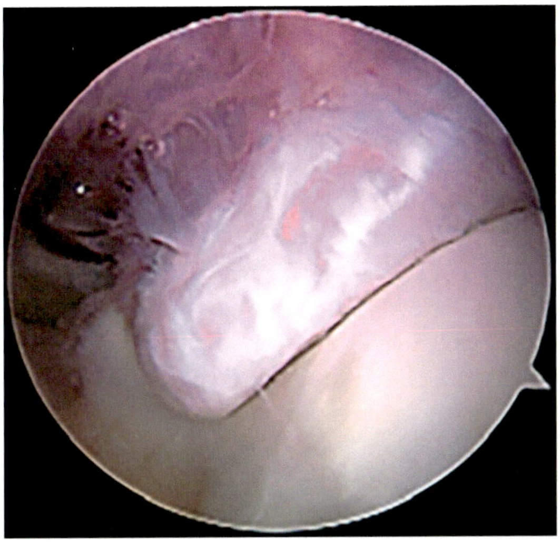

Fig. 6.6 Soft tissue and synovitis is debrided from the olecranon tip and olecranon fossa so that the entire bony margin of the olecranon tip can be visualized

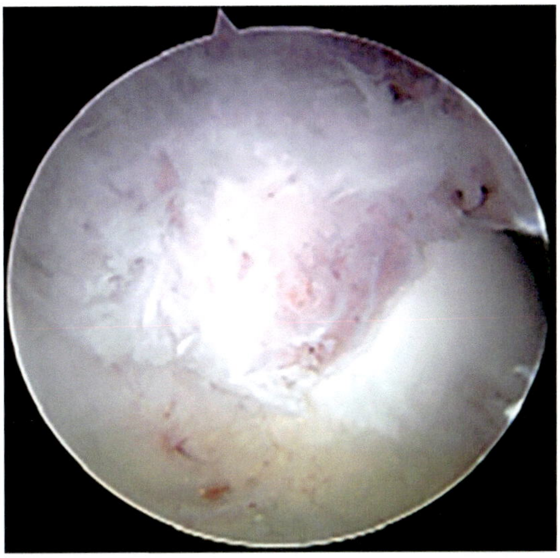

Fig. 6.7 Olecranon tip with bony hypertrophy preresection

Arthroscopic evaluation of the posterior compartment in throwers with VEO is of paramount importance as subtle olecranon osteophytes may not be visualized well on X-ray, but the margin of cartilage and bony hypertrophy is easily seen after adequate soft tissue debridement of the olecranon tip. The chondral injury on the posteromedial trochlea can also be easily identified and addressed. Loose cartilage margins and olecranon osteophytes are then excised with a sharp osteotome and 5.5-mm acromionizer burr. A small sharp osteotome is used to complete the osteophyte removal along the articular margin (Figs. 6.7 and 6.8). The small bone fragments are then removed with a grasper, typically through the straight posterior portal. Noticewala et al. suggest leaving some fibrous attachment to the osteophyte, debriding part of the fragment to decrease its size, and then detaching the fragment to facilitate its removal through a portal incision. They recommend removing the fragment via the posterior lateral portal due to fewer layers of surrounding tissue at this site [52]. The exact amount of olecranon osteophyte that can safely be excised is unknown. Typically ~3 mm of bone is resected [57–59]. This allows visualization into the articular space of the ulnohumeral joint and allows full elbow extension without impingement. A lateral radiograph is obtained intraoperatively to assess for adequate bone removal and to assure that no bone debris remains in the soft tissues around the elbow (Fig. 6.9). A compressive dressing is applied, and the arm is iced and elevated postoperatively [1, 2, 19, 21, 32, 44, 45, 55].

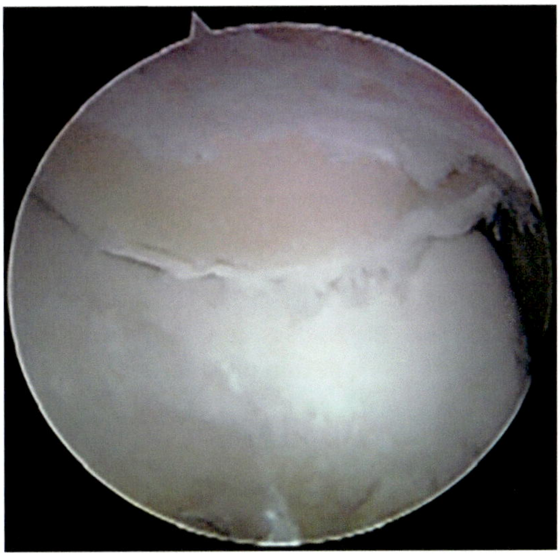

Fig. 6.8 Olecranon tip postresection of osteophytes

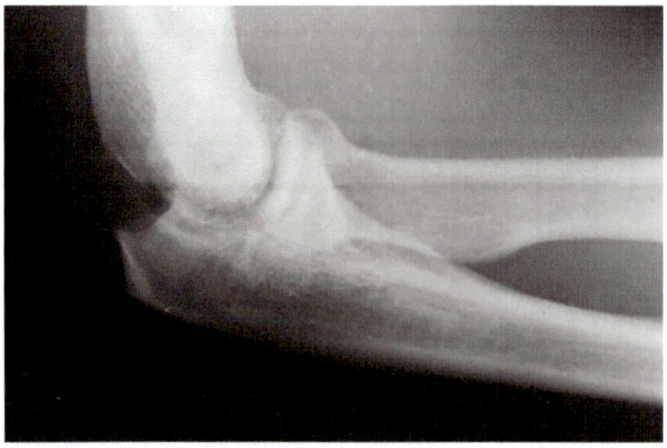

Fig. 6.9 Lateral radiograph obtained intraoperatively demonstrates adequate bone removal

Postoperative Management

The postoperative rehabilitation for elbow arthroscopy and osteophyte excision is focused on early ROM [60, 61]. The primary initial goal is to return to full motion; however, full elbow extension is often more difficult to obtain than with routine diagnostic elbow arthroscopy because of posterior osseous pain and synovitis. Gentle ROM is initiated on the day of surgery with the elbow in a soft dressing. The first 7–10 days are spent concentrating on active and active-assisted elbow ROM and wrist strengthening exercises. By 10 days after surgery, ROM is typically 15–100° flexion or better, and 5–10° to 115° flexion by 2 weeks postoperative. In most cases, full ROM (0–145°) returns by 3–4 weeks after surgery. The risk of an elbow flexion contracture may be minimized by early aggressive rehabilitation [60, 61].

Strengthening of the dynamic stabilizers of the arm is an important part of the rehabilitation process; these include forearm and wrist flexors such as biceps brachii, brachioradialis, and brachialis. These dynamic stabilizers play an integral part in controlling the valgus and rapid extension forces across the elbow during the throwing motion. Isometric strengthening is initiated during the first 10–14 days, followed by isotonic strengthening during weeks 3–6. Strengthening of the shoulder is started by week 6, with plyometrics and endurance exercises focused on the thrower's needs. In most cases, an interval-throwing program may begin at 10–12 weeks after surgery, with a return to competition after symptom-free completion of the throwing program [60–63].

Results

Multiple authors have retrospectively analyzed the results of arthroscopic posteromedial osteophyte excision in throwers, but no prospective, randomized data are currently available. Andrews and Timmerman reported the results of elbow surgery in 64 professional baseball players over a 5-year period [23], the most common procedure being arthroscopic debridement of posteromedial olecranon osteophytes (58%). Loose bodies were found in 27% of patients, and the authors noted poor sensitivity of both plain radiographs (27%) and CT arthrography (59%) for the preoperative diagnosis of loose bodies. Seventy-three percent of players were able to return to the same or higher level of play; however, 19 (32%) required subsequent surgical procedures, including 41% of patients initially treated with arthroscopic excision of an olecranon osteophyte [23]. The authors reported that in the high demand overhead athlete, these surgical procedures are often palliative treatments but may result in temporary relief of symptoms and successful return to play.

Reddy and colleagues [64] reported a large series performed at the Kerlan-Jobe clinic, in which the results of 187 arthroscopies were reviewed. The most common diagnoses were posterior impingement (51%), loose bodies (31%), and degenerative joint disease (22%) [64]. Ninety-two percent of 104 patients contacted had results rated as good or excellent at an average follow-up of 42 months, with the biggest improvement seen in pain scores when osteophytes were excised. Forty-seven of 55 baseball players (85%) were able to return to the same level of competition. The complication rate was 1.6% [64].

Park et al. reported on a small series (n = 13) of adolescent baseball players (mean age 15.4 year) with arthroscopically treated VEO syndrome and follow up of an average of 3.3 years. Patients reported a mean decrease in VAS score of 4.1–1.1, and the overall return to play rate was 85% (11 of 13). Four of the patients went on to have UCL reconstructions. The study suggests that adolescents who require surgical treatment of VEO have acceptable outcomes in the short term [65].

Summary

Posterior elbow pain is a common problem in the throwing athlete due to adaptive bony and soft tissue changes in response to VEO syndrome. The injury accounts for 2.9% of all injuries to players at the professional level. A thorough patient history and physical examination with appropriate diagnostic imaging are required to correctly identify the etiology of the elbow pain. It is important to recognize that VEO may occur in combination with other injuries in the elbow and specifically, an injury to the UCL with resultant micro or macro instability must be ruled out as the underlying cause. Osteophytes on the posteromedial olecranon that do not respond to rest and rehabilitation may require surgical excision, a procedure that may be performed arthroscopically with a low complication rate. The amount of olecranon tip that can safely be resected without placing additional stress on the UCL is thought to be less than 3 mm. Removing the least amount of olecranon tip while still adequately addressing the impingement lesions may offer the lowest risk of overloading the ulnar collateral ligament. With proper attention to anatomical landmarks for portal placement and meticulous surgical technique, arthroscopic evaluation and treatment of posterior elbow pain can be safely accomplished in the throwing athlete with minimal risk. Return to previous level of competition can be expected in a high percentage of cases; however, the incidence of additional future surgical procedures is as high as 30–40%.

References

1. O'Holleran JD, Altchek DW. The thrower's elbow: arthroscopic treatment of valgus extension overload syndrome. HSS J. 2006;2(1):83–93.
2. Cain ELJ, et al. Elbow injuries in throwing athletes: a current concepts review. Am J Sports Med. 2003;31(4):621–35.
3. Ciccotti MG, Pollack KM, Ciccotti MC, et al. Elbow injuries in professional baseball: epidemiological findings from the major league baseball injury surveillance system. Am J Sports Med. 2017;45(10):2319–28.
4. Hotchkiss RN, Weiland AJ. Valgus stability of the elbow. J Orthop Res. 1987;5(3):372–7.
5. Morrey BF. Applied anatomy and biomechanics of the elbow joint. Instr Course Lect. 1986;35:59–68.
6. Morrey BF, An KN. Articular and ligamentous contributions to the stability of the elbow joint. Am J Sports Med. 1983;11(5):315–9.
7. Morrey BF, An KN. Functional anatomy of the ligaments of the elbow. Clin Orthop Relat Res. 1985;Dec(201):84–90.
8. Regan WD, et al. Biomechanical study of ligaments around the elbow joint. Clin Orthop Relat Res. 1991;Oct(271):170–9.
9. Schwab GH, et al. Biomechanics of elbow instability: the role of the medial collateral ligament. Clin Orthop Relat Res. 1980;Jan–Feb(146):42–52.
10. Frangiamore SJ, Moatshe G, Kruckeberg BM, et al. Qualitative and quantitative analyses of the dynamic and static stabilizers of the medial elbow: an anatomic study. Am J Sports Med. 2018;46(3):687–94.
11. Schickendantz MS. Diagnosis and treatment of elbow disorders in the overhead athlete. Hand Clin. 2002;18(1):65–75.
12. Ball CM, Galatz LM, Yamaguchi K. Elbow instability: treatment strategies and emerging concepts. Instr Course Lect. 2002;51:53–61.
13. Rizio L, Uribe JW. Overuse injuries of the upper extremity in baseball. Clin Sports Med. 2001;20(3):453–68.
14. Fleisig GS, et al. Kinetics of baseball pitching with implications about injury mechanisms. Am J Sports Med. 1995;23(2):233–9.
15. Pappas AM, Zawacki RM, Sullivan TJ. Biomechanics of baseball pitching. A preliminary report. Am J Sports Med. 1985;13(4):216–22.
16. Wilson FD, et al. Valgus extension overload in the pitching elbow. Am J Sports Med. 1983;11(2):83–8.
17. Yocum LA. The diagnosis and nonoperative treatment of elbow problems in the athlete. Clin Sports Med. 1989;8(3):439–51.
18. Conway JE, et al. Medial instability of the elbow in throwing athletes. Treatment by repair or reconstruction of the ulnar collateral ligament. J Bone Joint Surg Am. 1992;74(1):67–83.
19. Ahmad CS, Conway JE. Elbow arthroscopy: valgus extension overload. Instr Course Lect. 2011;60:191–7.
20. Andrews JR, et al. Physical examination of the thrower's elbow. J Orthop Sports Phys Ther. 1993;17(6):296–304.
21. Dugas JR. Valgus extension overload: diagnosis and treatment. Clin Sports Med. 2010;29(4):645–54.
22. Osbahr DC, Dines JS, Breazeale NM, Deng XH, Altchek DW. Ulnohumeral chondral and ligamentous overload: biomechanical correlation for posteromedial chondromalacia of the elbow in throwing athletes. Am J Sports Med. 2010;38(12):2535–41.

23. Andrews JR, Timmerman LA. Outcome of elbow surgery in professional baseball players. Am J Sports Med. 1995;23(4):407–13.
24. Azar FM, et al. Operative treatment of ulnar collateral ligament injuries of the elbow in athletes. Am J Sports Med. 2000;28(1):16–23.
25. Beals RK. The normal carrying angle of the elbow. A radiographic study of 422 patients. Clin Orthop Relat Res. 1976;Sept(119):194–6.
26. King J, Brelsford HJ, Tullos HS. Analysis of the pitching arm of the professional baseball pitcher. Clin Orthop Relat Res. 1969;67:116–23.
27. Boone DC, Azen SP. Normal range of motion of joints in male subjects. J Bone Joint Surg Am. 1979;61(5):756–9.
28. Morrey BF, Askew LJ, Chao EY. A biomechanical study of normal functional elbow motion. J Bone Joint Surg Am. 1981;63(6):872–7.
29. Morrey BF, Chao EY. Passive motion of the elbow joint. J Bone Joint Surg Am. 1976;58(4):501–8.
30. Wagner C. Determination of the rotary flexibility of the elbow joint. Eur J Appl Physiol Occup Physiol. 1977;37(1):47–59.
31. Youm Y, et al. Biomechanical analyses of forearm pronation-supination and elbow flexion-extension. J Biomech. 1979;12(4):245–55.
32. Ahmad CS, NS EA. Valgus extension overload syndrome and stress injury of the olecranon. Clin Sports Med. 2004;23(4):665–76, x.
33. Spinner RJ, Goldner RD. Snapping of the medial head of the triceps and recurrent dislocation of the ulnar nerve. Anatomical and dynamic factors. J Bone Joint Surg Am. 1998;80(2):239–47.
34. Lee GA, Katz SD, Lazarus MD. Elbow valgus stress radiography in an uninjured population. Am J Sports Med. 1998;26(3):425–7.
35. Ellenbecker TS, et al. Medial elbow joint laxity in professional baseball pitchers. A bilateral comparison using stress radiography. Am J Sports Med. 1998;26(3):420–4.
36. DeHaven KE, Evarts CM. Throwing injuries of the elbow in athletes. Orthop Clin North Am. 1973;4(3):801–8.
37. Schwartz ML, et al. Ulnar collateral ligament injury in the throwing athlete: evaluation with saline-enhanced MR arthrography. Radiology. 1995;197(1):297–9.
38. Cohen SB, et al. Posteromedial elbow impingement: magnetic resonance imaging findings in overhead throwing athletes and results of arthroscopic treatment. Arthroscopy. 2011;27(10):1364–70.
39. Waris W. Elbow injuries of javelin -throwers. Acta Chir Scand. 1946;93(6):563–75.
40. Dines JS, Williams PN, ElAttrache N, et al. Platelet-rich plasma can be used to successfully treat elbow ulnar collateral ligament insufficiency in high-level throwers. Am J Orthop (Belle Mead NJ). 2016;45(5):296–300.
41. Podesta L, Crow SA, Volkmer D, Bert T, Yocum LA. Treatment of partial ulnar collateral ligament tears in the elbow with platelet-rich plasma. Am J Sports Med. 2013;41(7):1689–94.
42. Deal JB, Smith E, Heard W, O'Brien MJ, Savoie FH 3rd. Platelet-rich plasma for primary treatment of partial ulnar collateral ligament tears: mri correlation with results. Orthop J Sports Med. 2017;5(11):2325967117738238. Published 2017 Nov 13.
43. Byram IR, et al. Elbow arthroscopic surgery update for sports medicine conditions. Am J Sports Med. 2013;41(9):2191–202.
44. Levin JS, et al. Posterior olecranon resection and ulnar collateral ligament strain. J Shoulder Elb Surg. 2004;13(1):66–71.
45. O'Holleran JD, Altchek DW. Elbow arthroscopy: treatment of the thrower's elbow. Instr Course Lect. 2006;55:95–107.
46. Andrews JR, Baumgarten TE. Arthroscopic anatomy of the elbow. Orthop Clin North Am. 1995;26(4):671–7.
47. Day B. Elbow arthroscopy in the athlete. Clin Sports Med. 1996;15(4):785–97.
48. Moskal MJ, Savoie FH 3rd, Field LD. Elbow arthroscopy in trauma and reconstruction. Orthop Clin North Am. 1999;30(1):163–77.
49. O'Driscoll SW. Elbow arthroscopy for loose bodies. Orthopedics. 1992;15(7):855–9.
50. O'Driscoll SW, Morrey BF. Arthroscopy of the elbow. Diagnostic and therapeutic benefits and hazards. J Bone Joint Surg Am. 1992;74(1):84–94.
51. Stothers K, Day B, Regan WR. Arthroscopy of the elbow: anatomy, portal sites, and a description of the proximal lateral portal. Arthroscopy. 1995;11(4):449–57.
52. Noticewala MS, Vance DD, Trofa DP, Ahmad CS. Elbow arthroscopy for treatment of valgus extension overload. Arthrosc Tech. 2018;7(7):e705–10. Published 2018 Jun 4.
53. Barousse P, Saper M, Meijer K, Roth C, Andrews JR. Valgus extension overload: arthroscopic decompression in the supine-suspended position. Arthrosc Tech. 2016;5(4):e845–50. Published 2016 Aug 8.
54. Andrews JR, Carson WG. Arthroscopy of the elbow. Arthroscopy. 1985;1(2):97–107.
55. Andrews JR, St Pierre RK, Carson WGJ. Arthroscopy of the elbow. Clin Sports Med. 1986;5(4):653–62.
56. Field LD, Altchek DW. Evaluation of the arthroscopic valgus instability test of the elbow. Am J Sports Med. 1996;24(2):177–81.
57. Andrews JR, et al. Relationship of ulnar collateral ligament strain to amount of medial olecranon osteotomy. Am J Sports Med. 2001;29(6):716–21.
58. Kamineni S, et al. Medial collateral ligament strain with partial posteromedial olecranon resection. A biomechanical study. J Bone Joint Surg Am. 2004;86-A(11):2424–30.
59. Kamineni S, et al. Partial posteromedial olecranon resection: a kinematic study. J Bone Joint Surg Am. 2003;85-A(6):1005–11.

60. Wilk KE, Arrigo C, Andrews JR. Rehabilitation of the elbow in the throwing athlete. J Orthop Sports Phys Ther. 1993;17(6):305–17.
61. Wilk KE, Meister K, Andrews JR. Current concepts in the rehabilitation of the overhead throwing athlete. Am J Sports Med. 2002;30(1):136–51.
62. Leggin BG, Sheridan S, Eckenrode BJ. Rehabilitation after surgical management of the thrower's shoulder. Sports Med Arthrosc. 2012;20(1):49–55.
63. Wilk KE, et al. The advanced throwers ten exercise program: a new exercise series for enhanced dynamic shoulder control in the overhead throwing athlete. Phys Sportsmed. 2011;39(4):90–7.
64. Reddy AS, et al. Arthroscopy of the elbow: a long-term clinical review. Arthroscopy. 2000;16(6):588–94.
65. Park JY, Yoo HY, Chung SW, et al. Valgus extension overload syndrome in adolescent baseball players: clinical characteristics and surgical outcomes. J Shoulder Elb Surg. 2016;25(12):2048–56.
66. Andrews JR, Craven WM. Lesions of the posterior compartment of the elbow. Clin Sports Med. 1991;10(3):637–52.

7 Ulnohumeral Chondral and Ligamentous Overload

Rachel Faber, Christopher Garrett, Sheref E. Hassan, and Daryl C. Osbahr

Introduction

The concept of ulnohumeral chondral and ligamentous overload (UCLO) describes a complex pathological process associated with posteromedial impingement in the elbow that can occur in association with valgus instability secondary to ulnar collateral ligament (UCL) insufficiency throughout the entire throwing motion arc [1]. UCLO can subsequently lead to significant pathologic changes in the elbow. These pathological changes will typically manifest as posteromedial chondromalacia and osteophyte formation, which can result in persistent disability and inability to play in throwing athletes.

The elbow is subjected to tremendous valgus force during overhead activities. During the acceleration phase of the throwing motion, the valgus and extension forces placed on the elbow are resisted by the UCL and dynamic flexor-pronator musculature [2, 3]. If deceleration of the throwing motion is also not resisted by the UCL or flexor-pronator muscles at these low elbow flexion angles, repetitive valgus forces occur and result in posteromedial elbow impingement and a resultant spectrum of injuries [4, 5].

R. Faber (✉)
Department of Orthopaedics, Orlando Regional Medical Center, Orlando, FL, USA
e-mail: Rachel.faber@orlandohealth.com

C. Garrett
Department of Orthopaedics, Orlando Health, Orlando, FL, USA

S. E. Hassan
Orthopedic Surgery and Sports Medicine, Landa Spine and Orthopedic Center, Old Bridge, NJ, USA

D. C. Osbahr
Orlando Health Orthopedic Institute, Orlando, FL, USA

Functional Anatomy

The elbow is a hinged or ginglymus joint. It includes three articulations inside the same capsule—the ulnohumeral, radiohumeral (or radiocapitellar), and proximal radioulnar joints. The ulnohumeral joint provides the primary bony support. The greater sigmoid notch is linked to the distal humeral trochlea in a precise V-shaped articulation. This results in a highly constrained bony articulation stabilized anteriorly in flexion when the coronoid process on the ulna enters the humeral coronoid fossa and posteriorly in extension when the olecranon enters the humeral olecranon fossa. In full extension and at 90° of flexion, bony articulation provides approximately one-third of the total resistance to valgus stress. Through compressive lateral-based forces, the radiocapitellar joint also contributes to valgus stability to a lesser degree [6].

Elbow stability, therefore, relies on a complex interplay between both static and dynamic stabi-

J. S. Dines et al. (eds.), *Elbow Ulnar Collateral Ligament Injury*,
https://doi.org/10.1007/978-3-030-69567-5_7

lizers. The medial aspect of the elbow is reinforced by the UCL. The UCL is comprised of three fascicles. The anterior fascicle extends from the anteromedial aspect of the medial epicondyle to the coronoid process. The middle fascicle begins at the inferior aspect of the medial epicondyle and attaches to the medial aspect of the coronoid process and the medial ulna. Combined, these two fascicles comprise the anterior oblique bundle of the UCL as they coalesce into a fan-shaped single band. Posteriorly, the posterior band of the UCL is another fan-shaped fascicle that originates on the posteroinferior medial epicondyle and attaches on the medial aspect of the ulna. This bundle becomes taut as the elbow is flexed. The transverse band or Cooper's ligament completes the UCL as it extends from the base of the olecranon to the base of the coronoid process. Previous studies have demonstrated that the anterior bundle of the UCL remains under tension and serves as the primary static stabilizer against valgus stress in the elbow between 20 and 120° [6–10].

The muscles contributing to the dynamic stability of the elbow against valgus stress are the flexor-pronator mass. These muscles share an origin from the medial epicondyle and include the flexor carpi ulnaris, flexor digitorum superficialis, flexor carpi radialis, and pronator teres. Although the flexor-pronator mass as a whole is thought to be important to secondary stability to valgus stress of the elbow, biomechanical testing has shown the flexor carpi ulnaris to be the primary dynamic stabilizer to valgus stress [11].

Pathophysiology and Biomechanics

Posteromedial elbow impingement in the setting of UCL insufficiency has been classically described during low elbow flexion angles during the deceleration phase and was therefore termed valgus extension overload [5]. However, early reports in the literature have indirectly supported the concept of increased forces and posteromedial impingement throughout the entire throwing motion arc [5, 12–15]. More recent biomechanical analysis has confirmed the presence of increased contact forces in the posteromedial elbow in the UCL deficient elbow at 90° of flexion (late cocking/early acceleration phase), which suggests that UCL insufficiency may have an effect throughout the throwing arc [1]. The concept of UCLO describes this continuum of abnormal contact forces and resultant posteromedial ulnohumeral impingement throughout the entire arc of the throwing motion.

Biomechanical analysis has demonstrated that sectioning of the anterior bundle of the UCL causes a medial shift of the olecranon on the distal humeral trochlea. This shift was found to result in a significant increase in contact pressure and decrease in contact area concentrated in the posteromedial elbow. During the throwing, motion dynamic forces are generated as the elbow moves from flexion to extension under extreme speed, and torque may further increase this tremendous load in the posteromedial elbow [1].

Subtle shifts and changes in contact forces between the tip of the olecranon and distal humeral trochlea associated with UCL insufficiency may lead to pathologic changes in the posteromedial elbow, such as chondromalacia and osteophyte formation (Fig. 7.1; [1]). This "windshield wiper" effect as the olecranon tip translates medially on the humerus throughout the entire throwing motion may account for chondromalacia and osteophytosis observed in throwers with UCL insufficiency. These deviations in the biomechanics of the elbow result in UCLO and are in turn believed to occur as a direct result of valgus instability secondary to UCL insufficiency.

Although injury to the anterior bundle of the UCL has been implicated as the driving force for clinically apparent UCL insufficiency, there have been biomechanical studies suggesting isolated injury to the posterior bundle may also contribute to this "windshield wiper" effect. In a cadaveric study evaluating gapping between the medial epicondyle and proximal sigmoid notch before and after isolated posterior UCL transection, there was an average increase of at least 1.4 mm at all flexion angles tested [16].

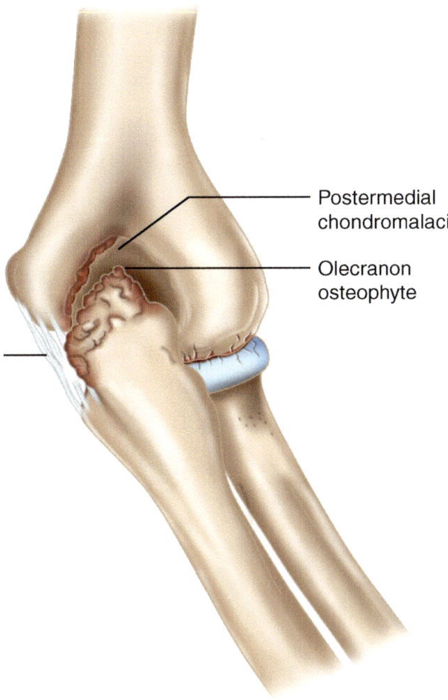

Fig. 7.1 Pathologic changes associated with UCLO include ulnar collateral ligament (*UCL*) insufficiency under valgus stress, ulnohumeral chondromalacia, and posteromedial olecranon osteophytes. (© 2013 Daryl C. Osbahr, all rights reserved)

Diagnosis

Clinical History

Injury from UCL insufficiency may occur as a result of an acute tear, a chronic tear causing abnormal biomechanics, or an acute on chronic tear in the setting of chronic UCL attenuation and suboptimal ligament infrastructure. Patients with acute tears may complain of acute onset of medial elbow pain, swelling, and instability with resultant decreased ability to throw at the preinjury level [5, 17, 18]. UCLO is more likely to occur with chronic symptomatology because posteromedial impingement and resultant chondromalacia and osteophyte formation may occur with progressive attenuation and failure of the UCL. It is possible that UCLO occurs subclinically and can present as an acute on chronic presentation where the patient may complain of acute onset of pain and instability in the setting of chronic changes such as posteromedial osteophytes and chondromalacia.

Physical Examination

In evaluating for UCL injury, a standard physical examination of the elbow is done noting range of motion, strength, neurovascular status, and special tests. Pain may be present at or near the UCL origin at the medial epicondyle or at the insertion at the sublime tubercle. Provocative tests that have been found to be useful in identifying UCL insufficiency include the milking maneuver, valgus stress test, the moving valgus stress test, and trochlear shear test; however, the clinician must consider that the athlete may not experience symptoms in the absence of throwing.

The valgus stress test involves placing the elbow at 20–30° to unlock the olecranon, externally rotating the humerus, and applying a valgus stress. Pain and/or laxity are considered a positive finding. The milking maneuver is performed by pulling on the patient's thumb with the forearm supinated and elbow flexed at 90° creating a valgus stress across the elbow. A positive test results in subjective apprehension, laxity, or pain at the UCL. The moving valgus stress test begins with the elbow in the same position as the milking maneuver, but a valgus stress is applied while the elbow is ranged through a full arc of motion from flexion to extension. A positive test results in subjective apprehension, laxity, or pain at the UCL between 70° and 120°. The moving valgus test is considered the most sensitive and specific of these provocative physical exam maneuvers [19]. The trochlear shear test is performed in the same manner as the moving valgus test but is considered positive when pain is present at elbow angles ≤60° (usually 10–40°). A positive trochlear shear test suggests posteromedial chondral erosion.

When considering the posteromedial impingement, the clinician must also consider the physical examination findings in addition to having a high index of suspicion from the clinical history. Patients with posteromedial impingement may often present with a lack of extension secondary to osteophyte formation [20]. In addition, the clinician should perform the posteromedial impingement test by placing a valgus force on a fully extended elbow and determining whether there is resultant pain to palpation at the posteromedial olecranon tip with or without crepitation. This test can detect symptoms secondary to the presence of posterior osteophytes and/or chondromalacia [20, 21]. Findings such as a positive posteromedial impingement test may be present in the subacute or chronic settings and may include posteromedial pain and/or crepitation during elbow extension [5, 17, 18, 20].

It is also critical to fully evaluate for concomitant pathology, including the ulnar nerve and flexor-pronator mass, because these problems may be an important component of the pathological disease, especially in athletes with chronic symptomatology. In addition to providing information regarding concomitant injuries, these findings may also help direct treatment through targeted rehabilitation or surgical interventions [21]. Testing for subluxation or hypermobility of the ulnar nerve can be performed by direct palpation along the posteromedial elbow within the cubital tunnel with arm abducted and externally rotated while moving the elbow through a range of motion. If tapping over the nerve within the cubital tunnel causes paresthesia or tingling (positive Tinel test), one must consider neuroma, compression, or traction injury secondary to instability associated with UCL insufficiency [21]. Flexor-pronator mass injury is assessed via direct palpation of its origin on the medial epicondyle and flexor-pronator mass attempting to elicit pain, which may indicate tendinosis versus tear. Furthermore, pain provoked with resisted forearm pronation may signify pronator teres injury, whereas pain with resisted wrist flexion may indicate wrist flexor pathology.

In addition to the physical examination targeted at the elbow, it is crucial to consider and evaluate the entire kinetic chain in the thrower. This examination includes a thorough analysis of shoulder, scapula, core, and lower extremity function. For example, an association with glenohumeral internal rotation deficit and UCL insufficiency has been described in baseball players [22]. Throwing slot has also been shown to play a role in the force across the UCL. Pitchers or throwers with a more overhead delivery reduces valgus torque across the elbow. A 13-degree decrease in arm slot (more horizontal delivery) was correlated to a 1 N-m increase in valgus torque across the UCL [23]. Therefore, abnormalities disrupting any of the components in the kinetic chain can ultimately cause abnormal throwing mechanics and excess stress on the UCL leading to attenuation and subsequent insufficiency, a decrease in performance, and onset of clinical symptoms.

Imaging

Although UCL insufficiency and posteromedial impingement are often clinical diagnoses, imaging may be necessary to further evaluate or rule out other concomitant pathology, including radiographs, magnetic resonance imaging (MRI), and/or dynamic ultrasound. Plain anteroposterior, lateral, and oblique radiographs of the elbow are often normal but may show evidence of ulnohumeral opening or posteromedial osteophytes. An olecranon axial view is very useful in elucidating posteromedial osteophytes that are not obvious on other radiographic views and is taken with the elbow at approximately 110° of flexion and the beam angled 45° to the ulna [5]. In addition, a valgus stress radiograph using a Telos device that demonstrate an increase in ulnohumeral widening in the injured elbow can be diagnostic of UCL insufficiency; however, standard normal values are not well established, although a difference >0.5 mm greater than the contralateral elbow has been proposed [24].

MRI with or without gadolinium enhancement may provide invaluable information relating to the diagnosis of UCLO and other concomitant pathology. UCL injuries are best visualized on the coronal T2 images on MRI, and findings may include complete and partial tears, edema, calcifications, or a thickened ligament indicating chronic injury (Fig. 7.2). An MRI arthrogram is usually diagnostic and can demon-

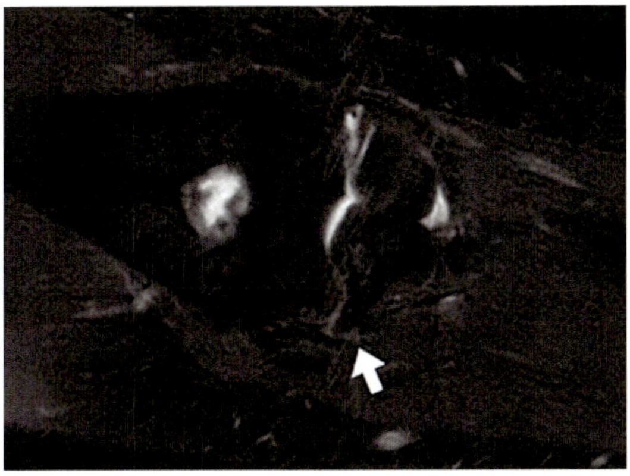

Fig. 7.2 Coronal T2 fat-suppressed image demonstrating distal complete tear of the UCL off of the sublime tubercle (*arrow*). (© 2013 Daryl C. Osbahr, all rights reserved)

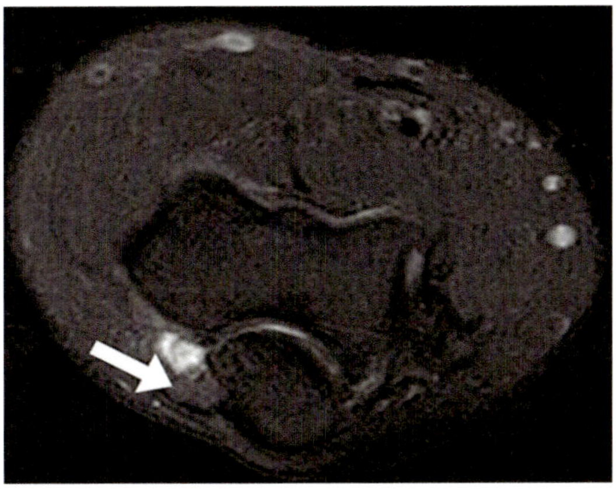

Fig. 7.3 Axial proton density fat-suppressed image demonstrating a posteromedial olecranon osteophyte (*arrow*) in the same patient with complete UCL tear. (© 2013 Daryl C. Osbahr, all rights reserved)

strate both full thickness and partial undersurface tears. For example, a "T-sign" with contrast extravasation along the distal insertion site of the UCL is classically described and observed in partial UCL tears involving the distal ulnar footprint at the sublime tubercle [25, 26].

In the setting of chronic UCL insufficiency with UCLO, a spectrum of MRI findings may be seen in the posteromedial elbow. This pattern may include edema in the subchondral bone, cartilage defects, loose bodies, and/or posteromedial olecranon osteophytes and spurring (Fig. 7.3). These MRI findings have been found to highly correlate with findings at arthroscopic evaluation [27].

Dynamic ultrasound is another useful evaluation option in which valgus stress is applied to the elbow and laxity is evaluated dynamically. Recently, thickening of the UCL on ultrasound has also been suggested to be an early sign of UCL injury [28].

Despite the multitude of imaging modalities used to evaluate pathology relating to UCLO, an approach utilizing a combination of clinical history, physical examination findings, and imaging must be carefully considered to determine appropriate treatment options. Multiple studies have shown imaging abnormalities and increased laxity in the dominant arm in asymptomatic throwers [24, 29]. Therefore, to successfully manage a throwing athlete, the surgeon should not treat based on the imaging findings alone.

Clinical Implications

From a clinical perspective, an athlete with symptoms related to UCLO may initially present with complaints reflective of UCL insufficiency. This includes pain over the medial elbow while throwing, especially during the late cocking and early acceleration phases. This in turn may result in a decrease in throwing velocity or loss of control and accuracy, which ultimately are devastating to the successful performance of a throwing athlete.

The clinical sequelae of UCLO may include chondromalacia, osteophyte formation, and ulnar neuritis, which may manifest in various clinical presentations. One study found an association between preinjury MRI findings of posteromedial impingement and future elbow surgery in asymptomatic professional baseball pitchers [30]. It is therefore essential to establish an early diagnosis before these pathological changes require operative intervention and further complicate recovery in the high-level throwing athlete. Upon identifying such posteromedial elbow pathology in a thrower, the clinician must have a high index of suspicion for UCL injury. In fact, one study noted that approximately 25% of professional baseball players who had previously undergone a posteromedial olecranon osteophyte excision required a subsequent UCL reconstruction [31]. This occurrence may be secondary to an unmasking of existing instability resulting from an insufficient UCL and highlights the importance of early recognition of UCL incompetence and associated conditions.

Treatment

Initially, treatment of UCLO should be focused on prevention. This includes early recognition of UCL insufficiency and prompt treatment. In the nonoperative setting, this may include a period of rest, followed by physical therapy that should include the lower extremity, core, scapula, shoulder, and elbow. Elbow rehabilitation should focus on the range of motion, flexibility, and flexor-pronator strengthening, as well as a well-constructed throwing mechanics program as symptoms resolve. A progressive interval throwing program is then subsequently implemented to gradually transition the athlete back to play. More recently, throwing athletes, especially pitchers, have been reintegrated back into full activities based upon a transition to play program relying on pitch and/or innings limit, so the throwing athlete is not overloaded within the initial return to play stages [32].

There has been a more recent trend to use biologics as an adjuvant to a structured rehabilitation program in the setting of UCL insufficiency with or without the other manifestations of UCLO. Several retrospective studies have shown improvements in the rates of return to play with the addition of PRP injections prior to beginning an interval throwing program in comparison to therapy alone [33, 34]. In addition, these athletes are returning to competition much faster than athletes who pursue UCL reconstructive surgery [35]. More recent research, however, has questioned the benefit of PRP injections in Major League Baseball (MLB) athletes. Chauhan et al. [36] used the MLB Health and Injury Tracking System to compare, in a matched cohort analysis, several outcomes measures, including return to play and return to throwing, between athletes who received PRP injections and those who did not for UCL injuries. This data suggested longer return to play and return to throwing times for athletes who received PRP injections, although there was significant variability in rehabilitation protocols and logistics of PRP use (23). While orthobiologics seem to present a viable alternative for returning throwing athletes to competition without requiring surgical intervention, more investigation into the type of injection, the amount injected, and the number of injections is required. Detailed rehabilitation protocols incorporating PRP injections have yet to be proposed, and randomized controlled trials are needed to determine the efficacy of this possible alternative. One common principal among these studies is the use of ultrasound guidance for injection near the UCL attachment. This modality allows better visualization of the degenerative area of tendon and ensures more accurate administration of the PRP injection (Fig. 7.4).

If an athlete fails a well-constructed nonoperative management plan, continued symptoms may warrant surgical management addressing UCL insufficiency and potentially other concomitant pathology. Specifically with UCLO, it is often necessary to address concomitant olecranon osteophytes and posteromedial chondromalacia. Posteromedial osteophytes and chondromalacia can be debrided either arthroscopically or via an open approach depending upon surgeon prefer-

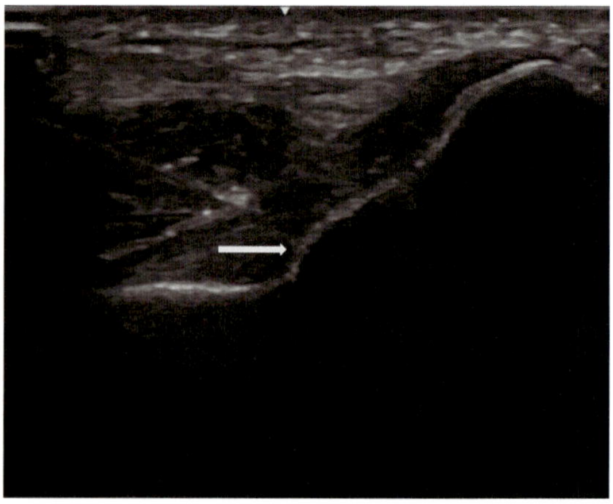

Fig. 7.4 Ultrasound imaging of PRP injection of proximal UCL attachment (*arrow*). (© 2020 Daryl C. Osbahr, all rights reserved)

ence. Although no long-term studies have evaluated the optimal method in addressing chondromalacia in this area of the elbow, viable options include observation, chondral debridement, and microfracture. These options should be dependent on the nature of the chondromalacia, but specific algorithms for optimal treatment have not been developed [20].

Overall, excision of an olecranon osteophyte has been shown to be reliably successful and is associated with good clinical outcomes [27, 37, 38]. A recent study highlighted the importance of addressing this concomitant pathology at the time of UCL reconstruction because the most common reason for reoperation was secondary to a posteromedial olecranon osteophyte [37]. Furthermore, care must be taken to avoid excessive excision of olecranon osteophytes in the overhead-throwing athlete because this may cause or unmask medial elbow instability [39].

Other concomitant pathology may need to be addressed at the time of surgery. Ulnar neuritis may require monitoring or surgical decompression with or without transposition. Debridement and/or reattachment of the flexor-pronator mass may be necessary depending on the degree of tendonosis or tearing, respectively. Combined flexor-pronator mass and UCL injuries should be suspected in baseball players over 30-years-old, and those patients should be counseled preoperatively that outcomes relating to this combined diagnosis carry a worse prognosis with an approximately 12.5% chance to return to prior level of play [38]. Similar to nonoperative treatment, an extensive rehabilitation and throwing program is gradually implemented, and a focus on prevention and proper throwing mechanics is emphasized.

Outcomes

Isolated treatment of UCL insufficiency via reconstruction has been shown to reliably allow athletes to return to their previous level of play 80–90% of the time [12, 15, 40–42]. Arthroscopic treatment of posteromedial impingement via debridement, olecranon osteophyte excision, and loose body removal has also been reported to allow for a high rate of return to play (85–89%) [26, 37, 43]. A clinical study with 2-year follow-up after olecranon osteophyte excision performed concurrently at the time of UCL reconstruction found comparable return to play rates compared with UCL reconstruction alone that did not require osteophyte excision (86 vs. 82%, respectively). Simultaneous treatment may be advisable in that reoperation for olecranon osteophyte excision after UCL reconstruction has been associated with a worse prognosis for return to the same or higher level of play when compared to having osteophytes excised during the index UCL reconstruction procedure (71 vs. 86%, respectively) [37]. In the setting of UCLO, the surgeon is also faced with the challenge of treating chondromalacia resulting from the posteromedial impingement that is likely secondary to UCL insufficiency. UCL reconstruction in association with posteromedial chondromalacia resulting from UCLO has also been found to result in a relatively low rate of return to the previous or higher level of play (76%) [20]. Therefore, better strategies for preventing, identifying, and treating posteromedial chondromalacia are needed to optimize clinical outcomes.

Studies also suggest that UCL reconstruction in patients with previous elbow surgery or combined flexor-pronator mass injuries results in a low rate for return to play (33 and 12.5%, respectively) [32, 44]. Careful patient selection and evaluation is therefore paramount as early recognition and treatment may portend a better prognosis if UCL insufficiency is treated earlier in the disease process, without other concomitant pathology, prior to the late chronic sequelae associated with UCLO.

Summary

UCLO is a dynamic phenomenon that occurs throughout the entire throwing motion arc in the setting of valgus instability secondary to UCL insufficiency and results in posteromedial impingement. This process can subsequently lead to pathologic changes that include posteromedial chondromalacia and osteophyte formation, which can result in persistent disability and inability to play in throwing athletes. UCLO treatment should first focus on early recognition and prevention in the overhead-throwing athlete. If nonoperative measures do not relieve symptoms and improve function, then surgical intervention may be indicated. In the setting of UCLO, UCL reconstruction is necessary to reestablish valgus stability, and the surgeon should also take great care in identifying and treating any concomitant pathology at the index procedure to optimize outcomes for a successful return to play.

References

1. Osbahr DC, Dines JS, Breazeale NM, Deng XH, Altchek DW. Ulnohumeral chondral and ligamentous overload: biomechanical correlation for posteromedial chondromalacia of the elbow in throwing athletes. Am J Sports Med. 2010;38:2535–41.
2. Fleisig GS, Barrentine SW, Escamilla RF, Andrews JR. Biomechanics of overhand throwing with implications for injuries. Sports Med. 1996;21:421–37.
3. Fleisig GS, Barrentine SW, Zheng N, Escamilla RF, Andrews JR. Kinematic and kinetic comparison of baseball pitching among various levels of development. J Biomech. 1999;32:1371–5.
4. Bennett GE. Shoulder and elbow lesions of the professional baseball pitcher. JAMA. 1941;117:510–4.
5. Wilson FD, Andrews JR, Blackburn TA, McCluskey G. Valgus extension overload in the pitching elbow. Am J Sports Med. 1983;11:83–8.
6. Morrey BF, An KN. Articular and ligamentous contributions to the stability of the elbow joint. Am J Sports Med. 1983;11:315–9.
7. Hotchkiss RN, Weiland AJ. Valgus stability of the elbow. J Orthop Res. 1987;5:372–7.
8. Morrey BF, Tanaka S, An KN. Valgus stability of the elbow. A definition of primary and secondary constraints. Clin Orthop. 1991;265:187–95.
9. Schwab GH, Bennett JB, Woods GW, Tullos HS. Biomechanics of elbow instability: the role of the medial collateral ligament. Clin Orthop. 1980;146:42–52.
10. Sojbjerg JO, Ovesen J, Nielsen S. Experimental elbow instability after transection of the medial collateral ligament. Clin Orthop. 1987;218:186–90.
11. Lin F, Kohli N, Perlmutter S, Lim D, Nuber GW, Makhsous M. Muscle contribution to elbow joint valgus stability. J Shoulder Elb Surg. 2007;16:795–802.
12. Dodson CC, Thomas A, Dines JS, Nho SJ, Williams RJIII, Altchek DW. Medial ulnar collateral ligament reconstruction of the elbow in throwing athletes. Am J Sports Med. 2006;34:1926–32.
13. Hyman J, Breazeale NM, Altchek DW. Valgus instability of the elbow in athletes. Clin Sports Med. 2001;20:25–45, viii.
14. Marshall KW, Marshall DL, Busch MT, Williams JP. Osteochondral lesions of the humeral trochlea in the young athlete. Skelet Radiol. 2009;38:479–91.
15. Vitale MA, Ahmad CS. The outcome of elbow ulnar collateral ligament reconstruction in overhead athletes: a systematic review. Am J Sports Med. 2008;36:1193–205.
16. Golan EJ, Shukla DR, Nasser P, Hausman M. Isolated ligamentous injury can cause posteromedial elbow instability: a cadaveric study. J Shoulder Elb Surg. 2016;25:2019–24.
17. Miller CD, Savoie FHIII. Valgus extension injuries of the elbow in the throwing athlete. J Am Acad Orthop Surg. 1994;2:261–9.
18. Moskal MJ. Arthroscopic treatment of posterior impingement of the elbow in athletes. Clin Sports Med. 2001;20:11–24.
19. O'Driscoll SW, Lawton RL, Smith AM. The "moving valgus stress test" for medial collateral ligament tears of the elbow. Am J Sports Med. 2005;33:231–9.
20. Osbahr DC, Dines JS, Rosenbaum AJ, Nguyen JT, Altchek DW. Does posteromedial chondromalacia reduce rate of return to play after ulnar collateral ligament reconstruction? Clin Orthop Relat Res. 2012;470:1558–64.
21. Andrews JR, Wilk KE, Satterwhite YE, Tedder JL. Physical examination of the thrower's elbow. J Orthop Sports Phys Ther. 1993;17:296–304.
22. Dines JS, Frank JB, Akerman M, Yocum LA. Glenohumeral internal rotation deficits in baseball players with ulnar collateral ligament insufficiency. Am J Sports Med. 2009;37:566–70.
23. Camp CL, Tubbs TG, Fleisig GS, Dines JS, Dines DM, Altchek DW, Dowling B. The relationship of throwing arm mechanics and elbow varus torque: within-subject variation for professional baseball pitchers across 82,000 throws. Am J Sports Med. 2017;45(13):3030–5.
24. Ellenbecker TS, Mattalino AJ, Elam EA, Caplinger RA. Medial elbow joint laxity in professional baseball pitchers. A bilateral comparison using stress radiography. Am J Sports Med. 1998;26:420–4.
25. Schwartz ML, al-Zahrani S, Morwessel RM, Andrews JR. Ulnar collateral ligament injury in the throwing athlete: evaluation with saline-enhanced MR arthrography. Radiology. 1995;197:297–9.
26. Timmerman LA, Schwartz ML, Andrews JR. Preoperative evaluation of the ulnar collateral ligament by magnetic resonance imaging and computed tomography arthrography. Evaluation in 25 baseball players with surgical confirmation. Am J Sports Med. 1994;22:26–31.
27. Cohen SB, Valko C, Zoga A, Dodson CC, Ciccotti MG. Posteromedial elbow impingement: magnetic resonance imaging findings in overhead throwing

athletes and results of arthroscopic treatment. Arthroscopy. 2011;27:1364–70.
28. Ciccotti MG, Nazarian L, Atanda A, Cohen SB, Homes L, Dodson C. Early anatomic abnormalities of the anterior band of the ulnar collateral ligament detected on dynamic elbow ultrasound in professional baseball pitchers age 17–21. Presented at the American Orthopaedic Society for Sports Medicine Meeting, Baltimore, Maryland, July, 2012 12–15.
29. Nazarian LN, McShane JM, Ciccotti MG, O'Kane PL, Harwood MI. Dynamic US of the anterior band of the ulnar collateral ligament of the elbow in asymptomatic major league baseball pitchers. Radiology. 2003;227:149–54.
30. Garcia GH, Gowd AK, Cabarcas BC, et al. Magnetic resonance imaging findings of the asymptomatic elbow predict injuries and surgery in major league baseball pitchers. Orthop J Sports Med. 2019;7(1):2325967118818413. Published 2019 Jan 29.
31. Andrews JR, Timmerman LA. Outcome of elbow surgery in professional baseball players. Am J Sports Med. 1995;23:407–13.
32. Axe M, Hurd W, Snyder-Mackler L. Data-based interval throwing programs for baseball players. Sports Health. 2009;1:145–53.
33. Deal, JB, Smith, E, Heard, W, O'Brien, MJ, Savoie, FH. Platelet-rich plasma for primary treatment of partial ulnar collateral ligament tears: MRI correlation with results. Orthop J Sports Med. 2017;5(11):1–6.
34. Podesta L, Crow SA, Volkmer D, Bert T, Yocum LA. Treatment of partial ulnar collateral ligament tears in the elbow with platelet-rich plasma. Am J Sports Med. 2013;41:1689–94.
35. Dines JS, Williams PN, ElAttrache N, et al. Platelet-rich plasma can be used to successfully treat elbow ulnar collateral ligament insufficiency in high-level throwers. Am J Orthop (Belle Mead NJ). 2016;45:296–300.
36. Chauhan A, McQueen P, Chalmers PN, Ciccotti MG, Camp CL, D'Angelo J, et al. Nonoperative treatment of elbow ulnar collateral ligament injuries with and without platelet-rich plasma in professional baseball players: a comparative and matched cohort analysis. Am J Sports Med. 2019;47(13):3107–19.
37. Cain ELJ, Andrews JR, Dugas JR, Wilk KE, McMichael CS, Walter JC, et al. Outcome of ulnar collateral ligament reconstruction of the elbow in 1281 athletes: results in 743 athletes with minimum 2-year follow-up. Am J Sports Med. 2010;38:2426–34.
38. Osbahr DC, Swaminathan SS, Allen AA, Dines JS, Coleman SH, Altchek DW. Combined flexor-pronator mass and ulnar collateral ligament injuries in the elbows of older baseball players. Am J Sports Med. 2010;38:733–9.
39. Inagaki K. Current concepts of elbow-joint disorders and their treatment. J Orthop Sci. 2013;18:1–7.
40. Conway JE, Jobe FW, Glousman RE, Pink M. Medial instability of the elbow in throwing athletes. Treatment by repair or reconstruction of the ulnar collateral ligament. J Bone Joint Surg Am. 1992;74:67–83.
41. Koh JL, Schafer MF, Keuter G, Hsu JE. Ulnar collateral ligament reconstruction in elite throwing athletes. Arthroscopy. 2006;22:1187–91.
42. Rohrbough JT, Altchek DW, Hyman J, Williams RJIII, Botts JD. Medial collateral ligament reconstruction of the elbow using the docking technique. Am J Sports Med. 2002;30:541–8.
43. Dines JS, Yocum LA, Frank JB, Elattrache NS, Gambardella RA, Jobe FW. Revision surgery for failed elbow medial collateral ligament reconstruction. Am J Sports Med. 2008;36:1061–5.
44. Reddy AS, Kvitne RS, Yocum LA, Elattrache NS, Glousman RE, Jobe FW. Arthroscopy of the elbow: a long-term clinical review. Arthroscopy. 2000;16:588–94.

Epidemiology of Elbow Ulnar Collateral Ligament Injuries

8

Lauren M. Fabian and Stan A. Conte

Introduction

Statistical analysis is nothing new to the sport of baseball. From box scores, batting average, and earned run average (ERA) to more complicated calculations such as on-base percentage plus slugging percentage (OPS) and walks plus hits allowed per inning pitched (WHIP), managers, and fans alike have been fascinated with the statistics of the game. More recently, the study of injury rates and their effect on the game and its players has received more attention, but few medical articles have examined the epidemiology of baseball from Little League to Major League Baseball.

The national pastime recruits a staggering number of participants across all levels. It has been estimated that two million children participate in youth baseball leagues, almost 500,000 at the high school level, 35,000 in National Collegiate Athletic Association (NCAA) competition, and over 7000 on professional teams (6500 minor league players and 750 in Major League Baseball). The length of the season, the high number of games and practices, and the repetitive nature of the sport place a great deal of stress on the upper extremity. Many authors have analyzed the biomechanics of the baseball throw, and how alterations to the complex nature of the overhead throwing motion and overuse can lead to injuries throughout the season [1, 2]. As medical and coaching personnel have begun to understand the limitations of the body, this has led to recommendations about structured resting, pitch count and pitch type limits on youth players, and the 5-day pitching cycle in Major League Baseball.

Since Frank Jobe first performed an ulnar collateral ligament reconstruction on Dodgers pitcher Tommy John in 1974, the term "Tommy John surgery" has joined the common vernacular of the sport. Perceptions among players, coaches, and fans reflect the trend that ulnar collateral ligament tears have become a more common injury in baseball through the years, and because of this there has even been a common misconception that prophylactic surgery is desirable [3, 4]. In the past 10 years, there has been a significant increase in the knowledge base about epidemiology of UCL injuries, particularly at the college and professional levels. Most of this is due to large centralized databases such as the NCAA Injury Surveillance System and detailed injury data reporting by Major League Baseball.

Analysis of this data on sports-related injuries can be used to measure comparative risk, identify risk factors, and predict the expected number of injuries over time. It allows coaches, trainers, and medical support personnel to treat expected

L. M. Fabian
Orthopaedic Specialty Group, Fairfield, CT, USA

S. A. Conte (✉)
Conte Sport Performance Therapy,
Scottsdale, AZ, USA

J. S. Dines et al. (eds.), *Elbow Ulnar Collateral Ligament Injury*,
https://doi.org/10.1007/978-3-030-69567-5_8

injuries and to prepare players for rehab and prognosis for return-to-play.

Ulnar Collateral Ligament Injuries in Other Sports

Although injuries to the ulnar collateral ligament of the elbow are most often associated with baseball, the first reported incident of ulnar collateral ligament injury was reported in an elite-level javelin thrower [5]. Ulnar collateral ligament injuries have been reported in a number of sports other than baseball, including javelin throwers, gymnastics, tennis, wrestling, and football [5–11]. The epidemiology of the injury in these groups is largely unknown, as the injuries are exceedingly rare, and often do not require surgery or extended lost time from sport.

Javelin throwers have been shown to place extreme valgus moments across their elbows after foot-strike as they bend their elbows during their throwing motion [12]. Despite the biomechanical risk these throwers place across their elbows, the relatively small number of elite-level javelin throwers and the infrequency of the injury has led to little epidemiologic data in the literature. At one major medical center, 9 out of 10 javelin throwers were able to return-to-play after undergoing ulnar collateral ligament (UCL) [7]. At another institution, 136 UCL injuries were collected over a 15-year period. Though the number of javelin injuries was low (5), the odds ratio for injury was highest among javelin throwers at 6.69 and baseball players 1.55 [13].

In youth gymnastics, the elbow is a weight-bearing joint; it often sees physiologic loads with valgus loads in the back handspring, uneven bars, and other maneuvers. Upper extremity injuries have been reported from 17% to 37% of injuries in different studies, though elbow injuries range from 4.1% to 8.5%. These elbow injuries include osteochondritis dessicans (OCD), elbow dislocations, and elbow "sprains." [14] While there is no literature that reports the epidemiology of UCL injuries specifically, there have been cases in the literature [6, 8]. In reports of UCL avulsions in collegiate gymnasts, the majority have been able to return to sport with conservative management [15]. Similarly, in wrestling, the elbow often becomes a weight-bearing joint. Traumatic injuries such as elbow dislocations occur, and UCL tears have been reported. In a comparison of high school versus college age wrestlers, 10.1% of the injuries seen in high school students were elbow injuries, whereas only 2.3% of the injuries college wrestlers sustained involved the elbow [11].

In respect to football, ulnar collateral ligament injuries tend to occur as a result of a contact mechanism. In data collected from the NCAA-ISP, 36 UCL sprains were identified in a 5-year period from 2009 to 2014, with an injury rate of 0.4 per 10,000 athletic exposures. Fewer than 2% required surgery [16]. Using data from the National Football League (NFL) Ketner et al. reported on medial collateral ligament (MCL) injuries during the 5-year period of 1991–1996. Mechanism of injury occurred with planted hand and valgus loads or contact during blocking for offensive and defensive line players, and contact while being tackled for skill players. None of the players required surgery, and all returned after missing 0–4 games [10]. Insight on the rate of UCL injury in pee-wee and high school players is not available, but is likely exceedingly rare.

Ulnar Collateral Ligament Injuries in Baseball

It is accepted that the overhead throwing motion in baseball places stress across the medial elbow. Extreme valgus stress across the medial elbow during the late-cocking and early acceleration phases of throwing among pitchers occurs during each throw, during which the anterior bundle of the UCL is subject to high tensile stress [17–21]. Over time, or in one single incident, these forces may lead to ligament attenuation and failure. Throwing in baseball, and specifically pitching is repetitive in nature, and the seasons become progressively longer with increasing numbers of games as players get older or progress to higher levels. Despite the vast literature about UCL injuries and reconstruction in baseball players, the true epidemiology of the injury is poorly defined in all major age groups.

Little League

There has been a trend in youth sports for athletes to start earlier and train harder. Early sports specialization have led adolescent baseball players to play year-round baseball, which has been shown to increase injuries [22, 23]. Young throwers often begin to complain about shoulder and elbow pain as early as little league. Injury trends in the National Electronic Injury Surveillance System showed that between 2006 and 2016, greater than 600,000 baseball injuries occurred annually, 17.7% of which involve the elbow and 16.2% involve the shoulder. Though overall incidence of baseball injuries has decreased, incidence of elbow injuries have become more prevalent [24]. In adolescent pitchers surveyed, 50% noted shoulder or elbow pain during the course of the season [25]. Twenty-eight percent of these youth pitchers experienced elbow pain at least once, and 7% of pitching outings resulted in an episode of elbow pain. Similarly, in a prospective cohort study of 198 youth pitchers over two seasons, 26% of players experienced elbow pain during the season [26]. Pitching mechanics, velocity, pitch counts, participation showcases, or on more than one team, and fatigue were all risk factors for increased pain and injury [17, 23, 25, 27].

Most elbow pain experienced by little league players spares the integrity of the UCL; however. Harada et al. examined 294 baseball players between the ages of 9 and 12 and found that of the 60 who had elbow injuries, most of the radiographic findings included medial epicondyle widening, fragmentation, and OCD of the capitellum. None of the players in this age group had ruptures of the UCL [28]. Similarly, Hang et al. did a radiographic study of 343 little leaguers in Taiwan and found that 58% of pitchers, 63% of catchers, and 48% of fielders complained of elbow soreness during the season. Almost all of the players showed radiographic evidence of medial epicondylar hypertrophy, and about half of the players had fragmentation of the epicondyle [29]. While these findings may be consistent with a valgus overload of the elbow while throwing, a.k.a. "little league elbow," magnetic resonance imaging (MRI) studies of throwers in this age group show no evidence of UCL rupture [30]. We may conclude in the skeletally immature elbow with open physes, injury to the UCL is exceedingly rare, even with exposure to repetitive valgus stress from throwing.

High School

According to the National Federation of State High School Associations, about eight million American high school students participate in interscholastic sports in the 2017–2018 season, and nearly 500,000 played baseball [31]. As the third most popular boys' sport, there is a large exposure to throwing in this age group, as an estimated ¼ of all high school players' pitch.

Over the course of a thrower's career, there is a cumulative risk of injury. In a 10-year longitudinal study of pitchers aged 9–14, Fleisig et al. demonstrated a 5% cumulative risk of serious shoulder or elbow injury, defined as surgery on either the shoulder or elbow, or retirement from the sport due to injury [23]. Data support that the level of play is commensurate with risk for elbow injury. Han et al. examined 490 baseball players undergoing rehab for shoulder and elbow injuries at one center. High school and college players were more likely than junior high school players to suffer from UCL injuries (33 and 38% vs. 27%) and were also more likely to have surgery for the condition [32]. UCL injuries were the most common injuries among the players treated (32.7%) followed by superior labral tear from anterior to posterior (SLAP) tears and OCD of the elbow. The vast majority (80%) of injured players with UCL tears were pitchers, whereas 11% were outfielders and 9% infielders.

Since Jobe reported on UCL reconstruction in 1986, the rate of high school aged players undergoing surgery for the condition has risen steadily [9]. Petty et al. reported on the rates of UCL reconstruction by a senior surgeon over the course of two separate 8-year periods and found that from 1988 to 1994, there were 85 baseball players who underwent UCL reconstruction, seven of which were in high school athletes (8%).

By contrast, between 1995 and 2003, 609 UCL reconstructions were done in baseball players, 77 of whom were high school athletes (13%) [33]. More recent research has shown that for the 2003–2014 period, UCL reconstruction rates in New York State increased by 343%, and 28% of the patients were high school age. Numbers are projected to increase significantly again by 2025 [34]. Reports of success rates of surgery in this age group is about equivalent to other age groups, with 74–89% of players returning to the same or higher level, and an average time to return to sport at 11.6 months [33, 35]. Risk factors for injury and surgery include velocity >80 mph, year-round throwing, and learning breaking pitches at early ages all of which have become more commonplace, the sport has become more competitive for younger athletes [33].

College

Collegiate baseball is extremely popular, and participation continues to grow. NCAA baseball participation has grown from 19,670 in the 1988–1989 season to 27,262 in the 2003–2004 season, and 35,460 in the 2017–2018 season [31]. Excellent data collection and monitoring systems have been put in place in NCAA competition via the Injury Surveillance System (ISS), leading to better information and understanding of the nature of collegiate injuries [36]. These databases may include the timing and location of injury events, including episodes during practice and game situations.

To calculate injury rates, McFarland and Wasik defined a "complaint" as a problem for which a player seeks evaluation or treatment from the medical team, an "injury" as any complaint that results in altered or lost participation in a practice or a game, and an "exposure" is defined as one athlete participating in one practice or one game [37]. Using these definitions, one may compare the injury rates across sports, seasons, levels, or different positions in a single sport.

Multiple studies have corroborated that injury rates in baseball players at the collegiate level, in general, are lower than other NCAA sports, including football, wrestling, soccer, and ice hockey [36]. The overall injury rate in baseball is fairly low, but athletes have an injury rate that is three times higher in games situations than in practice [36]. Injury rates in collegiate baseball vary across level of play, as Division I players have an higher injury rate when compared to Division II and II athletes, but across all divisions practice injury rates were the twice as high during preseason play as during the season [36]. In baseball, approximately 64% of game injuries and 42% of practice injuries are noncontact. Upper extremity injuries are the most common injuries among baseball players (45%), whereas they account for only for 18–21% injuries in NCAA sports in general [36]. According to Dick's NCAA study, while shoulder injuries remain the most common (23.4% of game, and 16% practice injuries), elbow injuries are still quite significant, at 9.3% of game and 10.8% of practice injuries. This is similar to McFarland and Wasik's findings that elbow injuries accounted for 14% of total injuries sustained [37]. Of the total number of elbow injuries associated with throwing, 78% occurred as a result of pitching.

Elbow ligament sprains, in particular, were three times more likely to occur in a game situation (0.18 per 1000 game exposures), than in practice (0.05 per 1000 exposures) [36]. Though the number of elbow ligament injuries appears low, they account for a significant amount of lost participation time. DeFroda et al. specifically examined UCL injuries through the NCAA Injury Surveillance Program in the academic years of 2009–2010 through 2013–2014 and found an overall incidence of 20 UCL injuries in 177,992 athletic exposures (1.12 per 10,000 AEs); 85% of these occurred during throwing and 15% were season ending, requiring surgery. For those who did not require surgery, all injuries resulted in lost playing time, as all injured players were out for 7 days or more [38]. Similarly, Rothermitch et al. examined the incidence of UCL injuries in NCAA Division I Baseball during the 2017 baseball season. They found that 134 players from 88 teams underwent surgery for the UCL, which is nearly 2.5% of all eligible athletes. Pitchers were much more likely to have UCL injury than nonpitchers (4.4/100 player-seasons for pitchers vs 0.7/100 player-seasons for nonpitchers), and underclassmen were more likely affected than upperclassmen [39].

Professional

The number of participants in professional baseball leagues in the USA includes over 7000 minor league players and 750 major league players. Roughly half of the players on a major league team at any given time are pitchers. Over the past 10 years, there has been a number of studies that have helped improve our understanding of epidemiology of ulnar collateral ligament injuries in professional baseball players. Using the disabled list as a proxy for injury rates in the sport, Conte et al. examined an 11-year period in Major League Baseball from 1988 to 1999 to ascertain injury rates in the sport. Defining an "injured player" as any player placed on the disabled list by his team, certified by a team physician, they found that both the number of injured players and the total number of disabled increased over the 11-year period studied [40]. With some perturbation in the trend, Posner et al. corroborated this finding while studying similar data over the 7-year period from 2002 to 2008 [41]. Despite improvements in training, conditioning, diagnosis, and surgical treatment methods, the incidence of injuries appears to be increasing over time in professional baseball.

The overall incidence rate for injuries in Major League Baseball is about 3.55 per 1000 exposures [41]. Similarly to the trend seen in college players, injury rates are significantly higher during Spring Training and the beginning of the season as the injury rate in April is 5.73 per 1000 exposures compared with 3.02–3.5 per 1000 exposures during the middle of the season [41]. Though the rates of elbow injuries and UCL tears have not been reported in this population, it stands to reason that the trend would be similar to the overall injury rate.

During these time periods, pitchers comprised an average of 48.4% of disabled list reports and 56.9% of disabled days. Over the course of Conte's 11-year study, both the number of pitchers and the number of disabled list days lost by pitchers increased [40]. By the time period covered in Posner's study, the percentage of disabled days reported for pitchers reached 62% [41]. Elbow injuries represent between 16% and 22% of the disabled days, and account for an average 4452 lost days during the Major League season. Looking specifically at pitchers, elbow injuries comprised 26% of all pitching disabled list days, second only to shoulder injuries, which were 30% [41].

In 2015, Conte et al. administered a questionnaire to all 30 Major League Baseball teams, and all six levels of their minor league affiliates to ascertain the prevalence of the injury. Of the 5088 athletes who responded, 53% were pitchers. In Major League Baseball, 25% of pitchers (96 of 382) had undergone UCL reconstruction, and 15% of Minor League pitchers had undergone UCL reconstruction (Fig. 8.1). Most pitchers at the Major League level (86%) had surgery as a professional, while most Minor League pitchers (61%) had surgery while in high school or college [42]. Interestingly, for players entering the amateur draft, those who had undergone UCL reconstruction before starting their professional careers were more likely to make it to the Major League level compared with their peers [43]. Recent studies have shown that rates of UCL reconstruction continue to climb in both Major League and Minor League Baseball (Fig. 8.1) [44]. Recent studies reproduced this data and showed a significant increase in the prevalence of UCL surgery in minor leagues pitchers from 15% to 19% (Figs. 8.2 and 8.3) [44, 45].

Surgical results have been reported at the professional level by a number of studies [44, 46–48]. For pitchers, return to play has been reported from 79% to 100% at any level, but notably 79–87% return to the same level of play [47]. Conte confirmed for all cases in MLB and Minor League Baseball that return to play was 83.7% overall and 72.8% to the same level of play within

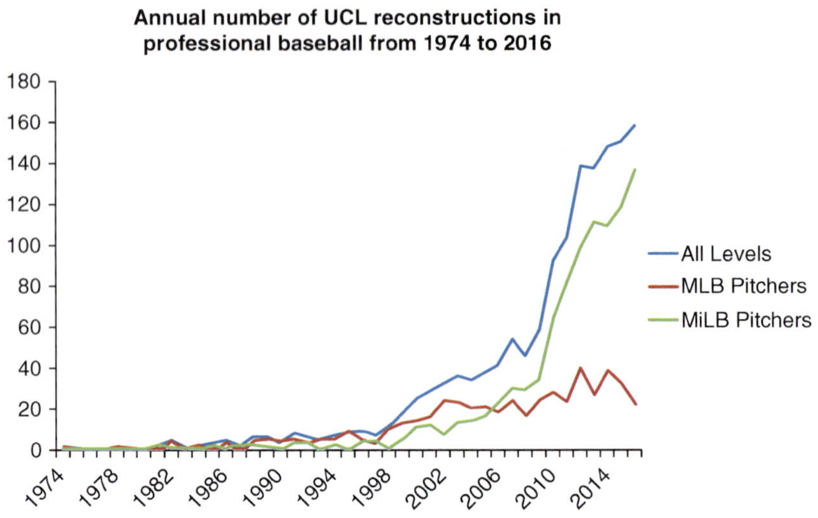

Fig. 8.1 Annual number UCL reconstruction in professional baseball. (From Camp et al. [44]; with permission)

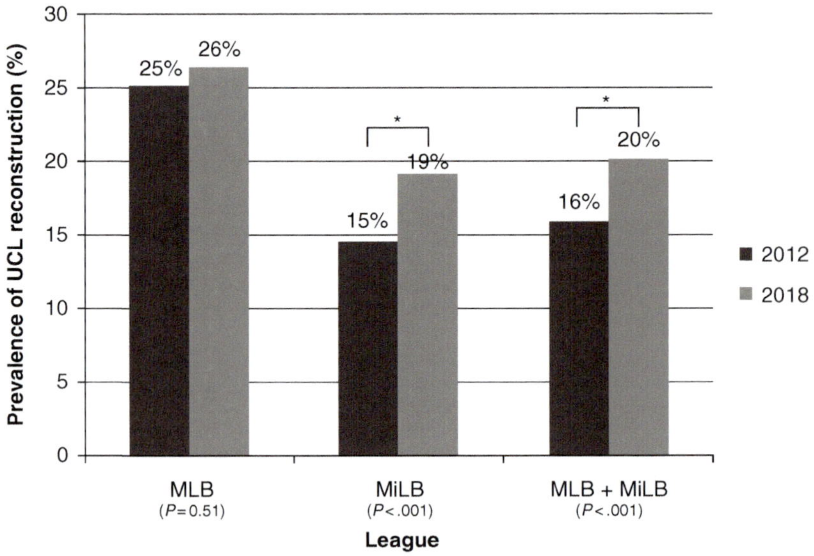

Fig. 8.2 Prevalence of ulnar collateral ligament (UCL) reconstruction among pitchers in Major League Baseball (MLB), Minor League Baseball (MiLB), and MLB + MiLB combined from 2012 to 2018 seasons. Statistically significant differences are denoted by an asterisk (*)

a mean of 506 days [42]. Several authors have noted that pitching statistics such as ERA, fastball velocity, and number of innings pitched all declined in major league pitchers who returned from UCL reconstruction [47].

The early UCL epidemiological studies at the professional level have been based on use of the Disabled List. These studies have a significant limitation in that the DL is not a true injury database but rather a roster management tool. The principal function of the DL is to replace injured players on the Major League roster. In addition, the players are required to stay on a minimum of 15 days even if they have fully recovered and can stay on for an unlimited amount of time thus the reporting number of DL days and placements may be manipulated to increase or decrease the lost time. To mitigate this, Major League developed an injury surveillance system called the Health and Injury Tracking System (HITS). HITS is the first comprehensive injury surveillance system developed to explore injuries among professional baseball players, whereby each team collects injury data on a daily basis [49].

The HITS database has been used in many professional baseball epidemiological studies

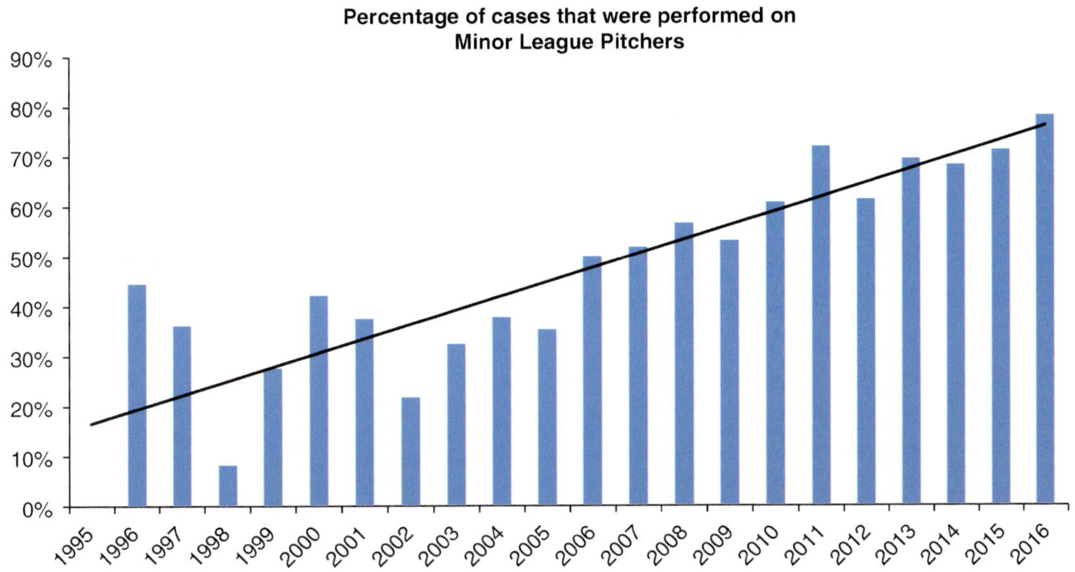

Fig. 8.3 Percentage UCL reconstructions in professional baseball performed on Minor League Pitchers, 1995–2016. (From Camp et al. [44]; with permission)

that have been published since 2011 [50, 51]. Camp et al. used the HITS database to study the increasing number of UCL reconstructions and identified 1429 UCL reconstructions on pitchers from 1974 to 2016. This is the largest sample size of any study on UCL reconstructions at any level. The results indicate that the annual rate of primary and revision UCL reconstructions are rising significantly. In addition, it was also noted that the main reason for the increase in incidence was due to younger, minor league pitchers increasingly undergoing UCL reconstructions. Other studies have found that reconstruction surgeries have a similar increase in incidence in younger pitchers [52, 53].

For pitchers who return to the same level of play after ligament reconstruction, survivorship has been defined as time to play without need for retirement or revision surgery. In Major League Baseball, there is a 9.4% revision rate (5.2% in Minor League), and mean survivorship is about 3.8 years [42]. Erickson et al. evaluated survivorship and reasons for retirement in MLB both in pitchers who had undergone UCL reconstruction and controls, and found that both cohorts had roughly the same career length (4.4 ± 4.7 years and 4.4 ± 3.5 years, respectively). Those who had undergone UCL reconstruction were more likely to be released during the season, while those without were more likely to retire due to shoulder injuries [54].

Perhaps the most surprising data in professional baseball comes from the evaluation of position players who suffer UCL injuries. While it is much less frequently seen in position players than in pitchers, the annual rate has increased from 1984 to 2015 and is proportionally higher in Minor League Baseball than in Major League baseball. Camp et al. evaluated outcomes in 168 position players and found an overall 75% return to play at 342 days overall, and only 58.6% return to play rate for catchers. Position players overall have a worse return to play rate than pitchers (83.7%), but usually a reduced time to return to play (342 days vs. 435 days) [55]. Performance of position players also seems to suffer after UCL reconstruction, and 48% of players are found to change to a different position. Players over 30 years of age have a decreased return rate, and catchers versus other position players have a significantly decreased postoperative career length (2.8±1.8 years vs. 6.1 ± 1.9 years) [56].

Conclusions

Significant progress has been made in the understanding of epidemiology and trends in UCL injuries and surgical outcomes at every level of play. While the odds ratio and risk seem to be highest for javelin throwers, the relative popularity and participation in baseball make this a phenomenon almost unique to the sport.

Elbow injuries, while increasingly common in little league players, seem to spare the UCL in terms of rupture, but show evidence of valgus overload. Once players reach the high school level, there are alarming trends toward increasing prevalence of UCL injuries and surgical intervention. Currently, it is quite commonplace among professional players with increasing incidence each year with younger players being the most affected. Continued preventative strategies and rehabilitation, and guidelines at all levels are needed to improve outcomes with regard to incidence and return-to-sport. These strategies and guidelines may help to stabilize an increasingly more common injury and its significant impact on players and the sport of baseball.

References

1. Chalmers PN, Wimmer MA, Verma NN, et al. The relationship between pitching mechanics and injury: a review of current concepts. Sports Health. 2017;9(3):216–21.
2. Erickson BJ, Sgori T, Chalmers PN, et al. The impact of fatigue on baseball pitching mechanics in adolescent male pitchers. Arthroscopy. 2016;32(5):762–71.
3. Ahmad CS, Grantham WJ, Greiwe RM. Public perceptions of Tommy John surgery. Phys Sportsmed. 2012;40(2):64–72.
4. Conte SA, Hodgins JL, ElAttrache NS, Patterson-Flynn N, Ahmad CS. Media perceptions of Tommy John surgery. Phys Sportsmed. 2015;43(4):375–80.
5. Waris W. Elbow injuries of javelin-throwers. Acta Chir Scand. 1946;93(6):563–75.
6. Cain EL Jr, Andrews JR, Dugas JR, et al. Outcome of ulnar collateral ligament reconstruction of the elbow in 1281 athletes: results in 743 athletes with minimum 2-year follow-up. Am J Sports Med. 2010;38(12):2426–34.
7. Dines JS, Jones KJ, Kahlenberg C, Rosenbaum A, Osbahr DC, Altchek DW. Elbow ulnar collateral ligament reconstruction in javelin throwers at a minimum 2-year follow-up. Am J Sports Med. 2012;40(1):148–51.
8. Grumet RC, Friel NA, Cole BJ. Bony avulsion of the medial ulnar collateral ligament in a gymnast: a case report. J Shoulder Elb Surg. 2010;19(7):e1–6.
9. Jobe FW, Stark H, Lombardo SJ. Reconstruction of the ulnar collateral ligament in athletes. J Bone Joint Surg Am. 1986;68(8):1158–63.
10. Kenter K, Behr CT, Warren RF, O'Brien SJ, Barnes R. Acute elbow injuries in the National Football League. J Shoulder Elb Surg. 2000;9(1):1–5.
11. Yard EE, Collins CL, Dick RW, Comstock RD. An epidemiologic comparison of high school and college wrestling injuries. Am J Sports Med. 2008;36(1):57–64.
12. Morriss C, Bartlett R. Biomechanical factors critical for performance in the men's javelin throw. Sports Med. 1996;21(6):438–46.
13. Zaremski JL, McClelland J, Vincent HK, Horodyski M. Trends in sports-related elbow ulnar collateral ligament injuries. Orthop J Sports Med. 2017;5(10):2325967117731296.
14. Caine D, Cochrane B, Caine C, Zemper E. An epidemiologic investigation of injuries affecting young competitive female gymnasts. Am J Sports Med. 1989;17(6):811–20.
15. Nicolette GW, Gravlee JR. Ulnar collateral ligament injuries of the elbow in female division I collegiate gymnasts: a report of five cases. Open Access J Sports Med. 2018;9:183–9.
16. Christopher ZK, Makovicka JL, Scott KL, et al. Elbow injuries in National Collegiate Athletic Association Football Players: an epidemiological study spanning 5 academic years. Orthop J Sports Med. 2019;7(9):2325967119867411.
17. Davis JT, Limpisvasti O, Fluhme D, et al. The effect of pitching biomechanics on the upper extremity in youth and adolescent baseball pitchers. Am J Sports Med. 2009;37(8):1484–91.
18. Fleisig GS, Andrews JR, Dillman CJ, Escamilla RF. Kinetics of baseball pitching with implications about injury mechanisms. Am J Sports Med. 1995;23(2):233–9.
19. Hutchinson MR, Wynn S. Biomechanics and development of the elbow in the young throwing athlete. Clin Sports Med. 2004;23(4):531–44, viii.
20. Olsen SJ 2nd, Fleisig GS, Dun S, Loftice J, Andrews JR. Risk factors for shoulder and elbow injuries in adolescent baseball pitchers. Am J Sports Med. 2006;34(6):905–12.
21. Schwab GH, Bennett JB, Woods GW, Tullos HS. Biomechanics of elbow instability: the role of the medial collateral ligament. Clin Orthop Relat Res. 1980;146:42–52.
22. Confino J, Irvine JN, O'Connor M, Ahmad CS, Lynch TS. Early sports specialization is associated with upper extremity injuries in throwers and fewer games played in Major League Baseball. Orthop J Sports Med. 2019;7(7):2325967119861101.

23. Fleisig GS, Andrews JR, Cutter GR, et al. Risk of serious injury for young baseball pitchers: a 10-year prospective study. Am J Sports Med. 2011;39(2):253–7.
24. Trofa DP, Obana KK, Swindell HW, et al. Increasing burden of youth baseball elbow injuries in US emergency departments. Orthop J Sports Med. 2019;7(5):2325967119845636.
25. Lyman S, Fleisig GS, Andrews JR, Osinski ED. Effect of pitch type, pitch count, and pitching mechanics on risk of elbow and shoulder pain in youth baseball pitchers. Am J Sports Med. 2002;30(4):463–8.
26. Lyman S, Fleisig GS, Waterbor JW, et al. Longitudinal study of elbow and shoulder pain in youth baseball pitchers. Med Sci Sports Exerc. 2001;33(11):1803–10.
27. Chambless KM, Knudtson J, Eck JC, Covington LA. Rate of injury in minor league baseball by level of play. Am J Orthop (Belle Mead NJ). 2000;29(11):869–72.
28. Harada M, Takahara M, Mura N, Sasaki J, Ito T, Ogino T. Risk factors for elbow injuries among young baseball players. J Shoulder Elb Surg. 2010;19(4):502–7.
29. Hang DW, Chao CM, Hang YS. A clinical and roentgenographic study of Little League elbow. Am J Sports Med. 2004;32(1):79–84.
30. Wei AS, Khana S, Limpisvasti O, Crues J, Podesta L, Yocum LA. Clinical and magnetic resonance imaging findings associated with Little League elbow. J Pediatr Orthop. 2010;30(7):715–9.
31. nfhs.org/media/1020205/2017-18_hs_participation_survey.pdf. Accessed.
32. Han KJ, Kim YK, Lim SK, Park JY, Oh KS. The effect of physical characteristics and field position on the shoulder and elbow injuries of 490 baseball players: confirmation of diagnosis by magnetic resonance imaging. Clin J Sport Med. 2009;19(4):271–6.
33. Petty DH, Andrews JR, Fleisig GS, Cain EL. Ulnar collateral ligament reconstruction in high school baseball players: clinical results and injury risk factors. Am J Sports Med. 2004;32(5):1158–64.
34. Mahure SA, Mollon B, Shamah SD, Kwon YW, Rokito AS. Disproportionate trends in ulnar collateral ligament reconstruction: projections through 2025 and a literature review. J Shoulder Elb Surg. 2016;25(6):1005–12.
35. Saper M, Shung J, Pearce S, Bompadre V, Andrews JR. Outcomes and return to sport after ulnar collateral ligament reconstruction in adolescent baseball players. Orthop J Sports Med. 2018;6(4):2325967118769328.
36. Hootman JM, Dick R, Agel J. Epidemiology of collegiate injuries for 15 sports: summary and recommendations for injury prevention initiatives. J Athl Train. 2007;42(2):311–9.
37. McFarland EG, Wasik M. Epidemiology of collegiate baseball injuries. Clin J Sport Med. 1998;8(1):10–3.
38. DeFroda SF, Goodman AD, Gil JA, Owens BD. Epidemiology of elbow ulnar collateral ligament injuries among baseball players: National Collegiate Athletic Association Injury Surveillance Program, 2009–2010 through 2013–2014. Am J Sports Med. 2018;46(9):2142–7.
39. Rothermich MA, Conte SA, Aune KT, Fleisig GS, Cain EL Jr, Dugas JR. Incidence of elbow ulnar collateral ligament surgery in collegiate baseball players. Orthop J Sports Med. 2018;6(4):2325967118764657.
40. Conte S, Requa RK, Garrick JG. Disability days in major league baseball. Am J Sports Med. 2001;29(4):431–6.
41. Posner M, Cameron KL, Wolf JM, Belmont PJ Jr, Owens BD. Epidemiology of Major League Baseball injuries. Am J Sports Med. 2011;39(8):1676–80.
42. Conte SA, Fleisig GS, Dines JS, et al. Prevalence of ulnar collateral ligament surgery in professional baseball players. Am J Sports Med. 2015;43(7):1764–9.
43. Camp CL, Conte S, D'Angelo J, Fealy SA, Ahmad CS. Effect of predraft ulnar collateral ligament reconstruction on future performance in professional baseball: a matched cohort comparison. Am J Sports Med. 2018;46(6):1459–64.
44. Camp CL, Conte S, D'Angelo J, Fealy SA. Epidemiology of ulnar collateral ligament reconstruction in Major and Minor League Baseball pitchers: comprehensive report of 1429 cases. J Shoulder Elb Surg. 2018;27(5):871–8.
45. Leland DP, Conte S, Flynn N, et al. Prevalence of medial ulnar collateral ligament surgery in 6135 current professional baseball players: a 2018 update. Orthop J Sports Med. 2019;7(9):2325967119871442.
46. Erickson BJ, Bach BR Jr, Bush-Joseph CA, Verma NN, Romeo AA. Medial ulnar collateral ligament reconstruction of the elbow in major league baseball players: where do we stand? World J Orthop. 2016;7(6):355–60.
47. Coughlin RP, Gohal C, Horner NS, et al. Return to play and in-game performance statistics among pitchers after ulnar collateral ligament reconstruction of the elbow: a systematic review. Am J Sports Med. 2019;47(8):2003–10.
48. Conte S, Camp CL, Dines JS. Injury trends in Major League Baseball over 18 seasons: 1998–2015. Am J Orthop (Belle Mead NJ). 2016;45(3):116–23.
49. Pollack KM, D'Angelo J, Green G, et al. Developing and implementing Major League Baseball's health and injury tracking system. Am J Epidemiol. 2016;183(5):490–6.
50. Ahmad CS, Dick RW, Snell E, et al. Major and Minor League Baseball hamstring injuries: epidemiologic findings from the Major League Baseball injury surveillance system. Am J Sports Med. 2014;42(6):1464–70.
51. Green GA, Pollack KM, D'Angelo J, et al. Mild traumatic brain injury in major and Minor League Baseball players. Am J Sports Med. 2015;43(5):1118–26.
52. Erickson BJ, Nwachukwu BU, Rosas S, et al. Trends in medial ulnar collateral ligament reconstruction in the United States: a retrospective review of a large

private-payer database from 2007 to 2011. Am J Sports Med. 2015;43(7):1770–4.
53. Hodgins JL, Vitale M, Arons RR, Ahmad CS. Epidemiology of medial ulnar collateral ligament reconstruction: a 10-year study in New York state. Am J Sports Med. 2016;44(3):729–34.
54. Erickson BJ, Ahn J, Chalmers PN, et al. Reasons for retirement following ulnar collateral ligament reconstruction among Major League Baseball pitchers. Orthop J Sports Med. 2017;5(12):2325967117745021.
55. Camp CL, Conte S, D'Angelo J, Fealy SA. Following ulnar collateral ligament reconstruction, professional baseball position players return to play faster than pitchers, but catchers return less frequently. J Shoulder Elb Surg. 2018;27(6):1078–85.
56. Jack RA 2nd, Burn MB, Sochacki KR, McCulloch PC, Lintner DM, Harris JD. Performance and return to sport after Tommy John surgery among Major League Baseball position players. Am J Sports Med. 2018;46(7):1720–6.

9 History and Physical Exam of the Thrower's Elbow

Brian Grawe, William Piwnica-Worms, Abigail Bacharach, and Joshua S. Dines

Introduction

Overhead athletes frequently sustain injuries to their dominant elbow secondary to the high valgus and extension forces of the throwing motion. The relatively unnatural motion of throwing can produce a myriad of pathological stresses on the structures about the elbow, namely tensile stresses medially, compression stresses laterally, and shear stresses posteromedially. Accurate diagnosis and treatment of elbow pain in the throwing athlete depend on a detailed history, methodical physical examination, and appropriate ancillary tests when needed, as any of the above-mentioned stresses may produce varying types of lesions in the elbow *joint*. The clinician must possess a thorough understanding of the functional anatomy and biomechanical characteristics of the complex elbow articulation to efficiently evaluate and diagnose such pathologies in the thrower's elbow.

This chapter reviews the proper components of a thorough history and physical examination on the elbow in the overhead athlete.

History

Evaluation of an athlete presenting with elbow pain must begin with a detailed throwing history, including onset and duration of symptoms, anatomical site of injury, temporal assessment of symptoms during the throwing motion, associated symptoms, previous treatment, and competition level/time of season [1].

Symptom Onset and Duration

Elbow pain in throwing athletes can often present as an acute event coinciding with a chronic overuse injury [1]. Pitchers are especially susceptible to acute-on-chronic injuries of the elbow due to the high volume and intensity of the overhead motion associated with pitching. Approximately 60% of throwers with ulnar collateral ligament (UCL) injury present with acute medial pain, frequently accompanied by an audible "pop" [2, 3]. These athletes recall the exact throw when they heard the "pop" and typically experience pain in their elbow immediately following the episode. Subsequently, the athlete will no longer be able to compete due to valgus instability of the elbow

B. Grawe
Department of Orthopaedics and Sports Medicine, University of Cincinnati Academic Health Center, Cincinnati, OH, USA

W. Piwnica-Worms · A. Bacharach
Orthopaedics Department, Hospital for Special Surgery, New York, NY, USA

J. S. Dines (✉)
Department of Orthopedic Surgery, Sports Medicine and Shoulder Service, Sports Medicine Institute, Hospital for Special Surgery, New York, NY, USA

J. S. Dines et al. (eds.), *Elbow Ulnar Collateral Ligament Injury*,
https://doi.org/10.1007/978-3-030-69567-5_9

during the throwing motion. Hemorrhage and edema in the elbow may cause symptoms of ulnar nerve irritation. If ulnar neuritis is suspected, special care must be taken during the ligamentous examination.

Many athletes, with or without the acute "pop," will experience concomitant prior medial elbow pain or treatment for flexor-pronator tendonitis or ulnar nerve neuritis. Incomplete healing of these pathologies may cause a subtle change in pitching mechanics that leads to long-term UCL attenuation. These problems may be viewed on a spectrum of overuse injuries to the elbow and are frequently the principal cause of pathology in the elbow of the overhead athlete. The clinician must be vigilant to assess for whether or not the athlete has had repeated or continuous bouts of medial elbow pain, responsive to conservative interventions. Such athletes often continue to throw with minor-to-moderate pain, but 50% demonstrate decreased command and velocity [4]. Kvitne and Jobe concluded that these players are typically unable to throw the ball at over 75% of their standard velocity due to pain [5]. Other complaints include early fatigue and inability to throw as many pitches per appearance.

Location of Injury

Injured athletes can often pinpoint the anatomic location of where they subjectively experience pain in the elbow during the overhead throwing cycle. The athlete's description of the location and intensity of pain will facilitate the clinician in formulating an early differential diagnosis that can be confirmed with a systematic physical examination of the injured elbow [6]. Pain on the medial aspect of the elbow can signify a host of different pathologic scenarios, namely, UCL insufficiency or tear, medial epicondylitis, ulnar nerve irritation or instability, flexor-pronator strain or tear, olecranon/ulnar stress fracture, or in the skeletally immature patient, avulsion fracture of the medial epicondyle. Medial epicondylitis presents with aching pain over the medial elbow and may chronically lead to subjective grip weakness. Point tenderness over the origin of the flexor mass, at the medial epicondyle, is the hallmark finding of medial epicondylitis. Ulnar nerve neuritis in the overhead athlete will produce similar symptoms to those seen in nonathletes who experience mononeuropathy of the ulnar nerve at the elbow; however, they are often exacerbated by or associated with throwing. The ulnar nerve lies in a precarious anatomic position and is very sensitive to traction injury as a result of even minor valgus instability. These symptoms may include medial joint-line pain, clumsiness or heaviness of the hand and fingers, numbness and tingling of the fourth and fifth digits, or medial pain that radiates along the forearm to the hand [6].

Lateral elbow pain, due to throwing, is often associated with radiocapitellar compression and associated chondral wear, lateral epicondylitis, olecranon stress fractures, a plica, or radial nerve entrapment syndrome. Posterior pain is often the direct result of valgus extension overload (VEO), and its differential diagnosis must include olecranon osteophyte formation, triceps tendonitis, or olecranon stress fracture [7]. Loose chondral bodies can lead to pain in the medial, lateral, and posterior aspects of the elbow and may manifest as a sensation of locking or catching. The athlete may also have to manipulate or snap the elbow in order to unlock or free the joint.

Timing During the Throwing Motion (Fig. 9.1)

A complete understanding of the phases that encompass the overhead throwing motion, and subsequent pathologic deviations, will enable the clinician to properly evaluate and diagnose injuries sustained by the overhead athlete during throwing. The phase at which the athlete experiences pain must be viewed as critical information and will aid during the process of performing a focused physical examination [8]. Three phases are historically connected with elbow pain in the throwing athlete—late cocking, acceleration, and deceleration. Nearly 85% of athletes with medial elbow instability complain of pain during the late cocking and acceleration phases of throwing,

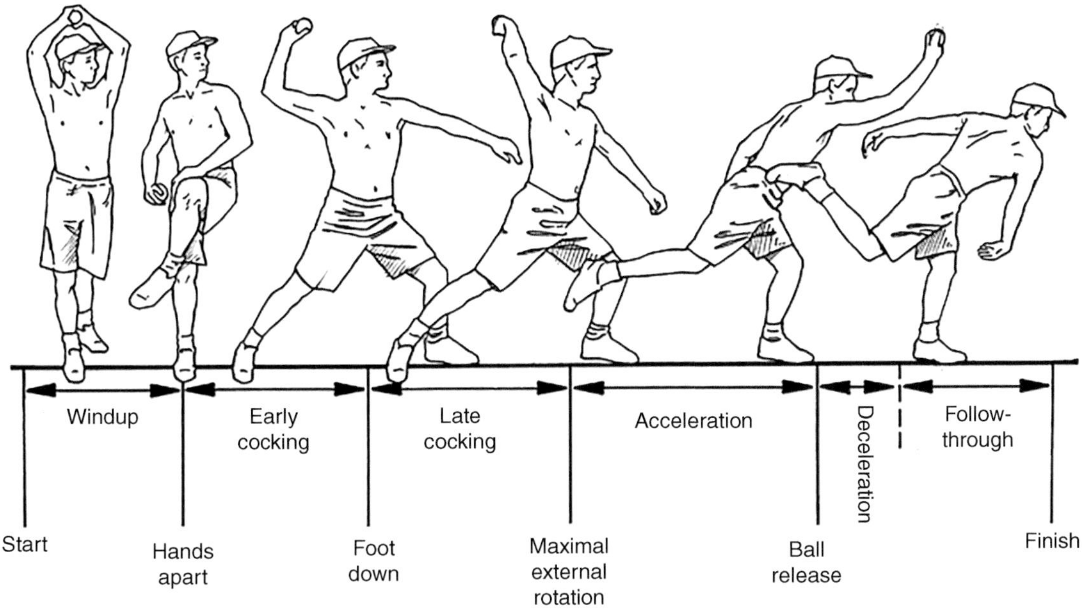

Fig. 9.1 The phases of the baseball pitch. (From [38]; with permission)

while less than 25% complain of pain during the deceleration phase [4]. Large tensile forces are generated on the medial aspect of the elbow which can result in pain, and they are ultimately the direct result of valgus torque seen during the late cocking and acceleration phases of throwing. When the athlete is experiencing pain during the deceleration phase, posterior pathology is often the culprit and is most often due to the large proximal forces that are generated during the overhead throwing motion (VEO, olecranon osteophyte formation, triceps tendonitis, loose bodies) [9, 10].

Associated Symptoms and Previous Treatment

Related symptoms during or in conjunction with throwing must be documented and further evaluated. Neurological or vascular complaints such as cold intolerance, numbness, or tingling in the hand or fingertips, sharp or shooting sensations radiating down the forearm, and fluctuating grip strength may be early indicators of significant neurovascular pathology [11]. Early fatigue or a chronic dull aching pain can signify early nerve compression, as a result of nerve entrapment or mononeuropathy. Complete motor loss or loss of precision with fine muscle movements of the hand often represents more severe nerve injury, and special care must be taken during the physical examination.

The physician should ask the athlete about any prior injuries or treatment to the throwing extremity. Previous treatment or surgery to the elbow or shoulder may give valuable information when determining the etiology of the athlete's current symptoms. It is not uncommon for the overhead athlete to develop elbow pain after a defined treatment period for shoulder pathology, and likewise those recovering from elbow pain may develop ipsilateral symptoms in the shoulder. The significance of the kinetic chain and its importance to injury prevention are well documented [12, 13]. Previous treatment for flexor tendinitis or ulnar nerve neuritis that continues to hinder the pitcher's performance may lead the physician to consider UCL attenuation as the origin of the pain generator [1].

All portions of the kinetic chain, which include the shoulder, back, hip, knee, and ankle, can subsequently produce undue kinematic effects in the elbow, and injuries that lead to deviations of successful execution of the kinetic chain in throwing must be closely evaluated [14]. Detailed analysis of the throwing motion has shown proximal-to-distal muscle activation, peak torque development, and force development radiation from the trunk to the elbow [15]. Proximal body segments provide dynamic mechanisms by which the forces generated by the overhead motion can be regulated to allow for minimal injury risk to the throwing elbow [14]. A more proximal injury could result in a functional change that leads to abnormal elbow kinematics and injury at the distal end of the kinetic chain. Glenohumeral internal rotation deficiency (GIRD) has also been linked with acute and chronic elbow problems in the throwing athlete. Morgan and colleagues analyzed the elbows of 20 symptomatic professional pitchers who presented with GIRD, defined as a loss of internal rotation greater than 25° compared to the contralateral shoulder, and determined that therapeutic correction of the arc of motion deficits can decrease subjective complaints of elbow pain in pitchers [16].

Level of Competition and Timing of Play

The athlete's level of competition and the temporal aspect of the athletic season are important considerations when discussing treatment options. Recreational athletes will not require the same aggressive treatment plan as high-level professional athletes, while younger athletes (the skeletally immature athlete) may consider less invasive treatment alternatives. Pitchers with improper mechanics or training regimens can present with medial elbow pain attributable to flexor-pronator tendonitis during preseason or spring training, whereas frank UCL injuries often occur in the middle or end of the season [3].

Excessive pitch counts, increased workload, insufficient rest between appearances, changing of arm slot, and the delivery of a large percentage of breaking balls are important factors when discussing modifiable elements that may prevent medial elbow injuries in the throwing athlete. In addition, catchers who throw back to the pitcher from their knees are not utilizing their kinetic chain properly and can also sustain injuries to their dominant elbow [17].

Physical Examination

It is important to perform a comprehensive and reproducible physical examination on overhead athletes who are experiencing elbow pain during throwing. A thorough exam can often allow the surgeon to properly diagnose the pathology without the necessity of further ancillary tests. The exam should be conducted methodically and include observation/inspection, palpation, neurovascular, and range of motion testing, and digressions from normal will then permit a more focused set of special tests to establish a conclusive diagnosis.

Observation/Inspection

It is imperative that all diagnostic maneuvers, throughout the entirety of the physical examination, be performed on both the affected and non-affected upper extremity, thus allowing for meaningful comparison of what should be considered a normal finding, an adaptive change, or overtly pathologic. A complete inspection of the elbow includes kinematic assessment of the ipsilateral shoulder and scapula [6]. The physician should note any subtle pathologic changes to the upper extremity and should recognize normal adaptive muscular hypertrophy in the throwing arm [18, 19]. Increased shoulder external rotation arc with a concomitant decrease in internal rotation, in comparison to the unaffected extremity, is not uncommon in the healthy throwers' arm. However, pathologic GIRD is associated with UCL insufficiency [13].

The carrying angle, defined as the angle between the long axis of the humerus and the long axis of the forearm in the coronal plane, should be measured and recorded. Normative values are typically reported as 11° and 13° of the valgus in males and females, respectively [20]. Many high-level athletes have carrying angles greater than 15°, and in the pitcher's arm, this angle may be 10–15° greater when compared to non-throwing extremity [19]. This phenomenon is likely due to the previous injury or developmental abnormalities from the repetitive stress put upon the elbow during throwing.

The soft tissues must always be evaluated for swelling or ecchymosis, which can indicate the acuity of any injuries to the structures of the elbow. Ecchymosis often develops in 24–72 h after sustaining an acute UCL injury. Bruising will occur along the medial elbow and proximal forearm in this setting. Significant swelling can also be seen in patients who rupture their flexor-pronator mass in conjunction with UCL tears. Chronic overuse UCL pathology will often exhibit a relatively normal soft-tissue envelope, and the clinician should more closely rely on manual maneuvers for an accurate diagnosis. Documentation of surgical scars, blanching due to vascular insufficiency, and olecranon swelling should be noted as well [21].

If UCL reconstruction is a possibility, the physician should also determine if the athlete has a palmaris longus tendon in the throwing or nonthrowing extremity. This is the most common tendon graft for UCL reconstruction and is found in only 80% of throwing athletes [3]. If the palmaris longus is not found in either forearm, the gracilis or plantaris tendons can function as viable options for autograft reconstruction alternatives.

Palpation

Palpation of the thrower's elbow should be conducted with a stepwise routine to discover the site of pain and rule out other pathologic conditions associated with throwing. The physician should palpate the injured elbow on the soft spot at the junction of the olecranon, capitellum, and radial head and compare it to the contralateral arm to assess for any joint effusion. The presence or absence of loose bodies must also be documented, as their significance can be quite dramatic, in terms of mechanical symptoms associated with the thrower's elbow.

With the elbow in approximately 50–70° flexion, palpation of the UCL should be performed. This flexion range moves the overlying flexor-pronator muscle mass anterior to the fibers of the UCL, giving the surgeon direct access to the ligament proper. Palpation should occur along the entire course of the UCL, moving proximal to distal from its origin at the inferior aspect of the medial epicondyle to its insertion onto the sublime tubercle of the proximal medial ulna. Athletes with UCL injury most often present with point tenderness about 2 cm distal to the medial epicondyle. Tenderness over the UCL may indicate ligament attenuation; however, it must be noted that pain over the UCL has an 81–94% sensitivity but only a 22% specificity for UCL tears [22].

The flexor-pronator muscle mass can be palpated to assess for medial epicondylitis by moving distal and slightly anterior to the medial epicondyle. Athletes most often feel pain associated with the pronator teres (PT) and flexor carpi radialis (FCR) tendons, which are located directly anterior to the course of the UCL [1]. Often, it can be difficult for the clinician to differentiate between medial epicondylitis and a UCL tear or avulsion due to their intimate anatomic relationship in the medial elbow. Resisted wrist flexion and forearm pronation may elicit greater pain in an athlete complaining of medial epicondylitis, compared to UCL injury [23]. More specific tests for the competency of the UCL, such as the valgus stress test, can help differentiate between these separate and often associated pathological conditions.

Neurovascular

The orthopedist must closely evaluate all neurovascular structure about the affected extremity, especially in athletes who complain of numbness or tingling. Gentle palpation of the ulnar nerve does not cause pain in the healthy elbow, but often causes discomfort in athletes with ulnar neuritis. The ulnar nerve must be evaluated throughout its entire course in the elbow startling just proximal to the medial epicondyle, through the cubital tunnel, and distally into the flexor carpi ulnaris muscle mass. Stability of the ulnar nerve must also be judged with gentle pressure applied on the nerve above the medial epicondyle, as the elbow is taken through a flexion-extension arc. Frank subluxation can often cause significant discomfort during hyperflexion and must be respected during the remainder of the exam. In some cases, the ulnar nerve dislocates anteriorly to the medial epicondyle, while the elbow is moved from extension to flexion, and this signifies moderate-to-severe ulnar nerve instability [24, 25].

Range of Motion

In normal controls, the range of motion (ROM) of the elbow is from 0° of extension to 140–150° of flexion, with 85° pronation and 90° supination [26, 27]. Both active and passive ROM should be determined, and intervals of pain during the arc of motion should be documented and further evaluated. Passive movement of the throwing arm should be checked for blockage or limitation of motion and compared to the contralateral arm [28, 29]. It is common for throwing athletes to demonstrate loss of elbow extension in the dominant extremity, which can either be an adaptive condition or an overt pathologic loss of motion. A flexion contracture of up to 20° may develop in a pitcher's throwing arm as well, but it is traditionally only considered pathologic if painful [1].

The physician should identify abnormalities in the attitude of the elbow joint at the end ranges of motion. At full extension, a bony stop occurs when the olecranon strikes the olecranon fossa, whereas terminal elbow flexion creates tissue approximation as the biceps brachia and wrist flexors approach one another [28, 30]. Pronation and supination should elicit a capsular end feel. The throwing arm should be compared to the nonthrowing arm as anything that varies from the contralateral side may indicate pathology. Osteophytic changes to either the proximal olecranon or coronoid tip can often produce asymmetric endpoints in extension and flexion arcs of the elbow, respectively.

Manipulative Tests

Assessing for the functional integrity of the UCL is a key to the diagnosis and is the most essential component of the physical examination. The difference between pathologic and healthy ligaments can be difficult to discern and, therefore, the clinician should always compare to the contralateral normal extremity.

The valgus stress (Fig. 9.2) test can be used to assess for injury to the anterior bundle of the UCL. With the elbow flexed to 30°, the physician stabilizes the athlete's humerus just above the humeral condyles and applies a valgus movement while grasping the athlete's pronated forearm [6]. UCL laxity in injured athletes is subtle and has been shown by Field and colleagues to only increase medial opening by 1–2 mm compared to the contralateral arm [31, 32]. Failure to maintain forearm pronation during the valgus pressure may cause subtle posterolateral instability that can resemble medial laxity.

The milking maneuver (Fig. 9.3) can also be used to evaluate valgus stability while the joint is in flexion. Theoretically the test, as originally described by Stephen O'Brien MD, isolates the

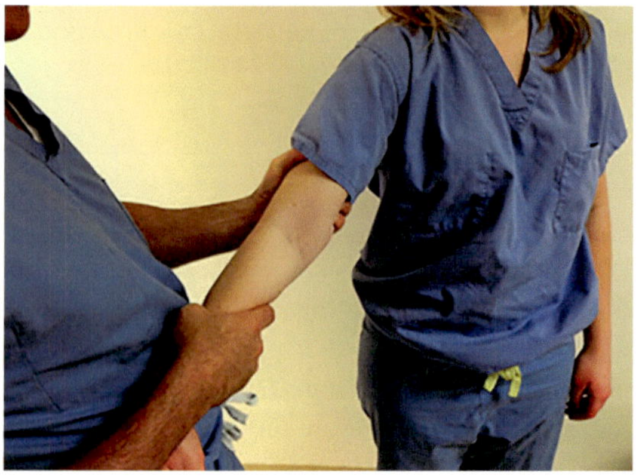

Fig. 9.2 Demonstrates the valgus stress test. Note the maintenance of pronation and the valgus pressure applied just above humeral condyles

posterior band of the anterior bundle of the UCL. The athlete flexes the throwing elbow beyond 90° and with the other arm reaches under the humerus and grabs the ipsilateral thumb, which exerts a valgus stress on the affected elbow [33]. The physician should then palpate along the course of the UCL to assess for tenderness and joint space opening.

It must be noted that modifications to the milking maneuver have also been described. At an angle greater than 120° flexion, the contribution of the bony anatomy makes evaluation of the ligament less sensitive, and consequently Safran and colleagues have described a variation that places the contralateral arm under the elbow being examined, eliminating the confounding factors associated with the osseous architecture that occurs during hyperflexion [6]. This position adducts the shoulder with maximal external rotation, which can be a problem with the original maneuver. The examiner then holds the throwing elbow at 70° flexion, which is the position of the greatest potential valgus laxity, as demonstrated in cadaveric studies [34–36]. Next, the examiner pulls down on the thumb with one arm and puts valgus stress on the elbow with the other, and with the hand imparting the valgus stress, the physician can still palpate the medial aspect with his thumb and assess for gapping or an increased joint space.

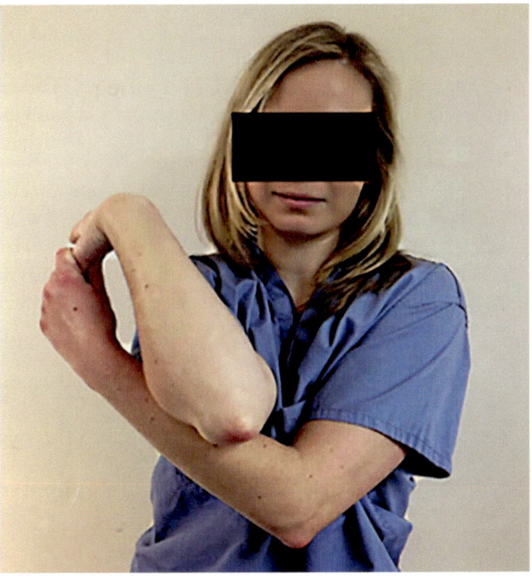

Fig. 9.3 Demonstrates the "milking maneuver." The examiner must palpate the medial portion of the ulnohumeral joint to discern the maximum point tenderness and whether there is medial opening

The moving valgus stress test (Fig. 9.4), described by O'Driscoll and Lawton, can also aid in the detection of UCL insufficiency [37]. The throwing shoulder is placed in an abducted and externally rotated position, while the physician takes the elbow through its flexion-extension limits under valgus pressure. In many athletes with UCL injury, pain is often felt at a specific point within the flexion arc of 80–120°, and this test aims to reproduce that pain because the shearing force applied to the ligament is similar to that applied during the late cocking/early acceleration phases of actual throwing [6]. It is important to note that while the authors documented 100% specificity during their initial study, in our experience, a positive result in the setting of UCL insufficiency, at times, depends on when the

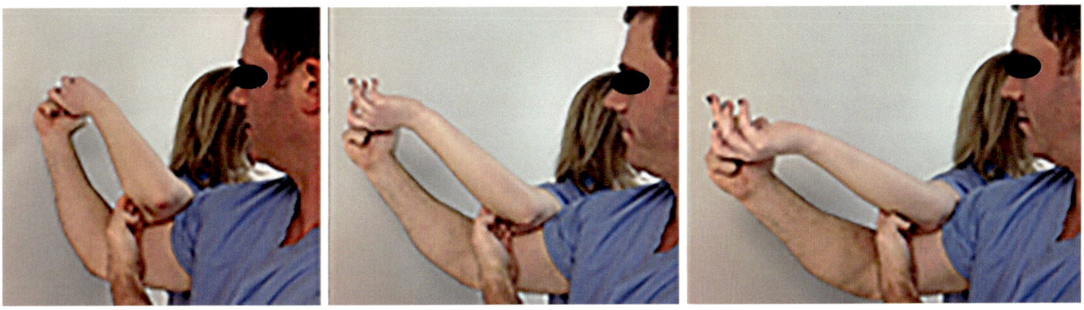

Fig. 9.4 Shows the moving valgus stress test as described by O'Driscoll and colleagues. It is important for the examiner to note where, during the arc of flexion, the test elicits pain

patient last threw. If athletes with UCL injury have not thrown a ball for weeks prior to their examination, they may not have pain with the moving valgus stress test.

If the athlete complains of posterior elbow pain, the VEO test may detect the presence of a posteromedial olecranon osteophyte or olecranon fossa overgrowth [1]. The examiner stabilizes the athlete's humerus with one hand, and pronates the forearm and applies a valgus force while quickly maximally extending the elbow with the other hand. The athlete may then experience pain in the posteromedial compartment of the elbow, as the olecranon tip osteophyte engages into the olecranon fossa.

Conclusion

Elbow injuries can be difficult to differentially diagnose in the overhead throwing athlete. The clinician must possess a comprehensive understanding of elbow anatomy and kinematics, along with the various stress demands applied to the elbow during the throwing motion. A detailed history and a thorough physical examination are essential in order to obtain an accurate diagnosis for the thrower that presents with elbow pain. Furthermore, an appropriate treatment plan will be multifaceted and involve the athlete's specific level of play and timing of the season. The role of imaging will be discussed in the subsequent chapter.

References

1. Cain EL, Dugas JR. History and examination of the thrower's elbow. Clin Sports Med. 2004;23:553–66.
2. Andrews JR, Timmerman LA. Outcome of elbow surgery in professional baseball players. Am J Sports Med. 1995;23:407–13.
3. Azar FM, Andrews JR, Wilk KE, et al. Operative treatment of ulnar collateral ligament injuries of the elbow in athletes. Am J Sports Med. 2000;28:16–23.
4. Conway JE, Jobe FW, Glousman RU, et al. Medial instability of the elbow in throwing athletes. J Bone Joint Surg Am. 1992;74:67–83.
5. Kvitne RS, Jobe RW. Ligamentous and posterior compartment injuries. In: Jobe FW, editor. Operative techniques in upper extremity sports injuries. St. Louis: Mosby; 1996. p. 411–30.
6. Safran MR. Ulnar collateral ligament injury in the overhead athlete: diagnosis and treatment. Clin Sports Med. 2004;23(4):643–63.
7. Wilson FD, Andrews JR, Blackburn TA, et al. Valgus extension overload in the pitching elbow. Am J Sports Med. 1983;11:83–7.
8. Fleisig GS, Andrews JR, Dillman CJ, et al. Kinetics of baseball pitching with implications about injury mechanisms. Am J Sports Med. 1995;23:233–9.
9. Loftice JW, Fleisig GS, Zheng N, et al. Biomechanics of the elbow in sports. Clin Sports Med. 2004;23:519–30.
10. Miller CD, Savoie FH III. Valgus extension injuries of the elbow in the throwing athlete. J Am Acad Orthop Surg. 1994;2:261–9.
11. Dugas JR, Weiland AJ. Vascular pathology in the throwing athlete. Hand Clin. 2000;16:477–85.
12. Burkhart SS, Morgan CD, Kibler WB. The disabled throwing shoulder: spectrum of pathology. Part 1, pathoanatomy and biomechanics. Arthroscopy. 2003;19:404–20.
13. Dines JS, Frank JB, Akerman M, Lewis MS, Yocum A. Glenohumeral internal rotation deficits in baseball players with ulnar collateral ligament insufficiency. Am J Sports Med. 2009;37:566–70.
14. Kibler WB, Sciascia A. Kinetic chain contributions to elbow function and dysfunction in sports. Clin Sports Med. 2004;23:545–52.
15. Hirashima M, Kadota H, Sakurai S, et al. Sequential muscle activity and its functional role in the upper extremity and trunk during overarm throwing. J Sports Sci. 2002;20:301–10.
16. Morgan CD. The relationship between elbow symptoms and shoulder internal rotation. Paper presented at: the closed meeting of the American Shoulder and Elbow Surgeons. Monterey, 10 Oct 2002.
17. Freehill MT, Safran MR. Diagnosis and management of ulnar collateral ligament injuries in throwers. Curr Sports Med Rep. 2011;10:271–8.
18. Andrews JR, Schemmel SP, Whiteside JA. Evaluation, treatment, and prevention of elbow injuries in throwing athletes. In: Nicholas JA, Hershman EB, editors. The upper extremity in sports medicine. Philadelphia: CV Mosby; 1990. p. 781–26.
19. King JW, Brelsford HI, Tullos HS. Analysis of the pitching arm of the professional baseball pitcher. Clin Orthop. 1969;67:1–16.
20. Beals BK. The normal carrying angle of the elbow. Clin Orthop. 1976;119:194–6.
21. Andrews JR, Wilk KE, Satterwhite YE, et al. Physical exam on the thrower's elbow. J Orthop Sports Phys Ther. 1993;17:296–304.
22. Timmerman LA, Schwartz ML, Andrews JR. Preoperative evaluation of the ulnar collateral ligament by magnetic resonance imaging and computed tomography arthrography. Evaluation in 25 baseball players with surgical confirmation. Am J Sports Med. 1994;22:26–31.
23. Lynch JR, Waitayawinyu T, Hanel DP, et al. Medial collateral ligament injury in the overhand-throwing athlete. J Hand Surg Am. 2008;33:430–7.

24. Childress HM. Recurrent ulnar nerve dislocation at the elbow. Clin Orthop. 1975;108:168–73.
25. Del Pizzo W, Jobe FW, Norwod L. Ulnar nerve entrapment syndrome in baseball players. Am J Sports Med. 1977;5:182–5.
26. Bennett B, Tullos HS. Ligamentous and articular injuries in the athlete. In: Morrey BF, editor. The elbow and its disorders. Philadelphia: WB Saunders; 1985. p. 502–22.
27. Kapandji IA. The physiology of the joints, upper limb, vol. I. 2nd ed. Williams & Wilkins Co: Baltimore; 1970.
28. Cyriax J. Diagnosis of soft tissue lesions. In: Textbook of orthopaedic medicine, vol. I. 8th ed. Balliere Tinell: New York; 1981. p. 52–4.
29. Hoppenfeld S. Physical examination of the spine and extremities. Nonvalk: Apple-Century-Crofts; 1976. p. 35–58.
30. Lobe FW, Fanton CS. Nerve injuries. In: Morrey BF, editor. The elbow and its disorders. Philadelphia: WB Saunders; 1985. p. 497–501.
31. Field LD, Altchek DW. Evaluation of the arthroscopic valgus instability test of the elbow. Am J Sports Med. 1996;24:177–81.
32. Field LD, Callaway GH, O'Brien SJ, et al. Arthroscopic assessment of the medial collateral ligament complex of the elbow. Am J Sports Med. 1995;23:396–400.
33. Veltri DM, O'Brien SJ, Field LD, Deutsch A, Altcher A, Potter H. The milking maneuver-a new test to evaluate the MCL of the elbow in the throwing athlete. Presented at the 10th open meeting of the American shoulder and elbow surgeons specialty day. New Orleans, 7 Feb 1994.
34. Callaway GH, Field LD, Deng XH, Torzilli PA, O'Brien SJ, Altchek DW, et al. Biomechanical evaluation of the medial collateral ligament of the elbow. J Bone Joint Surg. 1997;79:1223–31.
35. Floris S, Olsen BS, Dalstra M, Sojbjerg JO, Sneppen O. The medial collateral ligament of the elbow join: anatomy and kinematics. J Shoulder Elb Surg. 1998;7:345–51.
36. Sojbjerg JO, Overson J, Nielson S. Experimental elbow stability after transection of the medial collateral ligament. Clin Orthop. 1987;218:186–90.
37. O'Driscoll SW, Lawton RL. Moving valgus stress test. Presented at the 18th open meeting of the American shoulder and elbow surgeons. Dallas, 16 Feb 2002. p. 40.
38. Limpisvasti O, ElAttrache NS, Jobe FW. Understanding shoulder and elbow injuries in baseball. J Am Acad Orthop Surg. 2007;15:139–47.

10 Radiographic Imaging of the Elbow

Susie Muir and John V. Crues III

The elbow joint is a trochoginglymus joint that allows for flexion-extension and pronation-supination. Elbow range of motion extends from 0 to 140° with 75° of pronation and 85° of supination [1]. The elbow joint is contained within a capsule whose medial and lateral thickenings comprise the collateral ligaments; ligamentous injury may occur with or without injury to the adjacent flexor or extensor tendons. The ulnar collateral ligament (UCL) extends from the inferior surface to the anterior and posterior surface of the medial epicondyle and consists of three bands [2] as shown in Fig. 10.1.

The anterior band, which is the primary stabilizer of the elbow, is attached to the coronoid process at the sublime tubercle (Fig. 10.2a, b); a variation of ligamentous insertion is just inferior to the sublime tubercle (Fig. 10.2c). The fan-shaped posterior band extends from the medial condyle to the semilunar notch of the ulna and lies deep to the ulnar nerve forming the roof of the cubital tunnel (Fig. 10.3). It is a secondary stabilizer of the elbow when the joint is flexed beyond 90°. Between the anterior and posterior bands, a transverse band spans the notch and bridges the medial olecranon and the inferior medial coronoid process. The transverse band is universally regarded as an insignificant contributor to elbow stability.

The anterior band is the most discreet and well-defined band of the UCL. Its origin fans out and fibrofatty tissue or fibrofatty changes of the ligament often seen at its origin may mimic a tear (Fig. 10.4a). In such cases, posterior to anterior evaluation of the UCL fibers on sagittal sequences is necessary to assess for fiber disruption (Fig. 10.4b, c). Insertion on the sublime tubercle is tight; trace or no joint fluid lies between the ligament and the sublime tubercle in young individuals. In older individuals, the normal UCL attachment at the sublime tubercle often has a small groove that may also mimic a tear (Fig. 10.5; [3]). In adolescents, the anterior band of the UCL commonly originates from, and is an extension of, the periosteum bridging the physeal plate of the medial epicondyle (Fig. 10.6; [4]).

Functionally, the anterior band of the UCL is divided into anterior and posterior components [5]. These components are, however, not seen as separate structures on the magnetic resonance imaging (MRI) or at surgery. In valgus loading, the anterior portion is tense with elbow flexion (from 0 to 85°), whereas the posterior portion is taut (from 55° to full flexion). When under stress, beginning at 65° of flexion, the posterior bundle tightens [6]. This sequential tightening of the anterior band ensures that some portion of the band is taut during the entire arc of flexion making the UCL the primary stabilizer of the elbow

S. Muir (✉) · J. V. Crues III
RadNet, Inc., Los Angeles, CA, USA
e-mail: Susie.muir@radnet.com

J. S. Dines et al. (eds.), *Elbow Ulnar Collateral Ligament Injury*,
https://doi.org/10.1007/978-3-030-69567-5_10

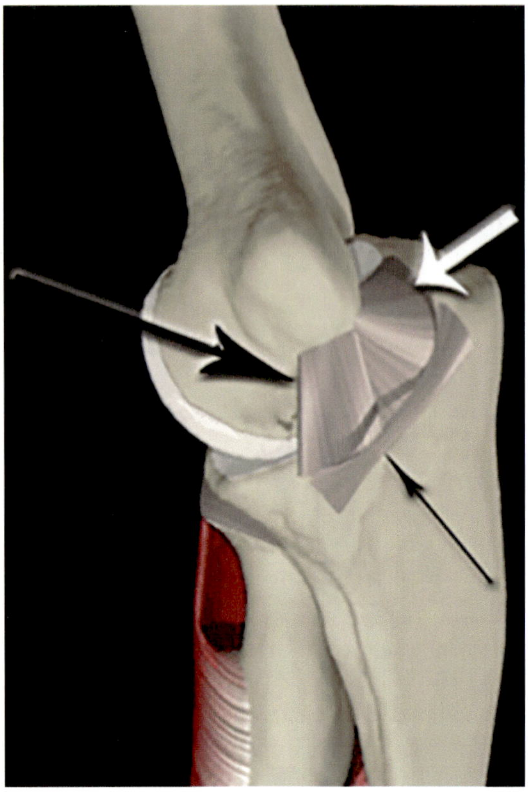

Fig. 10.1 Anatomy of the ulnar collateral ligament. Of the three recognized components of the ulnar collateral ligament, the anterior band (*large black arrow*) is the most important for elbow stability and is commonly injured in throwing athletes. The posterior band (*white arrow*) and transverse band (*small black arrow*) are of limited importance

against valgus stress [7, 8]. The UCL provides both static and dynamic stability to the elbow acting as the primary medial stabilizer in flexion; forces placed on the UCL during pitching are near the limits of the UCL tensile strength [9]. The tensile strength of the UCL is approximately 34 N m which exceeds the valgus stress placed on the medial elbow during pitching; a mean peak valgus torque of 120 N m has been reported for a professional population of pitchers [10]. The flexor–pronator mass is the dynamic, active stabilizer of the elbow and has been shown to be active

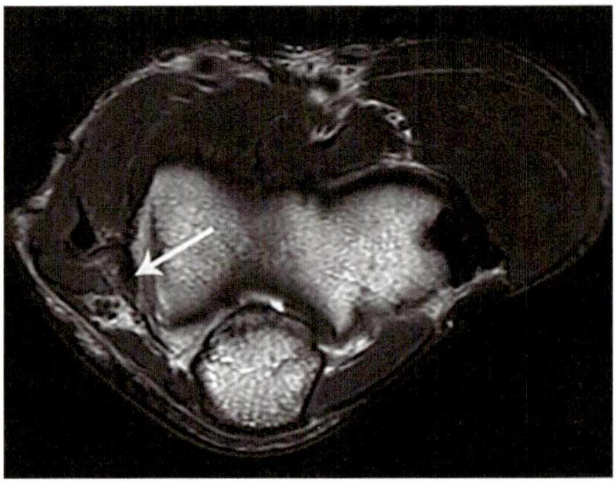

Fig. 10.3 The posterior band of the UCL lies deep to the ulnar nerve and forms the roof of the cubital tunnel

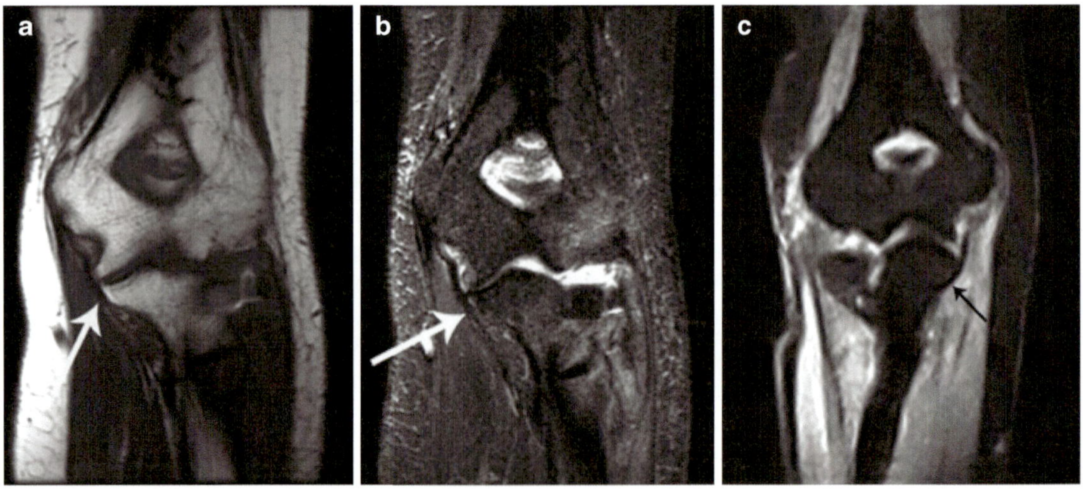

Fig. 10.2 Coronal T1-weighted (**a**) and coronal short tau inversion recovery (STIR) (**b**) images show the anterior band of the UCL as a continuous band of low-signal intensity extending from the inferior medial epicondyle to insert on the sublime tubercle of the coronoid (*arrows* show the attachment to the sublime tubercle). Variation of UCL anterior band attachment with insertion inferior to the sublime tubercle (*arrow*) (**c**)

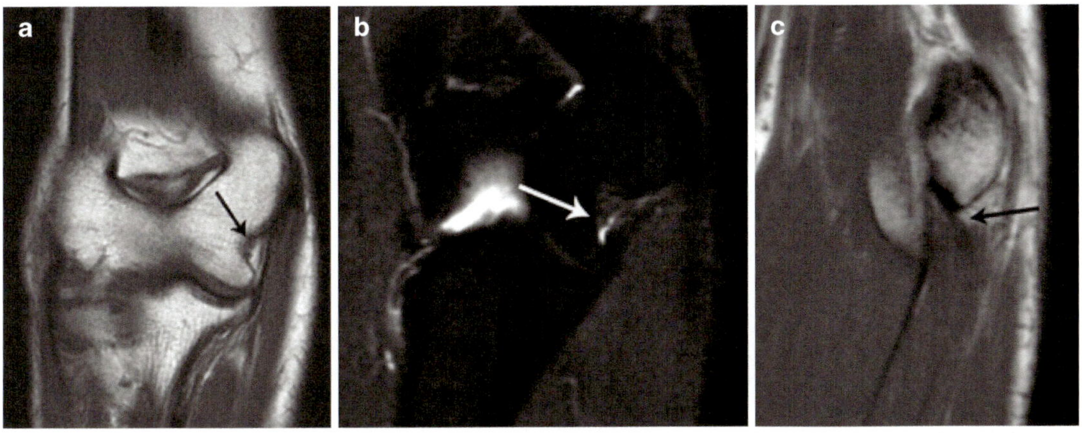

Fig. 10.4 (**a**) Coronal T1-weighted image shows high signal near the posterior origin of a normal anterior band. Fibrofatty changes can often be seen at the origin of the anterior band of the UCL (*arrow*) and should not be mistaken for a tear. (**b**) Coronal PDFS also shows increased signal at the posterior origin. (**c**) Sagittal T1-weighted image demonstrates an intact anterior band origin

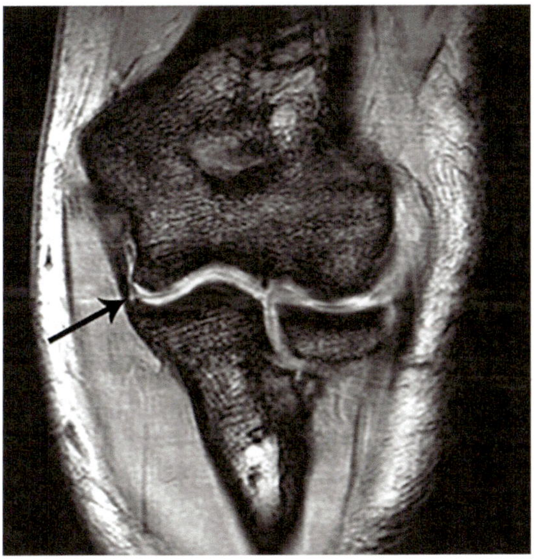

Fig. 10.5 The *arrow* points to the normal fissure of the sublime tubercle; the anterior band of the UCL is normal in its signal intensity, and there is no indication that the ligament is torn

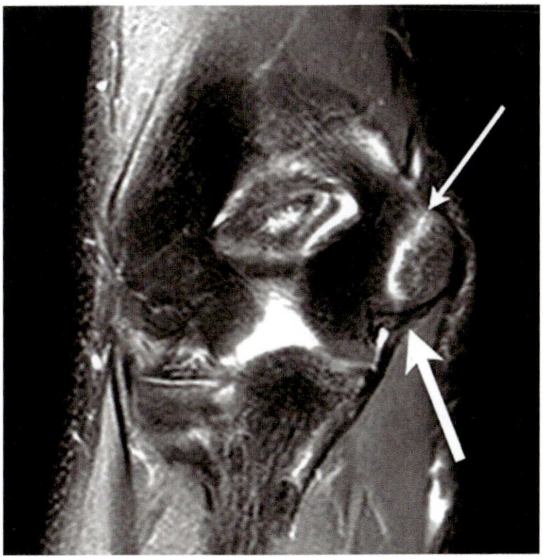

Fig. 10.6 In adolescents, the origin of the anterior band of the UCL (*large arrow*) commonly originates from the periosteum that bridges the physeal plate (*thin arrow*) of the medial epicondyle

during the late cocking and early acceleration phase of throwing.

Five stages of the pitching motion have been described: wind up, early cocking, late cocking, acceleration, and follow-through [11]. The late cocking and acceleration stages are those in which most UCL injuries occur as the greatest tensile stresses across the elbow develop during these specific stages. In the late cocking phase, the arm reaches maximal external rotation behind the trunk. The pitching arm can be in as much as 180° of external rotation. When the pitching arm has reached terminal external rotation, the acceleration phase begins. The arm internally rotates and extends at the elbow; the forearm pronates, the wrist flexes, and the fingers extend. A propul-

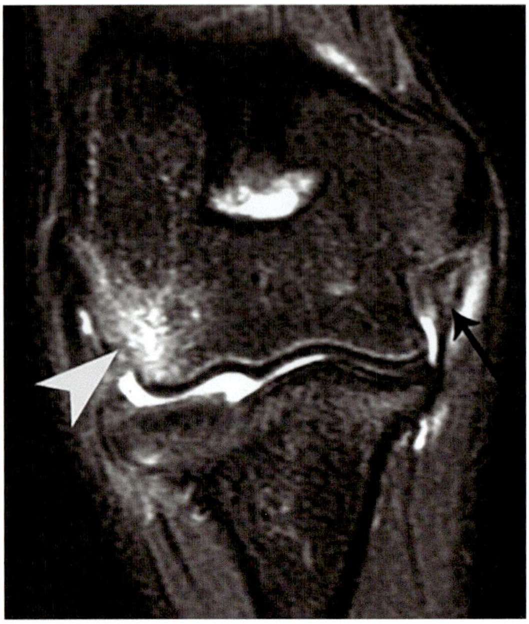

Fig. 10.7 Coronal STIR images demonstrate typical valgus injuries to the elbow. There is a proximal tear of the anterior band of the UCL (*arrow*) and microtrabecular bone injuries of the capitellum (*arrowhead*)

sive muscular force is transferred to the pitching hand and release of the ball. Ballistic stretching during the cocking phase preloads all involved muscles. Forces generated in the pitching motion are considerable and absorbed by muscles, tendons, bones, and ligaments. Repetitive pitching places tremendous demands upon the upper extremity they lead to cumulative trauma with at least 50% of baseball pitchers reporting injuries during their career [12, 13].

Overhead throwing subjects the elbow to tremendous valgus forces concentrated on the anterior bundle; a sudden valgus injury can lead to acute rupture of the ligament and typical capitellum microtrabecular bone injuries (Fig. 10.7). Patients may complain of a "pop" and medial elbow pain if this occurs. The majority of injuries to the UCL are the result of chronic overuse which leads to microtrauma and attenuation of the UCL. Acute injuries are the result of a sudden traumatic event. Patients with chronic injuries complain of insidious onset of pain, soreness, loss of control when pitching, and/or decrease in their ability to achieve high ball velocity when pitching. Complaints of ulnar neuritis, numbness, or paresthesia in the fourth and fifth digits are often reported in patients with UCL insufficiency; these patients may have symptoms of ulnar neuritis related to inflammation of the UCL with subsequent ulnar nerve compression or irritation [14].

The anterior band could be completely disrupted, yet valgus opening of the elbow may only occur to a very limited extent. Tensile stress on the medial aspect of the elbow produces compressive forces upon the radial head and capitellum; extension of the elbow during the acceleration phase causes the olecranon to forcefully make contact with the olecranon fossa and both of these actions may lead to osteophyte and loose body formation. This is most pronounced in the presence of valgus instability as a poorly aligned olecranon grates against the medial posterior aspect of the humerus in forced extension (Fig. 10.8) causing injury to the posteromedial articular cartilage and other signs of posterior impingement (Fig. 10.9). Occasionally, stress injuries of the olecranon (Fig. 10.10), or if there is continuous valgus stress, sublime tubercle avulsion injury (Fig. 10.11), or frank olecranon fracture (Fig. 10.12) may result.

Valgus forces produce distraction of the medial compartment, giving rise to tensile injuries of the UCL, flexor and pronator muscles, ulnar nerve, and medial epicondyle. Rupture of the UCL usually occurs in the flexed elbow under valgus stress. When a full-thickness tear of either the anterior or posterior band UCL occurs (Fig. 10.13), the disrupted ligament is often accompanied by extravasation of fluid or, if intra-articular contrast is injected, contrast material leaks into the surrounding soft tissues. Most tears occur in the midproximal or midsubstance fibers of the anterior bundle (Fig. 10.14) with distal anterior bundle UCL tears (Fig. 10.15) being less frequent. The injured ligament can demonstrate abnormal signal intensity, thickening and irregularity, ligamentous laxity, and poor definition [15]. Less frequently, avulsions occur proximally off the humerus or distally off the ulna. Rarely, an avulsion fracture of the sublime tubercle has been reported as a cause of UCL insufficiency.

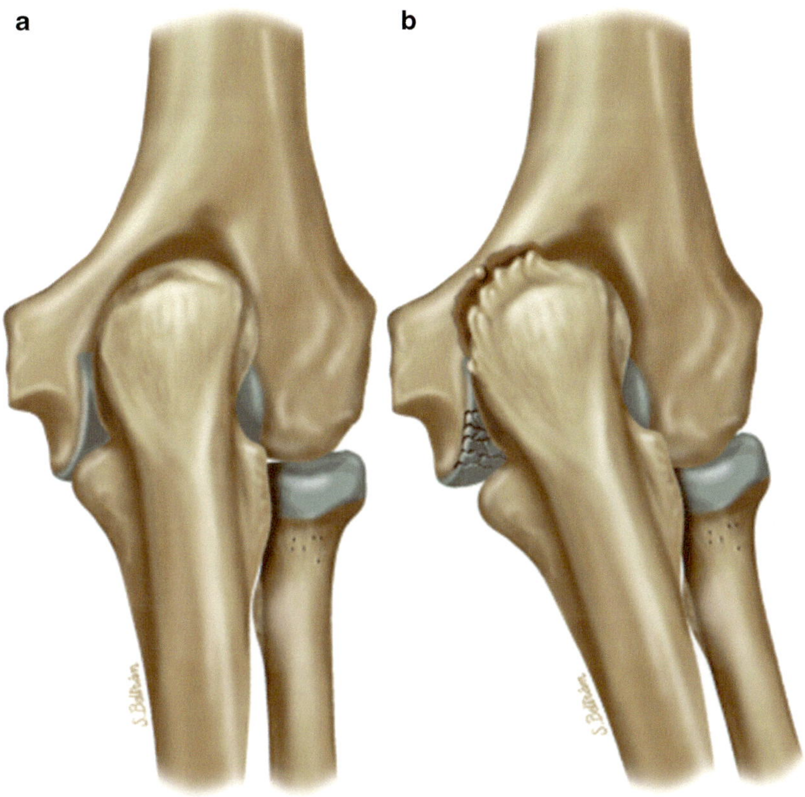

Fig. 10.8 Posterior valgus malalignment and impingement. (**a**) The ulna is centrally located in the posterior groove of the dorsal distal humerus in the normal elbow. (**b**) The medial olecranon grates against the dorsal medial humerus in valgus angulation injuring the articular cartilage and underlying bone resulting in osteophyte formation

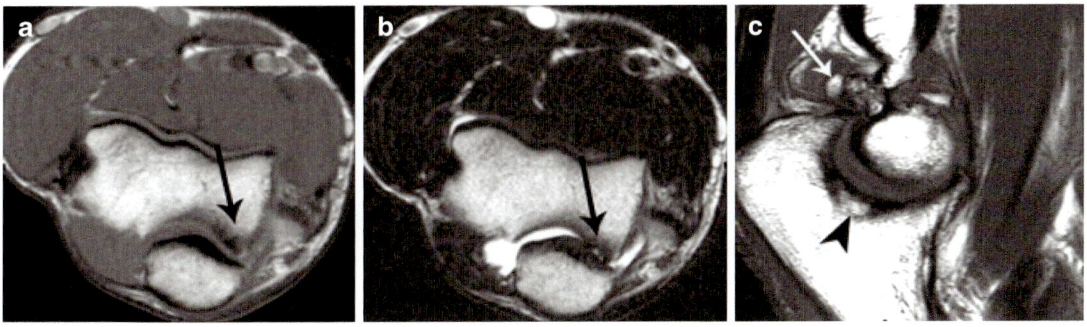

Fig. 10.9 (**a**) Axial T1- and (**b**) axial T2-weighted images show early articular cartilage injury and bone damage (*arrows*). Chronic extensive articular cartilage damage and osteophyte formation with posterior impingement and inability to fully extend the elbow. (**c**) Chronic extensive articular cartilage damage and osteophyte formation with posterior impingement and inability to fully extend the elbow (*white arrow* multiple loose bodies, *arrow head* degenerative osteophyte)

Partial-thickness tears are diagnosed when focal disruptions do not extend through the full thickness of the ligament and are best visualized if there is a fluid or contrast material adjacent to the ligament. A partial-thickness tear of the anterior bundle of the UCL that manifests at its insertion on the sublime tubercle with fluid or contrast extending medial to the sublime tubercle is described as the "T sign" [16] (Fig. 10.16). Lateral compartment bone contusions may be present in association with acute tears of the UCL. Overlying flexor tendon tears are also frequently seen. In chronic disease, the UCL may become significantly thickened with or without adjacent stress reaction within the sublime tubercle (Fig. 10.17). In the professional throwing athlete, single (Fig. 10.18a) or multiple ossicles may develop in the anterior band of the UCL or the anterior band itself may become almost entirely ossified (Fig. 10.18b, c).

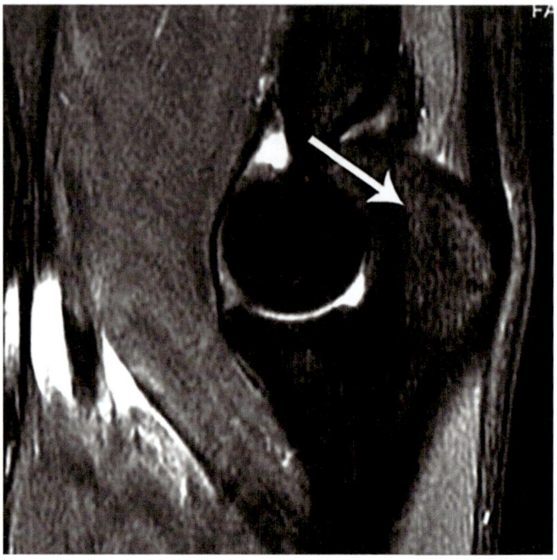

Fig. 10.10 Sagittal infrared (IR) image with stress injury of the ulna (*arrow*)

Injury to the UCL in the throwing athlete can be devastating because athletic performance is hindered due to pain and altered biomechanics. One looks for increased signal intensity within and adjacent to the ligament on MRI; this abnormal signal represents sprain, degeneration, hemorrhage, or edema due to microtears resulting from repetitive injury. Warning signs before UCL failure in pitchers include bone marrow edema in the medial epicondyle and sublime tubercle, loss of the fat pad with an intact anterior band of the UCL, bone marrow edema in the olecranon with intact triceps tendon and/or strains (edema) in the flexor, supinator, and brachialis muscles (Fig. 10.19).

MRI is the preferred imaging modality for evaluation of the soft-tissue structures of the elbow. Although contrast arthrography is commonly used to evaluate for UCL tears, it is not always necessary especially if the radiologist is experienced. Contrast MRI can potentially affect athlete performance for several days following intra-articular injection. In the setting of acute trauma magnetic resonance (MR),

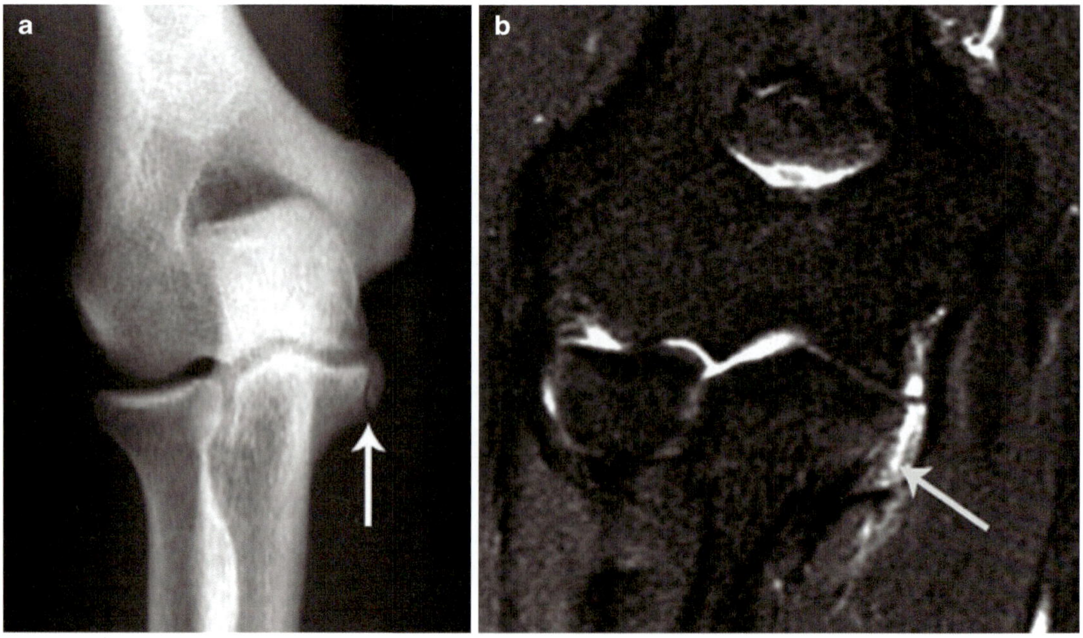

Fig. 10.11 Plain film (**a**) and coronal STIR (**b**) demonstrate avulsion injury of the sublime tubercle (*arrows*)

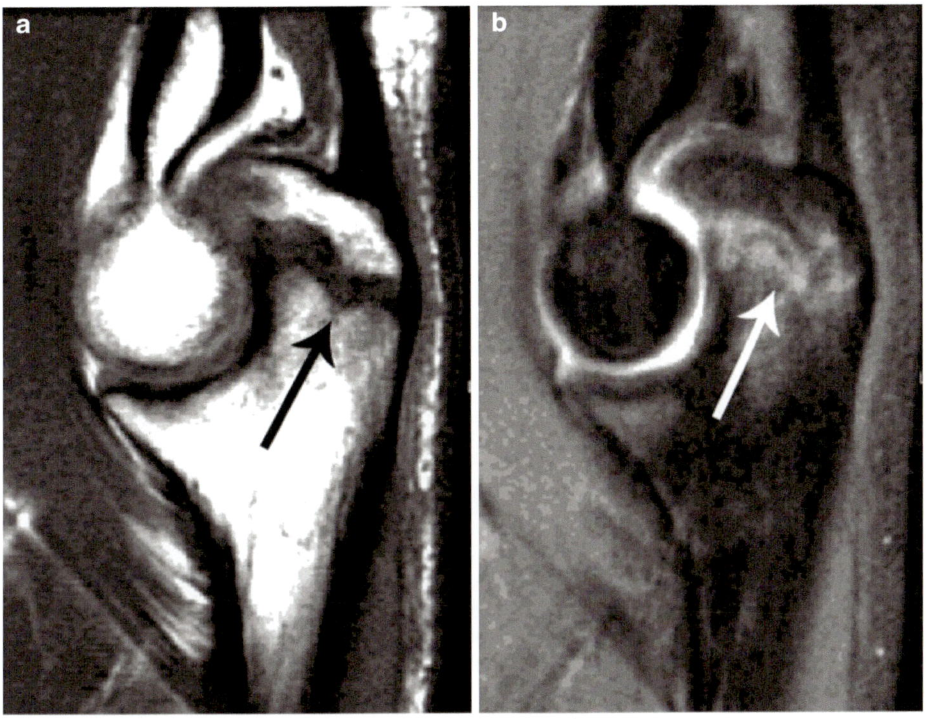

Fig. 10.12 Sagittal T1 (**a**) and STIR (**b**) images with noncomminuted fracture of the ulna (*arrows*)

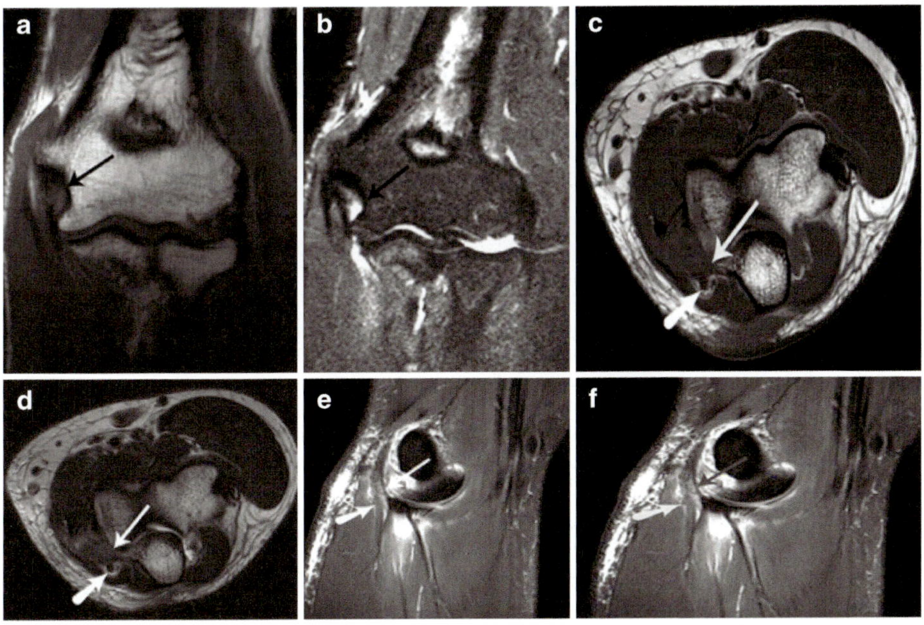

Fig. 10.13 Coronal T1-weighted (**a**) and coronal STIR (**b**) images demonstrate diffuse abnormal signal intensity adjacent to the anterior band of the UCL (*arrows*) with fluid extravasation at the sublime tubercle (*arrowhead*) related to a full-thickness tear of the anterior band. Axial T1-weighted (**c**) and axial T2-weighted (**d**) images demonstrating diffuse abnormal signal intensity within the posterior band of the UCL related to full-thickness tear of the posterior band (*straight arrows*) deep to the ulnar nerve (*rounded arrows*). Sagittal IR images (**e** and **f**) demonstrate the relationship of the course of the normal ulnar nerve (*rounded arrows*) and the torn posterior band (*straight arrows*)

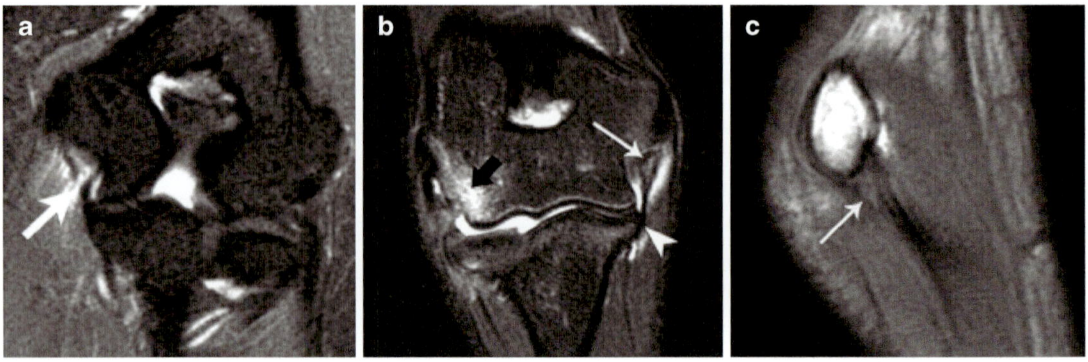

Fig. 10.14 STIR coronal (**a** and **b**) and STIR sagittal (**c**) images from different patients demonstrate discreet areas of high-signal intensity consistent with proximal to mid-substance tear of the anterior band of the UCL (**a**, **c** *white arrows*). (**b**) The *black* and the *white arrows* point to the valgus stress injury and the tear of the proximal UCL, respectively. The distal intact UCL is intact (*arrowhead*)

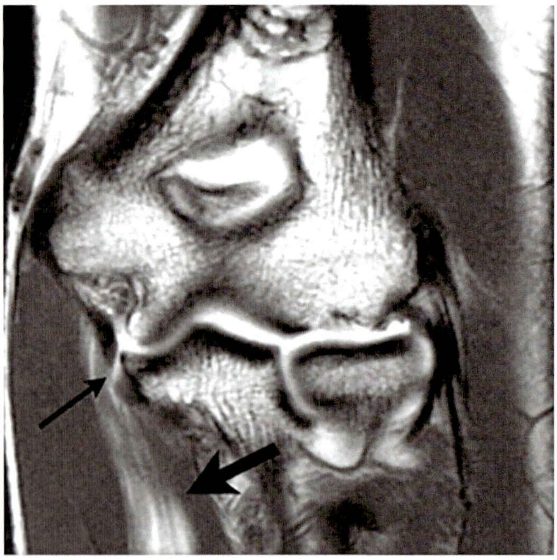

Fig. 10.15 T1 coronal MR arthrography. The *thin arrow* demonstrates a distal tear of the anterior band at its attachment to the sublime tubercle with extravasation of contrast into the surrounding soft tissues (*large arrow*)

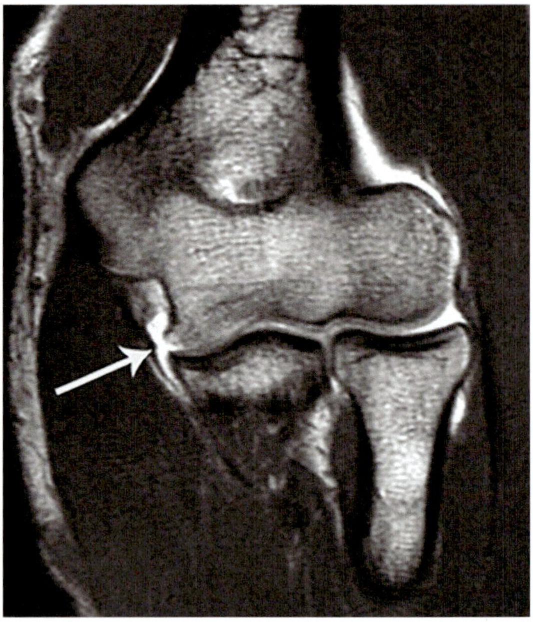

Fig. 10.16 Coronal IR image following elbow injury in a major baseball league pitcher. Partial-thickness tear of the anterior bundle of the UCL, described as the "T sign" (*arrow*), manifests at the insertion of the UCL onto the sublime tubercle. Following arthrography, contrast is seen extending medial to the sublime tubercle. The fluid takes the shape of a T as it tracks from the joint to the sublime tubercle

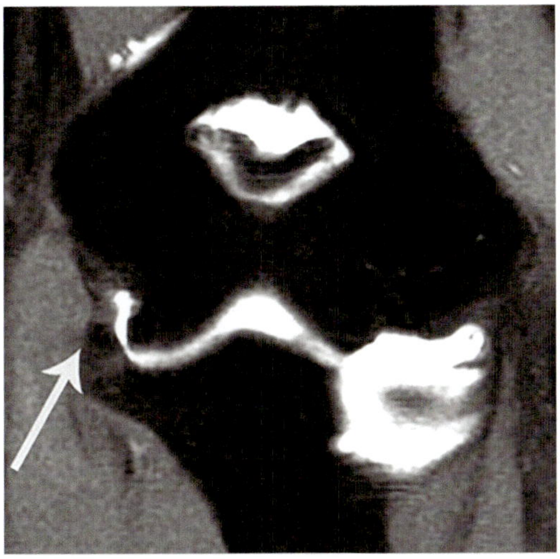

Fig. 10.17 Coronal T1-weighted image demonstrates marked thickening of the anterior band of the UCL seen in chronic injuries (*arrow*)

arthrography may help with the assessment of partial-thickness tears. Because the anterior band of the UCL is not well visualized arthroscopically, it must be carefully assessed on imaging.

More than half of adolescent pitching athletes experience elbow pain during a baseball season [17]. Adolescent injuries are more often associated with the relatively weak medial epicondyle apophyseal plate rather the UCL ligament injuries although chronic sprains may be seen (Fig. 10.20). The apophyseal plate is vulnerable to tensile forces related to contraction of the flexor–pronator muscles. Bone marrow edema and microtrabecular bone injuries of the sublime tubercle (Fig. 10.21), apophyseal widening and bone marrow edema of the medial epicondyle (Figs. 10.22 and

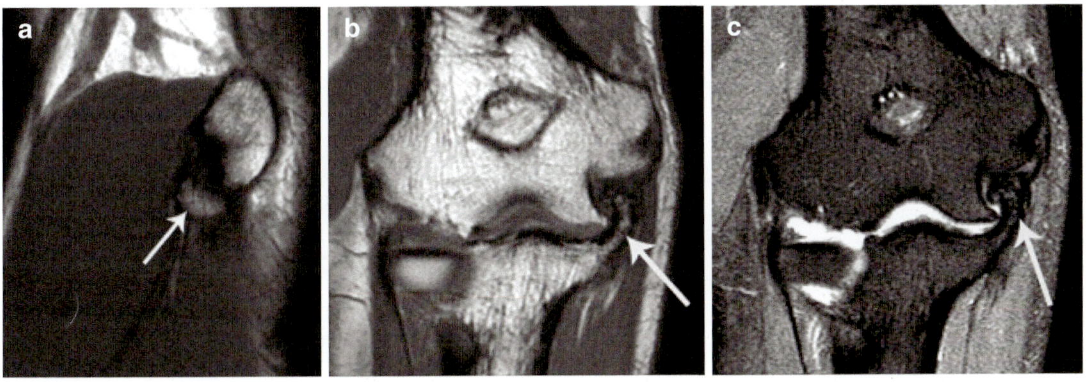

Fig. 10.18 Sagittal image demonstrates a single ossicle (*arrow*) in the anterior band of the UCL (**a**). Coronal T1-weighted (**b**) and coronal IR (**c**) images demonstrate diffuse, prominent thickening of the anterior band of the UCL which is partially ossified (*arrows*)

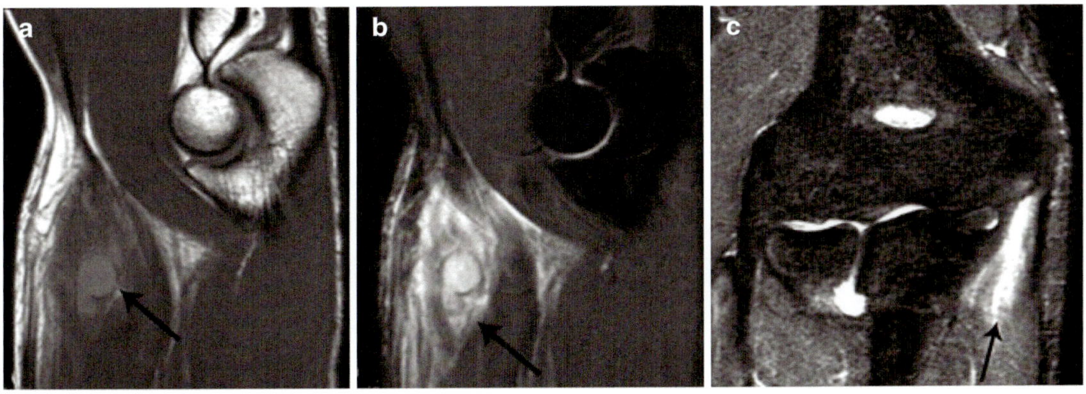

Fig. 10.19 Sagittal T1-weighted (**a**) and STIR (**b**) images demonstrate tears (*arrows*) of the proximal pronator teres muscle. Coronal STIE image (**c**) with tear of the flexor digitorum superficialis muscle (*arrow*). Axial T1 (**d**) and T2-weighted (**e**) images show strains of the triceps muscle

Fig. 10.19 (continued)

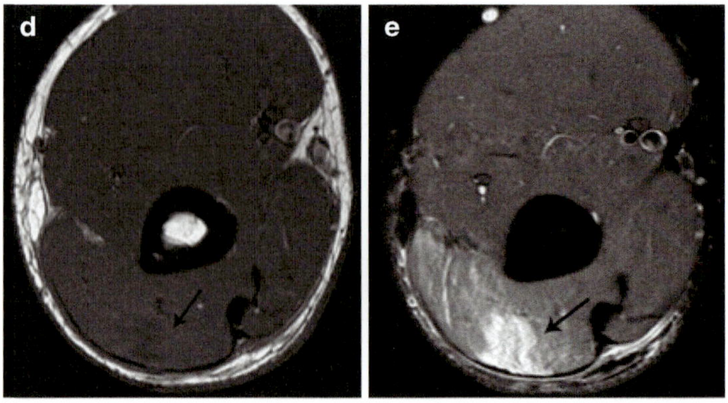

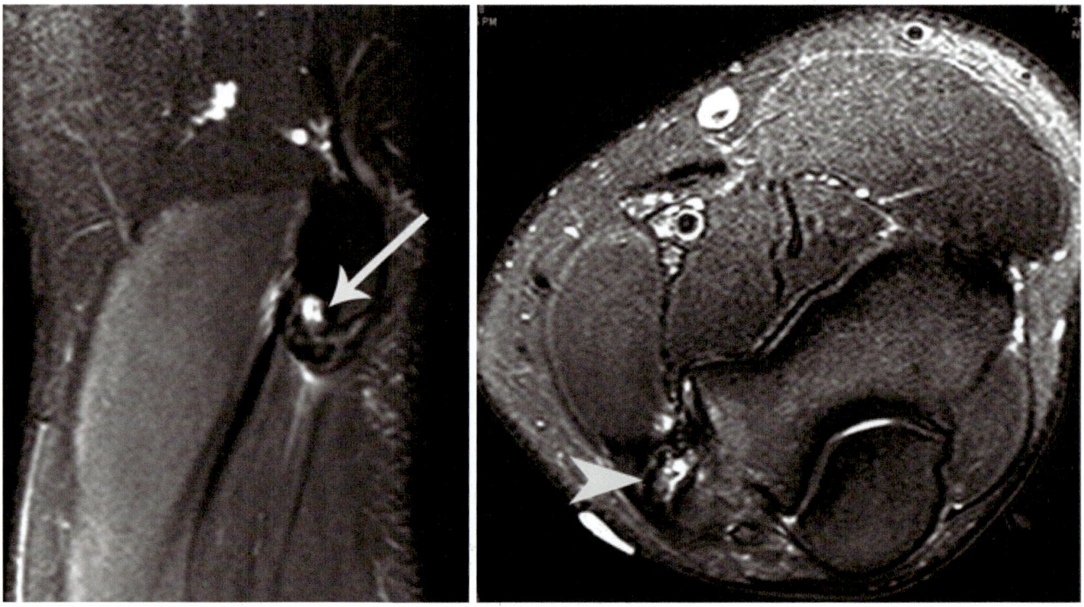

Fig. 10.20 Sagittal (*arrow*) and axial (*arrowhead*) images of a 16-year-old Little League pitcher elbow demonstrating a chronic sprain injury of the anterior band of the UCL

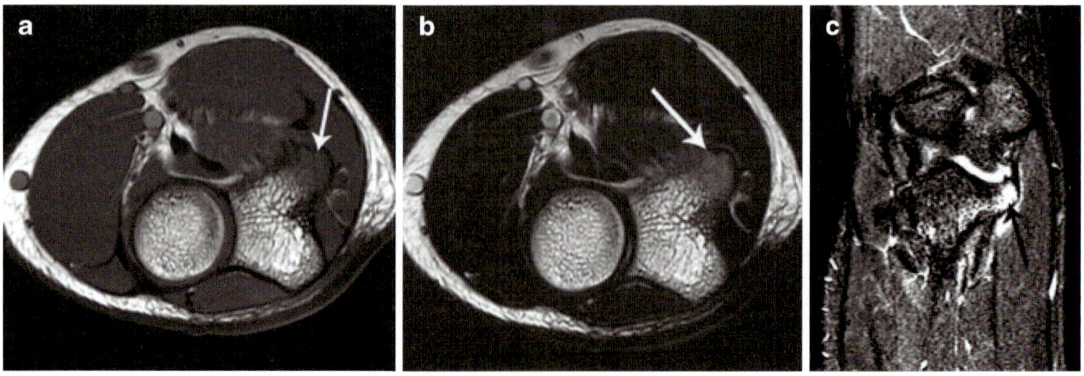

Fig. 10.21 Axial T1 (**a**) and axial T2 (**b**) images show early injury (*arrow*) to the sublime tubercle in a 14-year-old pitcher. Coronal IR image demonstrates (*arrow*) the intense bone marrow edema and microtrabecular bone injuries throughout the sublime tubercle; no UCL injuries or cortical fractures (**c**)

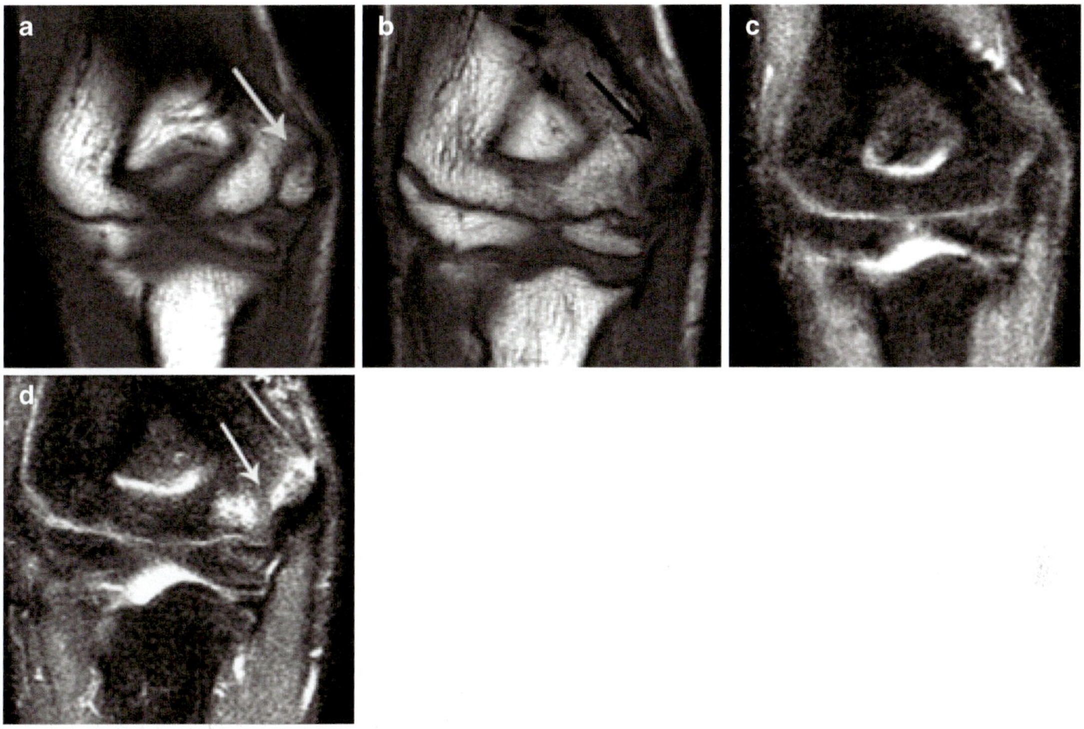

Fig. 10.22 (**a**) Coronal T1-weighted image of the asymptomatic elbow of a 15-year-old pitcher demonstrates normal signal intensity in the bone marrow (*arrow*) of the medial epiphysis. (**b**) The symptomatic elbow demonstrates abnormal signal consistent with edema and widening of the growth plate (*arrow*). (**c** and **d**) Abnormal STIR hyperintensity is seen in the symptomatic elbow (**c** normal, **d** symptomatic)

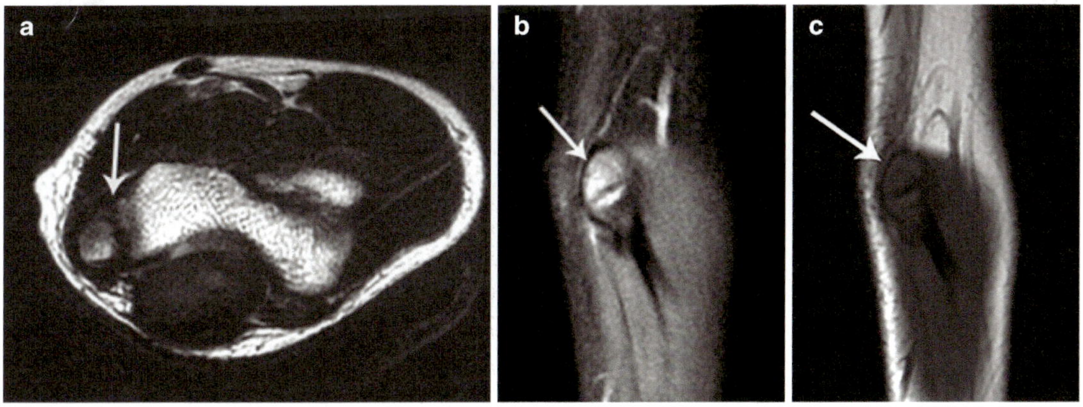

Fig. 10.23 A 9-year-old pitcher with sudden onset elbow pain. (**a**) Axial T1-weighted image shows irregularity and widening of the physis. (**b** and **c**) Sagittal images demonstrate intense edema within the medial epiphysis without cortical fracture. The UCL is intact

10.23) and/or fragmentation, epiphyseal hypertrophy and/or fragmentation or acute apophyseal avulsion (Fig. 10.24), that is, Salter-Harris I fracture, may occur, that is, "Little Leaguer's elbow" [18].

Following a "Tommy John" [19] procedure, postoperative MRI imaging is used to evaluate UCL graft integrity (Fig. 10.25).

Graft tears appear as high-signal intensity in the disrupted graft, similar to the native ligament

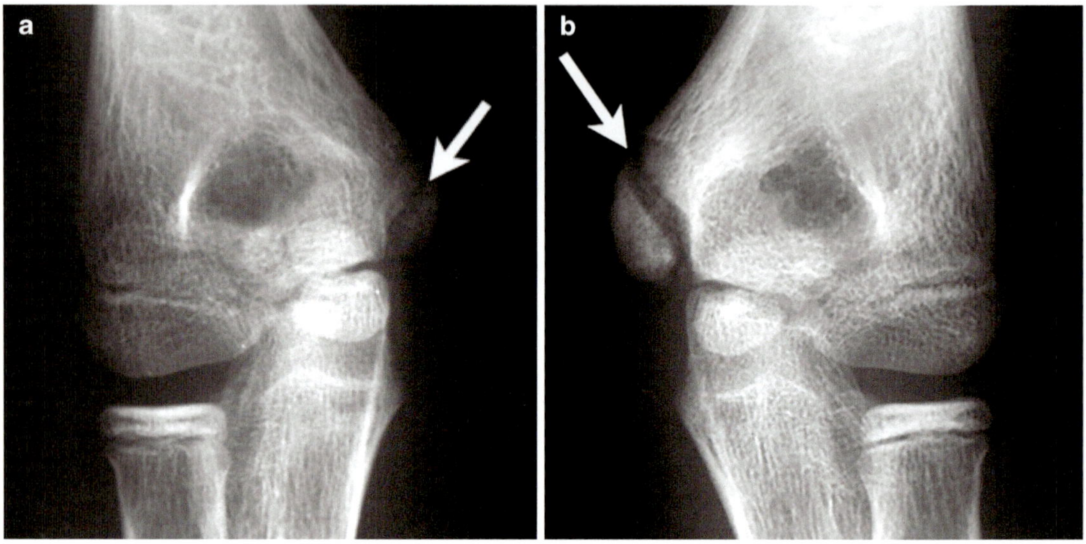

Fig. 10.24 (**a**) A 15-year-old pitcher with elbow pain. In the nonsymptomatic elbow, the medial growth plate is normal (*arrow*). (**b**) In the symptomatic elbow, apophyseal widening is evident (*arrow*)

Fig. 10.25 Major League baseball pitcher underwent a "Tommy John" procedure. Notice the tunnel in the medial epicondyle (*open arrow*) and the tunnel in the sublime tubercle (*closed arrow*) with low-intensity graft in between the two bony tunnels and loss of fat (*circle*) medial to the intact graft

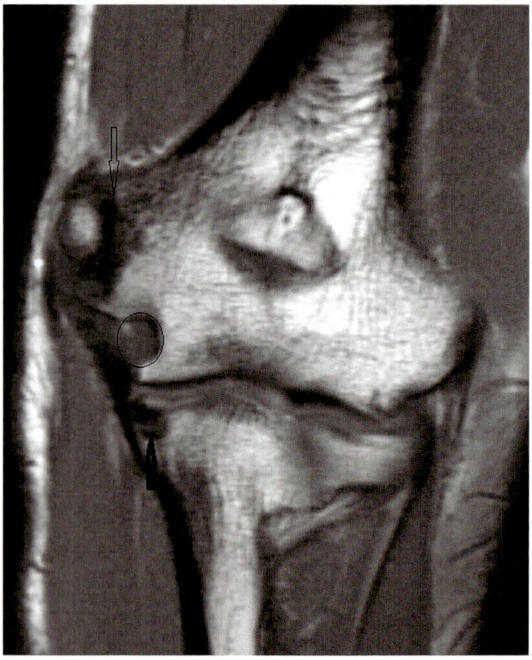

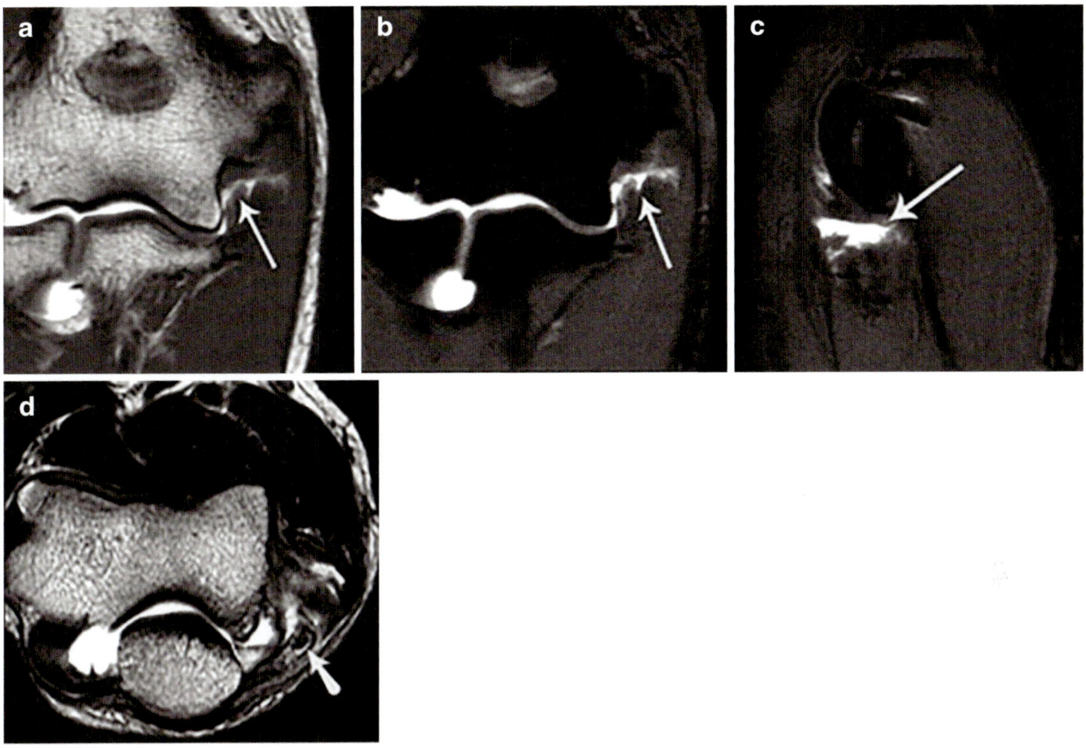

Fig. 10.26 Torn "Tommy John" graft in professional major league pitcher. Postarthrogram. Coronal axial T1 weighted (**a**). Coronal STIR (**b**) and sagittal STIR (**c**) images demonstrate distal graft tear with contrast extravasation through the tear (*arrows*). The position of the ulnar nerve (*rounded arrow*) lies in its normal relationship to the graft, that is, no ulnar nerve translocation (**d**)

(Fig. 10.26). Evaluation of the ulnar nerve is important in those patients who have undergone translocation of the nerve.

Summary

The UCL of the elbow, in particular, its anterior band, is the primary stabilizer to valgus stress at the elbow. Partial or full-thickness tears of the anterior band are commonly seen in throwing athletes, especially professional and amateur baseball pitchers, who by placing repetitive valgus stress injuries on the elbow during the late cocking and early acceleration phases of throwing frequently injure the UCL. Accurate interpretation of elbow imaging in these athletes requires intimate and detailed knowledge of the anatomy of the normal UCL and the spectrum of injuries to which it is subjected.

References

1. Johnston J, Plancher KD, Hawkins RJ. Elbow injuries to the throwing athlete. Clin Sports Med. 1996;15:307–29.
2. Fuss FK. The ulnar collateral ligament of the human elbow joint. Anatomy, function and biomechanics. J Anat. 1991;175:203–12.
3. Munshi M, Pretterklieber ML, Chung CB, Haghighi P, Cho J, Trudell DJ, Resnick D. Anterior bundle of ulnar collateral ligament: evaluation of anatomic relationships by using MR imaging, MR arthrography, and gross anatomic and histologic analysis. Radiology. 2004;231:797–803.
4. Sugimoto H, Ohsawa T. Ulnar collateral ligament in the growing elbow: MR imaging of normal development and throwing injuries. Radiology. 1994;192:417–22.
5. Morrey BF, An K. Functional anatomy of the ligaments of the elbow. Clin Orthop. 1985;201:84–90.
6. Regan WD, Korinek SL, Morrey BF, An K. Biomechanical study of ligaments around the elbow joint. Clin Orthop Relat Res. 1991;271:170–9.

7. Hotchkiss RN, Weiland AJ. Valgus stability of the elbow. J Orthop Res. 1987;5:372–7.
8. Sojbjerg JO, Oveson J, Nielson S. Experimental elbow instability after transection of the medial collateral ligament. Clin Orthop. 1987;218:186–90.
9. Fleisig GS, Andrews JR, Dillman CJ, Escamilla RF. Kinetics of baseball pitching with implications about injury mechanisms. Am J Sports Med. 1995;23:233–9.
10. Werner SL, Fleisig GS, Dillman CJ, Andrews JR. Biomechanics of the elbow during baseball pitching. J Orthop Sports Phys Ther. 1993;17:274–8.
11. Perry AM, Zawacki RM, Sullivan TJ. Biomechanics of throwing. In: Nicholas JA, Hershman EB, editors. The upper extremity in sports medicine. St Louis: C. V. Mosby Co.; 1990.
12. Posner M, Cameron KL, Wolf JM, Belmont PJ, Owens BD. Epidemiology of major league baseball injuries. Am J Sports Med. 2011;39:1676–80.
13. Langer P, Fadale P, Hulstyn M. Evolution of the treatment options of ulnar collateral ligament injuries of the elbow. Br J Sports Med. 2006;40:499–506.
14. Conway JE, Jobe FW, Glousman RE, Pink M. Medial instability of the elbow in throwing athletes. Treatment by repair or reconstruction of the ulnar collateral ligament. J Bone Joint Surg Am. 1992;76:67–83.
15. Mirowitz SA, London SL. Ulnar collateral ligament injury in baseball pitchers: MR imaging evaluation. Radiology. 1992;185:573–6.
16. Lin DJ, Kazam JK, Ahmed FS, Wong TT. Ulnar collateral ligament insertional injuries in pediatric overhead athletes: are MRI findings predictive of symptoms or need for surgery? AJR. 2019;212(4):867–73.
17. Lyman S, Fleisig GS, Andrews JR, Osinski ED. Effect of pitch type, pitch count and pitching mechanisms on risk of elbow and shoulder pain in youth baseball pitchers. Am J Sports Med. 2002;30:463–8.
18. Hang DW, Chao CM, Hang YS. A clinical and roentgenographic study of Little League elbow. Am J Sports Med. 2004;32:79–84.
19. Wear SA, Thornton DD, Schwartz ML, Weissmann RC, Cain EL, Andrews JR. MRI of the reconstructed ulnar collateral ligament. AJR. 2011;197(5):373–7.

MR Imaging in Patients with Ulnar Collateral Ligament Injury

11

Christin A. Tiegs-Heiden, Naveen S. Murthy, Brett Lurie, Jan Fritz, and Hollis G. Potter

Introduction

The ulnar collateral ligament (UCL), also referred to as the medial collateral ligament (MCL) of the elbow, may be injured acutely in the setting of a valgus load to the elbow or as a result of dislocation [1, 2]. In the athlete, the ligament may be chronically stressed by the high valgus loads that are repetitively imparted to the medial side of the elbow during the late cocking phase of throwing. Diagnosing UCL injury in the patient with medial elbow pain can be challenging both clinically and arthroscopically, highlighting the need for accurate diagnostic imaging [3, 4]. MRI offers unparalleled soft-tissue contrast resolution, direct multiplanar imaging capabilities, and high-spatial resolution, allowing for reproducible, accurate, preoperative diagnosis of UCL abnormalities. MRI is also useful postoperatively to assess the integrity of ligament reconstruction and to diagnose potential re-injury.

C. A. Tiegs-Heiden · N. S. Murthy (✉)
Department of Radiology, Mayo Clinic, Rochester, MN, USA
e-mail: Murthy.naveen@mayo.edu

B. Lurie · J. Fritz · H. G. Potter
Radiology and Imaging, MRI Division, Hospital for Special Surgery, New York, NY, USA

Technique

MRI of the elbow should be performed at field strengths of 1.5 T or higher, with 3.0 T being preferred. The elbow is typically imaged either in the "superman" position or with the patient in the supine position with the elbow extended at the side and the forearm supinated. Imaging in this position tensions the anterior bundle of the MCL, allowing for more accurate assessment of ligament integrity. If clinically indicated, the posterior bundle of the UCL can be assessed with the elbow in flexion. A phased array surface coil is used to obtain the best possible signal-to-noise ratio [5, 6]. A circumferential coil is necessary to obtain sufficient signal from the posterior elbow structures [7].

The multiplanar capabilities of MRI are extremely valuable for obtaining true sagittal and true coronal images of the obliquely oriented elbow joint [8]. We recommend obtaining three planes of T1 or PD and fluid-sensitive sequences, with a minimum of one T1-weighted sequence. Cartilage and fluid-sensitive pulse sequences are essential for adequate evaluation of all patients. If the elbow is imaged at the patient's side, inversion recovery sequences are recommended over frequency-selective fat-suppressed sequences due to the magnetic field inhomogeneities encountered away from the isocenter of the bore [7].

High-resolution (512 × 320 matrix, 1.5–2.5 mm slice thickness) intermediate echo time fast spin

J. S. Dines et al. (eds.), *Elbow Ulnar Collateral Ligament Injury*,
https://doi.org/10.1007/978-3-030-69567-5_11

echo (FSE) imaging performed in the coronal plane is used to assess the signal intensity of ligaments and tendons as well as regional cartilage status. A high-spatial resolution (512 × 224 matrix, 1.7-mm slice thickness) small field of view gradient recalled echo (GRE) pulse sequence in the coronal plane yields an in-plane resolution of 300 microns, thus diminishing partial volume and signal averaging, and is useful for assessment of ligament and tendon morphology. Axial and sagittal high-resolution (sagittal 512 × 320 matrix) FSE images with intermediate echo time and slightly increased slice thickness (3.5 mm) are obtained as well to aid in the assessment of the remainder of the elbow structures. Fat-suppressed GRE sequences, which are sensitive to the cartilage of unfused physes, are added for the characterization of growth plates of skeletally immature patients.

Some authors advocate the use of magnetic resonance (MR) arthrography using an intra-articular injection of a gadolinium-based contrast agent or intra-articular saline to aid in the detection of partial tears of the UCL [3, 9]. Distension of the joint capsule with fluid may improve visualization of structures which are normally closely opposed [10]. At the authors' institutions, elbow imaging is performed without the use of intra-articular contrast, preserving MRI as a noninvasive, painless, time efficient, and cost-effective examination. Close attention to high-spatial resolution, noncontrast MRI technique obviates the need for intra-articular contrast [8, 11]. We believe that noncontrast MRI is superior to arthrography for assessment of cartilage, taking advantage of the inherent magnetization transfer contrast provided by intermediate echo time FSE, and that synovitis and patterns of synovial proliferation are better assessed without the confounding factor of a joint distended with contrast material.

Imaging Anatomy

The UCL is a cord-like structure, which averages 27 mm in length and 4–5 mm in width [12]. The three components of the UCL are the anterior bundle, posterior bundle, and transverse bundle [13]. The anterior bundle is further divided into biomechanically distinct anterior and posterior bands, which are taut at different degrees of flexion and extension and serve as the primary restraint to valgus stress [14–16]. The anterior bundle originates on the undersurface of the medial epicondyle and inserts on the ulna at or within 1–2 mm of the anteromedial facet of the coronoid process, the sublime tubercle [17]. The posterior bundle forms the floor of the cubital tunnel and is more of a thickening of the posterior capsule than a distinct ligament [13]. The transverse bundle runs between the tip of the olecranon and the coronoid process and does not contribute significantly to elbow stability. Neither the posterior nor the transverse bundles are routinely assessed on standard MR imaging with the elbow in extension.

Normal Appearance of the UCL

The UCL is best assessed on coronal images using the GRE and FSE sequences to assess morphology and the STIR and FSE sequences to assess signal intensity.

The intact UCL is thin, vertically oriented, and uniformly low-signal intensity reflecting its composition of highly organized type I collagen (Fig. 11.1; [18]). A normal infolding of synovium may be identified deep to the humeral origin of the posterior band of the anterior bundle, which should not be misinterpreted as a tear [1, 3, 4]. Interdigitation of fat can also be seen at the origin of the posterior band of the anterior bundle, resulting in a slightly striated appearance to the ligament in some patients [17, 19]. The humeral origin of the anterior bundle is fairly broad, with convergence of the ligament as it approaches its insertion on the ulna, where the ligament is continuous with the ulnar periosteum [6, 17, 20]. The deep muscle fibers of the flexor digitorum superficialis are closely apposed to the outer surface of the UCL.

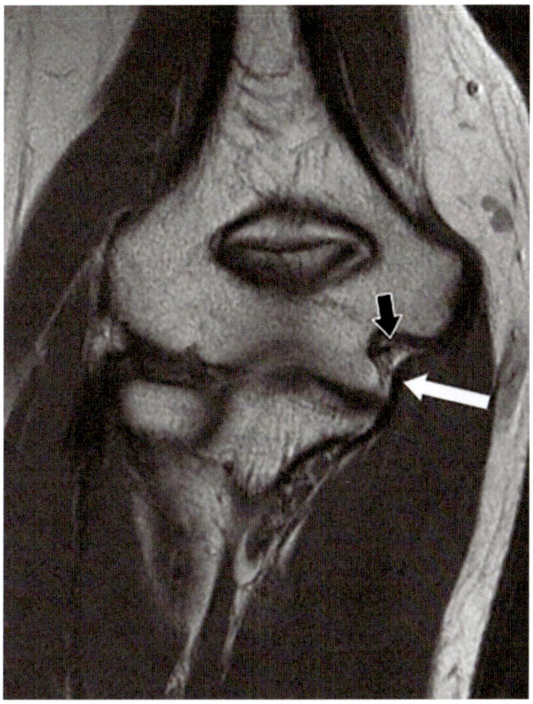

Fig. 11.1 Coronal intermediate echo time FSE MR image of a normal thin, vertically oriented and hypointense UCL (*white arrow*). Note the normal infolding of synovium and fat deep to the ligament (*black arrow*)

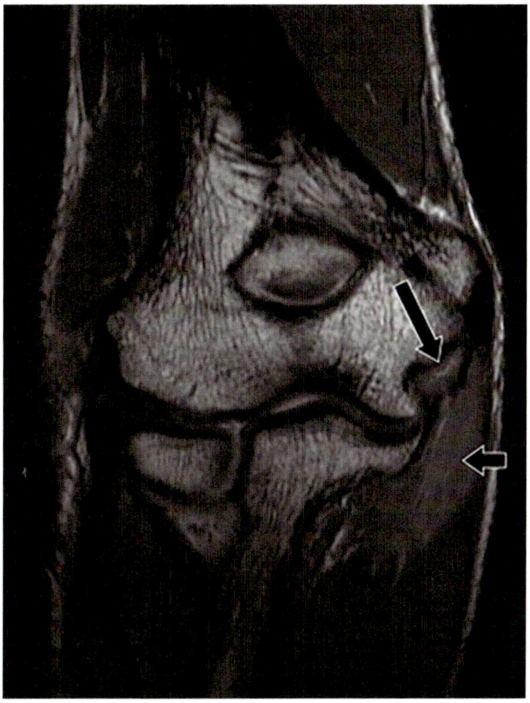

Fig. 11.2 Coronal FSE MR image demonstrating acute on chronic injury to the UCL. The *long black arrow* indicates a complete tear of the thickened posterior band of the anterior bundle. Adjacent soft-tissue edema is noted within the flexor pronator muscles (*short arrow*)

MR Findings in UCL Injury

Acute Injury

Acute injuries to the UCL are seen as areas of altered signal intensity, altered morphology, or indistinctness of the normally hypointense, vertically oriented ligament [1, 4]. There may be a discontinuity of some or all of the fibers of the UCL with or without retraction (Fig. 11.2; [6]). Adjacent soft-tissue edema as well as injury to the flexor pronator origin may serve as additional evidence of an acute injury (Fig. 11.3).

Tears of the UCL are most commonly at the humeral origin of the ligament, while midsubstance and distal tears are less common (Fig. 11.4; [5]). Avulsion fractures of the sublime tubercle or of traction osteophytes may also be seen (Fig. 11.5; [11]).

Partial thickness tears of the UCL are further classified as high-grade partial or low-grade partial, which are differentiated based on the involvement of more or less than 50% of the ligament thickness, respectively (Fig. 11.6; [21]). A focal defect in the ligament may be seen, but more commonly, partial thickness tears are diagnosed on the basis of ligament indistinctness and hyperintensity. Fluid imbibition can help to delineate an acute tear, but the absence of this sign does not exclude injury to the ligament (Fig. 11.7).

The "T-sign" describes the appearance of fluid extending distally between the ulna and the UCL due to stripping of deep fibers of the ligament off the sublime tubercle (Fig. 11.8; [3]). While originally described with computed tomography (CT) and MR arthrography, a T-sign can be observed in nonarthrographic MRI provided that close attention is paid to MR technique. It is commonly held that nonarthrographic MRI has a relatively low sensitivity for the detection of partial thickness tears, somewhere in the order of 57% [3]. The use of high-resolution, fluid-sensitive inter-

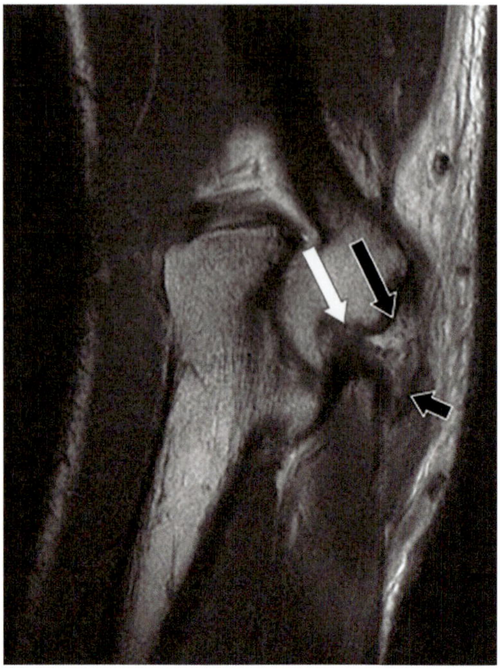

Fig. 11.3 Coronal FSE image shows an acute complete tear of the flexor pronator origin (*long black arrow*) with retraction (*short black arrow*). The UCL ligament appears high signal and slightly ill-defined reflecting concomitant low-grade injury to the UCL (*white arrow*)

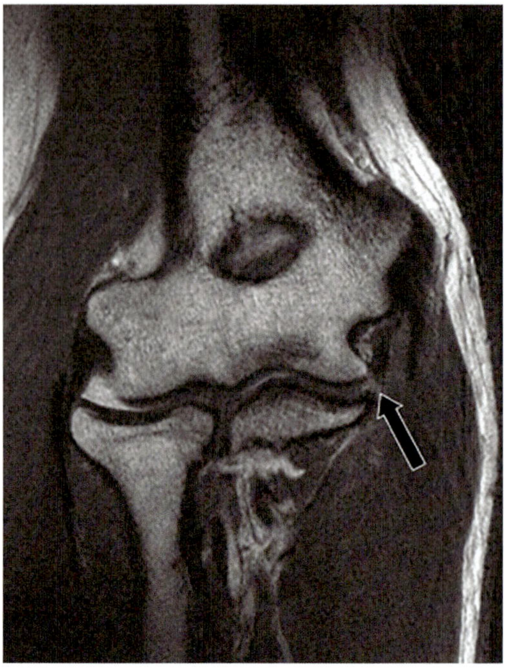

Fig. 11.4 Coronal FSE MR image shows a complete tear of the anterior band of the anterior bundle of the UCL off its ulnar insertion (*arrow*)

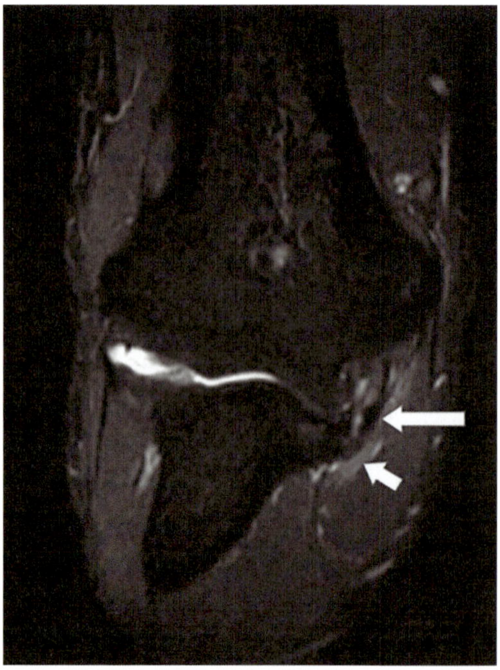

Fig. 11.5 Coronal STIR image shows an avulsion fracture of an osteophyte arising off the ulna (*long arrow*). Adjacent soft-tissue edema is indicated by the *short arrow*

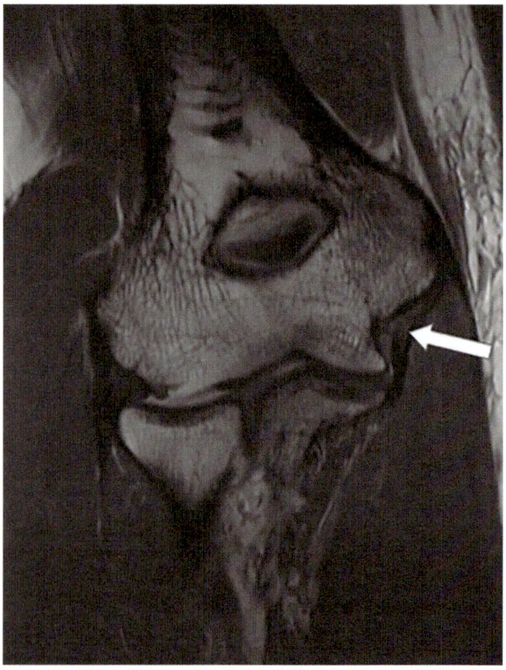

Fig. 11.6 Coronal FSE MR image demonstrating intrasubstance high signal (*arrow*) indicative of a low-grade interstitial partial tear at the humeral origin of the posterior band of the anterior bundle of the UCL

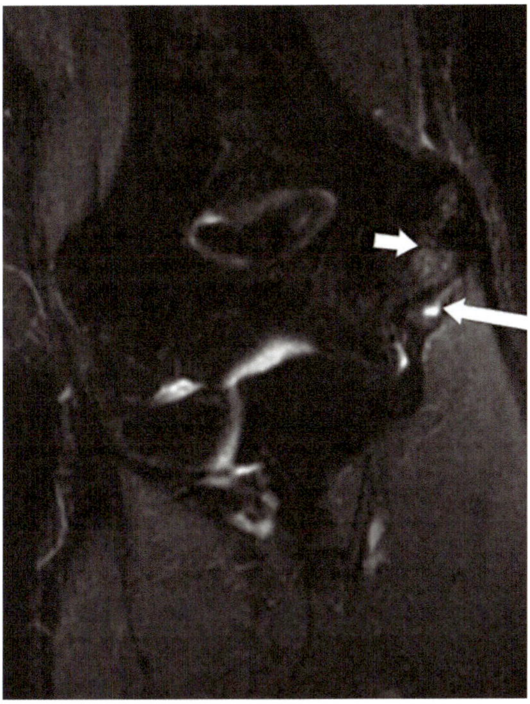

Fig. 11.7 Coronal STIR image shows a high-grade partial tear of the posterior band of the anterior bundle of the UCL (*long arrow*). A reactive marrow edema pattern is seen within the medial epicondyle reflecting a stress reaction (*short arrow*)

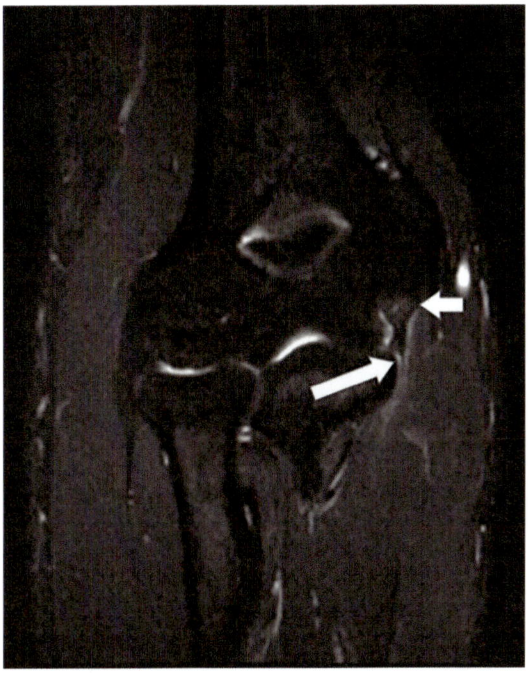

Fig. 11.8 Coronal STIR MR image shows fluid between the UCL and the sublime tubercle (*T-sign*) indicating avulsion of deep fibers of the UCL off the ulna in the setting of an undersurface partial tear (*long arrow*). The *short arrow* shows edema at the humeral origin of the chronically thickened UCL

mediate echo time FSE sequences allows for the diagnosis of partial tears with much higher sensitivity than is typically quoted in the literature for nonarthrographic studies [6, 11].

The term interstitial load can be applied to ligaments that appear stretched, mildly attenuated, and diffusely hyperintense reflecting the presence of interstitial microtears caused by an acute distracting force, without a well-defined partial thickness tear (Fig. 11.9).

MRI-based classification systems for UCL injuries have been proposed. A 6-stage classification system was described by Ramkumar et al. based on the location (proximal, midsubstance, or distal) and degree of tear (partial or complete) [22]. This system demonstrated very good reliability and may aid in decision-making as complete and distal tears are more likely to require operative management [22, 23].

Chronic Injury

Ligaments subject to chronic repetitive stress may remodel resulting in asymmetric ligament thickening and altered signal intensity, even in the asymptomatic patient (Fig. 11.10; [5, 24]). The chronically stressed UCL may demonstrate plastic deformation appearing lax, redundant, or indistinct [8, 12]. Associated mild ligament hyperintensity has been attributed to the presence of chronic microtears leading to intraligamentous hemorrhage and edema [25]. Foci of intraligamentous calcification or heterotopic ossification may also be identified in the chronically overloaded and repetitively injured UCL (Fig. 11.11).

Osseous stress reactions are also commonly seen and may manifest as a focal bone marrow edema pattern, either at the humerus or at the coronoid process. Chronic valgus stress may also

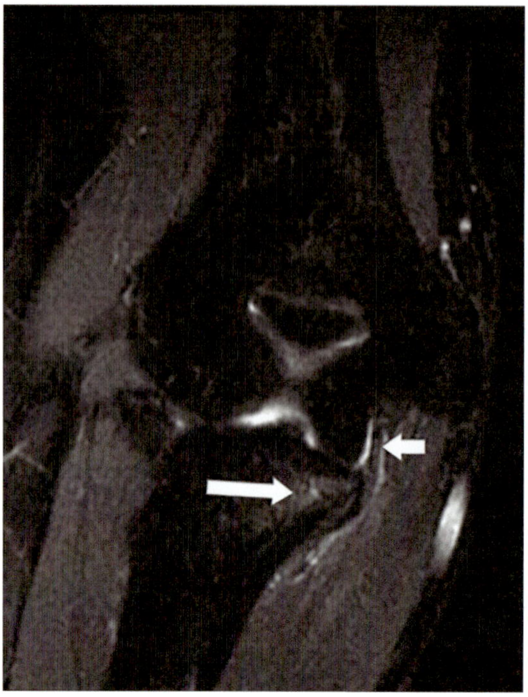

Fig. 11.9 Coronal STIR MR image demonstrates diffuse hyperintensity of the posterior band of the anterior bundle of the UCL without focal discontinuity (*short arrow*) indicating the effects of an acute interstitial load. A focal bone marrow edema pattern is seen at the ulna reflecting a mild stress reaction (*long arrow*)

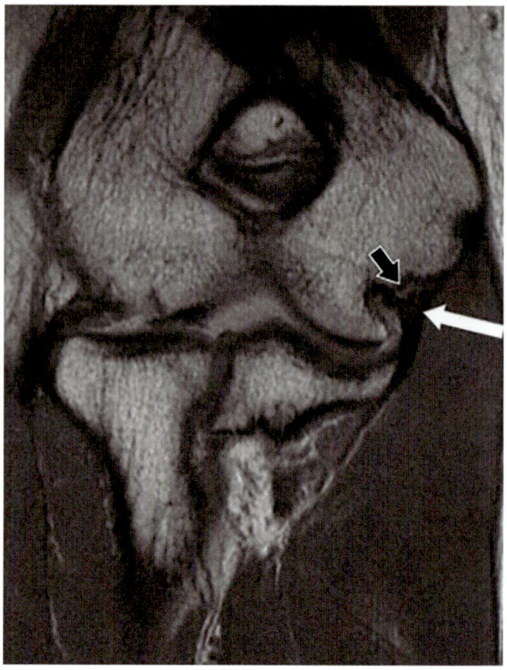

Fig. 11.10 Coronal FSE MR image of a chronically remodeled UCL ligament in a pitcher (*white arrow*). The ligament is thicker than usual but is still uniformly hypointense. A small traction spur is noted arising off the slightly bulbous medial epicondyle (*black arrow*)

result in osseous remodeling on the medial side of the elbow resulting in traction osteophytes, which may be subject to fracture or avulsion in the setting of acute on chronic injury.

Associated Elbow Findings in Chronic Valgus Overload

Chronic valgus overload to the elbow results in attritional attenuation of the UCL leading to laxity and eventual ligament failure [25]. Prior to ligament failure, the chronically stressed elbow will develop osteoarthritic changes as a result of excessive posteromedial joint contact. Subchondral sclerosis may be observed over the posteromedial aspect of the ulna and the corresponding posterior aspect of the trochlea, reflecting the presence of subchondral bony remodeling (Fig. 11.12). Another early sign of posteromedial impingement is prominent synovitis within the

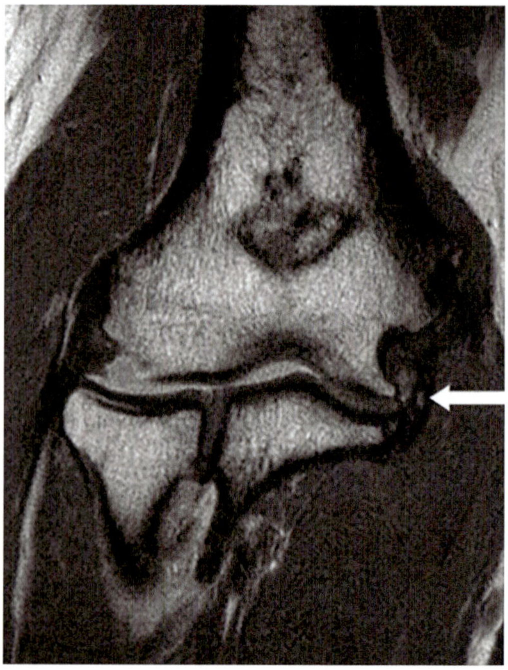

Fig. 11.11 Coronal FSE MR image demonstrates a focus of intraligamentous ossification in a chronically injured UCL (*arrow*)

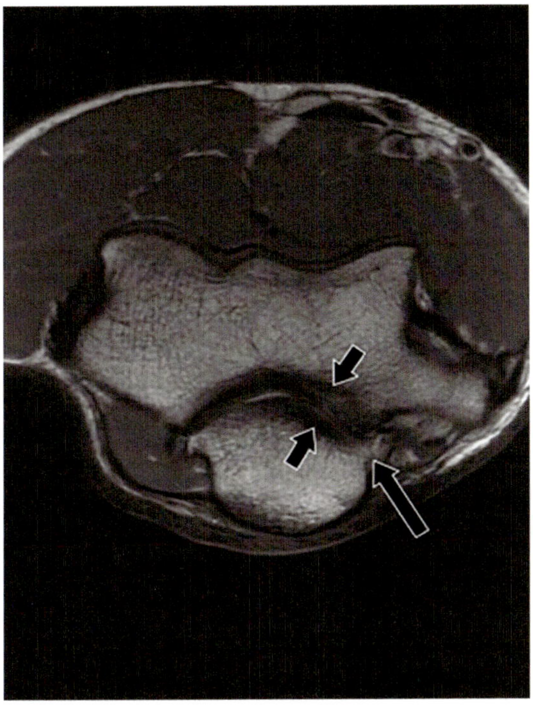

Fig. 11.12 Axial FSE MR image demonstrating features of posteromedial impingement in the setting of chronic valgus extension overload. The *short arrows* indicate subchondral sclerosis, chronic bony remodeling, and partial cartilage wear in the posteromedial humeroulnar compartment. The *long arrow* shows a developing osteophyte off the medial aspect of the olecranon process

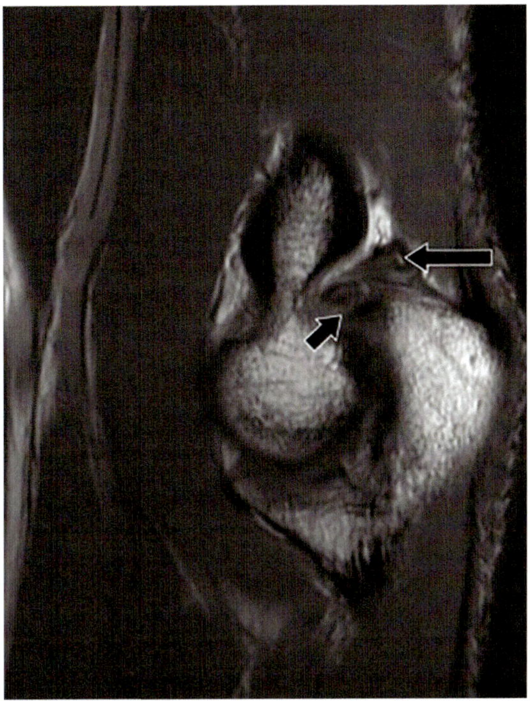

Fig. 11.13 Sagittal FSE MR image shows additional findings of posteromedial impingement with marked synovial scarring at the posteromedial aspect of the elbow joint surrounding a loose body (*long arrow*). The *short arrow* indicates a chronic fracture through an olecranon osteophyte

posteromedial joint capsule, which is most easily appreciated on sagittal and axial FSE images (Fig. 11.13). As posteromedial impingement continues, chondral thinning may be observed at the posteromedial ulnohumeral articulation, leading to the development of osteophytes usually on the olecranon [24]. In chronic posteromedial impingement, there may also be intra-articular loose bodies due to chondral injury. Fractured osteophytes are also commonly seen and can be visualized on the far posterior images of the coronal series or on axial images. A lateral radiograph in maximum flexion is also efficacious in defining the osteophytes. The inability to obtain full extension of the elbow should prompt a search for additional evidence of posteromedial impingement.

Flexor Tendinopathy and Tears

An acute valgus load to the elbow is frequently accompanied by contusion or tears of the flexor pronator origin with extensive soft-tissue edema [2]. Excessive tension on the medial elbow soft tissues in the setting of chronic valgus extension overload may also lead to the development of tendinosis and tears, most commonly affecting the pronator teres and the flexor carpi radialis [1]. Tendinosis manifests on MRI as intermediate to increased T2 signal intensity within the tendon, often with focal enlargement (Fig. 11.14). The observed areas of increased signal intensity correspond to areas of collagen disruption, mucoid or hyaline degeneration, and neovascularization [26]. Areas of heterotopic ossification or dystro-

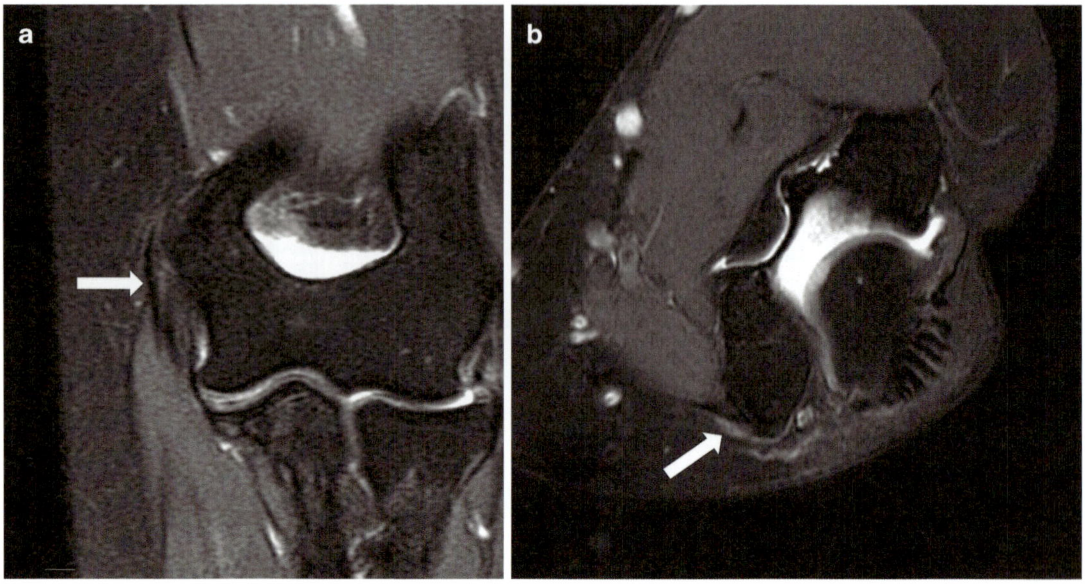

Fig. 11.14 Coronal (**a**) and axial (**b**) T2 FSE MR images with fat saturation demonstrating mild increased signal and focal enlargement of the flexor carpi radialis origin compatible with mild tendinopathy (*arrows*)

phic calcification may also be observed at the origin of previously injured or chronically degenerated tendons.

Ulnar Neuropathy

Ulnar neuritis may manifest on MRI as nerve or fascicular enlargement within or more typically proximal to the cubital tunnel. The normal fascicular architecture of the nerve can be disrupted, and the nerve may appear hyperintense on both FSE and inversion recovery pulse sequences (Fig. 11.15). Masses, osteophytes, ganglia, and accessory muscles may all cause impingement of the ulnar nerve in the cubital tunnel [27], but in the throwing athlete, ulnar neuritis is more frequently a result of chronic traction caused by excessive valgus laxity. Morphological and signal alterations within the ulnar nerve are a frequent finding even in the asymptomatic patient, highlighting the importance of interpreting the MR findings in the context of clinical symptoms.

Radiocapitellar Osteochondral Defects

Injury to the cartilage of the radiocapitellar compartment can occur in the setting of an acute valgus load or following dislocation due to direct impaction of the radius against the capitellum. Capitellar osteochondral lesions may also develop in the context of valgus extension overload (Fig. 11.16). The possibility of associated osteochondral lesions in the setting of acute and chronic UCL injury underscores the importance of cartilage-sensitive imaging in all patients, as these lesions reflect a primary ischemic insult to subchondral bone and the overlying cartilage represents the "innocent bystander" of the process [8]. Mild chondral hyperintensity and subchondral flattening may serve as early evidence of an osteochondral lesion, formerly termed osteochondritis dissecans [28]. As changes progress, there may be frank subchondral collapse, cystic resorption of subchondral bone, fluid imbibition between the osteochondral lesion and the parent bone, or a loose osteochondral fragment.

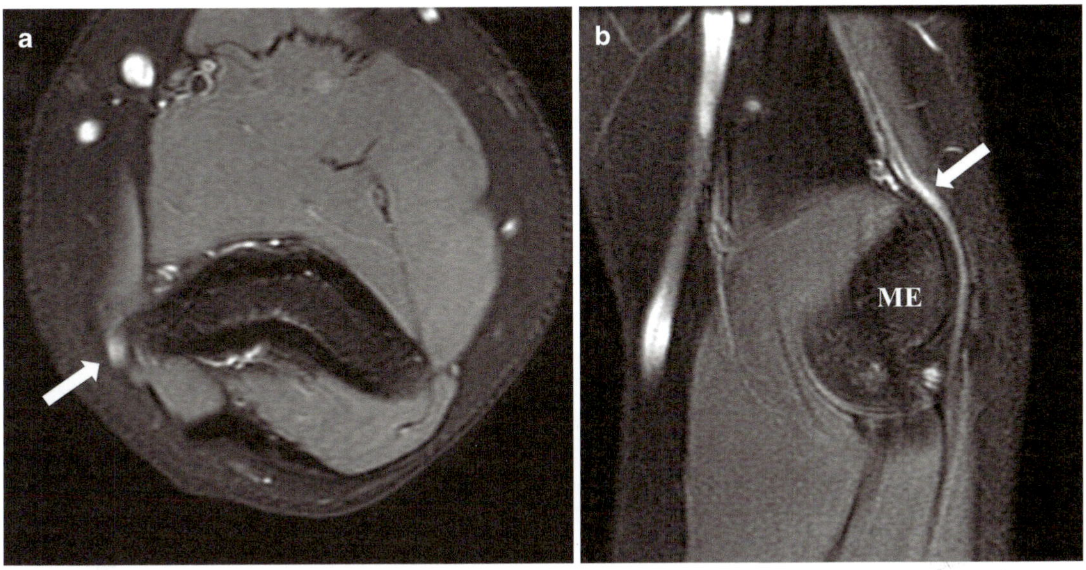

Fig. 11.15 Overhead throwing athlete with recalcitrant ulnar neuropathy despite conservative management. Axial (**a**) and sagittal (**b**) T2 FSE MR images with fat saturation showing mild increased signal and enlargement of the ulnar nerve just proximal to the cubital tunnel (*arrows*). ME, medial humeral epicondyle

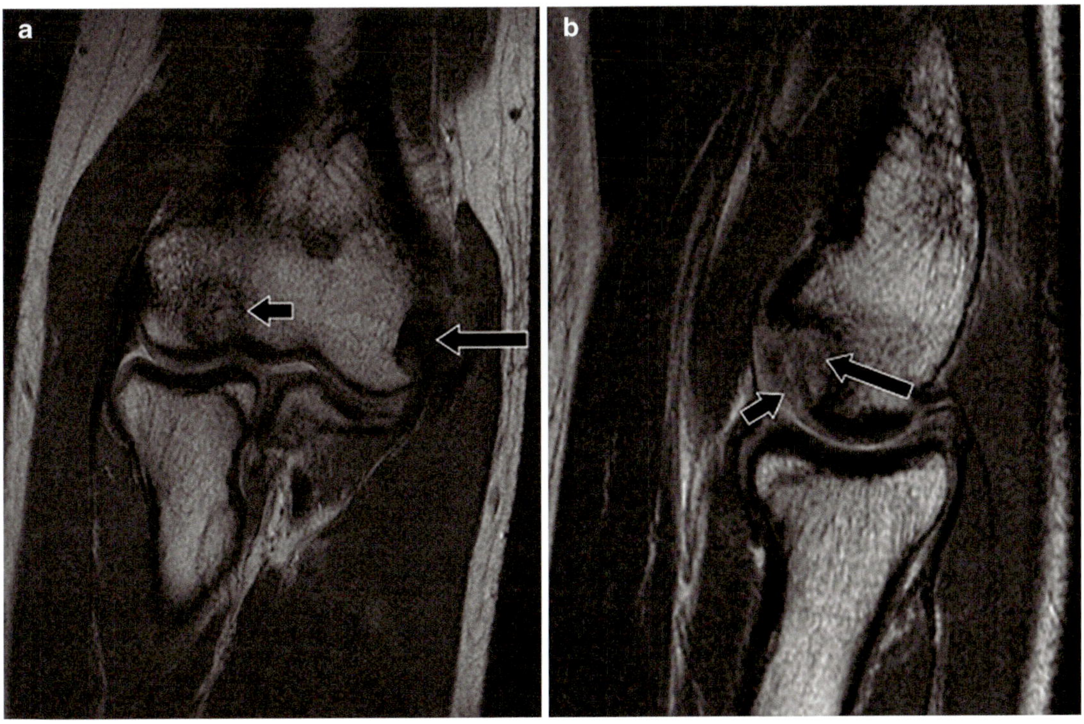

Fig. 11.16 (**a**) Coronal FSE image demonstrates chronic thickening of the UCL in a throwing athlete (*long arrow*). The *short arrow* indicates a capitellar osteochondral lesion. (**b**) Sagittal FSE image in the same patient demonstrates a capitellar osteochondral lesion (*long arrow*) with loss of the tidemark, subchondral collapse, cystic resorption of subchondral bone, and early fragmentation. The overlying cartilage (*short arrow*) is markedly hyperintense

Apophyseal Injury

In the skeletally immature athlete, acute and chronic stresses to the UCL are preferentially transmitted to the medial epicondylar apophysis with relatively little observable change in the ligament itself [29]. A Salter Harris I fracture may occur with variable degrees of separation of the medial epicondylar apophysis (Fig. 11.17). Associated bone marrow edema patterns may be present in the apophysis. In the chronic setting, a traction apophysitis may be seen with widening of the growth plate or fragmentation of the epicondylar apophysis [5]. The observation of a bulbous contour to the medial epicondyle may serve as evidence of remote apophyseal injury prior to physeal fusion.

Postsurgical Elbow

UCL reconstruction is the primary procedure available to restore medial elbow stability and relieve elbow pain in patients with injury to the UCL [30]. MRI following ligament reconstruction is technically challenging due to the presence of metallic debris and associated susceptibility artifact (Fig. 11.18). This is particularly prominent on gradient recalled sequences due to the lack of a 180° rephasing pulse, limiting the utility of this sequence in the postoperative setting [6]. Interpreting the postoperative MRI is also diagnostically challenging due to the wide spectrum of "normal" postoperative appearances and varying approaches to ligament reconstruction.

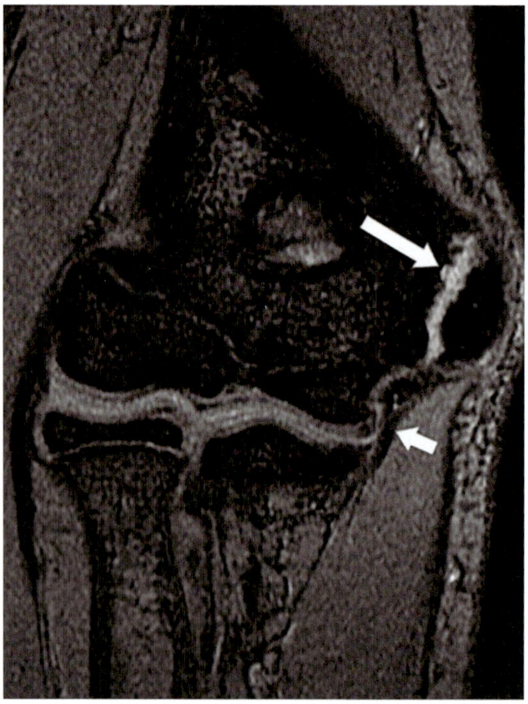

Fig. 11.17 Coronal GRE image demonstrating chronic widening of the unfused medial epicondylar apophysis in a skeletally immature pitcher (*long arrow*). The UCL ligament (*short arrow*) is mildly thickened but otherwise unremarkable in appearance reflecting the preferential transmission of valgus force to the apophysis

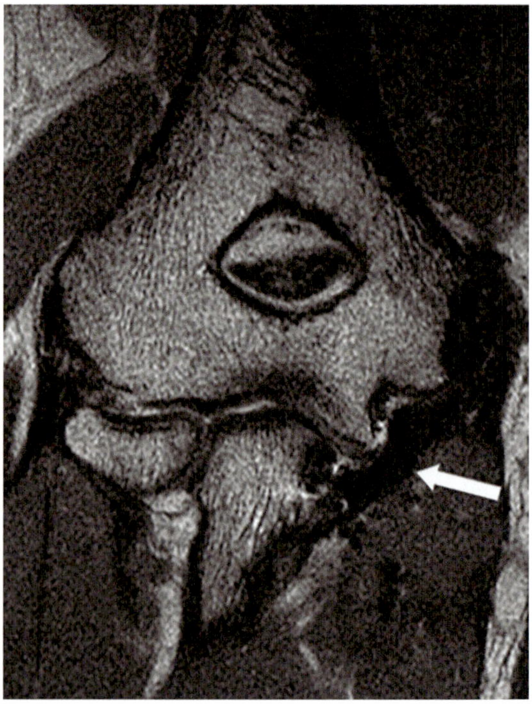

Fig. 11.18 Coronal FSE image in a patient following UCL ligament reconstruction. The *white arrow* indicates a normal appearing graft, which is thicker than the native ligament but demonstrates uniform hypointensity and appears taut in extension. Note the small foci of magnetic susceptibility adjacent to the sublime tubercle

MRI in the postoperative elbow is useful for the assessment of the integrity of the reconstruction, detecting stress fractures, for the visualization of the transposed and nontransposed ulnar nerve, for the assessment of cartilage integrity, and for the evaluation of the remainder of the elbow and adjacent soft tissues (Fig. 11.19; [31]).

The reconstructed UCL is much thicker than the native UCL reflecting the double bundle nature of most grafts and the remnant native UCL. The well-functioning graft should appear taut in extension [31]; graft dysfunction may be suspected when the graft appears lax or redundant. Graft signal intensity is more difficult to interpret as the signal may vary depending on the time since surgery and the degree of remodeling. Heterotopic ossification may be seen within and adjacent to a reconstructed UCL, rarely resulting in bony bridging or fibrous bridging at the humerus or the ulna (Fig. 11.20a). A partial or complete re-tear of the graft can be confidently diagnosed when there is linear fluid imbibition into a focal discontinuity of the graft (Fig. 11.20b). Interstitial partial tearing may also be seen as redundancy or outward bowing of the graft or new high signal within a graft [32]. On the rare occasion when heterotopic ossification is extensive, a re-tear may be identified as a fracture through a fibrous union between the ossified ligament and the humerus or ulna.

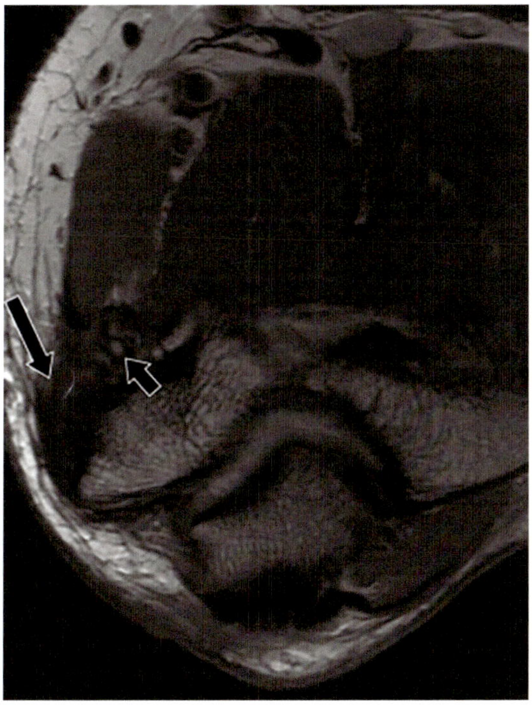

Fig. 11.19 Axial FSE image in patient following repair of the flexor pronator origin (*long arrow*) shows a transposed ulnar nerve which is encased in hypertrophic scar (*short arrow*). The nerve is hyperintense with marked enlargement of individual nerve fascicles reflecting ulnar neuritis

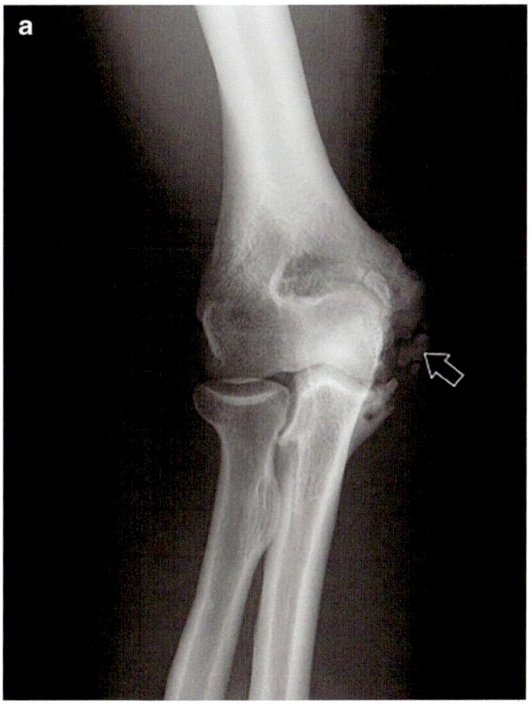

Fig. 11.20 (**a**) AP radiograph demonstrates multiple foci of heterotopic ossification within a reconstructed UCL (*arrow*). (**b**) Corresponding FSE MRI demonstrates the appearance of heterotopic ossification on MRI (*short arrow*). A near complete tear of the reconstruction is indicated by fluid imbibition into a defect in the partially ossified ligament (*long arrow*)

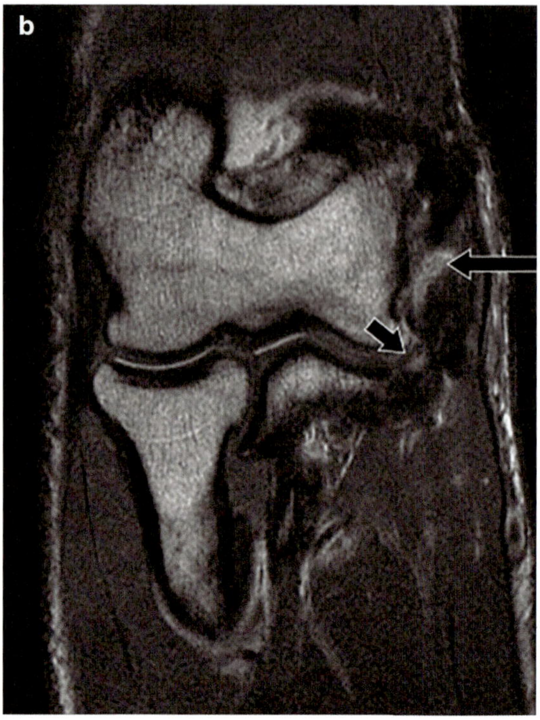

Fig. 11.20 (continued)

Conclusion

MR imaging of the elbow allows for accurate and early diagnosis of acute, chronic, and acute on chronic injuries to the UCL. Optimized high-spatial resolution and high soft-tissue contrast MR imaging may reveal several abnormalities that could potentially contribute to elbow pain and dysfunction, particularly in the throwing athlete. The importance of a thorough history, clinical examination, and a good working relationship between the interpreting radiologist and the referring clinician cannot be overstated.

References

1. Kijowski R, Tuite M, Sanford M. Magnetic resonance imaging of the elbow. Part II: abnormalities of the ligaments, tendons, and nerves. Skeletal Radiol. 2004;34(1):1–18.
2. Richard MJ. Traumatic valgus instability of the elbow: pathoanatomy and results of direct repair. J Bone Joint Surg Am. 2008;90(11):2416.
3. Timmerman LAL, Schwartz MLM, Andrews JRJ. Preoperative evaluation of the ulnar collateral ligament by magnetic resonance imaging and computed tomography arthrography. Evaluation in 25 baseball players with surgical confirmation. Am J Sports Med. 1994;22(1):26–32.
4. Gaary EA, Potter HG, Altchek DW. Medial elbow pain in the throwing athlete: MR imaging evaluation. AJR Am J Roentgenol. 1997;168(3):795–800. (PubMed—NCBI).
5. Potter HG, Ho ST, Altchek DW. Magnetic resonance imaging of the elbow. Semin Musculoskelet Radiol. 2004;8(1):5–16. (Copyright© 2004 by Thieme Medical Publishers, Inc., 333 Seventh Avenue, New York, NY 10001, USA).
6. Kaplan LJ, Potter HG. MR imaging of ligament injuries to the elbow. Radiol Clin N Am. 2006;44(4):583–94.
7. Johnson D, Stevens KJ, Riley G, Shapiro L, Yoshioka H, Gold GE. Approach to MR imaging of the elbow and wrist: technical aspects and innovation. Magn Reson Imaging Clin N Am. 2015;23(3):355–66.
8. Potter HG. Imaging of posttraumatic and soft tissue dysfunction of the elbow. Clin Orthop Relat Res. 2000;(370):9–18.
9. Magee T. Accuracy of 3-T MR arthrography versus conventional 3-T MRI of elbow tendons and ligaments compared with surgery. AJR Am J Roentgenol. 2015;204(1):W70–5.
10. LiMarzi GM, O'Dell MC, Scherer K, Pettis C, Wasyliw CW, Bancroft LW. Magnetic resonance arthrography of the wrist and elbow. Magn Reson Imaging Clin N Am. 2015;23(3):441–55.
11. Salvo JP, Rizio L, Zvijac JE, Uribe JW, Hechtman KS. Avulsion fracture of the ulnar sublime tubercle in overhead throwing athletes. Am J Sports Med. 2002;30(3):426–31.
12. Mirowitz SAS, London SLS. Ulnar collateral ligament injury in baseball pitchers: MR imaging evaluation. Radiology. 1992;185(2):573–6.
13. Bryce CDC, Armstrong ADA. Anatomy and biomechanics of the elbow. Orthop Clin North Am. 2008;39(2):141–54.
14. Hotchkiss RN, Weiland AJ. Valgus stability of the elbow. J Orthop Res. 1987;5(3):372–7.
15. Callaway GH, Field LD, Deng XH, Torzilli PA, O'Brien SJ, Altchek DW, et al. Biomechanical evaluation of the medial collateral ligament of the elbow. J Bone Joint Surg Am. 1997;79(8):1223–31.
16. Morrey BF, An K. Functional anatomy of the ligaments of the elbow. Clin Orthop Relat Res. 1985;201:84–90.
17. Munshi M, Pretterklieber ML, Chung CB, Haghighi P, Cho JH, Trudell DJ, et al. Anterior bundle of ulnar collateral ligament: evaluation of anatomic relationships by using MR imaging, MR arthrography, and gross anatomic and histologic analysis. Radiology. 2004;231(3):797–803.
18. Gustas CN, Lee KS. Multimodality imaging of the painful elbow: current imaging concepts and image-

guided treatments for the injured Thrower's elbow. Radiol Clin N Am. 2016;54(5):817–39.
19. Husarik DB, Saupe N, Pfirrmann CWA, Jost B, Hodler J, Zanetti M. Ligaments and plicae of the elbow: normal MR imaging variability in 60 asymptomatic subjects. Radiology. 2010;257(1):185–94.
20. Sugimoto H, Ohsawa T. Ulnar collateral ligament in the growing elbow: MR imaging of normal development and throwing injuries. Radiology. 1994;192(2):417–22.
21. Kim NR, Moon SG, Ko SM, Moon W-J, Choi JW, Park J-Y. MR imaging of ulnar collateral ligament injury in baseball players: value for predicting rehabilitation outcome. Eur J Radiol. 2011;80(3):e422–6.
22. Ramkumar PN, Frangiamore SJ, Navarro SM, Lynch TS, Forney MC, Kaar SG, et al. Interobserver and intraobserver reliability of an MRI-based classification system for injuries to the ulnar collateral ligament. Am J Sports Med. 2018;46(11):2755–60.
23. Ramkumar PN, Haeberle HS, Navarro SM, Frangiamore SJ, Farrow LD, Schickendantz MS. Prognostic utility of an magnetic resonance imaging-based classification for operative versus nonoperative management of ulnar collateral ligament tears: one-year follow-up. J Shoulder Elb Surg. 2019;28(6):1159–65.
24. Hurd WJ, Eby S, Kaufman KR, Murthy NS. Magnetic resonance imaging of the throwing elbow in the uninjured, high school-aged baseball pitcher. Am J Sports Med. 2011;39(4):722–8.
25. Dodson CC, Thomas A, Dines JS, Nho SJ, Williams RJ, Altchek DW. Medial ulnar collateral ligament reconstruction of the elbow in throwing athletes. Am J Sports Med. 2006;34(12):1926–32.
26. Potter HGH, Hannafin JAJ, Morwessel RMR, DiCarlo EFE, O'Brien SJS, Altchek DWD. Lateral epicondylitis: correlation of MR imaging, surgical, and histopathologic findings. Radiology. 1995;196(1):43–6.
27. Hash T, Bogner E. Nerve entrapment and compression syndromes of the elbow. Semin Musculoskelet Radiol. 2010;14(4):438–48.
28. Sofka CM, Potter HG. Imaging of elbow injuries in the child and adult athlete. Radiol Clin N Am. 2002;40(2):251–65.
29. Benjamin HJH, Briner WW Jr. Little league elbow. Clin J Sport Med. 2005;15(1):37–40.
30. Jobe FWF, Stark HH, Lombardo SJS. Reconstruction of the ulnar collateral ligament in athletes. J Bone Joint Surg Am. 1986;68(8):1158–63.
31. Wear SA, Thornton DD, Schwartz ML, Weissmann RC III, Cain EL, Andrews JR. MRI of the reconstructed ulnar collateral ligament. Am J Roentgenol. 2011;197(5):1198–204.
32. Daniels SP, Mintz DN, Endo Y, Dines JS, Sneag DB. Imaging of the post-operative medial elbow in the overhead thrower: common and abnormal findings after ulnar collateral ligament reconstruction and ulnar nerve transposition. Skelet Radiol. 2019;48:1843–60.

Ultrasound Imaging of Ulnar Collateral Ligament Injury

12

Michael C. Ciccotti, Levon N. Nazarian, and Michael G. Ciccotti

Introduction

Overhead throwing athletes subject the medial elbow to tremendous forces during the late cocking and early acceleration phases of the throwing motion [1]. It has been documented that up to 97% of elbow complaints in pitchers involve medial elbow symptoms [2]. The ulnar collateral ligament (UCL), particularly the anterior band of the UCL, serves as the primary stabilizer of the elbow against valgus forces and is the most commonly injured soft tissue structure of the elbow in this athletic population [2]. These forces result in a predictable pattern of stresses across the elbow including tension medially, compression laterally, and shear posteriorly, and a predictable pattern of resultant pathology. Traditionally, diagnosis of UCL injury has relied heavily on history and physical exam. However, physical exam findings may be unimpressive or nonspecific. Although they remain crucial to arriving at a correct diagnosis, even a thorough history and physical examination may yield a broad differential diagnosis including ulnar collateral ligament (UCL) injury, flexor-pronator injury, peri-elbow soft tissue contracture, ulnar nerve irritation, olecranon or medial epicondyle stress fracture/apophysitis, posterior medial impingement with olecranon osteophytes, radiocapitellar osteochondral injury, and associated loose bodies/free osteochondral fragments [2, 3]. Thus, conventional imaging modalities such as plain X-ray, stress radiography, magnetic resonance imaging, and arthrography have played traditionally significant roles in the diagnosis of this clinically challenging entity [3–10]. Imaging allows the identification of pathologic changes such as bony changes (medial UCL ossification, radiocapitellar flattening/osteochondral defects [OCD], olecranon/coronoid spurring), musculotendinous changes (flexor-pronator and extensor tendon degeneration/fraying/tearing), ligamentous changes (UCL degeneration/fraying/tearing), and nerve changes (ulnar nerve edema/scarring/subluxation) [11–15]. Unfortunately, conventional imaging is accompanied by limitations such as significant time, cost, exposure to ionizing radiation, and static imaging. Although initially described in 1978, ultrasonography (US) of the elbow, including stress ultrasonography (SUS),

M. C. Ciccotti
Orthopaedics Sports Medicine Fellow, The Steadman Clinic and Steadman Philippon Research Institute, Vail, CO, USA

L. N. Nazarian
The William E. Conrady, MD Professor of Radiology, Sidney Kimmel Medical College of Thomas Jefferson University, Philadelphia, PA, USA

M. G. Ciccotti (✉)
The Everett J. and Marian Gordon Professor of Orthopaedic Surgery, Division of Sports Medicine, The Rothman Institute, Thomas Jefferon University, Philadelphia, PA, USA
e-mail: Michael.ciccotti@rothmanortho.com

J. S. Dines et al. (eds.), *Elbow Ulnar Collateral Ligament Injury*,
https://doi.org/10.1007/978-3-030-69567-5_12

has become an increasingly important adjunct to the management of elbow pathology in an athletic population. US/SUS provides the clinician with a rapid, low-cost, noninvasive, radiation-free, high-resolution imaging modality. With the added utility of dynamic/functional assessment, that can increase the accuracy of diagnosis and guide the clinician in recommendation of optimal treatment.

Science of Ultrasonography

Ultrasonography has become increasingly ubiquitous in clinical settings ranging from emergency departments to outpatient clinics and athletic training rooms in addition to radiology departments. A variety of health-care providers including athletic trainers, ultrasound technologists/sonographers, and physicians in multiple specialties now perform this diagnostic procedure on a routine basis. Both increased access and growing expertise have accelerated the application of ultrasonography to a broad spectrum of pathology to supplement and/or supplant more traditional imaging modalities by leveraging the unique capabilities of ultrasonography. The past 15–20 years in particular have witnessed a notable increase in the application of ultrasonography to musculoskeletal medicine, including significant interest in the evaluation of the athlete's elbow and ulnar collateral ligament injury.

Musculoskeletal ultrasonography (US) is a real-time imaging modality that utilizes reflected pulses of high-frequency (ultrasonic) sound waves to visualize and assess tendons, ligaments, muscles, nerves, vessels, joints, cartilage, bone surfaces, soft tissue masses, and fluid containing structures. The intensity of the reflected ultrasound echo from a given structure is depicted utilizing a gray scale, and the time it takes for the reflected echo to return to the transducer determines the depth of that structure on the image that is created.

The ultrasound equipment utilized in musculoskeletal medicine is essentially the same as equipment used for other medical applications (Fig. 12.1). Linear array rather than curved transducers are typically preferred for musculoskeletal applications. Modern ultrasound machines are equipped with multifrequency/broadband transducers in the range of 5–10 MHz, 7.5–13 MHz, or higher. Higher frequency (and thus a shorter wavelength) translates to better axial resolution of the acquired ultrasound image. The trade-off is that higher frequency transducers come at the sacrifice of tissue penetration. However, tissue penetration is not a major issue at the elbow joint due to the limited subcutaneous adipose tissue, such that high-frequency transducers can be used successfully. Ultrasound transducers typically used for musculoskeletal imaging have an axial resolution of 0.15 mm at 10 MHz and 0.04 mm at 20 MHz. This superb axial resolution enables ultrasonography to depict fine anatomic changes that are difficult to depict with any other imaging modality, increasing the diagnostic value of musculoskeletal ultrasonography.

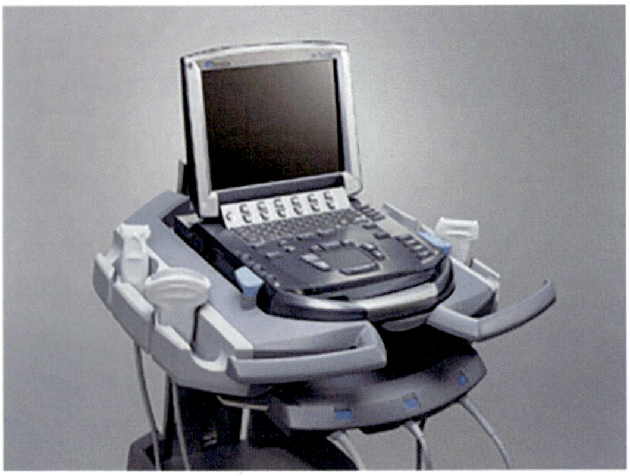

Fig. 12.1 A multifrequency, broadband ultrasound transducer with monitor

A variety of common imaging artifacts can be seen with ultrasonography. Anisotropy is an imaging artifact of hypoechogenicity commonly seen with tendons (and to a lesser degree with muscles, nerves, and ligaments) due to reflection of the ultrasound beam into another plane if the beam is not perpendicular to the tendon surface. If the beam is reflected into a different plane, echoes will not be available to return to the transducer and contribute to image formation. Acoustic shadowing is the inability to visualize anything behind intact bone or dense calcifications due to absorption and nearly complete reflection of sound waves. Other common artifacts include acoustic enhancement, by which the zone deep to a structure that does not absorb much of the ultrasound beam, such as a cyst, appears brighter than the adjacent soft tissues; reverberation, by which the bouncing of the sound wave between the transducer and metal structures like prostheses, implants, or needles generates multiple echoes; and edge shadows, by which hypoechoic areas can be seen behind spherical, fluid-filled structures.

The image visualized via ultrasound is dependent upon the orientation of the transducer. A transverse orientation, or short-axis view, yields images similar to axial views obtained by computed tomography (CT) or magnetic resonance (MR) imaging. A longitudinal transducer orientation yields a long-axis view similar to a coronal or sagittal sequence. Echogenicity is dependent upon both the characteristics of the tissues visualized and the frequency of transducer utilized. However, standard characteristics have been defined for musculoskeletal tissues when imaged with transducer frequencies from 5 to 15 MHz, the range of most commonly available ultrasound transducers. Bone surface is typically hyperechoic (white) and demonstrates posterior acoustic shadowing (Fig. 12.2). Articular cartilage is typically anechoic (black) with a smooth surface (Fig. 12.3); however, degenerative cartilage may have increased echogenicity and demonstrates irregular surface. In contrast, fibrocartilage such as that of the glenoid labrum is hyperechoic. Synovium demonstrates an intermediate echogenicity while synovial fluid is anechoic, lacks a Doppler signal, and is displaceable and compressible on examination. The joint capsule can be visualized as the boundary between the hypoechoic synovium and anechoic synovial fluid. Tendons characteristically display a fine internal fibrillar pattern and are slightly hyperechoic when perpendicular to the probe (Fig. 12.2); it is important to note that tendons may demonstrate anisotropy. Nerves have similar echogenicity to tendons but are slightly hypoechoic, with a less tightly packed fascicular pattern compared to the fibrillar pattern of tendons (Fig. 12.4). Muscles are predominantly hypoechoic, dependent upon trans-

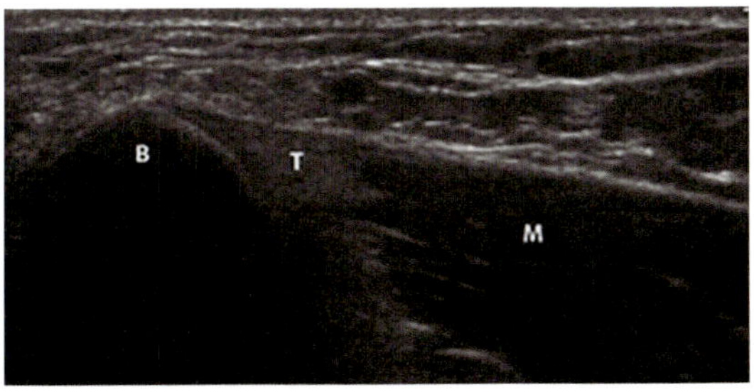

Fig. 12.2 Longitudinal ultrasound view of the medial elbow showing the medial epicondyle of the humerus (B), the common flexor-pronator tendon (T), and the flexor-pronator muscle (M)

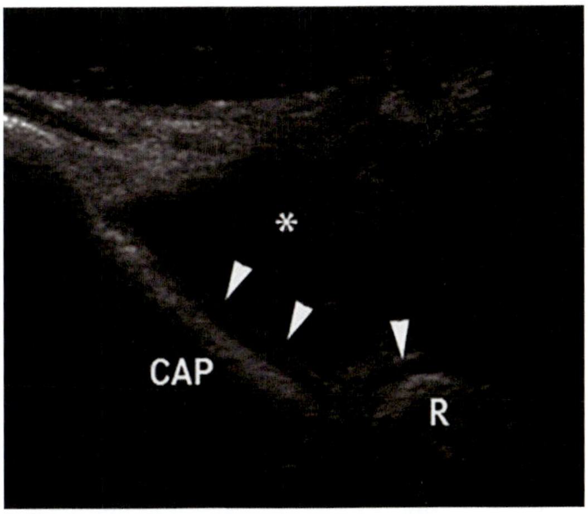

Fig. 12.3 Longitudinal ultrasound view of the lateral elbow showing the articular cartilage (arrowheads) of the capitellum (CAP) and radius (R). Joint fluid is marked with the asterisk

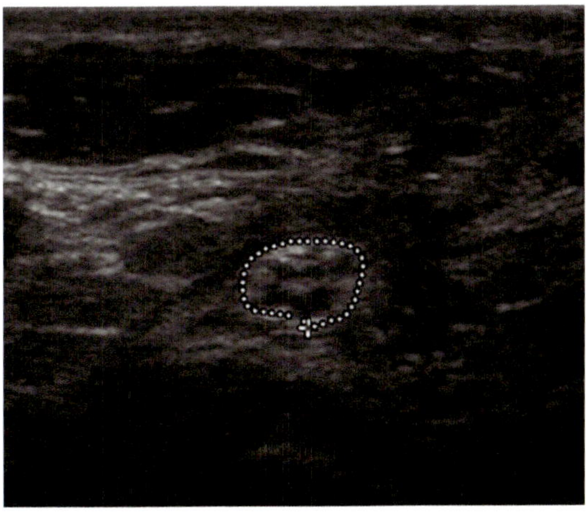

Fig. 12.4 Cross-sectional ultrasound view of the ulnar nerve (encircled by cursors) at the level of the cubital tunnel showing the characteristic fascicular pattern

ducer orientation, with hyperechoic lines within the muscle substance indicating peri- and epimysium and thicker hyperechoic lines indicating septae and investing fascia (Fig. 12.2). Bursae are visualized as hypoechoic or anechoic. Finally, ligaments have similar echotexture to tendons but consist of several layers with fibrillar patterns running in different directions (Fig. 12.5).

Abnormal ultrasound findings are common in the overhead throwing athlete and may be symptomatic or asymptomatic. Such findings include thickening of the anterior band of the UCL in the dominant arm compared to the nondominant arm. Ultrasound may reveal calcification (Fig. 12.6) as hyperechogenicity within the substance of the ligament with or without acoustic shadowing, or conversely pathology may manifest as hypoechoic foci (Fig. 12.7a, b). Tears of the UCL can be visualized as disruption of the substance of the UCL with anechoic fluid within the tear (Fig. 12.8).

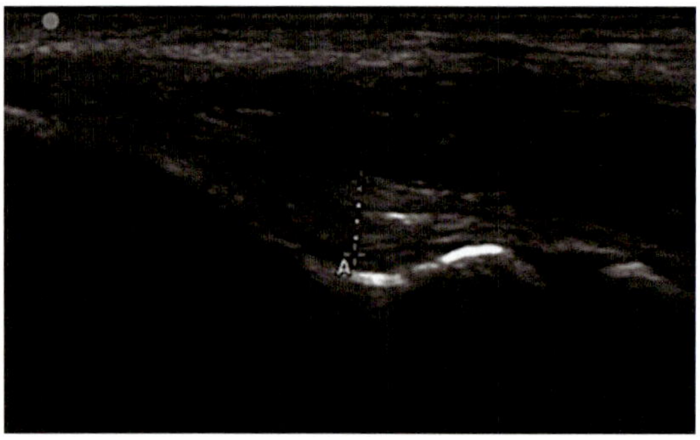

Fig. 12.5 Longitudinal ultrasound view of the anterior band (A) of a normal ulnar collateral ligament of the elbow. The thickness of the ligament is represented by the cursors

Ultrasound for the Evaluation of the UCL

The unique capabilities of ultrasonography as a low-cost, noninvasive, nonradiating, real-time imaging modality allowing dynamic evaluation with applied stress address a number of deficiencies of traditional imaging. Plain radiography can define bony changes including osteophytes, cystic changes, joint space narrowing, and loose bodies; however, it lacks the ability to provide direct evidence of soft tissue injury [4, 7, 8]. Additionally, it is a static test with the elbow in one position for each view obtained. In 2007, Wright et al. used plain radiographs to examine the elbows of 56 asymptomatic professional

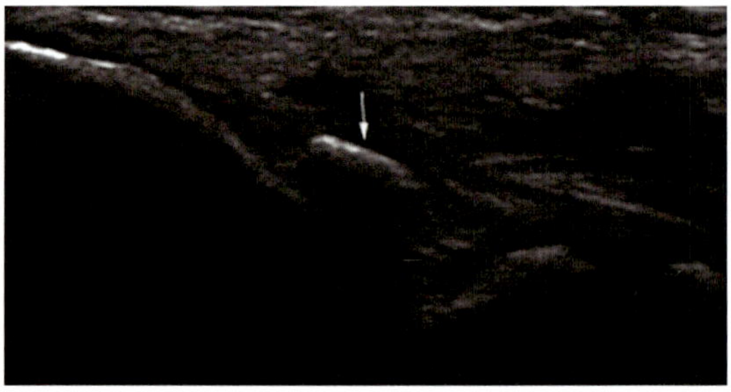

Fig. 12.6 Longitudinal ultrasound view showing calcification (arrow) in the ulnar collateral ligament of a pitcher

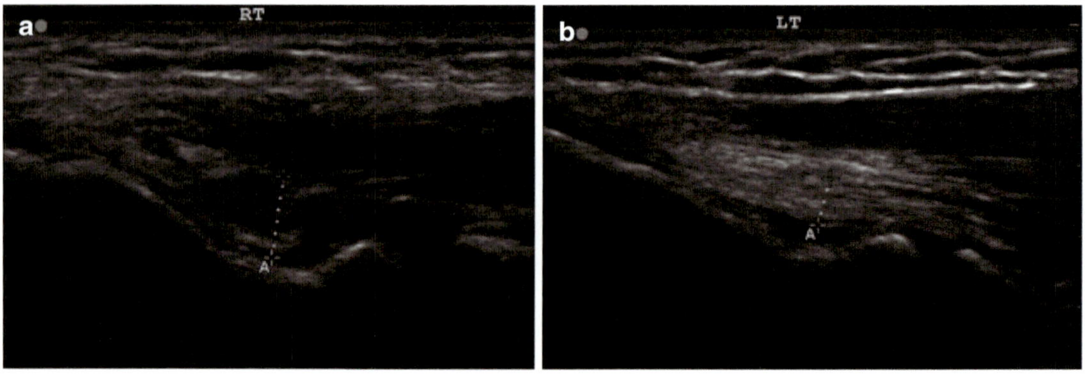

Fig. 12.7 Longitudinal ultrasound view of (**a**) a hypoechoic signal (cursors) in the anterior band (A) of the ulnar collateral ligament of a pitcher, (**b**) compared to the normal anterior band (A) of the contralateral ligament (cursors)

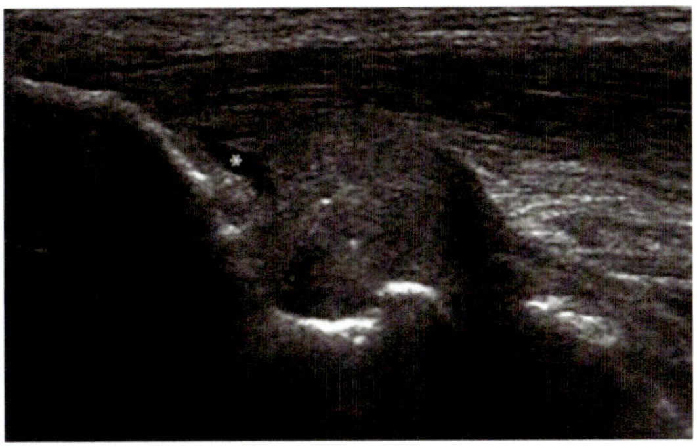

Fig. 12.8 Longitudinal ultrasound view of the thickened anterior band of the ulnar collateral ligament with a focal tear (*)

baseball pitchers [9]. Although they did find that degenerative changes developed over time, these changes correlated poorly to time spent on the Major League Baseball disabled list or risk of future injury, showing limited prognostic value for plain radiography. Some authors have advocated the use of stress radiography to more precisely evaluate functional UCL laxity [10, 16, 17]. However, this modality also does not provide direct assessment of the ligament, may be cumbersome to employ, and is provider dependent [18]. Rijke et al. described the use of a calibrated device to produce a valgus stress during radiography to evaluate patients with UCL injuries as a valuable contribution to the field [17]. Lee et al. utilized radiography to compare the amount of ulnohumeral joint space gapping with and without stress in "normal" individuals [16]. They demonstrated a significant difference in the amount of gapping when 5 lbs of valgus stress was applied at both 0° and 30° of elbow flexion. However, there was no difference in gapping whether they looked at the nondominant or dominant elbow. Ellenbecker et al. reported the results of a similar study, but in a more specific population of uninjured, professional baseball pitchers [10]. They found a significantly greater difference in the amount of ulnohumeral joint space widening with stress when comparing the dominant to nondominant elbows. They concluded that increased medial elbow laxity exists in the dominant arms of uninjured pitchers. Despite providing a more functional evaluation of the ulnohumeral joint space, these plain radiography studies cannot comment directly on the UCL or surrounding soft tissue structures.

Although conventional MR imaging provides excellent visualization of acute, complete ruptures of the UCL, it may be less accurate for the diagnosis of partial thickness injury [19, 20–23]. Numerous studies have demonstrated the ability of conventional MR imaging to provide excellent visualization of complete tears of the UCL, heterotopic calcification, flexor-pronator inflammation, and associated bony edema [7, 8, 20, 22, 23]. MR arthrography has been advocated as a more accurate technique for both partial and chronic UCL injury, but MR arthrography is expensive, time-consuming, and invasive such that patient reluctance has limited its routine use in elite-level pitchers [18, 21–23]. Quite often elite-level pitchers are extremely reluctant to have contrast injected into their injured, dominant elbow. Although it may visualize clear irregularities in the UCL, MR arthrography nonetheless fails to provide a dynamic assessment of ligament laxity as the patient's elbow remains in one position throughout the procedure. In contrast, stress ultrasonography (SUS) provides the clinician with soft tissue visualization akin to MRI as well as the ability to functionally assess the elbow with applied stress akin to stress radiography. Specifically, SUS has been utilized to diagnose clinically significant UCL injury with associated valgus instability.

Although the earliest description of the application of ultrasonography to musculoskeletal medicine was published in 1978, literature exploring the application of this technology to ulnar collateral ligament injury has only proliferated in the past decade [24]. In 2002, DeSmet et al. were the first to report on two cases of collegiate-level baseball pitchers with medial elbow pain and laxity evaluated via dynamic ultrasonography (DUS) [25]. In both cases, DUS was able to identify injury to the UCL and the authors described their ability to measure the amount of joint widening occurring with valgus stress during DUS examination. A case report in 2010 from Wood et al. (one patient) corroborated these findings by similarly demonstrating the ability of DUS to assess medial valgus instability while stressing the elbow with ultrasound of the contralateral elbow performed for comparison [26]. In all cases, UCL injury detected at DUS was later confirmed at the time of surgical reconstruction. One of the key observations by DeSmet et al. was the need for additional research to determine an optimal method for applying reproducible, standardized stress to the ligament.

In 2002, Sasaki et al. reported on DUS evaluations of 30 asymptomatic, collegiate baseball players [27]. Their work demonstrated that the ulnohumeral joint space of the dominant elbow was significantly wider than that of the nondominant elbow with that additional laxity occurring with application of valgus stress. Their DUS methods were slightly different than we employ: They placed the elbow in 90 degrees of flexion, used gravity stress instead of manual stress by standardized device, and did not comment on the qualitative characteristics of the UCL. In addition, only 12 of the 30 players in their cohort were pitchers.

In 2003, Jacobson et al. also reported on the characterization of the anterior band of the UCL using ultrasound in four cadavers (eight elbows) [28]. The elbows were blindly evaluated using ultrasound by a single musculoskeletal radiologist with the findings compared to standard arthrography, MR arthrography, and anatomic slices by two musculoskeletal radiologists. Abnormality of the UCL was defined as contrast material extension into the substance of the ligament or fiber discontinuity, by MR arthrography or anatomic slices. The UCL was determined to be unequivocally normal in three specimens, abnormal in two specimens, and the remaining three specimens were excluded for failing to meet either criteria. Ultrasound findings of the normal UCL included a fibrillar appearance and hyperechoic signal between the medial epicondyle and proximal ulna. The two abnormal ligaments demonstrated areas of hypoechogenicity and ligament fiber disruption.

Review of Stress Ultrasound and the UCL: A 15+ Year Experience

Although significant literature exists regarding the use of ultrasonography in musculoskeletal medicine, the senior authors identified the deficiencies of traditional static imaging for ulnar collateral ligament injury and recognized the dearth of focused literature in this area. They sought to apply ultrasonography to address the shortcomings of conventional imaging and more thoroughly evaluate the elbow in a functional manner by leveraging the unique capabilities of the modality described above. Furthermore, they surmised that stress ultrasonography (SUS) could identify ulnohumeral joint space gapping as compared to the contralateral arm and thereby indicate significant UCL injury in patients with equivocal physical exam and/or conventional imaging. A preliminary cadaveric investigation was carried out to define technique and applicability of this imaging modality. This led to the significant amount of prospective published and submitted [26] clinical data acquired on elite throwing athletes by these authors [18, 29].

In 2003, the senior authors published a study utilizing stress ultrasound to evaluate the ulnar collateral ligament in 26 asymptomatic Major League Baseball pitchers [18]. Ultrasonography was performed on both the dominant and nondominant elbows of these pitchers at spring training with a multifrequency 13-MHz linear array transducer. The thickness of the anterior band of the UCL and the width of the ulnohumeral joint were measured at 30° of flexion, at rest, and with an applied valgus stress (Fig. 12.9a, b) The anterior band of the UCL was found to be significantly thicker at rest in the dominant arm (6.3 mm ± 1.1) compared to the nondominant arm (5.3 mm ± 1.0, $p < 0.01$), as well as with an applied valgus stress (6.3 mm ± 1.4 vs. 4.8 mm ± 0.19, $p < 0.001$). With stress applied, the width of the ulnohumeral joint space was also significantly different with greater laxity in the dominant arm (4.2 mm ± 1.5) compared to the nondominant arm (3 mm ± 1.0, $p < 0.01$). Hypoechoic foci were more common in the UCL of the dominant arm (69% vs. 12%, $p < 0.001$) as

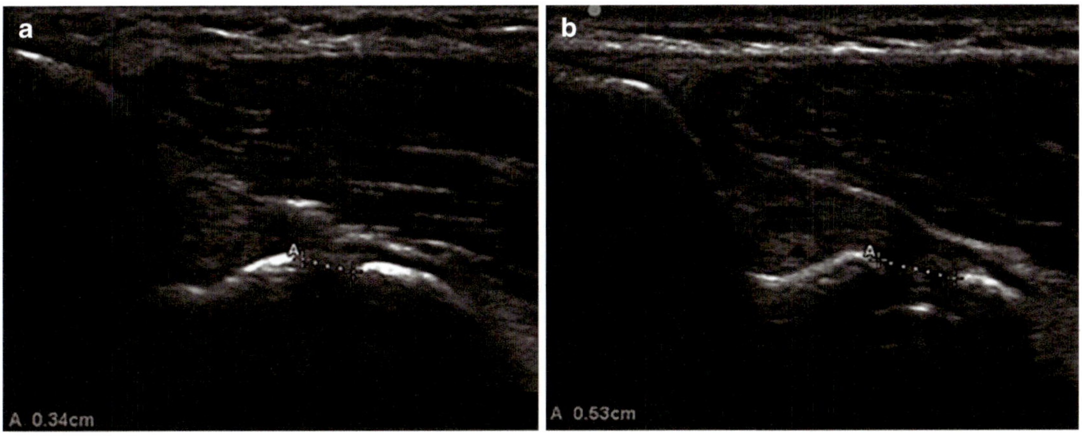

Fig. 12.9 Stress ultrasound demonstrating (**a**) the width of the ulnohumeral joint at rest; (**b**) the width of the ulnohumeral joint with applied valgus stress

were calcifications (35% vs. 0%, $p < 0.001$). The average length of time for bilateral ultrasound was 10.4 minutes. Stress ultrasound provided a rapid means of evaluating the UCL in professional pitchers. In the dominant elbows of these athletes, the UCL was thicker, more likely to have hypoechoic foci and/or calcifications, and demonstrated increased laxity on valgus stress.

In a continuing, prospective evaluation, the senior authors performed routine, annual SUS on professional baseball pitchers from 2002 to 2012 during Major League Baseball Spring Training camp [29]. A total of 736 SUS studies were performed on the dominant and nondominant elbows of 368 pitchers over the 10-year period. SUS was performed by a single, experienced musculoskeletal radiologist using a 13-MHz linear array transducer (Fig. 12.10) with the arm at 30° of flexion. Images were acquired of the dominant and nondominant elbows both with the elbow at rest and with a 15-lb stress applied using a standardized instrumented device (Telos, Marburg, Germany). Measurements included thickness of the ligament, width of the ulnohumeral joint space at rest and with applied stress, and any abnormal echotextural findings within the ligament. A longitudinal comparison was made for all players with more than one SUS performed during the 10-year study period in order to determine if there were any progressive changes with continued time pitching. Players with a subsequent UCL injury had their prior SUS findings compared to the asymptomatic group. Statistical analysis was carried out in order to determine if early abnormal findings were associated with an increased relative risk of future UCL injury. As noted in the senior authors' original 2003 study, the mean thickness of the UCL was greater in the dominant/pitching arm (6.15 mm vs. 4.82 mm, $P < 0.0001$). Although joint space width at rest was not significantly different, with applied stress, the dominant elbow demonstrated significantly greater gapping (4.56 mm vs. 3.72 mm, $p < 0.02$). Similar to previous studies, the dominant arm was also significantly more likely to demonstrate hypoechoic changes (28% vs. 3.5%,

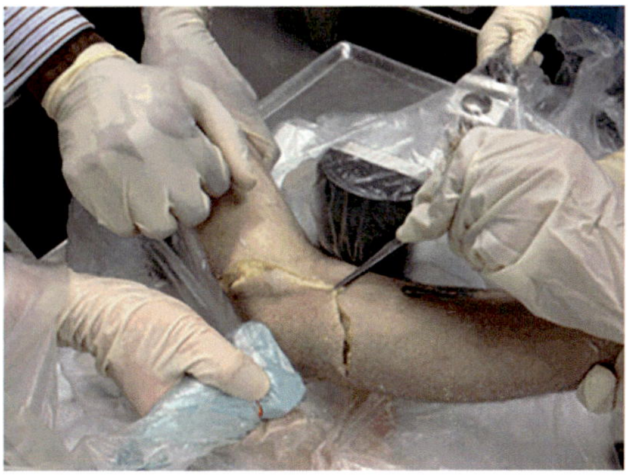

Fig. 12.10 A multifrequency US transducer applied to a cadaveric elbow within a Telos machine for application of standardized valgus stress

$p < 0.001$) and calcifications (24.9% vs. 1.6%, $p < 0.001$). During the 10-year study period, 131 players had multiple SUS evaluations with an average increase in dominant arm ulnohumeral joint gapping of 0.78 mm. Of the 368 pitchers, 12 sustained subsequent ulnar collateral ligament injury during the study period, all of which required surgical reconstruction. When this UCL-injured subgroup was compared to the remaining asymptomatic players, these pitchers had differences trending toward significance in ligament thickness (6.84 mm vs. 6.11 mm), ulnohumeral joint gapping (4.5 mm vs. 4.09 mm), proportion with hypoechoic foci (42% vs. 29.4%), and calcifications (25% vs. 24%). As with the 2003 study, SUS provided a rapid, noninvasive, functional assessment of the UCL in elite pitchers. This study noted that the UCL in the dominant elbow of this patient population is thicker, more likely to have hypoechoic foci and/or calcifications, and is more lax with valgus stress than the nondominant elbow. SUS indicated that a large percentage of these athletes showed increased joint space gapping with stress over time. Furthermore, SUS indicated that pitchers incurring a UCL injury may have increased abnormalities in their dominant elbow compared to asymptomatic players. The 10-year follow-up period did not provide enough UCL injuries to identify a statistically significant difference from dominant to nondominant elbows with respect to the delta between stressed and unstressed ulnohumeral joint gapping. These findings suggest that further longitudinal follow-up with SUS evaluation may ultimately be able to identify athletes with an increased relative risk of future UCL injury.

Our institution has investigated US/SUS for throwing elbow complaints in the youth and adolescent pitching population as well. Atanda et al. have published SUS findings in asymptomatic professional pitchers aged 17–21, divided by both age and experience [30]. In this population, they reported increasing UCL thickness by number of years of professional pitching. Atanda et al. have also published the results of SUS in a youth and adolescent pitching population. In that study, 102 youth and adolescent athletes were divided into two groups based on age (aged 12–14 vs. aged 15–18) [31]. As in the previous study, a thicker UCL on US/SUS correlated with greater time pitching and more pitches per appearance. Cumulatively, these studies suggest that UCL thickening may represent the earliest adaptive or pathologic change to occur in response to the significant stresses of pitching.

The authors have also sought to validate these techniques by performing a series of cadaveric studies. The first cadaveric study performed sequential medial soft-tissue sectioning of 12 freshly frozen cadaveric elbows to determine the relative contribution of each medial elbow stabilizer to valgus elbow stability [13]. The same SUS methodology as utilized in vivo was applied. Medial soft tissue stabilizers including the anterior bundle of the anterior band of the UCL, the posterior bundle of the anterior band of the UCL, the posterior band of the UCL, the transverse band of the UCL, and the flexor-pronator muscle mass were evaluated. The largest change in ulnohumeral joint width with applied valgus stress was measured with the release of the entire anterior band of the UCL (mean 3.4 mm increased in joint space width). Release of either the anterior or posterior bundles of the anterior band of the UCL resulted in an increase in joint space width >1.4 mm. This was significantly greater than the increase in joint space width seen with sectioning of the posterior band of the UCL, the transverse band of the UCL, or the flexor-pronator mass when other stabilizers remained intact. As a result, the authors have adopted a threshold of >1.4 mm of increased joint space width with applied stress in the dominant compared to non-dominant, uninjured extremity to suggest clinically significant injury in vivo.

Using freshly frozen cadavers and the same SUS methodology as the previous study, the authors simulated patterns of partial tearing seen clinically on MRI at different anatomic locations within the anterior band of the UCL. SUS measurements were performed with the elbow fully intact, the anterior band of the UCL partially torn, and the anterior band of the UCL completely torn. Location of the simulated partial tear resulted in different degrees of increased joint space width with applied valgus stress. Some partial tears more closely approximated the intact state whereas others behaved similarly to complete tears. This joins a growing volume of literature suggesting that some partial tear patterns based on anatomic location may be indicated for a trial of nonoperative treatment, while others are indicated for early reconstruction [32–44].

Finally, our institution has reported results of a combined diagnostic approach in 144 baseball players at all levels of competition who had both MRA and SUS preoperatively [45]. The imaging findings of MRA and SUS individually as well as in combination were correlated with surgical findings as the gold standard for diagnosis. MRA alone resulted in sensitivity, specificity, and accuracy for UCL injury of 81%, 91%, and 88%. SUS alone resulted in sensitivity, specificity, and accuracy of 96%, 81%, and 87% for UCL injury. The combination of MRA and SUS results significantly increased sensitivity, specificity, and accuracy for UCL injury to 96%, 99%, and 98%. As a result, we have adopted this combined approach in our own practice.

Algorithm Utilizing Ultrasound for UCL Injury

Evaluation for possible UCL injury in a throwing athlete should always begin with a thorough history and a comprehensive physical examination including the entirety of the kinetic chain. History indicative of UCL injury includes both sudden and insidious medial elbow pain/discomfort and/or decreased throwing effectiveness in terms of velocity and/or control. Physical examination findings consistent with UCL injury include tenderness to palpation along the course of the anterior band of the UCL, a positive moving valgus stress test, and a positive milking test. Plain radiographs remain as an important initial screening tool to rule out acute or chronic osseous injury. If additional imaging is warranted on the basis of history, exam, and initial radiographs, we utilize a combined approach utilizing both MRI/MRA and stress ultrasound to maximize diagnostic accuracy as discussed above. With SUS, we utilize either manual valgus stress with an assistant or a standardized instrumented device (Telos, Marburg, Germany) applying a reproducible 15 decaNewton valgus force across the elbow. The width of the ulnohumeral joint space is measured both with and without this applied valgus stress and compared to the contralateral extremity. In our experience, this is rapid and well tolerated by the patient. Our ultrasonographic examination of the medial elbow begins by seating the patient across from the examiner at a well-padded table such that the arm can be comfortably placed on the table. The arm is positioned semi-extended with a padded bump or rolled towel placed proximal to the elbow as a support. The ultrasound machine is placed on the same side of the table as the patient so that the examiner can easily view the screen. We begin with the arm fully supinated and the probe oriented in the long-axis view at the medial epicondyle. The origin of the common flexor tendon is visualized in both the long-axis and short-axis views to evaluate the full length and width of the tendon and identify the presence of any calcifications, tendinopathy, or tears. The probe is then moved distally to evaluate for edema, hematoma, or muscle tearing within the flexor-pronator muscles. Next, the anterior band of the UCL is identified running from the base of the medial epicondyle to insert broadly on the sublime tubercle of the ulna, viewing it in both the long-axis and short-axis views along its entire length. The thickness of the ligament can be measured as well as the presence of calcifications or hypoechoic foci. The ulnohumeral joint space is measured without stress in a reproducible manner as the distance from the trochlea to the sublime tubercle in the long axis. The use of consistent landmarks is critical for meaningful comparison of the joint space in the unstressed and stressed states. The elbow is then raised off the table and the probe is placed in the short-axis view to bridge across the olecranon and medial epicondyle so that the ulnar nerve can be identified between them. With this orientation, the ulnar nerve appears as an oval structure with a honeycomb or stippled appearance. The elbow can be dynamically flexed and extended while continuing to visualize the nerve in order to identify any subluxation. The long-axis view can then identify constriction as areas of narrowing of the nerve fascicles that result in an hourglass appearance.

The stress ultrasound portion of the examination next assesses medial elbow stability and thus the functional competency of the UCL by measuring the ulnohumeral joint space with an applied valgus stress. This is particularly useful when UCL injury is suspected by history and physical examination, but conventional imaging remains inconclusive or equivocal. This portion of the examination benefits from an assistant to stress the arm. We perform joint space measurements in 30 degrees of elbow flexion where the anterior band of the UCL has been demonstrated to become the primary restraint against valgus stress. Both the dominant and nondominant arms are measured in this manner for comparison. Based on our prior research, the mean ulnohumeral joint space under stress in the nondominant elbow of a pitcher is 3.72 mm, while the dominant arm tends to have a wider mean joint space under stress of 4.56 mm [29]. As noted above, we begin by measuring the joint space in the unstressed state using standardized landmarks in the long-axis view. Next, a 15 daN valgus stress is applied across the elbow utilizing a standardized device (Telos, Marburg, Germany) or manually by an assistant if a standardized device is unavailable. Joint space width in the unstressed and stressed states is measured three times for each elbow and mean values are calculated. The change in joint space width between the unstressed and stressed states, the delta, is calculated by subtracting the mean joint space in the unstressed state from the mean joint space under valgus stress. Based on our previous in vivo and cadaveric experience, we utilize a cutoff value for the delta greater than 1.5 mm and a substantial difference between arms as suggestive of UCL injury.

Based on our institution's cumulative experience on imaging of the elbow in the throwing athlete, the authors have established a clinical algorithm (Fig. 12.11) for the diagnosis and management of medial elbow injury in this population.

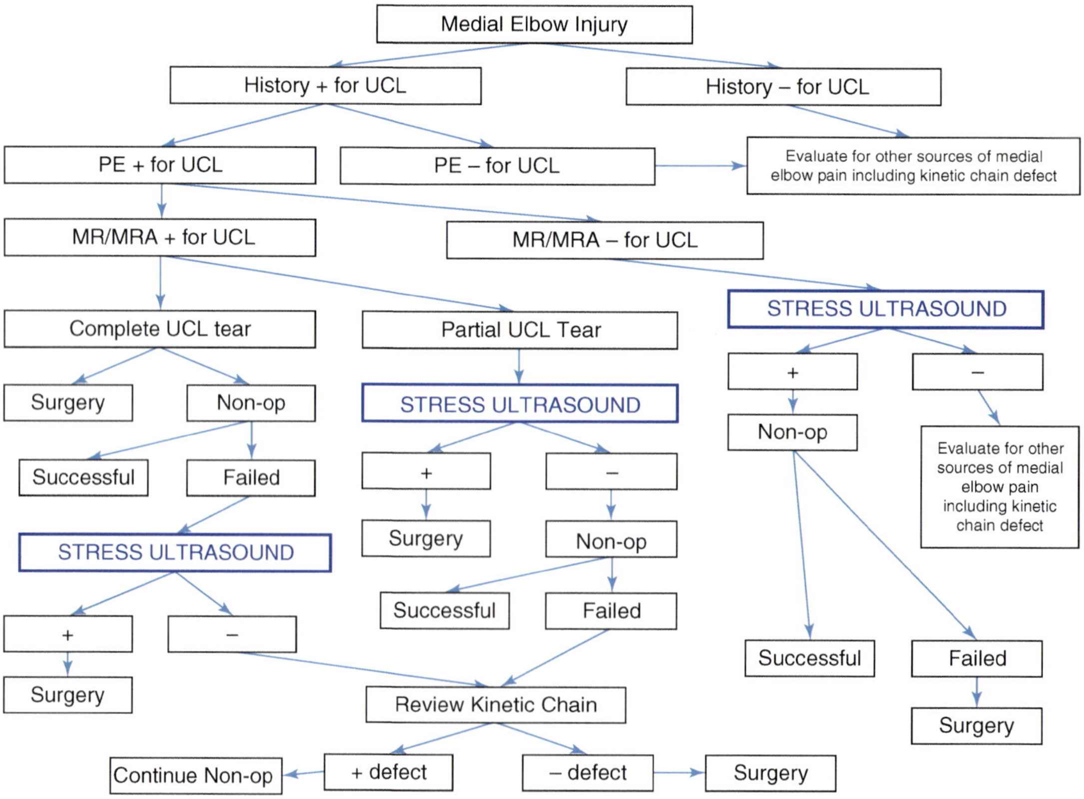

Fig. 12.11 Clinical algorithm for the diagnosis and management of ulnar collateral ligament injury including appropriate use of stress ultrasound (SUS)

Case Examples

Acute, Partial UCL Tear

A 25-year-old, right-hand dominant Minor League Baseball player had 6 months of progressive, right medial elbow pain and stiffness. He did not miss any scheduled pitching starts, but noted a progressive increase in symptoms. During his last outing, he noted a sharp increase in medial elbow pain and was unable to continue. Examination of the involved elbow revealed mild swelling with range of motion from 7° to 135° with full pronation and supination. Resisted wrist flexion and forearm pronation caused no significant increased tenderness. He was neurovascularly intact with a negative Tinel's sign at the cubital tunnel and a negative elbow flexion test. He had increased pain with valgus stress at 30° and a moderately positive dynamic milking test. Plain X-rays showed no significant abnormalities while MR arthrogram showed a partial tear of the deep portion of the anterior band of the UCL (Fig. 12.12). SUS was performed and showed an increase in dominant elbow ulnohumeral joint space width of 3.3 mm with stress from the resting, unstressed position (Fig. 12.13a, b). The nondominant elbow had an increase in ulnohumeral joint space width of 0.1 mm with stress from the resting position (Fig. 12.13c, d). The dominant to nondominant difference was 3.2 mm. Because of the acute and chronic history of a partial UCL tear with clear-cut instability on exam and positive ultrasound findings, surgical treatment was recommended. At the time of surgery, he was found to have a significant undersurface tear of the anterior band of the UCL of the elbow.

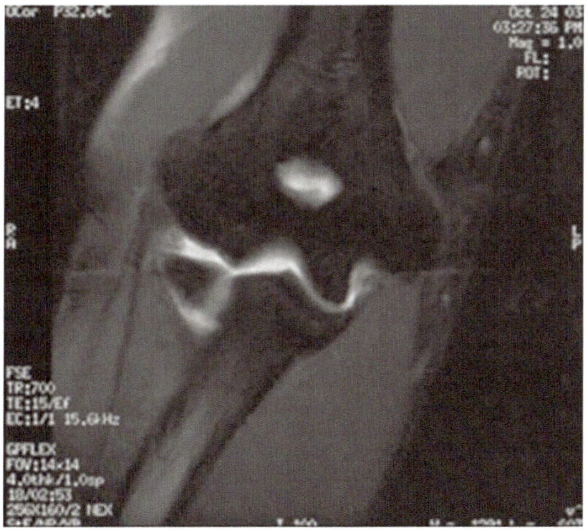

Fig. 12.12 MR arthrogram demonstrating partial tear of the deep portion of the anterior band of the UCL

Failure of Nonoperative Treatment for UCL Tear

An 18-year-old, right-hand dominant elite high school pitcher noted the acute onset of right medial elbow pain while pitching. He was unable to continue pitching. His examination revealed minimal swelling, range of motion from 10° to 130° with 80° of pronation and supination. Resisted wrist flexion and forearm pronation caused minimal increased tenderness. He was neurovascularly intact with a negative Tinel's sign at the cubital tunnel and a negative elbow flexion test. He had increased pain with valgus stress at 30° and a positive dynamic milking test. Plain X-rays were normal, and MRI revealed a partial tear of the anterior band of the UCL (Fig. 12.14). Nonoperative treatment was initiated including 6 weeks of no throwing and a focused shoulder, core, lower extremity, and aerobic conditioning program. A tossing program was begun at 6 weeks, and he progressed until developing recurrent pain while throwing from the mound. A stress ultrasound was performed and demonstrated an increase in dominant elbow ulnohumeral joint space width of 3.7 mm with stress from the resting, unstressed position (Fig. 12.15a, b). The nondominant elbow had an increase in ulnohumeral joint space width of 0.3 mm with stress from the resting position (Fig. 12.15c, d). The dominant to nondominant difference was 3.4 mm. Because of the failure of nonoperative treatment with positive stress ultrasound findings, surgical treatment was recommended. At the time of surgery, he was found to have a significant undersurface tear of the anterior band of the UCL of the elbow.

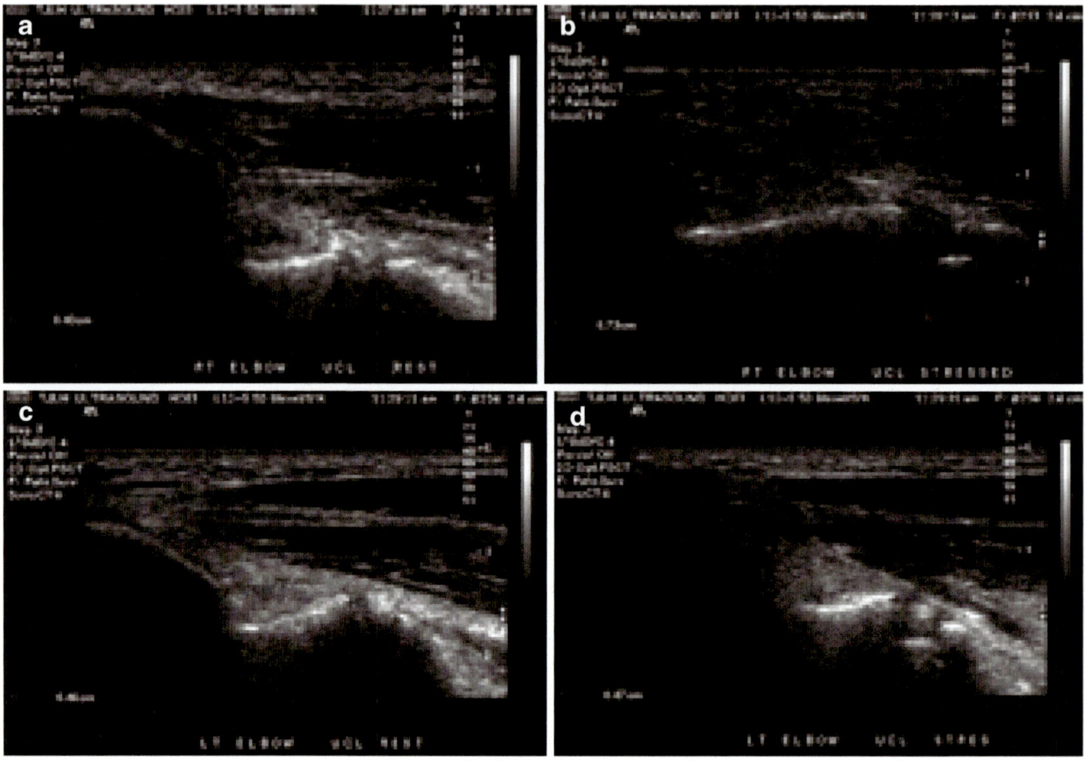

Fig. 12.13 Stress ultrasound demonstrating (**a**), ulnohumeral joint space width in the injured, dominant elbow at rest (4.0 mm); (**b**) significant increased ulnohumeral joint gapping (7.3 mm, delta = 3.3 mm) in the injured, dominant elbow with the application of valgus stress; (**c**) ulnohumeral joint space width in the nondominant elbow at rest (4.6 mm); (**d**) minimal increased ulnohumeral joint gapping (4.7 mm, delta = 0.1 mm) in the nondominant elbow with valgus stress

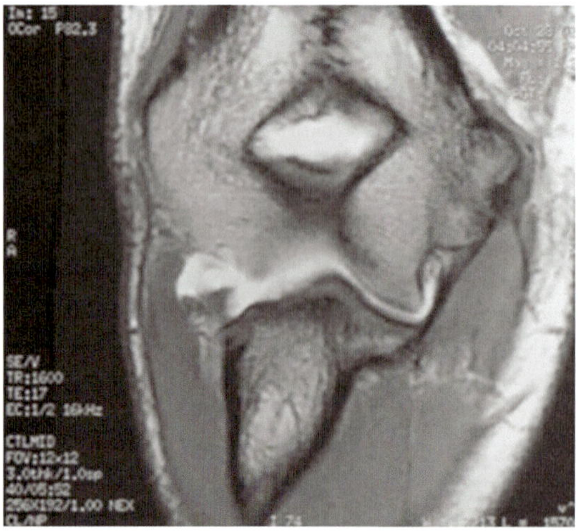

Fig. 12.14 MR arthrogram demonstrating partial tear of the deep portion of the anterior band of the UCL

Revision UCL with Post-op Pain Secondary to Kinetic Chain Deficits

A 19-year-old, right-hand dominant elite college javelin thrower developed acute right medial elbow pain while throwing in an international competition. He was unable to complete the competition. His examination revealed moderate swelling, with a range of motion from 12° to 125° and with 60° of pronation and supination. Resisted wrist flexion and forearm pronation caused moderate increased tenderness. He was neurovascularly intact with a negative Tinel's sign at the cubital tunnel and a negative elbow flexion test. He had significantly increased pain with valgus stress at 30° and a positive dynamic milking test. Plain X-rays were normal and MRI revealed a

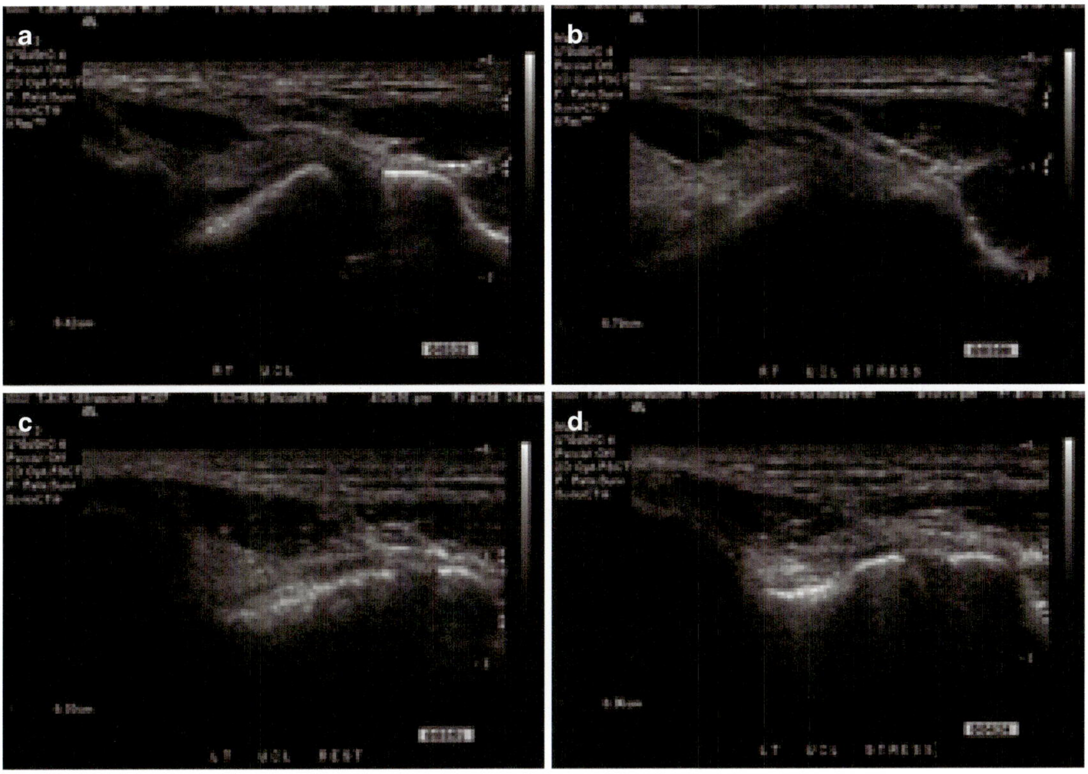

Fig. 12.15 Stress ultrasound demonstrating (**a**) ulnohumeral joint space width in the injured, dominant elbow at rest (4.2 mm); (**b**) significant increased ulnohumeral joint gapping (7.9 mm, delta = 3.7 mm) in the injured, dominant elbow with the application of valgus stress; (**c**) ulnohumeral joint space width in the nondominant elbow at rest (3.3 mm); (**d**) minimal increased ulnohumeral joint gapping (3.6 mm, delta = 0.3 mm) in the nondominant elbow with valgus stress

complete tear of the anterior band of the UCL. He underwent a right elbow UCL reconstruction and his initial rehabilitation progressed smoothly. At 8 months postoperatively, he developed vague recurrent right medial elbow pain while tossing. On examination, he had no significant swelling. His range of motion was from 5° to 145°, and he had no tenderness with resisted wrist flexion and forearm pronation. He was neurovascularly intact with a negative Tinel's sign and flexion pronator test. He had no significant pain with valgus stress at 30° and an equivocal milking test. An MR arthrogram demonstrated no clear-cut recurrent injury (Fig. 12.16). A stress ultrasound was performed and demonstrated an increase in dominant elbow ulnohumeral joint space width of 0.6 mm

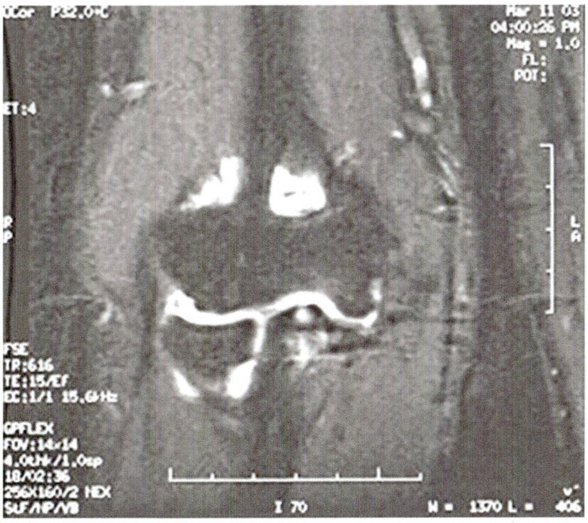

Fig. 12.16 MR arthogram demonstrating no recurrent injury to the UCL reconstruction

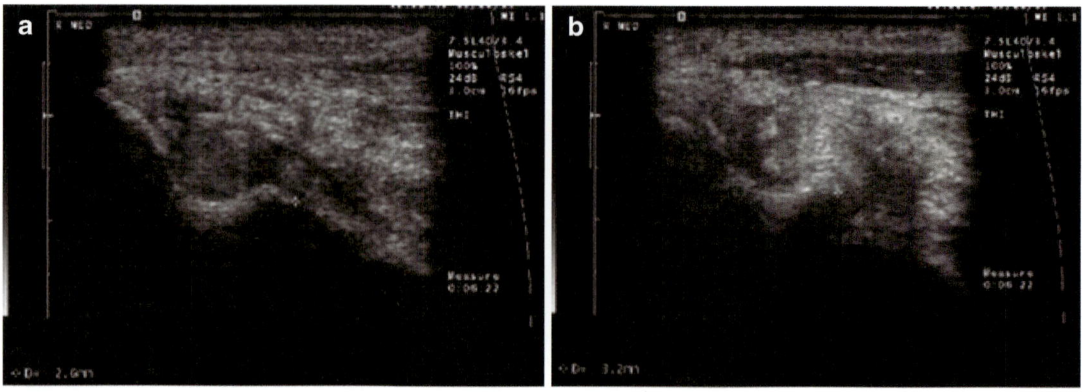

Fig. 12.17 Stress ultrasound demonstrating (**a**) ulnohumeral joint space width of 2.6 mm in the reconstructed elbow at rest; (**b**) minimal increased ulnohumeral joint gapping in the reconstructed elbow to 3.2 mm with the application of valgus stress (delta of 0.6 mm)

with stress from the resting, unstressed position (Fig. 12.17a) to the stressed position (Fig. 12.17b). The nondominant elbow had an increase in ulnohumeral joint space width of 0.3 mm with stress from the resting position. The dominant to nondominant difference was 0.3 mm. Because of the nonfocal nature of his complaints and the nonspecific findings on exam and normal SUS, nonoperative treatment was continued. A thorough evaluation identified deficiencies in the kinetic chain and after focused shoulder, core, lower extremity, aerobic conditioning, and a throwing mechanics program, his symptoms resolved. He was subsequently able to successfully return to competition at an elite level.

Summary

Injury of the ulnar collateral ligament is common in overhead throwing athletes leading to significant functional limitations and disability. The treatment of UCL injury requires a lengthy rehabilitation prior to return to full activity. Unfortunately, UCL injury can be diagnostically challenging for even the most experienced orthopedic surgeon. Traditionally, orthopedists have utilized static imaging studies such as plain X-ray, stress radiography, and MRI/MRA, but these are time-consuming, costly, and may be accompanied by radiation exposure. Ultrasonography complements conventional imaging by providing a rapid, low-cost, noninvasive, dynamic assessment of medial elbow stability including visualization and evaluation of the anterior band of the UCL. Currently, stress ultrasound can be particularly beneficial when evaluating partial tears of the UCL, athletes who have failed nonoperative treatment, or in the setting of recurrent injury. Stress ultrasonography adds to the diagnostic evaluation of ulnar collateral ligament injury in the overhead throwing athlete. Furthermore, continued use and long-term evaluation of stress ultrasonography may allow it to be used as a predictor of possible risk for ulnar collateral ligament injury in currently asymptomatic patients.

References

1. Aguinaldo AL, Chambers H. Correlation of throwing mechanics with elbow valgus load in adult baseball pitchers. Am J Sports Med. 2009;37(10):2043–8. https://doi.org/10.1177/0363546509336721.
2. Chen F, Rokito A, Jobe F. Medial elbow problems in the overhead-throwing athlete. J Am Acad Orthop Surg. 2001;9(2):99–113.
3. Timmerman LA, Schwartz ML, Andrews JR. Preoperative evaluation of the ulnar collateral ligament by magnetic resonance imaging and computed tomography arthrography. Am J Sports Med. 1994;22(1):26–32. https://doi.org/10.1177/036354659402200105.

4. Bowerman JW, McDonnell EJ. Radiology of athletic injuries: baseball. Radiology. 1975;116(3):611–5. https://doi.org/10.1148/116.3.611.
5. Cain EL, Dugas JR, Wolf RS, Andrews JR. Elbow injuries in throwing athletes: a current concepts review. Am J Sports Med. 2003;31(4):621–35. https://doi.org/10.1177/03635465030310042601.
6. Ciccotti MG. Medial collateral ligament instability and ulnar neuritis in the athlete's elbow. Instr Course Lect. 1999;48:383–91.
7. Mulligan SA, Schwartz ML, Broussard MF, Andrews JR. Heterotopic calcification and tears of the ulnar collateral ligament. Am J Roentgenol. 2000;175(4):1099–102. https://doi.org/10.2214/ajr.175.4.1751099.
8. Popovic N, Ferrara MA, Daenen B, Georis P, Lemaire R. Imaging overuse injury of the elbow in professional team handball players: a bilateral comparison using plain films, stress radiography, ultrasound, and magnetic resonance imaging. Int J Sports Med. 2002;22(01):60–7. https://doi.org/10.1055/s-2001-11333.
9. Wright RW, Steger-May K, Klein SE. Radiographic findings in the shoulder and elbow of Major League Baseball pitchers. Am J Sports Med. 2007;35(11):1839–43. https://doi.org/10.1177/0363546507304493.
10. Ellenbecker TS, Mattalino AJ, Elam EA, Caplinger RA. Medial elbow joint laxity in professional baseball pitchers. Am J Sports Med. 1998;26(3):420–4. https://doi.org/10.1177/03635465980260031301.
11. Joyner PW, Bruce J, Hess R, Mates A, Mills FB IV, Andrews JR. Magnetic resonance imaging–based classification for ulnar collateral ligament injuries of the elbow. J Shoulder Elb Surg. 2016;25(10):1710–6. https://doi.org/10.1016/j.jse.2016.05.006.
12. Cohen SB, Valko C, Zoga A, Dodson CC, Ciccotti MG. Posteromedial elbow impingement: magnetic resonance imaging findings in overhead throwing athletes and results of arthroscopic treatment. Arthrosc J Arthrosc Relat Surg. 2011;27(10):1364–70. https://doi.org/10.1016/j.arthro.2011.06.012.
13. Ciccotti MC, Hammoud S, Dodson CC, Cohen SB, Nazarian LN, Ciccotti MG. Stress ultrasound evaluation of medial elbow instability in a cadaveric model. Am J Sports Med. 2014;42(10):2463–9. https://doi.org/10.1177/0363546514542805.
14. Gustas CN, Lee KS. Multimodality imaging of the painful elbow. Imaging Athlete. 2016;54(5):817–39. https://doi.org/10.1016/j.rcl.2016.04.005.
15. Sampath SC, Sampath SC, Bredella MA. Magnetic resonance imaging of the elbow: a structured approach. Sports Health. 2013;5(1):34–49. https://doi.org/10.1177/1941738112467941.
16. Lee GA, Katz SD, Lazarus MD. Elbow Valgus stress radiography in an uninjured population. Am J Sports Med. 1998;26(3):425–7. https://doi.org/10.1177/03635465980260031401.
17. Rijke AM, Goitz HT, McCue FC, Andrews JR, Berr SS. Stress radiography of the medial elbow ligaments. Radiology. 1994;191(1):213–6. https://doi.org/10.1148/radiology.191.1.8134574.
18. Nazarian LN, McShane JM, Ciccotti MG, O'Kane PL, Harwood MI. Dynamic US of the anterior band of the ulnar collateral ligament of the elbow in asymptomatic Major League Baseball pitchers. Radiology. 2003;227(1):149–54. https://doi.org/10.1148/radiol.2271020288.
19. Brunton LM, Anderson MW, Pannunzio ME, Khanna AJ, Chhabra AB. Magnetic resonance imaging of the elbow: update on current techniques and indications. J Hand Surg Am. 2006;31(6):1001–11. https://doi.org/10.1016/j.jhsa.2006.04.006.
20. Fritz RC. MR imaging of the elbow. An update. Radiol Clin North Am. 1997;35(1):117–44.
21. Cotten A, Jacobson J, Brossmann J, et al. Collateral ligaments of the elbow: conventional MR imaging and MR arthrography with coronal oblique plane and elbow flexion. Radiology. 1997;204(3):806–12. https://doi.org/10.1148/radiology.204.3.9280264.
22. Kaplan LJ, Potter HG. MR imaging of ligament injuries to the elbow. Imaging Up Extrem. 2006;44(4):583–94. https://doi.org/10.1016/j.rcl.2006.04.007.
23. Schwartz ML, al-Zahrani S, Morwessel RM, Andrews JR. Ulnar collateral ligament injury in the throwing athlete: evaluation with saline-enhanced MR arthrography. Radiology. 1995;197(1):297–9. https://doi.org/10.1148/radiology.197.1.7568841.
24. Cooperberg PL, Tsang I, Truelove L, Knickerbocker WJ. Gray scale ultrasound in the evaluation of rheumatoid arthritis of the knee. Radiology. 1978;126(3):759–63. https://doi.org/10.1148/126.3.759.
25. De Smet AA, Winter TC, Best TM, Bernhardt DT. Dynamic sonography with valgus stress to assess elbow ulnar collateral ligament injury in baseball pitchers. Skelet Radiol. 2002;31(11):671–6. https://doi.org/10.1007/s00256-002-0558-0.
26. Wood N, Konin JG, Nofsinger C. Diagnosis of an ulnar collateral ligament tear using musculoskeletal ultrasound in a collegiate baseball pitcher: a case report. N Am J Sports Phys Ther. 2010;5(4):227–33.
27. Sasaki J, Takahara M, Ogino T, Kashiwa H, Ishigaki D, Kanauchi Y. Ultrasonographic assessment of the ulnar collateral ligament and medial elbow laxity in college baseball players. J Bone Joint Surg Am. 2002;84(4):525–31.
28. Jacobson JA, Propeck T, Jamadar DA, Jebson PJL, Hayes CW. US of the anterior bundle of the ulnar collateral ligament: findings in five cadaver elbows with MR arthrographic and anatomic comparison—initial observations. Radiology. 2003;227(2):561–6. https://doi.org/10.1148/radiol.2272020462.
29. Ciccotti MG, Atanda A, Nazarian LN, Dodson CC, Holmes L, Cohen SB. Stress sonography of the ulnar collateral ligament of the elbow in professional baseball pitchers. Am J Sports Med. 2014;42(3):544–51. https://doi.org/10.1177/0363546513516592.
30. Atanda A, Buckley PS, Hammoud S, Cohen SB, Nazarian LN, Ciccotti MG. Early anatomic changes

of the ulnar collateral ligament identified by stress ultrasound of the elbow in young professional baseball pitchers. Am J Sports Med. 2015;43(12):2943–9. https://doi.org/10.1177/0363546515605042.
31. Atanda A, Averill LW, Wallace M, Niiler TA, Nazarian LN, Ciccotti MG. Factors related to increased ulnar collateral ligament thickness on stress sonography of the elbow in asymptomatic youth and adolescent baseball pitchers. Am J Sports Med. 2016;44(12):3179–87. https://doi.org/10.1177/0363546516661010.
32. Hurwit DJ, Garcia GH, Liu J, Altchek DW, Romeo A, Dines J. Management of ulnar collateral ligament injury in throwing athletes: a survey of the American Shoulder and Elbow Surgeons. J Shoulder Elb Surg. 2017;26(11):2023–8. https://doi.org/10.1016/j.jse.2017.08.005.
33. Deal JB, Smith E, Heard W, O'Brien MJ, Savoie FH 3rd. Platelet-rich plasma for primary treatment of partial ulnar collateral ligament tears: MRI correlation with results. Orthop J Sports Med. 2017;5(11):2325967117738238. https://doi.org/10.1177/2325967117738238.
34. Dines J, Williams P, ElAttrache N. Platelet-rich plasma can be used to successfully treat elbow ulnar collateral ligament insufficiency in high-level throwers. Am J Orthop. 2016;45(4):296–300.
35. Ford GM, Genuario J, Kinkartz J, Githens T, Noonan T. Return-to-play outcomes in professional baseball players after medial ulnar collateral ligament injuries: comparison of operative versus nonoperative treatment based on magnetic resonance imaging findings. Am J Sports Med. 2016;44(3):723–8. https://doi.org/10.1177/0363546515621756.
36. Podesta L, Crow SA, Volkmer D, Bert T, Yocum LA. Treatment of partial ulnar collateral ligament tears in the elbow with platelet-rich plasma. Am J Sports Med. 2013;41(7):1689–94. https://doi.org/10.1177/0363546513487979.
37. Rettig AC, Sherrill C, Snead DS, Mendler JC, Mieling P. Nonoperative treatment of ulnar collateral ligament injuries in throwing athletes. Am J Sports Med. 2001;29(1):15–7. https://doi.org/10.1177/03635465010290010601.
38. Frangiamore SJ, Lynch TS, Vaughn MD, et al. Magnetic resonance imaging predictors of failure in the nonoperative management of ulnar collateral ligament injuries in professional baseball pitchers. Am J Sports Med. 2017;45(8):1783–9. https://doi.org/10.1177/0363546517699832.
39. Ramkumar PN, Frangiamore SJ, Navarro SM, et al. Interobserver and intraobserver reliability of an MRI-based classification system for injuries to the ulnar collateral ligament. Am J Sports Med. 2018;46(11):2755–60. https://doi.org/10.1177/0363546518786970.
40. Ramkumar PN, Haeberle HS, Navarro SM, Frangiamore SJ, Farrow LD, Schickendantz MS. Clinical utility of an MRI-based classification system for operative versus nonoperative management of ulnar collateral ligament tears: a 2-year follow-up study. Orthop J Sports Med. 2019;7(4):2325967119839785. https://doi.org/10.1177/2325967119839785.
41. Ramkumar PN, Haeberle HS, Navarro SM, Frangiamore SJ, Farrow LD, Schickendantz MS. Prognostic utility of a magnetic resonance imaging-based classification for operative versus nonoperative management of ulnar collateral ligament tears: one-year follow-up. J Shoulder Elb Surg. 2019;28(6):1159–65. https://doi.org/10.1016/j.jse.2018.11.063.
42. Buckley PS, Morris ER, Robbins CM, et al. Variations in blood supply from proximal to distal in the ulnar collateral ligament of the elbow: a qualitative descriptive cadaveric study. Am J Sports Med. 2019;47(5):1117–23. https://doi.org/10.1177/0363546519831693.
43. Frangiamore SJ, Morris ER, Scibetta AC, et al. Evaluation of endothelial and vascular-derived progenitor cell populations in the proximal and distal UCL of the elbow: a comparative study. Orthop J Sports Med. 2018;6(6):2325967118777825. https://doi.org/10.1177/2325967118777825.
44. Frangiamore SJ, Bigart K, Nagle T, Colbrunn R, Millis A, Schickendantz MS. Biomechanical analysis of elbow medial ulnar collateral ligament tear location and its effect on rotational stability. J Shoulder Elb Surg. 2018;27(11):2068–76. https://doi.org/10.1016/j.jse.2018.05.020.
45. Roedl JB, Gonzalez FM, Zoga AC, et al. Potential utility of a combined approach with US and MR arthrography to image medial elbow pain in baseball players. Radiology. 2016;279(3):827–37. https://doi.org/10.1148/radiol.2015151256.

13 The Conservative Treatment of Ulnar Collateral Ligament Injuries

Frank J. Alexander, Fiona E. Nugent, and Christopher S. Ahmad

Introduction

Nonoperative treatment is often the first step in the management of ulnar collateral ligament (UCL) injuries, though many factors influence decision-making. Specific features of the clinical history, injury mechanism, physical exam, and imaging help guide the decision to pursue nonoperative treatment. Education, injury prevention, and realistic patient expectations should be emphasized as important counselling aspects of nonoperative treatment.

Treatment is aimed at reducing pain and inflammation prior to initiating active rehabilitation. A period of throwing cessation may be combined with biologic treatment to accelerate and/or improve UCL healing and associated injuries such a flexor muscle strain. Rehabilitation for UCL injuries involves global conditioning of the entire kinetic chain with correction of modifiable UCL injury risk factors. Throwing athletes should undergo a supervised program of progressive throwing that emphasizes proper mechanics and technique. The outcomes of nonoperative management of UCL injury are often satisfactory in well-selected patients with optimal injury features.

Treatments typically include physical therapy, anti-inflammatory medications, and the use of biologic injections. Biologic use has become a popular treatment in the athletic population but with controversial evidence. Physical exam, imaging, seasonal/career timing, and a player's future aspirations are just a few criteria that factor into decision-making. In the setting of recurrent sprains or failure of nonoperative treatment, the desire to continue playing, surgical intervention is indicated.

Clinical History

The majority of patients who experience medial elbow pain and are overhead throwers sustain UCL injury due to the repetitive valgus stress on the medial elbow. Pitchers can exert a valgus load of up to 60–65 Nm on their UCL during cocking and acceleration phases of pitching which approaches or exceeds normal UCL strength [1]. As such, baseball players injure their UCL often and are unable to return to high-effort throwing if their UCL is compromised.

Throwers may present with different features of medial elbow pain. Some may complain of a

F. J. Alexander (✉) · F. E. Nugent
Center for Shoulder, Elbow, and Sports Medicine, Columbia University Irving Medical Center, New York, NY, USA
e-mail: Fa2366@cumc.columbia.edu

C. S. Ahmad
New York Yankees, Center for Shoulder, Elbow, and Sports Medicine, Columbia University Irving Medical Center, New York, NY, USA

J. S. Dines et al. (eds.), *Elbow Ulnar Collateral Ligament Injury*,
https://doi.org/10.1007/978-3-030-69567-5_13

single pop at the medial elbow, whereas others may have slow progressive stiffness and/or difficulty warming up. They may describe pain in the acceleration phase of pitching, often associated with tingling in their fingers, and loss of command and/or velocity. Additionally, players may describe the inability to throw at higher effort levels and "not being able to hit the next gear."

History taking should ascertain modifiable risk factors that may be managed as part of the nonoperative treatment. Examples include fastball velocity, recent increase in throwing volume, change in throwing mechanics, working on new types of pitches, use of velocity enhancement programs and weighted balls, and injury to other areas in their body that may affect kinetic chain.

Physical Examination

Global musculoskeletal assessment of the patient must be emphasized as problems in the kinetic chain are intimately connected to the upper extremity. A general physical examination of the upper extremity should include cervical spine and bilateral shoulder range of motion, strength testing, and provocative maneuvers including Spurling's and O'Brien's. Additionally, the extremities should be examined for posture, asymmetry, atrophy, edema, or ecchymosis. The examiner should take time to evaluate the scapula for periscapular muscular tone and bulk as well as normal scapulothoracic rhythm during functional shoulder motion. Scapular dysfunction is commonly found in throwing athletes and should be addressed during rehabilitation [2]. Furthermore, the shoulder should be evaluated for glenohumeral internal rotation deficit (GIRD), which has been identified as a significant risk factor associated with UCL injury [3]. Any deficits in shoulder rotation should be corrected through rehabilitation and reassessed in conjunction with conservative treatment of UCL injury.

The bilateral elbows should be examined for active and passive range of motion. Painful limitations in motion can be indicative of posterior–medial impingement, loose bodies, or contracture and may alter the treatment plan. Provocative testing such as an arm bar or bounce test should be performed toward the end of the examination as they may elicit increased pain and compromise the remainder of the exam. Laterally, the radiocapitellar joint should be palpated and assessed for crepitus, as youth baseball players are susceptible to osteochondritis dissecans.

At the medial elbow, the ulnar nerve should be located, assessed for hypermobility, and for full motor and sensory function. The UCL originates at the medial epicondyle proximally, and inserts at the sublime tubercle distally. These anatomic sites along with the midsubstance of the ligament should be palpated, as tenderness may be indicative of pathology. The moving valgus stress test may indicate partial or complete tear of the UCL [1]. Injury to the flexor mass may produce pain anterior and distal to the medial epicondyle, and may elicit pain and weakness with resisted forearm pronation. Recently, Hodgins et al. [4] concluded that flexor mass injuries may be a significant risk factor for subsequent upper extremity injuries including UCL tears.

Imaging

Patients should receive standard elbow anteroposterior (AP), lateral, and oblique radiographs. Radiographs can identify avulsion fractures at either the medial epicondyle or the sublime tubercle, which have a poor prognosis with nonoperative care [5, 6]. Radiographs can also evaluate for chronic UCL insufficiency as evidenced by calcifications within the ligament (Fig. 13.1) and posterior–medial olecranon osteophytes. Osteophytes at the olecranon can be suggestive of ligament insufficiency due to valgus extension overload [7, 8]. If injury to the UCL is suspected, valgus stress radiographs can evaluate for the presence of ulnohumeral medial joint gapping [9, 10]. Gapping of greater than 0.5 mm when compared to the contralateral elbow has been shown in complete and large partial tears [11]. Valgus stress testing is more commonly performed with ultrasound currently.

Patients with suspected UCL injury benefit from magnetic resonance imaging (MRI) of the

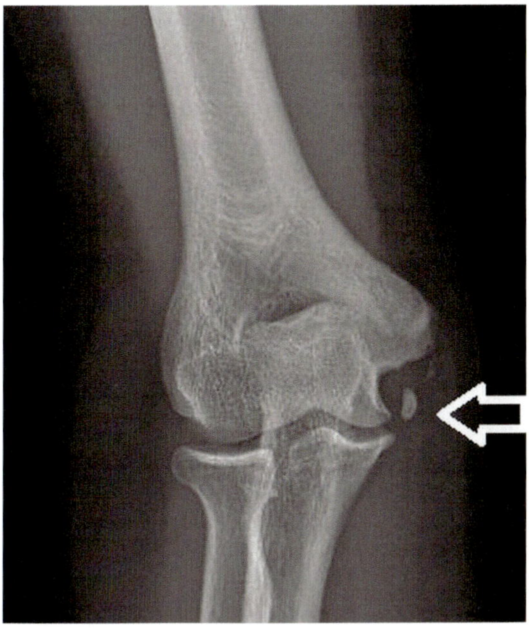

Fig. 13.1 X-ray demonstrating calcification within the UCL (arrow), indicative of chronic changes

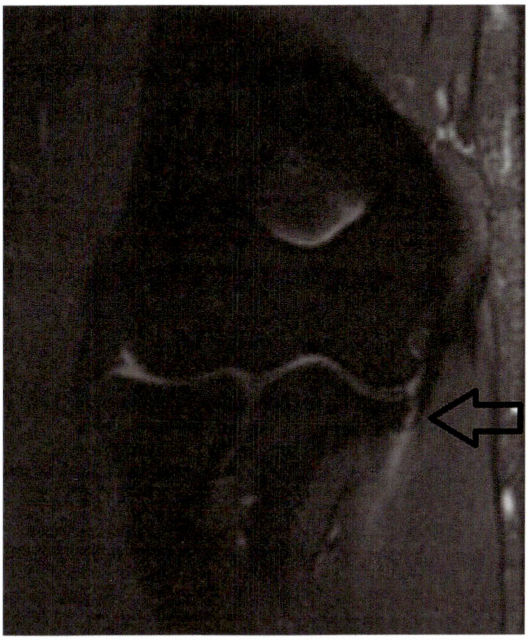

Fig. 13.2 MRI scan indicating a distal tear of the UCL at the sublime tubercle (arrow)

elbow to allow for evaluation of chronic changes and characterization of the UCL [12]. In addition to the presence of partial- and full-thickness tears of the UCL, MRI also reveals concomitant pathology such as loose bodies, flexor-pronator tendinopathy, and posteromedial ulnohumeral chondromalacia [13]. MRI can also identify chronic changes to the UCL including ligament thickening and signal changes [10, 14]. Furthermore, MRI can identify tear patterns with a poor prognosis, such as sublime tubercle avulsions (Fig. 13.2) [15]. MRI has also been shown to aid in predicting the outcome of nonoperative treatment. A study by Kim et al. [16] demonstrated that low-grade partial tears and tears-in-continuity—specifically, those with low/intermediate MR signal intensity of the UCL on fat-suppressed T2-weighted images—were associated with successful nonsurgical rehabilitation in a cohort of 39 baseball players. MR arthrography can improve the diagnosis of partial undersurface tears [17, 18].

Patients with a history and physical examination suggestive of a UCL injury can be evaluated under dynamic stress ultrasound. Ultrasound allows for the application of dynamic forces to evaluate ulnar humeral gapping with valgus stress, and is both cost and time effective [19–22]. Ultrasound can evaluate for morphologic changes of the UCL, such as ligament thickening and ligament calcification, and can determine UCL incompetence. Dynamic stress ultrasound has demonstrated that athletes with medial-sided elbow pain were more likely to have increased ulnohumeral gapping than those athletes without elbow pain and as compared to the contralateral side [19, 23].

Treatment Options

Injection Treatments

The use of corticosteroid injections is highly discouraged for treatment of UCL injuries due to the concern for its detrimental effect on tissue integrity. The literature has widely favored biologic augmentation, specifically the use of platelet-rich plasma (PRP) for the treatment of UCL pathology.

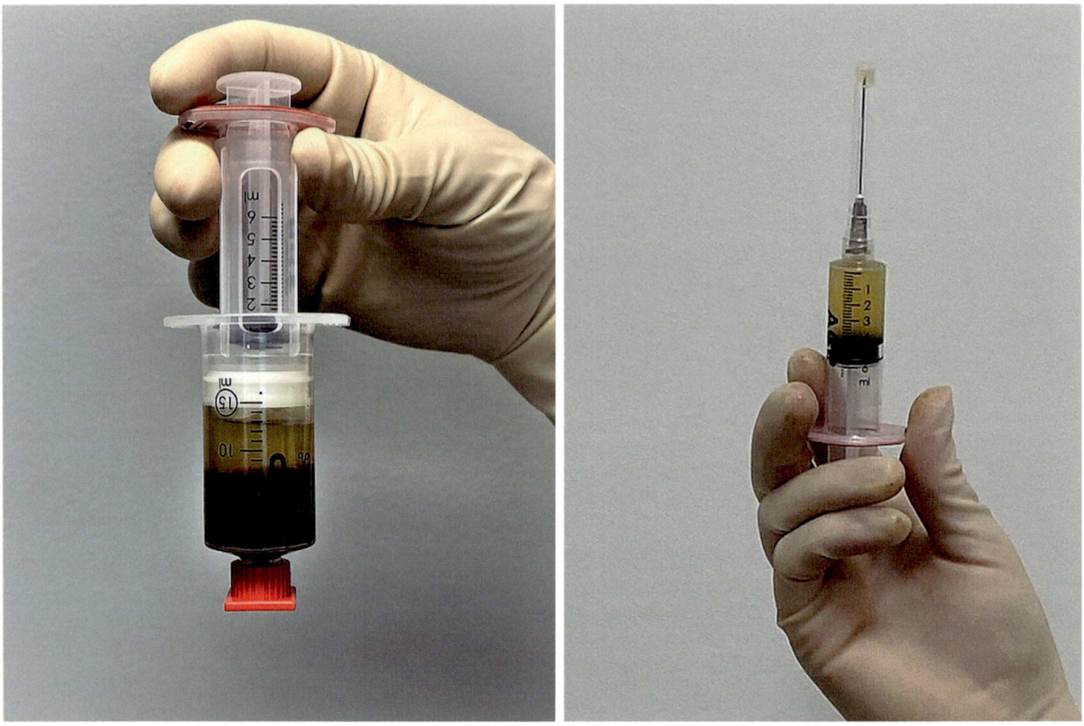

Fig. 13.3 PRP separated from the oxygen-carrying red blood cells

PRP uses autologous platelets in high concentrations that are injected over an area of injury, affecting the release of growth factors and biologic factors to stimulate healing. The process of a PRP injection can be performed in a same-day office visit. Blood is drawn from the patient and spun in a centrifuge. The PRP is separated from the oxygen-carrying red blood cells (Fig. 13.3). PRP is then injected over the superficial aspect of the damaged portion of the ligament, bathing it in the solution under ultrasound guidance for accuracy (Fig. 13.4).

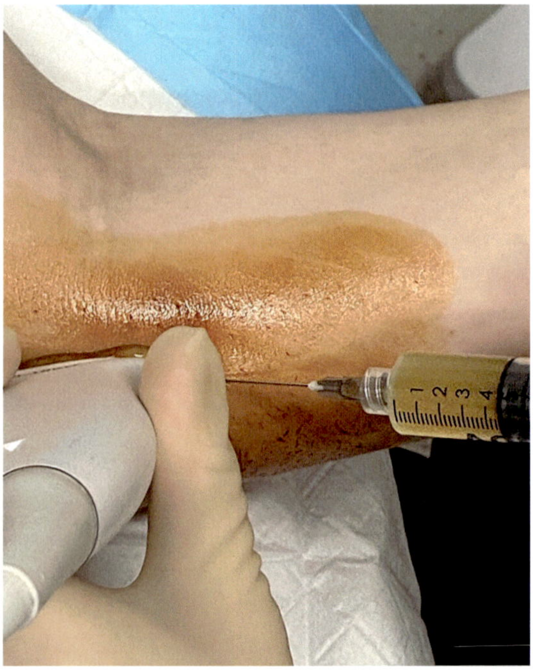

Fig. 13.4 A PRP injection being administered to the UCL with ultrasound guidance

Few complications have been reported with the use of PRP injections and it is readily available, making it a favorable treatment modality for athletes. Consensus is lacking regarding the ideal number of PRP injections necessary or which family of PRP is most beneficial. Different variations of PRP include pure platelet-rich plasma, leukocyte- and platelet-rich plasma, pure platelet-rich fibrin, or leukocyte- and platelet-rich fibrin [24]. Kato et al. [25] favored the use of pure platelet-rich plasma to avoid the anabolic and catabolic effects associated with leukocyte use which may cause ligament and tendon degradation.

There is little evidence supporting the use of mesenchymal stem cells for orthopedic injuries in humans. A study in rat models published in 2016 did have promising results with primed mesenchymal stem cells injected into the medial collateral ligament (MCL) that resulted in improved ligament healing compared to control groups [26]. Much more research and evidence are needed before mesenchymal stem cells are utilized as a treatment modality for UCL injuries.

Principles of Rehabilitation

Physical therapy performed during nonoperative treatment of UCL injuries follows a similar construct to a rehab program following UCL surgery. The primary goals are to decrease pain and inflammation and increase elbow range of motion and strength. Throughout the rehab process, special attention is also paid to the throwing shoulder. The entire kinetic chain is enhanced by identifying and correcting any flaws that may be present.

Physical therapists and athletic trainers initially select exercises that avoid valgus stress but increase the strength of the flexor pronator mass. As the rehab progresses, exercises, such as plyometric (plyo) ball tossing into a trampoline, are incorporated to amplify the demand on the medial elbow. These exercises are used with the intention of focusing on strength and endurance rather than velocity enhancement. It is imperative that the athlete knows the difference.

The phases of rehab are typically broken down into 6-week intervals with athletes progressing at different paces. Various studies have identified rest periods of 6 weeks, 6–8 weeks, and 8–12 weeks [15, 27]. The first week includes complete rest, anti-inflammatory medications, stretching, and elbow range-of-motion exercises. To limit valgus stress in the immediate phases of rehab, a hinged brace may be utilized until the elbow is pain-free [27, 28]. Once pain-free and there is minimal tenderness to the UCL, exercises can progress.

Weeks 2 through 4 incorporate more intense strengthening with a progression to isotonic elbow, wrist, and forearm work [29]. Rotator cuff and periscapular muscle strengthening is also initiated. Eccentric movements are emphasized, manual resistance for shoulder proprioceptive neuromuscular facilitation (PNF), diagonal patterns, and wrist and forearm movements are also included [29]. It has been recommended that PNF patterns should be performed with a more proximal lever to reduce force with a progression to distal forces [29].

Advanced strengthening can be implemented in weeks 4 through 6. This phase of the therapy program is directed at preparing the athlete for a throwing progression. Exercises including two- and one-handed plyo-ball tosses are added to the program with the goal of increasing the intensity by decreasing the contact time, thus preparing the athlete for higher-level throwing activities [28].

Throughout the process, modalities are incorporated into the programming. Modalities such as electric stimulation, soft tissue mobilization, massage, scraping, ultrasound, and laser therapies have been shown to aid in recovery [30]. Recently, blood flow restriction (BFR) has gained significant popularity and has been incorporated in physical therapy clinics and athletic training rooms alike. BFR was initially applied during exercise to create a metabolic environment capable of altering neuromuscular activity [31]. A restrictive device, typically a tourniquet, is placed at the proximal portion of the extremity with the purpose of reducing both the amount of arterial blood flow and venous return. BFR has been shown to be effective with lower load required to elicit a response [31]. Moreover, it has shown to increase skeletal muscle size, strength, and possibly induce positive vascular and bone adaptations as well [31]. BFR can be used with low-load, high-repetition exercises such as prone horizontal abduction (Fig. 13.5) and internal and external rotation (Figs. 13.6 and 13.7).

In addition to shoulder, elbow, and wrist strengthening, the core and lower extremity should not be neglected. Failure to address insufficiencies in the entire kinetic chain may compromise and undermine the recovery process [32].

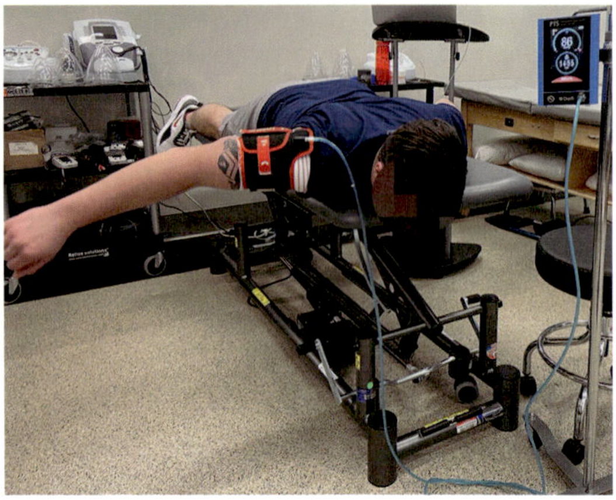

Fig. 13.5 Blood Flow Restriction (BFR) is utilized during a prone horizontal abduction exercise

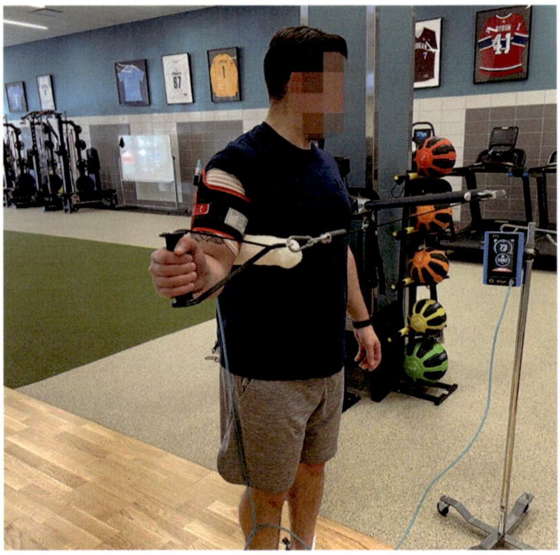

Fig. 13.7 Shoulder external rotation performed with BFR

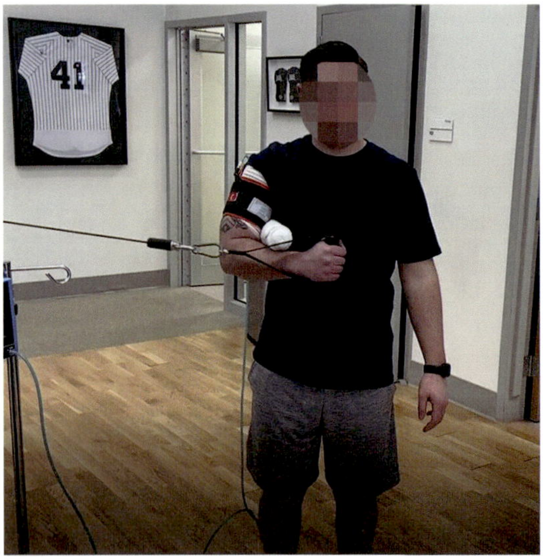

Fig. 13.6 Shoulder internal rotation performed with BFR

Furthermore, proprioceptive training may also play a role in the rehabilitative process as it may help prevent future elbow injuries since impaired balance has been associated with UCL injures at higher levels of competition [32, 33].

Athletic trainers and physical therapists should also take time to assess the athlete's lower extremity for hip and knee range of motion, and assess for strength deficits in the core, hamstrings, quads, and adductors. There is a correlation between the incidence of a hip or groin injury and UCL injury. One study demonstrated that of 145 MLB pitchers with UCL pathology, 40% had suffered a hip, hamstring, or groin injury [34]. Thus, hip injuries can lead to compensatory changes within the kinetic chain that could result in elbow injury. Any deficits in these areas should be addressed while the athlete is rehabilitating to reduce the incidence of UCL injuries.

Once the athlete has demonstrated that they have full, pain-free range of motion, normal clinical exam, and adequate strength of the shoulder and elbow, a throwing progression may be initiated. If, at any point, symptoms return throughout the rehab progression, then the player needs to be shut down immediately. Once symptoms resolve, the program may be reinitiated at the point prior to the recurrence of symptoms. Should symptoms not resolve, surgical intervention should be considered. In some cases, the healthcare team may prefer to accelerate or slow the player's rehab progression based on factors such as lingering or absence of symptoms and seasonal or career timing.

Thrower's Assessment

Return to Sport (RTS) assessments are becoming increasingly popular prior to an athlete returning to competition following injury and reconstruc-

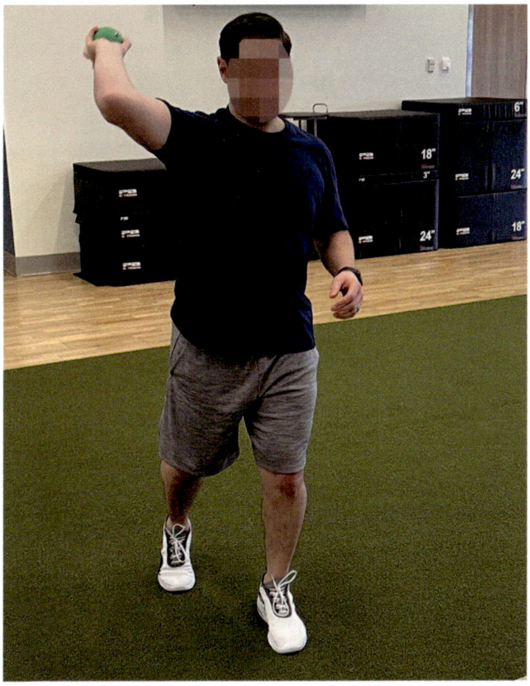

Fig. 13.8 Plyometric ball tossing into a trampoline or rebounder to emphasize dynamic mobility and control

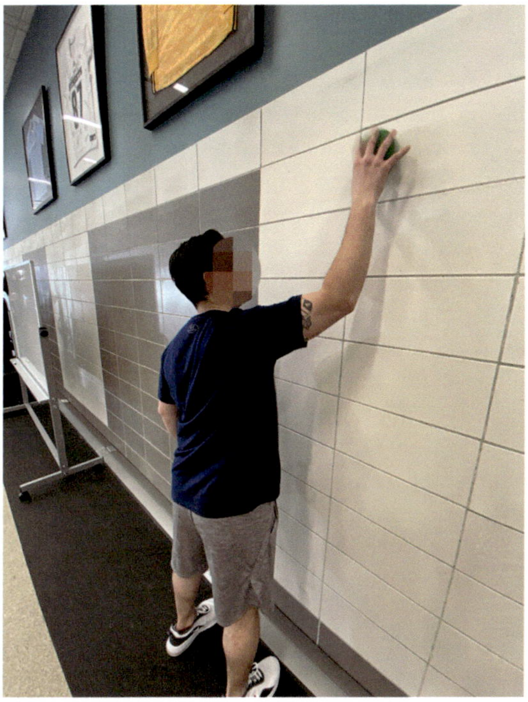

Fig. 13.9 Plyometric wall taps with a ball are performed for a predetermined period of time to increase dynamic mobility and endurance

tive surgery, especially so for anterior cruciate ligament reconstructions in the knee. RTS assessments are comprised of a battery of tests that are designed to safely return an athlete to sport without increasing their risk for re-injury. These assessments are typically employed at the final stages of rehabilitation to clear the athlete [35].

In the lower extremity, RTS assessments have varied with regard to battery content; however, the tests are designed to include a number of risk factor domains [35]. It has been described that assessments should include various strength testing and should assess the quality of range of motion; for patients coming off of returning to play from knee surgery, hop testing has also been included [35]. For the upper extremity, strength testing and range of motion quality are also imperative to be included in the assessment. Additionally, shoulder and elbow dynamic mobility (Fig. 13.8) and endurance (Fig. 13.9) should also be assessed as players will be required to throw multiple efforts in a given practice or game.

As Webster and Hewett [35] expertly stated, the true value of any RTS assessment is the ability to assess whether patients have returned to their prior level of sport at a high-performance level while also reducing the risk for a second injury. Therefore, testing athletes who have been treated nonoperatively for UCL injuries could reduce the risk of further injury propagation leading to surgery. While a UCL RTS assessment is currently being implemented and validated at our institution, it has not been clearly defined in the UCL literature as of this writing.

Progressive Throwing Program

In order for a player to start a throwing program, they must have already demonstrated a normal clinical exam and have adequate shoulder and elbow strength. Furthermore, increasing literature exists that a functional assessment should be incorporated prior to initiating a return to sport progression to decrease the likelihood of re-injury [35]. The length of the throwing progression is typically based on the length of time that the athlete is sidelined for. Should a player undergo a 6-week rehab program, then the throwing program should also be for 6 weeks.

Throwing progressions are performed in a gradual fashion and steps should not be skipped. However, seasonal timing may lend itself to an accelerated or decelerated progression. For instance, an athlete being treated nonoperatively at the beginning of the off-season will be managed differently than one who sustained their injury in the middle of the regular season.

A typical progression has 3 days of throwing separated by off days which may include physical therapy, treatment sessions, and/or arm care. It is our recommendation that players do not perform their exercises prior to throwing, so that should they fatigue, they know exactly the cause. A warm-up may include riding a stationary bike or a light jog around the field to increase core temperature.

Throwing distances typically include 60, 90, and 120 feet. Each week of the progression increases the number of throws or the distance throws are performed at. The player's ability to progress relies upon the successful completion of each phase without pain or recurring symptoms. A general principle is that the rehabilitating athlete should throw with enough effort to reach their partner. Rehab throwing should not be a maximal effort event. Players may exceed 120 feet but evidence exists that suggests throwing longer distances changes kinematic and kinetic forces [36]. Longer throws also produced greater elbow and shoulder torques, which may attenuate the healing ligament; therefore, a throwing progression should focus on mechanics while progressively loading the UCL [36].

Injury Prevention

Injury prevention starts at the youth level and should continue throughout a player's career. As the amount of injury risk factors continues to rise, so too do the number of prevention programs. Such programs include pitch counts, decreasing sport specialization, and arm care programs (i.e., the Thrower's Ten). In conjunction with conservative treatment of UCL injury, it is important to educate patients and families regarding injury prevention, focusing on age-specific guidelines for safe activity level and proper pitching mechanics. It is imperative to elicit opportunities for rest and activity modification when chronic overuse is suspected, and emphasize that the strongest correlation to upper extremity injury is the total amount of throwing [34].

Pitch Counts and Off-Days

In 2007, Little League Baseball implemented its pitch count rule. Prior to this implementation, there was an innings limit, which is less precise as pitchers could dramatically vary in number of pitches thrown in a given inning. Being as pitch counts have been linked to injury rates in adolescent baseball players [37], in addition to Little League Baseball, Major League Baseball (MLB) established a task force to reduce the amount of injuries at the youth level, called the Pitch Smart Initiative. This task force has made recommendations for pitch counts and mandated off-days based on age [38]. It is recommended that players not only keep a log of their single-game pitch count but also their season-long pitch and inning counts. Fleisig et al. [39] found that if a youth player throws over 100 innings per season, they are at a higher risk for shoulder and elbow injury.

Aside from the recommendations set forth by MLB Pitch Smart, researchers have concluded that pitching on back-to-back days without rest is also an injury risk factor for youth baseball players [39]. The guidelines are not based solely on age, but also by number of pitches thrown [39]; however, pitch type has not been established. Furthermore, pitchers who also play a catcher should not play either battery position on consecutive days [40]. Pitchers should not be removed and put in the catcher position in the same game and vice versa to decrease the amount throws a player is required to make in a given game.

Sport Diversification

Recently, there has been a push for players to specialize in a single sport year round in hopes that they gain a competitive advantage and succeed in their given sport [37]. Padaki et al. [41] surveyed 235 youth athletes with a mean age of about 14 years regarding sport specialization. The authors found that players started specializing around 8 years of age and 31% played a single sport with 60% of the athletes playing a single sport for 9 or more months per year [41]. Shockingly, one-third of players were instructed by a coach to not play other sports; this was significantly higher in the athletes who specialized [41].

Sport specialization is also of interest in players who have made it to the most elite levels of their sport. Confino et al. [42] studied first- and second-round MLB draft picks over a 9-year span. Professional baseball players who participated in multiple sports in high school played in more Major League games than those who specialized. Moreover, the players who did not specialize experienced lower injury rates than their specializing counterparts [42].

Education

Prevention also includes the education of not only the players but also their parents, coaches, and all others involved in a player's development, as they are just as impactful on a player's career decisions. This is extremely true due to the misperceptions of UCL surgery. In a survey of players, coaches, and parents, 51% of high school players, 26% of college players, 37% of parents, and 30% of coaches believed that Tommy John Surgery should be performed in the absence of injury in order to enhance performance [43]. With regard to pitch counts, 31% of coaches, 28% of player, and 25% of parents did not believe that pitch count is a factor in UCL injuries [43]. These misperceptions are among many reasons to educate the public on UCL injuries and various treatment options.

Seasonal Timing Considerations

Seasonal timing should be a consideration in determining a patient's treatment options. The average return to play with conservative treatment is 12 weeks [26–28]. A conversation with the patient around timing to have the patient ready for spring baseball may influence their pursuance of conservative measures. It is in the player's best interest to not miss two consecutive seasons recovering from the same injury, if at all possible.

RTS timelines may be affected by career timing, which can impact a single or multiple seasons. An athlete in their junior year of high school may need to be ready for a college recruitment showcase and the protocol will be adjusted to get them ready instead of adhering to a traditional timeline. Nonetheless, symptoms and kinetic chain kinematics in physical therapy dictate if the player is ready or not to initiate a throwing program in spite of how quickly they wish to RTS. The player's health should not be compromised at the expense of a quicker return to sport.

Extrinsic factors such as parents, coaches, and advisors may add additional pressures for athletes to return to the field quicker. Regardless of pressures and perceived need to RTS, it should be the common goal of the sports medicine team to return the player safely without exacerbating the injury.

Outcomes

The likelihood of success with nonoperative treatment is heavily influenced by the location of tear, grade, and severity of the tear [40]. In general, distal tears are 12.40 times more likely to fail nonoperative treatment [44]. Another study concluded that a high-grade tear at the distal aspect of the ligament has an 88% chance of failure with conservative measures [15]. Outside of baseball, football players also have excellent return-to-play rates. One report on quarterbacks demonstrated 90% success rate of nonoperative treatment and a mean RTS of 26 days [45].

Conservative management of grade 1 partial UCL tears is heavily supported by the existing literature [15, 28, 44, 46, 47]. A retrospective study of baseball players with isolated symptomatic partial UCL tears treated with platelet-rich plasma yielded favorable outcomes. Dines et al. [47] reported on 44 athletes treated with PRP, 15 returned to play with excellent outcomes and 17 returned to play with good outcomes. Furthermore, four of the six professional athletes included in the study were able to return to professional play. The mean time to return to throwing was 5 weeks, and the mean return to competition was 12 weeks. These results favor the use of PRP treatment for isolated UCL injury in symptomatic throwers who wish to avoid the risks and lengthy recovery of reconstructive surgery.

Similarly, a study of 34 baseball players with partial or complete UCL tears that were treated with PRP injection resulted in 26 athletes being able to return to preinjury level of play within 6 months [25]. The authors reported a range of return-to-play time between 10 and 18 weeks and an average of 12.4 weeks [25].

Conclusions

Seasonal timing is an important consideration when deciding to move forward with conservative versus surgical management. The treating provider should have a conversation with the patient to discuss the athlete's goals and desires to return to sport, and set reasonable expectations for return to play. Ideally, an athlete should avoid missing two seasons due to injury. The sports medicine team and the athlete should also consider the athlete's potential for future career in baseball when deciding on conservative treatment.

References

1. Redler LH, Watling JP, Ahmad CS. 5 points on physical examination of the throwing Athlete's elbow. Am J Orthop. 2015;44(1):13–8.
2. Ben Kibler W, Sciascia A. Kinetic chain contributions to elbow function and dysfunction in sports. Clin Sports Med. 2004;23(4):545–52, viii.
3. Dines JS, et al. Glenohumeral internal rotation deficits in baseball players with ulnar collateral ligament insufficiency. Am J Sports Med. 2009;37(3):566–70.
4. Hodgins JL, Trofa DP, Donohue S, Littlefield M, Schuk M, Ahmad CS. Forearm flexor injuries among Major League Baseball players: epidemiology, performance and associated injuries. Am J Sports Med. 2018;46(9):2154–60. https://doi.org/10.1177/0363546518778252.
5. Grumet RC, Friel NA, Cole BJ. Bony avulsion of the medial ulnar collateral ligament in a gymnast: a case report. J Shoulder Elb Surg. 2010;19(7):e1–6.
6. Osbahr DC, et al. Does posteromedial chondromalacia reduce rate of return to play after ulnar collateral ligament reconstruction? Clin Orthop Relat Res. 2012;470(6):1558–64.
7. Ahmad CS, Park MC, Elattrache NS. Elbow medial ulnar collateral ligament insufficiency alters posteromedial olecranon contact. Am J Sports Med. 2004;32(7):1607–12.
8. Cain EL, Dugas JR, Wolf RS, Andrews JR. Elbow injuries in throwing athletes: a current concepts review. Am J Sports Med. 2003;31(4):621–35.
9. Rijke AM, Goitz HT, McCue FC, Andrews JR, Berr SS. Stress radiography of the medial elbow ligaments. Radiology. 1994;191(1):213–6.
10. Ciccotti MC, Bishop M, Ciccotti MG. MRI and ultrasound imaging of the throwing Athlete's elbow. Baseball Sports Med. 2018;6:52–65.
11. Bruce JR, Hess R, Joyner P, Andrews JR. How much valgus instability can be expected with ulnar collateral ligament injuries? A review of 273 baseball players with UCL injuries. J Shoulder Elb Surg. 2014;23(10):1521–6.
12. Sugimoto H, Ohsawa T. Ulnar collateral ligament in the growing elbow: MR imaging of normal development and throwing injuries. Radiology. 1994;192(2):417–22.
13. Shahabpour M, et al. The effectiveness of diagnostic imaging methods for the assessment of soft tissue and articular disorders of the shoulder and elbow. Eur J Radiol. 2008;65(2):194–200.
14. Kaplan LJ, Potter HG. MR imaging of ligament injuries to the elbow. Imaging Upper Extremity. 2006;44(4):583–94.
15. Frangiamore SJ, Lynch TS, Vaughn MD, et al. Magnetic resonance imaging predictors of failure in the nonoperative management of ulnar collateral ligament injuries in professional baseball pitchers. Am J Sports Med. 2017;45(8):1783–9. April:363546517699832.
16. Kim NR, et al. MR imaging of ulnar collateral ligament injury in baseball players: value for predicting rehabilitation outcome. Eur J Radiol. 2011;80(3):e422–6.
17. Munshi M, et al. Anterior bundle of ulnar collateral ligament: evaluation of anatomic relationships by using MR imaging, MR arthrography, and

gross anatomic and histologic analysis. Radiology. 2004;231(3):797–803.
18. Hill NB Jr, et al. Magnetic resonance imaging of injury to the medial collateral ligament of the elbow: a cadaver model. J Shoulder Elb Surg. 2000;9(5):418–22.
19. Ciccotti MG, Atanda A Jr, Nazarian LN, Dodson CC, Holmes L, Cohen SB. Stress sonography of the ulnar collateral ligament of the elbow in professional baseball pitchers: a 10-year study. Am J Sports Med. 2014;42(3):544–51. https://doi.org/10.1177/0363546513516592.
20. Lee KS, Rosas HG, Craig JG. Musculoskeletal ultrasound: elbow imaging and procedures. Semin Musculoskelet Radiol. 2010;14:449–60.
21. Martinoli C, Bianchi S, Giovagnorio F, Pugliese F. Ultrasound of the elbow. Skelet Radiol. 2001;30:605–61.
22. Tran N, Chow K. Ultrasonography of the elbow. Semin Musculoskelet Radiol. 2007;11:105–16.
23. Sasaki J, Takahara M, Ogino T, Kashiwa H, Ishigaki D, Kanauchi Y. Ultrasonographic assessment of the ulnar collateral ligament and medial elbow laxity in college baseball players. J Bone Joint Surg Am. 2002;84:525–31.
24. Kobayashi Y, Saita Y, Nishio H, Ikeda Y, Takazawa Y, Nagao M, et al. Leukocyte concentration and composition in platelet-rich plasma (PRP) influences the growth factor and protease concentrations. J Orthop Sci. 2016;21(5):683–9.
25. Kato Y, Yamada S, Chavez J. Can platelet-rich plasma therapy save patients with ulnar collateral ligament tears from surgery? Regen Ther. 2019;10:123–6.
26. Seather EE, Chamberlain CS, Aktas E, et al. Primed mesenchymal stem cells alter and improve rat medial collateral ligament healing. Stem Cell Rev Rep. 2016;12(1):42–53.
27. Rettig AC, Sherrill C, Snead DS, et al. Nonoperative treatment of ulnar collateral ligament injuries in throwing athletes. Am J Sports Med. 2001;29(1):15–7.
28. Smucny M, Westermann RW, Winters M, Mark SS. Non-operative management of ulnar collateral ligament injuries in the throwing athlete. Phys Sportsmed. 2017;45(3):234–8.
29. Wilk KE, Macrina LC, Cain EL, Dugas JR, Andrews JR. Rehabilitation of the overhead Athlete's elbow. Sports Health. 2012;4(5):404–14.
30. Ford G, Genuario J, Kinkartz J, Githens T, Noonan T. Return-to-play outcomes in professional baseball players after medial ulnar collateral ligament injuries: comparison of operative versus nonoperative treatment based on magnetic resonance imaging findings. Am J Sports Med. 2016;44(3):723–8. https://doi.org/10.1177/0363546515621756.
31. Jessee MB, Mattocks KT, Buckner SL, et al. Mechanisms of blood flow restriction: the new testament. Tech Orthop. 2018;33:72–9.
32. Rebolledo BJ, Dugas JR, Bedi A, et al. Avoiding Tommy John surgery: what are the alternatives? Am J Sports Med. 2017;4(13):3143–8.
33. Kadri OM, Okoroha KR, Patel RB, et al. Nonoperative treatment of medial ulnar collateral ligament injuries in the throwing athlete: indications, evaluation, and management. JBJS. 2019;7(1):e6.
34. Kantrowitz DE, Trofa DP, Woode DR, Ahmad CS, Lynch TS. Athletic hip injuries in Major League Baseball pitchers associated with ulnar collateral ligament tears. Orthop J Sports Med. 2018;6(10) https://doi.org/10.1177/2325967118800704.
35. Webster KE, Hewett TE. What is the evidence for and validity of return-to-sport testing after anterior cruciate ligament reconstruction surgery? A systematic review and meta-analysis. Sports Med. 2019;49:917–29. https://doi.org/10.1007/s40279-019-01093-x.
36. Fleisig GS, Bolt B, Fortenbaugh D, Wilk KE, Andrews JR. Biomechanical comparison of baseball pitching and long-toss: implications for training and rehabilitation. J Orthop Sports Phys Ther. 2011;41(4):296–303.
37. Erickson BJ, Chalmers PN, Ahmad CS, Andrews JR. Injury prevention in youth baseball. In: Ahmad CS, Romeo AA, editors. Baseball sports medicine. 1st ed. Philadelphia: Wolters Kluwer; 2019.
38. Smart MP. Guidelines for youth and adolescent pitchers. Available at http://m.mlb.com/pitchsmart/pitching-guidelines/. Accessed 20 Feb 2020.
39. Fleisig GS, Andrews JR, Cutter GR, et al. Risk of serious injury for young baseball pitchers: a 10-year prospective study. Am J Sports Med. 2011;39(2):253–7.
40. Fleisig GS, Andrews JR. Prevention of elbow injuries in youth baseball pitchers. Sports Health. 2012;4(5):419–24.
41. Padaki AS, Popkin CA, Hodgins JL, Kovacevic D, Lynch TS, Ahmad CS. Factors that drive youth sport specialization. Sport Health. 2017;9(6):532–6. https://doi.org/10.1177/1941738117734149.
42. Confino J, Irvine JN, O'Connor M, Ahmad CA, Lynch TS. Early sports specialization is associated with upper extremity injuries in throwers and fewer games played in Major League Baseball. Orthop J Sports Med. 2019;7(7) https://doi.org/10.1177/2325967119861101.
43. Ahmad CS, Grantham WJ, Greiwe RM. Public perceptions of Tommy John surgery. Phys Sportsmed. 2012;40(2):54–72.
44. Clark NJ, Desai VS, Dines JD, Morrey ME, Camp CL. Nonreconstruction options for treating medial ulnar collateral ligament injuries of the elbow in overhead athletes. Curr Rev Musculoskelet Med. 2018;11(1):48–54. https://doi.org/10.1007/s12178-018-9458-3.
45. Dodson CC, Slenker N, Cohen SB, et al. Ulnar collateral ligament injuries of the elbow in professional football quarterbacks. J Shoulder Elb Surg. 2010;19(8):1276–80.
46. Cascia N, Uhl T, Hettirch C. Return to play following nonoperative treatment of partial ulnar collateral ligament injuries in professional baseball players: a critically appraised topic. J Sport Rehabil. 2019;28:660–4.
47. Dines JS. Platelet rich plasma can be used to successfully treat elbow ulnar collateral ligament insufficiency in high-level throwers. Am J Orthop. 2016;5:2016.

The Role of Biologics in Ulnar Collateral Ligament Injuries

14

John M. Apostolakos, Joshua Wright-Chisem, Joshua S. Dines, David W. Altchek, James B. Carr II, Michael E. Angeline, John M. Zajac, and Albert O. Gee

Introduction

The throwing motion places an extreme demand on the shoulder and elbow of overhead throwing athletes. An injury can occur within this cycle when either the throwing shoulder or elbow is subject to applied stresses at a rate that exceeds the tissues' maximum load to failure [1]. This is especially true for the medial ulnar collateral ligament (MUCL) [2]. Anatomically, the MUCL is composed of three bundles: anterior, posterior, and oblique [2]. The anterior bundle is the primary static stabilizer to valgus stress from 20° to 120° of elbow flexion and can be injured due to the large amount of valgus torque generated during the late cocking phase of throwing. The anterior bundle originates from the anteroinferior edge of the medial humeral epicondyle and inserts onto the sublime tubercle of the ulna where it is divided into an anterior and posterior band [3, 4]. Histologically, the anterior bundle is composed of two separate layers: a deep layer, which consists of collagen bundles contained within the capsule, and a superficial layer that is a distinct ligamentous structure separate from the underlying joint capsule [5]. When medial ligamentous insufficiency develops from repetitive valgus loads, the athlete may have chronic, disabling elbow pain or have an inability to throw effectively [6, 7]. The combination of improved diagnostic capabilities, earlier participation in competitive sports, and prolonged athletic seasons have led to an increased incidence of MUCL injuries in overhead throwers of all ages across all levels of competition [8–14]. Management of these injuries includes both operative and nonoperative options. Ultimately, the treatment decision is multifactorial and must include evaluation of location (proximal, midsubstance, or distal) and degree of tear (complete vs partial), previous treatments, injury acuity, age of patient, and level of competitive sport.

J. M. Apostolakos (✉) · J. Wright-Chisem
J. S. Dines · D. W. Altchek
Department of Orthopedic Surgery, Sports Medicine and Shoulder Service, Sports Medicine Institute, Hospital for Special Surgery, New York, NY, USA

J. B. Carr II
Sports Medicine Institute, Hospital for Special Surgery, West Palm Beach, FL, USA

M. E. Angeline
Mercy Health System, Janesville, WI, USA

J. M. Zajac
New York Mets Baseball Club, Flushing, NY, USA

A. O. Gee
Orthopaedics and Sports Medicine, University of Washington Medical Center, Seattle, WA, USA

J. S. Dines et al. (eds.), *Elbow Ulnar Collateral Ligament Injury*,
https://doi.org/10.1007/978-3-030-69567-5_14

Management Decision-Making

The current gold-standard management for full thickness, attritional, midsubstance tears in high-demand or professional throwing athletes is surgical reconstruction [8, 15]. Since the original description by Jobe, there have been several modifications for ligament reconstruction with return to play rates as high as 80–95% and mean return to play time in Major League Baseball (MLB) players being between 11.6 and 16.8 months [16–32]. Given the prolonged recovery period after surgical intervention, other avenues for successful treatment of MUCL insufficiency have been explored including potential injections into the ligament. Conservative treatment can be considered for select patients as nonoperative management provides the potential for a quicker return to sport without jeopardizing outcomes in appropriately selected patients. Nonoperative protocols are utilized in nearly all cases of partial ulnar collateral ligament (UCL) tears and typically involve rest, anti-inflammatory medications, and a structured rehabilitation program with a gradual return to competitive throwing once asymptomatic. Nonoperative options must also be considered for skeletally immature patients with full thickness tears and amateur-level athletes without plans for future competitive play [8, 15]. Despite strides in our understanding of UCL injuries and a general consensus for operative management of full thickness tears and injuries in professional athletes, Hurwit et al. [33] reported a survey of the American Shoulder and Elbow Surgeons (ASES) indicating a lack of consensus regarding management of partial tears and non-professional athletes. Overall, 36.3% of respondents reported using platelet-rich plasma (PRP) in their treatment protocols while 8% reported using stem cell augmentation. This study revealed the lack of clarity regarding management of partial tears and amateur athletes in addition to the variable use of biological augmentation in UCL injuries.

A crucial aspect of patient evaluation includes a critical evaluation of advanced imaging. Frangiamore et al. [34] evaluated magnetic resonance imaging (MRI) findings in 32 professional pitchers who initially underwent conservative management of their UCL injury. The investigators defined successful management as return to at least the same level of play at a minimum of 1 year and failure as recurrent pain or weakness when attempting a return to throwing rehabilitation program after a minimum of 3 months rest. The authors found 34% (11/32) failed conservative management prompting operative reconstruction and 64% (21/32) successfully returned to play without operative intervention. Of those that failed conservative management, 82% (9/11) had tears of the distal UCL. Of the patients successfully managed nonoperatively, 81% (17/21) had tears of the proximal UCL. After adjusting for confounding variables they reported a 12.4 time greater likelihood of failing nonoperative management with a distal UCL tear. The study highlights the importance of tear location in predicting successful outcomes in nonoperative management. The findings may be explained by a cadaveric investigation by Buckley et al. [35] reporting a more robust blood supply to the proximal UCL as compared to the distal UCL while also noting a potential osseous contribution from the medial epicondyle. These investigations highlight the importance of critically evaluating MRI examinations to precisely determine the anatomic location of the injury, as this may help predict the potential success of nonoperative management.

Biologic Augmentation

There are several options for nonoperative treatment protocols that commonly include a combination of rest, bracing, and physical therapy. Injection of biologic agents is an emerging field that is commonly used in nonoperative protocols for MUCL partial tears, and this will be the main focus of the current chapter. Corticosteroids are not utilized for an acute ligamentous injury, as they have been shown to have a negative effect on ligament healing. In a study by Walsh and colleagues, an acute injection of betamethasone into a transected rabbit medial collateral ligament (MCL) was shown to negatively impact the biomechanical and histological properties as compared to control ligaments that did not have an injection [36]. These effects were observed for up to 3 months following the injury and steroid injection. Due to the negative influence of corticosteroids on acute ligamentous injuries, other potential options for an injection have been explored including platelet-rich plasma (PRP) and autologous stem cells.

The natural tendon and ligamentous healing response involves a cascade of events including inflammation, repair, and remodeling. In general, tendons and ligaments display a poor intrinsic healing potential, which has ignited an interest in biological agents to augment the healing process [8, 37–44]. During the repair phase, there is an increased expression of growth factors that help enable cellular proliferation and matrix production [45]. Many of these growth factors and cytokines have been shown to potentiate the effects of other factors within the repair phase of healing. When platelet-derived growth factor (PDGF) has been combined with insulin-like growth factor-1 (IGF-1), the two have been shown to work synergistically and potentiate the tendon- and ligament-healing response through matrix formation, cell proliferation, and differentiation [46]. In addition, platelet derived growth factor-BB (PDGF-BB) has been shown to increase the expression of vascular endothelial growth factor (VEGF), which results in an increased angiogenic response via the targeting of endothelial cells [47]. These findings suggest that an increased concentration of these growth factors/cytokines may lead to a potential for an augmented healing response through enhanced endothelial cell, stem cell, and tenocyte recruitment. PRP is the most researched biologic agent in the setting of UCL injuries. It has an autologous, ultra-concentrate, whole blood product within a small volume of plasma with a higher concentration of platelets [8, 38, 39, 48–52]. PRP has been shown to contain over 300 distinct cytokines and growth factors including PDGF, VEGF, IGF, transforming growth factor (TGF) beta-1, and basic fibroblast growth factor, creating an environment thought to promote healing [8, 48–50].

Platelet-rich plasma is not without limitations, most notably cost and variability in the preparation process. In regard to cost, it is currently not covered by insurance companies, which can limit the availability in cases where the patient deems it to be cost-prohibitive. Furthermore, there can be a significant variability in the content of PRP based on the preparation process. The specific bioavailability of various growth factors can theoretically be altered by formulation changes such as leukocyte-rich (LR-PRP) versus leukocyte-poor (LP-PRP) preparations and methods of activation [49, 50]. As of 2019, over 16 commercially available PRP systems were on the market with variable collection and preparation protocols and without a precise understanding of clinical implications [49]. In addition, variability exists even within an individual as platelet, cell, and growth factor levels have been shown to fluctuate regardless of the collection and formulation protocol, making it challenging to accurately assess and compare PRP effectiveness between studies [50, 53].

Current research into the use of PRP within the field of orthopedics is varied. In general, there is evidence supporting the use of LR-PRP for lateral epicondylitis of the elbow and patellar tendinopathy, LP-PRP for osteoarthritis of the knee, and support for PRP injections over corticosteroids for the treatment of plantar fasciitis [49, 54–60]. Investigations into other musculoskeletal pathologies including rotator cuff disease, Achilles tendinopathy, osteoarthritis of the hip, donor site pain in anterior cruciate ligament (ACL) reconstruction, and ankle sprains remain unclear [49, 61–69].

The use of PRP for chronic elbow tendinosis and lateral epicondylitis of the elbow has also been investigated. A 2006 investigation by Mishra and colleagues demonstrated that patients treated with a PRP injection for chronic elbow tendinosis had significantly reduced pain as compared to a control group treated with a bupivacaine injection alone [70]. In a series of two studies in 2010 and 2011, randomized controlled trials comparing the effectiveness of PRP to corticosteroid injections in patients with chronic lateral epicondylitis confirmed the benefit of PRP for elbow tendinosis [71, 72].

Recently, there have been a few notable reports on the management of UCL injuries using PRP. Posdesta et al. [73] prospectively reported on the use of PRP in 34 athletes with MRI-confirmed partial UCL injuries. Each athlete underwent 2 months of nonoperative management followed by a failed attempt at return to play. Each patient then received a single LR-PRP injection under ultrasound guidance followed by a formal physical therapy program. At a mean follow-up of 70 weeks, 88% (30/34) patients returned to the same level of play without complaints at an average of 12 weeks. It should be noted that this study was limited by a lack of MRI follow-up or comparison to a control group.

A 2016 report by Dines et al. [74] also investigated the effects of PRP injection on partial UCL tears in high-level throwing athletes. This retrospective review of 44 baseball players (6 professional, 14 college, 24 high school players) with MRI-confirmed partial tears reported an excellent outcome in 15 patients (34%), a good outcome in 17 patients (39%), a fair outcome in 2 patients (5%), and a poor outcome in 10 patients (23%). A total of four out of six professional athletes returned to professional play. The mean time from injection to return to throwing was 5 weeks with a mean time to return to competition of 12 weeks. While the results were promising, the study was limited by a variable amount of PRP injections and lack of a control group.

Deal et al. [75] also conducted an investigation on 23 patients with MRI-confirmed, primary grade II UCL tears. This 2017 study utilized a series of two LR-PRP injections administered 2 weeks apart. The injections were augmented with bracing, a physical therapy program, and a structured throwing program. Twenty-two patients (96%) returned to play at the same level of competition or higher with repeated MRIs revealing full ligament reconstitution in 91% (20/22). The mean return to athletic competition was 82 days.

The most recent investigation into PRP use in UCL injuries was conducted in 2019 by Chauhan et al. [76]. This was the first comparative study performed in a homogenous cohort of professional baseball players treated nonoperatively with and without PRP injections. The authors utilized the Major League Baseball (MLB) Health and Injury Tracking System to identify 544 professional baseball players who had been treated nonoperatively for UCL injuries between 2011 and 2015. Overall, 133 of these players received PRP injections prior to their treatment program while 411 did not. To reduce bias, the authors performed a 1:1 matched comparison between groups. The overall results found a 54% rate of return to play. The PRP group experienced a significantly longer delay in return to throwing and return to play. Pitchers in the MLB and Minor League Baseball (MiLB) leagues who managed without PRP had a significantly faster rate of return to throwing. MiLB pitchers without PRP also experienced a statistically faster return to play. In this comparative analysis, PRP did not improve return to play outcomes although the authors did note variability between PRP preparations, injection protocols, time from injury to injection, and specific rehabilitation protocols.

More recently, interest has increased in the use of autologous stem cells in various orthopedic pathologies, including the UCL. The goal of this therapy is for cells to differentiate into healthy tissue and to secrete factors to promote an environment of healing. An understanding of the current state of stem cell therapy requires clear definitions of these therapies. Stem cells are progenitor cells classified by their ability to self-renew and differentiate into various tissue lines with long-term viability [37, 77]. Stem cells are affected by multiple variables, creating a significant heterogeneity within the literature. The term "stem cell" is a broad term which can be more specifically defined as adult versus embryonic, pluripotent versus multipotent, dedifferentiated versus predifferentiated, pure stem cell versus bone marrow concentrate, and connective tissue progenitors versus mesenchymal stem cells. Further classifications can be made based on harvest sites such as bone marrow, adipose, vascular, or muscular derived. These terms and definitions can create confusion for patients and even providers when discussing "stem cell therapy." A mesenchymal stem cell, as generally defined by the International Society for Cell Therapy (ISCT), must display the ability to be plastic adherent when maintained in standard culture conditions, display tri-lineage differentiation under standard in vitro differentiating conditions, and must have a specific cell surface marker profile [78, 79]. To be defined as a mesenchymal stem cell, the cells must have the ability to differentiate into osteocytes, tenocytes, chondrocytes, and adipocytes under specific environmental stimuli [37, 80].

Due to ethical considerations related to the harvesting of embryonic stem cells, adult sources are typically utilized in the field of orthopedic surgery. Orthopedic literature includes investigations reporting cell procurement from bone marrow, adipose tissue, peripheral blood, and the subacromial bursa [37, 80–85]. Cell-based therapy has been investigated in the management of rotator cuff repairs, anterior cruciate ligament reconstruction, lateral epicondylitis, patellar tendinopathy, and bone healing in fractures and nonunions without conclusive evidence to support efficacy [40–44, 52, 86, 87]. One of the more common cell-based formulations utilized in orthopedics is bone marrow aspirate concentrate (BMAC). BMAC has been reported to be harvested from multiple sites including the iliac crest, distal femur, and proximal humerus [87–92]. The aspiration is then mixed with an anticoagulant and centrifuged to isolate cells. As with PRP, a lack of standardization during this process leads to significant variability. Additionally, based on the formal criteria, the concentration of stem cells in BMAC is low with reports indicating yields of 0.001% to 0.01%. Therefore, it is unknown if the efficacy related to BMAC is related to other aspects of its composition including PDGF, TGF-ß, bone morphogenic protein BMP-2, and BMP-7 [78, 87, 93–95].

The only published report on the efficacy of cell-based therapy in the management of UCL injuries was by Hoffman et al. [96] in 2015. This case report described the treatment of a 25-year-old professional baseball pitcher with UCL instability and ulnar neuritis. The patient underwent operative intervention consisting of a dermal allograft, PRP, and mesenchymal stem cells (MSCs) with ulnar nerve decompression. Following a postoperative course of occupational therapy, 6 weeks of bracing, and progressive range of motion with strengthening exercises, the patient began a throwing program after 4 months. At 21 months postoperatively the patient reported no signs of ulnar neuropathy or instability and successfully returned to throwing.

Currently there is no consensus regarding the use of PRP or cell-based therapies in the setting of UCL injuries. The current literature reports mixed results regarding the use of PRP which may be partly explained by the significant variability pertaining to PRP preparations, injection protocols, rehabilitation protocols, injury patterns, and indications for use. The use of cell-based therapies remains primitive, with a need for further research to better define indications and treatment protocols.

Our Preferred Treatment Algorithm

We consider a potential PRP injection in athletes with physical examination and imaging findings (Fig. 14.1), consistent with grade I or grade II proximal partial MUCL insufficiency, especially if a trial of conservative management has been unsuccessful. We do not consider a PRP injection for patients with complete MUCL insufficiency (i.e., grade III tear) regardless of tear location. In the setting of a low-grade partial distal MUCL tear, we will consider a possible PRP injection depending on the patient's preference based on age, level of play, and timing within the season. However, the role of PRP injections in the management of distal partial tears is especially ambiguous due to the poor healing potential of the distal MUCL. Therefore, we have a much lower threshold to offer surgical management to patients with a distal MUCL tear who have failed conservative management.

The PRP solution is prepared according to manufacturer's guidelines and typically a total of 3 ml of PRP is injected into the ligament under ultrasound guidance. After the injection, patients use acetaminophen and ice for pain control. Anti-inflammatory medications are avoided for a minimum of 2 weeks after the injection in order to allow a maximum inflammatory healing response.

Following the injection, our preferred conservative treatment plan includes rest, activity modification, anti-inflammatory medications, and physical therapy followed by an attempt to return

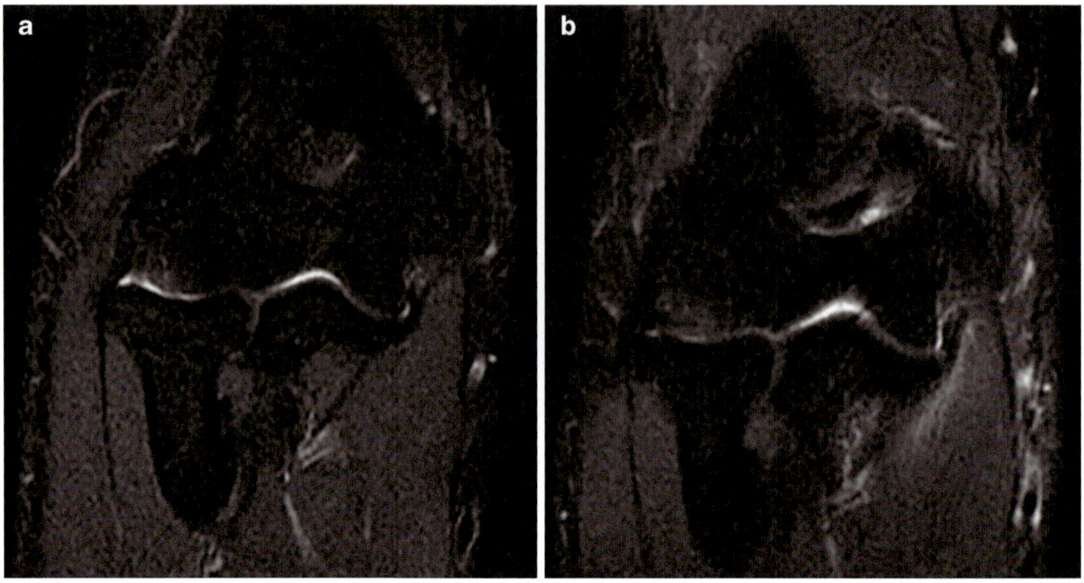

Fig. 14.1 Magnetic resonance imaging (MRI) of the right elbow in a professional pitcher, from (**a**) 04/2009 to (**b**) 04/2012, utilizing coronal fast inversion recovery that demonstrates a progressive partial tear of the posterior band of the anterior bundle of the medial collateral ligament with recent injury to the ulnar attachment without complete discontinuity

to throwing using an interval throwing program. Most patients require at least 1 month off from throwing, followed by a return to play around 12–16 weeks once an interval throwing program can be successfully completed.

Once the injection has been performed, the athlete is progressed through a criterion-based rehabilitation program. This includes a focus on range of motion (ROM) for the shoulder and elbow, good overall rotator cuff and scapular stabilizer strength, and the ability to tolerate a double arm then single arm plyometric program. Additionally, the athlete should demonstrate good glenohumeral joint proprioceptive awareness. Axe and colleagues have reported a rehabilitation program for the overhead athlete that involves a gradual restoration of ROM, strength, muscular endurance, dynamic stabilization, and neuromuscular control [97]. Reinold et al. have also described treatment guidelines for an overhead athlete involved in a rehabilitation program for the shoulder all of which can be applied to an MUCL injury [98]. These guidelines require maintaining appropriate ROM for the thrower, developing acceptable glenohumeral and scapular strength, emphasizing dynamic stabilization and neuromuscular control, and enhancing core and lower body strengthening.

After the athlete has completed these phases of the rehabilitation program, an interval throwing program can be started to prepare the athlete for return to competition. For the overhead athlete, an interval throwing program should be considered to be the final and necessary phase of rehabilitation before return to regular competition. There is modest evidence in the literature describing interval throwing programs for baseball athletes and none specifically described for those athletes who have received a PRP injection for an MUCL injury. Axe and colleagues provide data-based interval throwing programs for baseball players based on position (pitchers, catchers, infielders, and outfielders), age, and level of play [97]. In addition, program progression is broken down into whether the injury is tendon/ligament or bruise/bony in nature, involvement of the dominant or nondominant arm, or if recovering from surgery. This may serve as a helpful guide in returning the athlete back to competition after a PRP injection for an MUCL injury.

Our interval throwing program, Table 14.1, is a modification of our MUCL surgical reconstruc-

Table 14.1 Interval throwing program

Phase I: Long-toss program	
45' stage	Warm-up throwing
	25 throws
	15-min rest
	Warm-up throwing
	25 throws
60' stage	Warm-up throwing
	25 throws
	15-min rest
	Warm-up throwing
	25 throws
90' stage	Warm-up throwing
	25 throws
	Rest 15'
	Warm-up throwing
	25 throws
120' stage	Warm-up throwing
	25 throws
	Rest 15'
	Warm-up throwing
	25 throws
150' stage	Warm-up throwing
	25 throws
	Rest 15'
	Warm-up throwing
	25 throws
180' stage	Warm-up throwing
	25 throws
	Rest 15'
	Warm-up throwing
	25 throws
Throwing performed every other day (phase I and phase II)	
Pre- and post-throwing exercises must be performed (phase I and phase II)	
Each stage should be 1 week	
If pain occurs during any stage, back up to previous stage	
Begin throwing from mound or to respective position once completed	
Phase II: Throwing off the mound	
Stage I: Fastballs only	
Step 1	Interval throwing
	15 throws from mound (50%)
Step 2	Interval throwing
	30 throws from mound (50%)
Step 3	Interval throwing
	45 throws from mound (50%)
Stage II: Fastballs only	
Step 4	Interval throwing
	60 throws from mound (60%)
Step 5	Interval throwing
	30 throws from mound (75%)
Step 6	30 throws from mound (75%)
	45 throws from mound (50%)
Stage III: Fastballs only	
Step 7	45 throws from mound (75%)
	15 throws from mound (50%)
Step 8	60 throws from mound (75%)
Stage IV: Fastballs only	
Step 9	45 throws from mound (75%)
	15 throws in batting practice

tion program. The starting point for an athlete within the program is determined by when an athlete last participated in significant overhead throwing. Many athletes who have had less down time from throwing would therefore require less time in the shorter distances and could be progressed more quickly than a player who has not been throwing for a longer period of time.

Conclusion

Platelet-rich plasma injections for the MUCL may play a role in the management of young overhead athletes who have acute damage to an isolated part of the ligament, and in those athletes who are unwilling or unable to undergo the extended rehabilitation required after surgical reconstruction of the ligament. Despite promising clinical results, the significant variability within PRP formulations, timing and number of injections, and postinjection rehabilitation protocols makes it difficult to determine the true efficacy. Even more so than PRP, the efficacy of cell-based therapy remains unclear in the setting of an UCL injury as research investigating its general utility in the field of orthopedic surgery remains primitive.

While PRP and cell-based augmentation can be considered in the setting of MUCL insufficiency, further research is needed in order to clarify indications. Specifically, future investigations to determine optimal procurement and formulation protocols, timing and number of injections, and appropriate clinical application of these biological augmentations are needed.

Disclosure The authors did not receive any outside funding or grants in support of the research for or preparation of this work.

References

1. Kvitne RS, Jobe FW. The diagnosis and treatment of anterior instability in the throwing athlete. Clin Orthop Relat Res. 1993;291:107–23.
2. Jones KJ, Osbahr DC, Schrumpf MA, Dines JS, Altchek DW. Ulnar collateral ligament reconstruction in throwing athletes: a review of current concepts. AAOS exhibit selection. J Bone Joint Surg Am. 2012;94(8):e49.
3. Floris S, Olsen BS, Dalstra M, Sojbjerg JO, Sneppen O. The medial collateral ligament of the elbow joint: anatomy and kinematics. J Shoulder Elb Surg. 1998;7(4):345–51.
4. Dugas JR, Ostrander RV, Cain EL, Kingsley D, Andrews JR. Anatomy of the anterior bundle of the ulnar collateral ligament. J Shoulder Elb Surg. 2007;16(5):657–60.
5. Timmerman LA, Andrews JR. Histology and arthroscopic anatomy of the ulnar collateral ligament of the elbow. Am J Sports Med. 1994;22(5):667–73.
6. Miller CD, Savoie FH 3rd. Valgus extension injuries of the elbow in the throwing athlete. J Am Acad Orthop Surg. 1994;2(5):261–9.
7. Wilson FD, Andrews JR, Blackburn TA, McCluskey G. Valgus extension overload in the pitching elbow. Am J Sports Med. 1983;11(2):83–8.
8. Clark NJ, Desai VS, Dines JD, Morrey ME, Camp CL. Nonreconstruction options for treating medial ulnar collateral ligament injuries of the elbow in overhead athletes. Curr Rev Musculoskelet Med. 2018;11(1):48–54.
9. Cain EL Jr, Dugas JR, Wolf RS, Andrews JR. Elbow injuries in throwing athletes: a current concepts review. Am J Sports Med. 2003;31(4):621–35.
10. Hodgins JL, Vitale M, Arons RR, Ahmad CS. Epidemiology of medial ulnar collateral ligament reconstruction: a 10-year study in New York state. Am J Sports Med. 2016;44(3):729–34.
11. Li NY, Goodman AD, Lemme NJ, Owens BD. Epidemiology of elbow ulnar collateral ligament injuries in throwing versus contact athletes of the National Collegiate Athletic Association: analysis of the 2009-2010 to 2013–2014 seasons. Orthop J Sports Med. 2019;7(4):2325967119836428.
12. Conte SA, Fleisig GS, Dines JS, et al. Prevalence of ulnar collateral ligament surgery in professional baseball players. Am J Sports Med. 2015;43(7):1764–9.
13. Conte S, Camp CL, Dines JS. Injury trends in Major League Baseball over 18 seasons: 1998–2015. Am J Orthop (Belle Mead NJ). 2016;45(3):116–23.
14. Erickson BJ, Nwachukwu BU, Rosas S, et al. Trends in medial ulnar collateral ligament reconstruction in the United States: a retrospective review of a large private-payer database from 2007 to 2011. Am J Sports Med. 2015;43(7):1770–4.
15. Rebolledo BJ, Dugas JR, Bedi A, Ciccotti MG, Altchek DW, Dines JS. Avoiding Tommy John surgery: what are the alternatives? Am J Sports Med. 2017;45(13):3143–8.
16. Jobe FW, Stark H, Lombardo SJ. Reconstruction of the ulnar collateral ligament in athletes. J Bone Joint Surg Am. 1986;68(8):1158–63.
17. Thompson WH, Jobe FW, Yocum LA, Pink MM. Ulnar collateral ligament reconstruction in athletes: muscle-splitting approach without transposition of the ulnar nerve. J Shoulder Elb Surg. 2001;10(2):152–7.
18. Andrews JR, Timmerman LA. Outcome of elbow surgery in professional baseball players. Am J Sports Med. 1995;23(4):407–13.
19. Azar FM, Andrews JR, Wilk KE, Groh D. Operative treatment of ulnar collateral ligament injuries of the elbow in athletes. Am J Sports Med. 2000;28(1):16–23.
20. Petty DH, Andrews JR, Fleisig GS, Cain EL. Ulnar collateral ligament reconstruction in high school baseball players: clinical results and injury risk factors. Am J Sports Med. 2004;32(5):1158–64.
21. Cain EL Jr, Andrews JR, Dugas JR, et al. Outcome of ulnar collateral ligament reconstruction of the elbow in 1281 athletes: results in 743 athletes with minimum 2-year follow-up. Am J Sports Med. 2010;38(12):2426–34.
22. Dugas JR, Bilotta J, Watts CD, et al. Ulnar collateral ligament reconstruction with gracilis tendon in athletes with intraligamentous bony excision: technique and results. Am J Sports Med. 2012;40(7):1578–82.
23. Rohrbough JT, Altchek DW, Hyman J, Williams RJ 3rd, Botts JD. Medial collateral ligament reconstruction of the elbow using the docking technique. Am J Sports Med. 2002;30(4):541–8.
24. Dodson CC, Thomas A, Dines JS, Nho SJ, Williams RJ 3rd, Altchek DW. Medial ulnar collateral ligament reconstruction of the elbow in throwing athletes. Am J Sports Med. 2006;34(12):1926–32.
25. Paletta GA Jr, Wright RW. The modified docking procedure for elbow ulnar collateral ligament reconstruction: 2-year follow-up in elite throwers. Am J Sports Med. 2006;34(10):1594–8.
26. Koh JL, Schafer MF, Keuter G, Hsu JE. Ulnar collateral ligament reconstruction in elite throwing athletes. Arthroscopy. 2006;22(11):1187–91.
27. Bowers AL, Dines JS, Dines DM, Altchek DW. Elbow medial ulnar collateral ligament reconstruction: clinical relevance and the docking technique. J Shoulder Elb Surg. 2010;19(2 Suppl):110–7.
28. Dines JS, ElAttrache NS, Conway JE, Smith W, Ahmad CS. Clinical outcomes of the DANE TJ technique to treat ulnar collateral ligament insufficiency of the elbow. Am J Sports Med. 2007;35(12):2039–44.
29. Kodde IF, Rahusen FT, Eygendaal D. Long-term results after ulnar collateral ligament reconstruction of the elbow in European athletes with interference screw technique and triceps fascia autograft. J Shoulder Elb Surg. 2012;21(12):1656–63.

30. Hechtman KS, Zvijac JE, Wells ME, Botto-van Bemden A. Long-term results of ulnar collateral ligament reconstruction in throwing athletes based on a hybrid technique. Am J Sports Med. 2011;39(2):342–7.
31. Savoie FH 3rd, Morgan C, Yaste J, Hurt J, Field L. Medial ulnar collateral ligament reconstruction using hamstring allograft in overhead throwing athletes. J Bone Joint Surg Am. 2013;95(12):1062–6.
32. Makhni EC, Lee RW, Morrow ZS, Gualtieri AP, Gorroochurn P, Ahmad CS. Performance, return to competition, and reinjury after Tommy John surgery in Major League Baseball pitchers: a review of 147 cases. Am J Sports Med. 2014;42(6):1323–32.
33. Hurwit DJ, Garcia GH, Liu J, Altchek DW, Romeo A, Dines J. Management of ulnar collateral ligament injury in throwing athletes: a survey of the American Shoulder and Elbow Surgeons. J Shoulder Elb Surg. 2017;26(11):2023–8.
34. Frangiamore SJ, Lynch TS, Vaughn MD, et al. Magnetic resonance imaging predictors of failure in the nonoperative management of ulnar collateral ligament injuries in professional baseball pitchers. Am J Sports Med. 2017;45(8):1783–9.
35. Buckley PS, Morris ER, Robbins CM, et al. Variations in blood supply from proximal to distal in the ulnar collateral ligament of the elbow: a qualitative descriptive cadaveric study. Am J Sports Med. 2019;47(5):1117–23.
36. Walsh WR, Wiggins ME, Fadale PD, Ehrlich MG. Effects of a delayed steroid injection on ligament healing using a rabbit medial collateral ligament model. Biomaterials. 1995;16(12):905–10.
37. Fralinger DJ, Kaplan DJ, Weinberg ME, Strauss EJ, Jazrawi LM. Biological treatments for tendon and ligament abnormalities: a critical analysis review. JBJS Rev. 2016;4(6).
38. Cook CS, Smith PA. Clinical update: why PRP should be your first choice for injection therapy in treating osteoarthritis of the knee. Curr Rev Musculoskelet Med. 2018;11(4):583–92.
39. Barber FA. PRP as an adjunct to rotator cuff tendon repair. Sports Med Arthrosc Rev. 2018;26(2):42–7.
40. Hernigou P, Flouzat Lachaniette CH, Delambre J, et al. Biologic augmentation of rotator cuff repair with mesenchymal stem cells during arthroscopy improves healing and prevents further tears: a case-controlled study. Int Orthop. 2014;38(9):1811–8.
41. Silva A, Sampaio R, Fernandes R, Pinto E. Is there a role for adult non-cultivated bone marrow stem cells in ACL reconstruction? Knee Surg Sports Traumatol Arthrosc. 2014;22(1):66–71.
42. Connell D, Datir A, Alyas F, Curtis M. Treatment of lateral epicondylitis using skin-derived tenocyte-like cells. Br J Sports Med. 2009;43(4):293–8.
43. Singh A, Gangwar DS, Singh S. Bone marrow injection: a novel treatment for tennis elbow. J Nat Sci Biol Med. 2014;5(2):389–91.
44. Pascual-Garrido C, Rolon A, Makino A. Treatment of chronic patellar tendinopathy with autologous bone marrow stem cells: a 5-year-followup. Stem Cells Int. 2012;2012:953510.
45. Angeline ME, Rodeo SA. Biologics in the management of rotator cuff surgery. Clin Sports Med. 2012;31(4):645–63.
46. Oliva F, Via AG, Maffulli N. Role of growth factors in rotator cuff healing. Sports Med Arthrosc Rev. 2011;19(3):218–26.
47. Hollinger JO, Hart CE, Hirsch SN, Lynch S, Friedlaender GE. Recombinant human platelet-derived growth factor: biology and clinical applications. J Bone Joint Surg Am. 2008;90 Suppl 1:48–54.
48. Hall MP, Band PA, Meislin RJ, Jazrawi LM, Cardone DA. Platelet-rich plasma: current concepts and application in sports medicine. J Am Acad Orthop Surg. 2009;17(10):602–8.
49. Le ADK, Enweze L, DeBaun MR, Dragoo JL. Platelet-rich plasma. Clin Sports Med. 2019;38(1):17–44.
50. Murray IR, LaPrade RF. Platelet-rich plasma: renewed scientific understanding must guide appropriate use. Bone Joint Res. 2016;5(3):92–4.
51. Kia C, Baldino J, Bell R, Ramji A, Uyeki C, Mazzocca A. Platelet-rich plasma: review of current literature on its use for tendon and ligament pathology. Curr Rev Musculoskelet Med. 2018;11(4):566–72.
52. Ellera Gomes JL, da Silva RC, Silla LM, Abreu MR, Pellanda R. Conventional rotator cuff repair complemented by the aid of mononuclear autologous stem cells. Knee Surg Sports Traumatol Arthrosc. 2012;20(2):373–7.
53. Mazzocca AD, McCarthy MB, Chowaniec DM, et al. Platelet-rich plasma differs according to preparation method and human variability. J Bone Joint Surg Am. 2012;94(4):308–16.
54. Mishra AK, Skrepnik NV, Edwards SG, et al. Efficacy of platelet-rich plasma for chronic tennis elbow: a double-blind, prospective, multicenter, randomized controlled trial of 230 patients. Am J Sports Med. 2014;42(2):463–71.
55. Dragoo JL, Wasterlain AS, Braun HJ, Nead KT. Platelet-rich plasma as a treatment for patellar tendinopathy: a double-blind, randomized controlled trial. Am J Sports Med. 2014;42(3):610–8.
56. Vetrano M, Castorina A, Vulpiani MC, Baldini R, Pavan A, Ferretti A. Platelet-rich plasma versus focused shock waves in the treatment of jumper's knee in athletes. Am J Sports Med. 2013;41(4):795–803.
57. Yang WY, Han YH, Cao XW, et al. Platelet-rich plasma as a treatment for plantar fasciitis: a meta-analysis of randomized controlled trials. Medicine (Baltimore). 2017;96(44):e8475.
58. Singh P, Madanipour S, Bhamra JS, Gill I. A systematic review and meta-analysis of platelet-rich plasma versus corticosteroid injections for plantar fasciopathy. Int Orthop. 2017;41(6):1169–81.
59. Smith PA. Intra-articular autologous conditioned plasma injections provide safe and efficacious treatment for knee osteoarthritis: an FDA-sanctioned, ran-

domized, double-blind, placebo-controlled clinical trial. Am J Sports Med. 2016;44(4):884–91.
60. Shen L, Yuan T, Chen S, Xie X, Zhang C. The temporal effect of platelet-rich plasma on pain and physical function in the treatment of knee osteoarthritis: systematic review and meta-analysis of randomized controlled trials. J Orthop Surg Res. 2017;12(1):16.
61. de Vos RJ, Weir A, van Schie HT, et al. Platelet-rich plasma injection for chronic Achilles tendinopathy: a randomized controlled trial. JAMA. 2010;303(2):144–9.
62. de Vos RJ, Weir A, Tol JL, Verhaar JA, Weinans H, van Schie HT. No effects of PRP on ultrasonographic tendon structure and neovascularisation in chronic midportion Achilles tendinopathy. Br J Sports Med. 2011;45(5):387–92.
63. Boesen AP, Hansen R, Boesen MI, Malliaras P, Langberg H. Effect of high-volume injection, platelet-rich plasma, and sham treatment in chronic midportion Achilles tendinopathy: a randomized double-blinded prospective study. Am J Sports Med. 2017;45(9):2034–43.
64. de Jonge S, de Vos RJ, Weir A, et al. One-year follow-up of platelet-rich plasma treatment in chronic Achilles tendinopathy: a double-blind randomized placebo-controlled trial. Am J Sports Med. 2011;39(8):1623–9.
65. Kesikburun S, Tan AK, Yilmaz B, Yasar E, Yazicioglu K. Platelet-rich plasma injections in the treatment of chronic rotator cuff tendinopathy: a randomized controlled trial with 1-year follow-up. Am J Sports Med. 2013;41(11):2609–16.
66. Rha DW, Park GY, Kim YK, Kim MT, Lee SC. Comparison of the therapeutic effects of ultrasound-guided platelet-rich plasma injection and dry needling in rotator cuff disease: a randomized controlled trial. Clin Rehabil. 2013;27(2):113–22.
67. Shams A, El-Sayed M, Gamal O, Ewes W. Subacromial injection of autologous platelet-rich plasma versus corticosteroid for the treatment of symptomatic partial rotator cuff tears. Eur J Orthop Surg Traumatol. 2016;26(8):837–42.
68. Dallari D, Stagni C, Rani N, et al. Ultrasound-guided injection of platelet-rich plasma and hyaluronic acid, separately and in combination, for hip osteoarthritis: a randomized controlled study. Am J Sports Med. 2016;44(3):664–71.
69. Doria C, Mosele GR, Caggiari G, Puddu L, Ciurlia E. Treatment of early hip osteoarthritis: ultrasound-guided platelet rich plasma versus hyaluronic acid injections in a randomized clinical trial. Joints. 2017;5(3):152–5.
70. Mishra A, Pavelko T. Treatment of chronic elbow tendinosis with buffered platelet-rich plasma. Am J Sports Med. 2006;34(11):1774–8.
71. Peerbooms JC, Sluimer J, Bruijn DJ, Gosens T. Positive effect of an autologous platelet concentrate in lateral epicondylitis in a double-blind randomized controlled trial: platelet-rich plasma versus corticosteroid injection with a 1-year follow-up. Am J Sports Med. 2010;38(2):255–62.
72. Gosens T, Peerbooms JC, van Laar W, den Oudsten BL. Ongoing positive effect of platelet-rich plasma versus corticosteroid injection in lateral epicondylitis: a double-blind randomized controlled trial with 2-year follow-up. Am J Sports Med. 2011;39(6):1200–8.
73. Podesta L, Crow SA, Volkmer D, Bert T, Yocum LA. Treatment of partial ulnar collateral ligament tears in the elbow with platelet-rich plasma. Am J Sports Med. 2013;41(7):1689–94.
74. Dines JS, Williams PN, ElAttrache N, et al. Platelet-rich plasma can be used to successfully treat elbow ulnar collateral ligament insufficiency in high-level throwers. Am J Orthop (Belle Mead NJ). 2016;45(5):296–300.
75. Deal JB, Smith E, Heard W, O'Brien MJ, Savoie FH 3rd. Platelet-rich plasma for primary treatment of partial ulnar collateral ligament tears: MRI correlation with results. Orthop J Sports Med. 2017;5(11):2325967117738238.
76. Chauhan A, McQueen P, Chalmers PN, et al. Nonoperative treatment of elbow ulnar collateral ligament injuries with and without platelet-rich plasma in professional baseball players: a comparative and matched cohort analysis. Am J Sports Med. 2019;47(13):3107–19.
77. Hevesi M, LaPrade M, Saris DBF, Krych AJ. Stem cell treatment for ligament repair and reconstruction. Curr Rev Musculoskelet Med. 2019;12(4):446–50.
78. Carr JB 2nd, Rodeo SA. The role of biologic agents in the management of common shoulder pathologies: current state and future directions. J Shoulder Elb Surg. 2019;28(11):2041–52.
79. Dominici M, Le Blanc K, Mueller I, et al. Minimal criteria for defining multipotent mesenchymal stromal cells. The International Society for Cellular Therapy position statement. Cytotherapy. 2006;8(4):315–7.
80. Randelli P, Randelli F, Ragone V, et al. Regenerative medicine in rotator cuff injuries. Biomed Res Int. 2014;2014:129515.
81. Ahmad Z, Wardale J, Brooks R, Henson F, Noorani A, Rushton N. Exploring the application of stem cells in tendon repair and regeneration. Arthroscopy. 2012;28(7):1018–29.
82. Mazzocca AD, McCarthy MB, Chowaniec D, et al. Bone marrow-derived mesenchymal stem cells obtained during arthroscopic rotator cuff repair surgery show potential for tendon cell differentiation after treatment with insulin. Arthroscopy. 2011;27(11):1459–71.
83. Perdisa F, Gostynska N, Roffi A, Filardo G, Marcacci M, Kon E. Adipose-derived mesenchymal stem cells for the treatment of articular cartilage: a systematic review on preclinical and clinical evidence. Stem Cells Int. 2015;2015:597652.
84. Dragoo JL, Samimi B, Zhu M, et al. Tissue-engineered cartilage and bone using stem cells from human infrapatellar fat pads. J Bone Joint Surg Br. 2003;85(5):740–7.

85. Saw KY, Anz A, Siew-Yoke Jee C, et al. Articular cartilage regeneration with autologous peripheral blood stem cells versus hyaluronic acid: a randomized controlled trial. Arthroscopy. 2013;29(4):684–94.
86. Clarke AW, Alyas F, Morris T, Robertson CJ, Bell J, Connell DA. Skin-derived tenocyte-like cells for the treatment of patellar tendinopathy. Am J Sports Med. 2011;39(3):614–23.
87. Lin K, Rodeo S. Tendon and ligament healing. In: Wolters Kluwer. 2020.
88. Beitzel K, McCarthy MB, Cote MP, et al. Comparison of mesenchymal stem cells (osteoprogenitors) harvested from proximal humerus and distal femur during arthroscopic surgery. Arthroscopy. 2013;29(2):301–8.
89. Hernigou P, Poignard A, Beaujean F, Rouard H. Percutaneous autologous bone-marrow grafting for nonunions. Influence of the number and concentration of progenitor cells. J Bone Joint Surg Am. 2005;87(7):1430–7.
90. Hernigou P, Mathieu G, Poignard A, Manicom O, Beaujean F, Rouard H. Percutaneous autologous bone-marrow grafting for nonunions. Surgical technique. J Bone Joint Surg Am. 2006;88 Suppl 1 Pt 2:322–7.
91. Mazzocca AD, McCarthy MB, Chowaniec DM, Cote MP, Arciero RA, Drissi H. Rapid isolation of human stem cells (connective tissue progenitor cells) from the proximal humerus during arthroscopic rotator cuff surgery. Am J Sports Med. 2010;38(7):1438–47.
92. Beitzel K, McCarthy MB, Cote MP, et al. Rapid isolation of human stem cells (connective progenitor cells) from the distal femur during arthroscopic knee surgery. Arthroscopy. 2012;28(1):74–84.
93. Pittenger MF, Mackay AM, Beck SC, et al. Multilineage potential of adult human mesenchymal stem cells. Science. 1999;284(5411):143–7.
94. Chahla J, Mannava S, Cinque ME, Geeslin AG, Codina D, LaPrade RF. Bone marrow aspirate concentrate harvesting and processing technique. Arthrosc Tech. 2017;6(2):e441–5.
95. Martin DR, Cox NR, Hathcock TL, Niemeyer GP, Baker HJ. Isolation and characterization of multipotential mesenchymal stem cells from feline bone marrow. Exp Hematol. 2002;30(8):879–86.
96. Hoffman JK, Protzman NM, Malhotra AD. Biologic augmentation of the ulnar collateral ligament in the elbow of a professional baseball pitcher. Case Rep Orthop. 2015;2015:130157.
97. Axe M, Hurd W, Snyder-Mackler L. Data-based interval throwing programs for baseball players. Sports Health. 2009;1(2):145–53.
98. Reinold MM, Gill TJ, Wilk KE, Andrews JR. Current concepts in the evaluation and treatment of the shoulder in overhead throwing athletes, part 2: injury prevention and treatment. Sports Health. 2010;2(2):101–15.

15 Evolution of Surgical Reconstruction of the Medial Ulnar Collateral Ligament of the Elbow

Andrew R. Jensen, Matthew D. LaPrade, and Christopher L. Camp

Introduction

Medial ulnar collateral ligament (MUCL) tears were once known as devastating injuries for overhead athletes, particularly for baseball pitchers. However, in 1974, Dr. Frank Jobe invented a novel surgical technique to reconstruct the anterior bundle of the MUCL, and this new procedure allowed many athletes to return to their high levels of competition [1–3]. This surgery, known as the "Tommy John" procedure, revolutionized the surgical management of MUCL tears.

Since the initial description of MUCL reconstruction surgery was published in 1986, there have been many subsequent modifications to the initial technique, many of which have themselves been altered further over time [4]. Currently, the phrase "Tommy John surgery" actually refers to a heterogenous population of surgical techniques, all of which ultimately reconstruct the anterior bundle of the MUCL but with technical differences according to soft tissue management and graft fixation methods.

In this chapter, we will review this evolution of MUCL reconstructive surgery. MUCL repair techniques are discussed elsewhere in this book. Although we have included a chronologic listing of published techniques (Table 15.1) [5–18], our aim is to describe the evolutionary process of the surgical technique (Fig. 15.1) and to emphasize not only what changes were instituted with each new surgical technique, but the reasons for those changes.

MUCL Reconstruction Techniques – Figure of Eight Constructs (Fig. 15.2)

Jobe Technique (1986)

Dr. Jobe's original technique involved releasing the flexor-pronator mass off of the medial epicondyle and used a submuscular transposition for the ulnar nerve for complete visualization of the MUCL [5]. For osseous graft fixation, a V-shaped bone tunnel was drilled into the ulna at the level of the sublime tubercle and a Y-shaped bone tunnel was drilled into the medial epicondyle [5]. The common, distal aspect of the medial epicondyle's bone tunnel was wide enough to accommodate both strands of the eventual graft, while the two proximal tunnels were just wide enough for one limb each. Of the two proximal humeral drill holes, one was directed posteriorly toward the ulnar nerve, so ulnar nerve transposition was performed prior to drilling [5]. The tendon graft was then passed through the two ulnar and

A. R. Jensen (✉)
Department of Orthopaedic Surgery, University of California, Los Angeles, Santa Monica, CA, USA

M. D. LaPrade · C. L. Camp
Department of Orthopedic Surgery, Mayo Clinic, Rochester, MN, USA

J. S. Dines et al. (eds.), *Elbow Ulnar Collateral Ligament Injury*, https://doi.org/10.1007/978-3-030-69567-5_15

Table 15.1 Introduction of MUCL reconstruction techniques by year

Year	Technique name	Authors	Construct family
1986	Jobe	Jobe et al. [5]	Figure of 8
1995	American Sports Medicine Institute (ASMI)	Andrews et al. [6]	Figure of 8
1998	Hybrid	Hechtman et al. [7]	Triangular
2001	Modified Jobe	Thompson et al. [8]	Figure of 8
2002	Docking	Rohrbough et al. [9]	Triangular
2003	Dual interference screw	Ahmad et al. [10]	Linear
2005	EndoButton	Armstrong et al. [11]	Linear
2006	DANE TJ	Conway [12]	Linear
2006	Three-strand docking	Koh et al. [13]	Triangular
2006	Four-strand docking	Paletta et al. [14]	Triangular
2007	Double docking	Furukawa et al. [15]	Linear
2013	Docking plus	McGraw et al. [16]	Figure of 8
2013	GraftLink	Lynch et al. [17]	Linear
2013	TightRope	Lynch et al. [17]	Linear
2019	Anatomic	Camp et al. [18]	Linear

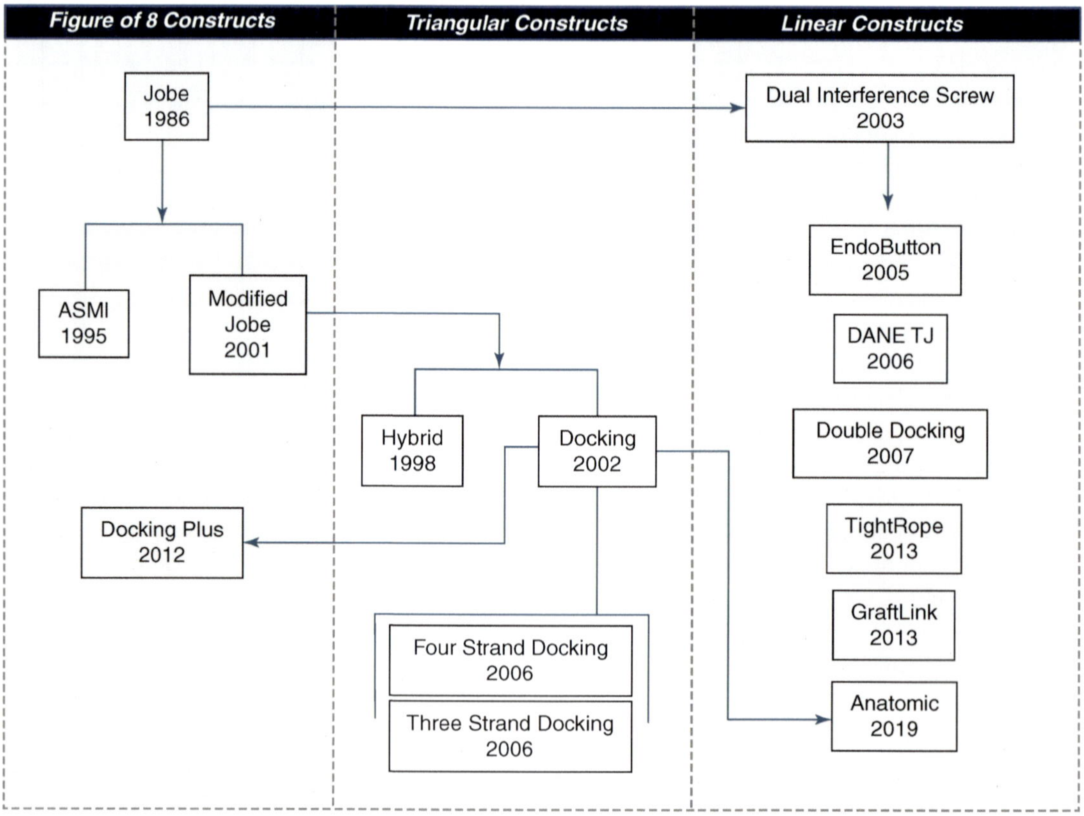

Fig. 15.1 MUCL reconstruction evolution flowchart

humeral bone tunnels and sutured onto itself, creating a figure of eight construct [5].

In Dr. Jobe's initial study, 63% of his 16 patients were able to return to preinjury level of competition [5]. However, 31% experienced postoperative ulnar neuropathy (including Tommy John himself) [5]. Another study of 56 patients found that 68% returned to preinjury

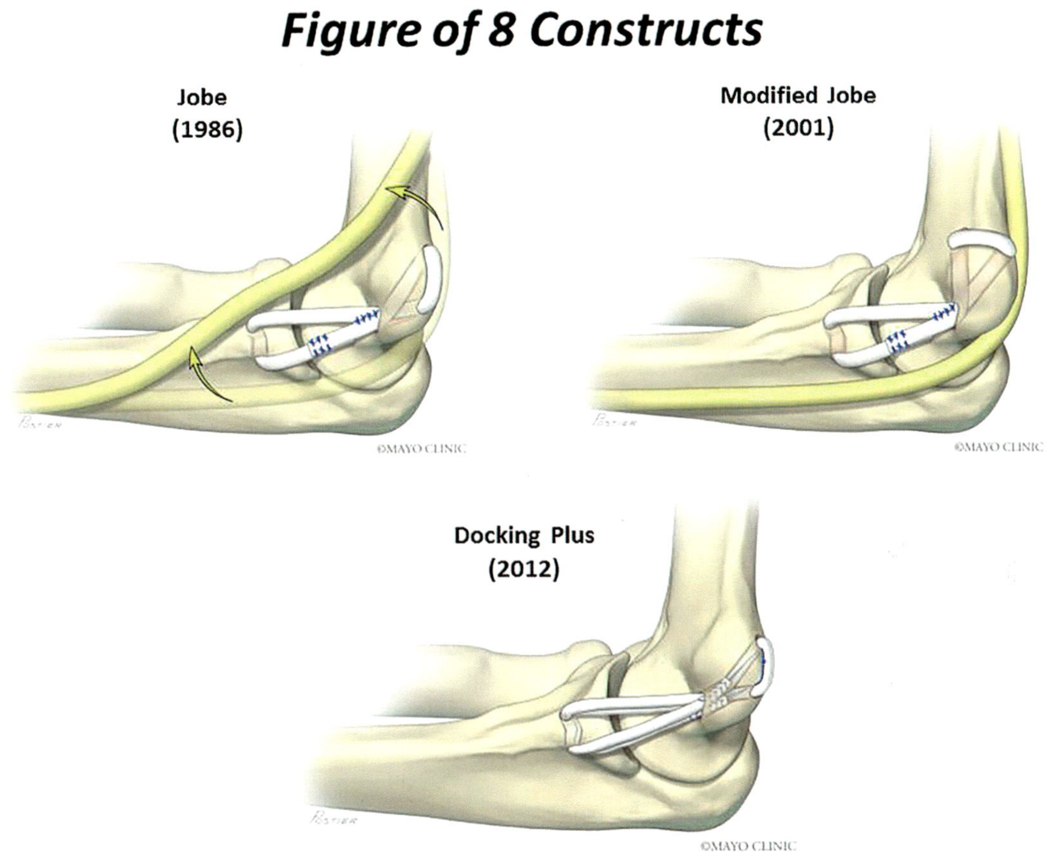

Fig. 15.2 Figure of eight MUCL reconstruction constructs

level of competition but, again, there was a high rate of ulnar neuropathy (25%) [19].

Although these return to play rates are much lower than those of most modern techniques, these results represented an incredible improvement for athletes with MUCL tears at that time.

American Sports Medicine Institute (ASMI) Technique (1995)

Due to the high rates of ulnar neuropathy in Dr. Jobe's cohort of patients, Drs. Andrews and Timmerman of the ASMI proposed a modification of the Jobe technique which became known as the ASMI technique [6]. This first evolution of Tommy John surgery sought to decrease ulnar neuropathy rates by minimizing manipulation of the soft tissues and the ulnar nerve. The ASMI technique therefore utilized a flexor carpi ulnaris (FCU) split instead of flexor-pronator mass detachment and performed a subcutaneous transposition in place of a submuscular one [6]. The osseous graft fixation method was not modified from the Jobe technique [6].

A large study published by the ASMI group in 2010 demonstrated that their technique resulted in excellent results for 83% of their patients with just a 16% ulnar neuropathy rate, which was typically self-resolving by 6 weeks [20]. Both of these values represented notable improvements over those from the original Jobe technique, marking these soft tissue changes of the ASMI technique a successful adaptation of the Tommy John surgery.

Modified Jobe Technique (2001)

A cadaveric study published in 1996 showed that a "muscle-splitting" approach to the MUCL, through a raphe between the ulnar-innervated FCU and the median-innervated common flexor mass, did not violate branches of either nerves [21]. Based on this work, Drs. Thompson and Jobe published a modification of their technique in 2001, which became known as the modified Jobe technique [8]. Three modifications were adopted in this technique in an effort to decrease ulnar neuropathy rates: in addition to using the muscle-splitting approach in lieu of the flexor-pronator mass release, the authors moved the proximal humeral tunnels so that both exited away from the ulnar nerve, and the ulnar nerve was protected but not dissected or routinely transposed as it previously had been [8].

Using the modified Jobe technique for MUCL reconstruction, the authors found that 94% of patients had good or excellent clinical results and just 15% had self-resolving postoperative ulnar neuropathy [8]. A systematic review on the use of the muscle-splitting approach, as compared to the flexor-pronator mass detachment, found a 17% increase in excellent clinical results and decrease in ulnar neuropathy rates from 14% to 5% [22]. Ultimately, these three changes to Tommy John surgery have improved clinical outcomes and decreased complication rates from previous iterations of the surgery.

Docking Plus Technique (2012)

After the docking technique, which will be discussed in the Triangular Construct section, was described in 2002, the docking plus technique was created in 2013. Also a figure of eight construct, the impetus behind the docking plus technique was to hold tension on the tendon graft during osseous fixation and to allow entire graft utilization without having to remove redundant graft, as occurs with the docking technique [16]. To achieve these goals, one of the graft limbs is sutured back onto the graft after being passed through the ulnar tunnel. They are then docked together into the common humeral tunnel, leaving the other graft limb free to be passed through the two proximal humeral tunnels, as in the other figure of eight construct methods, and through the ulnar tunnel again, all while tension is held [16].

A retrospective study of the docking plus technique found 88% good or excellent Conway scores [23]. However, it is currently unclear if the evolutionary changes of the docking plus technique represent true clinically relevant improvements to the traditional docking technique, as clinical results thus far have been equivalent.

MUCL Reconstruction Techniques – Triangular Constructs (Fig. 15.3)

Docking Technique (2002)

The docking technique, developed by Dr. David Altchek and first published in 2002, marked the first major change to graft construct orientation in Tommy John surgery [9]. Instead of a figure of eight graft construct, the docking technique and its evolutionary descendants utilize a triangular graft construct [9]. The main purpose of this change was to minimize bone loss from the medial epicondyle during humeral tunnel preparation [9].

Instead of drilling three 3.2-mm tunnels in a Y-configuration in the medial epicondyle as occurs in the Jobe technique, the docking technique uses a single 4.0-mm common humeral tunnel into which graft is "docked" and two proximal 2.0-mm connecting tunnels through which sutures only are passed [9]. After the graft has been cut to length and docked into the common humeral tunnel, thus creating the triangular graft construct, the suture limbs are retrieved out of the smaller proximal humeral tunnels and tied over a bone bridge on the medial epicondyle [9].

The docking technique modifications of MUCL reconstruction surgery addressed many perceived technical weaknesses of previous techniques. Multiple clinical studies have found close to or greater than 90% return to play rates and very low rates of ulnar neuropathy with use of the

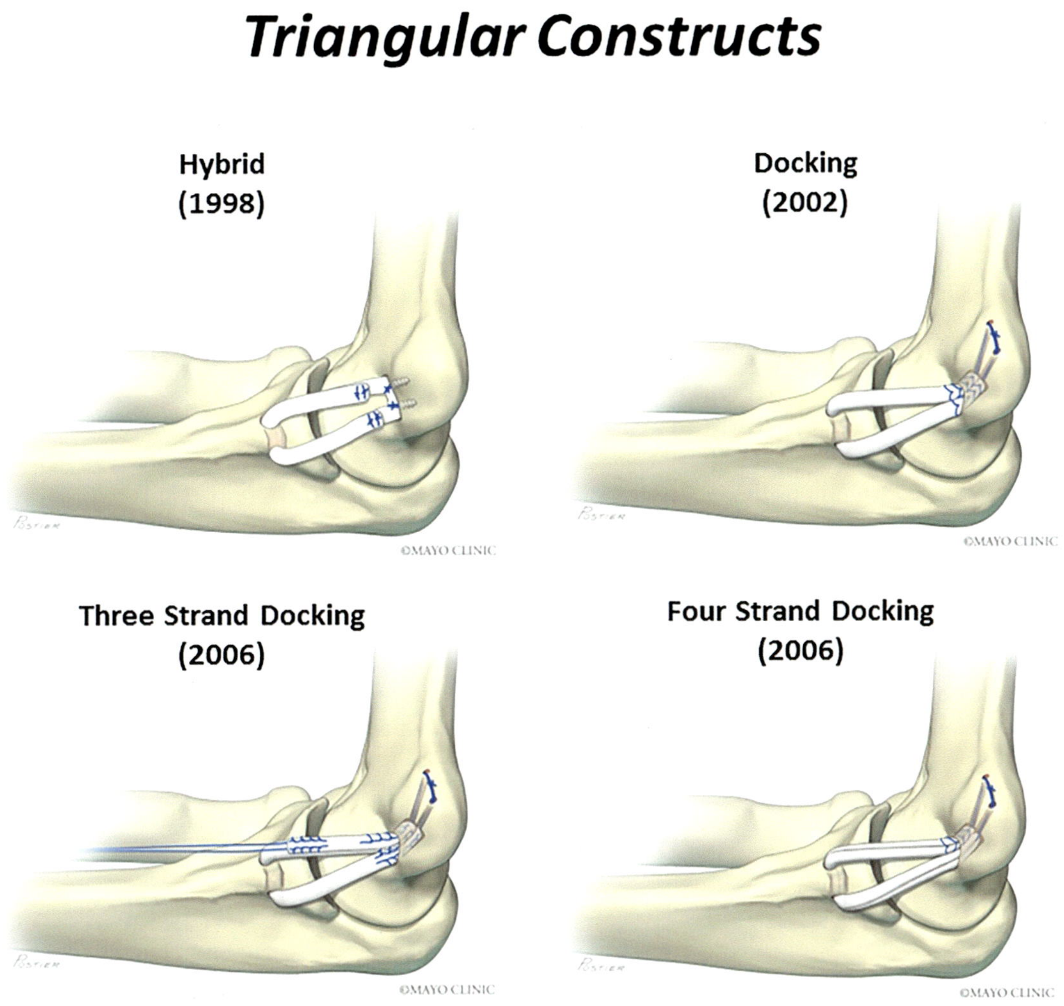

Fig. 15.3 Triangular MUCL reconstruction constructs

docking technique [9, 24–27]. Accordingly, the docking technique has become the most commonly performed variant of Tommy John surgery for professional baseball players [28].

Three- and Four-Strand Docking Techniques (2006)

One perceived weakness of the docking technique is that excess graft is removed prior to docking the graft, thus decreasing the potential collagen content of the ultimate construct. To address this perceived weakness, the three-strand and four-strand docking techniques were separately described, both in 2006.

In the three-strand docking technique, the anterior limb of the graft is folded back on itself after being passed through the ulnar tunnel [13]. This results in two anterior limbs and one posterior limb being docked into the medial epicondyle [13]. In the four-strand docking technique, the entire length of graft is first folded and then passed through the ulnar tunnel, such that there are two anterior and two posterior limbs to be docked into the medial epicondyle [14]. In both situations, excess tendon graft is incorporated into the final construct rather than being excised.

Clinical studies on the two techniques have demonstrated greater than 90% excellent clinical outcomes and very low rates of ulnar neuropathy [13, 29, 30], results that are comparable to those of the docking technique. These evolutions of the docking technique appear to increase collagen content of the graft construct without compromising clinical results, but whether these changes lead to clinical improvements for patients is not known.

Hechtman's Hybrid Technique (1998)

Dr. Hechtman's Hybrid technique was published in 2011 as an attempt to minimize soft tissue dissection and more closely approximate normal MUCL anatomy than is seen with the Jobe technique [7]. The first iteration of this Hybrid technique initially utilized dual suture anchor fixation on both the humeral and ulnar ends, resulting in a rectangular shaped construct, but was ultimately changed to a triangular shaped construct with Jobe-style tunnels instead of suture anchors for the ulnar fixation [31].

Excellent clinical results have been found in 85% of patients undergoing the Hybrid technique for MUCL reconstruction, with just one case of ulnar neuropathy reported [31]. Thus, compared to the Jobe technique from which it was derived, the Hybrid technique has been a successful improvement in clinical results and complication rates.

MUCL Reconstruction Techniques – Linear Constructs (Fig. 15.4)

In 2002, a cadaveric study demonstrated that the central fibers of the anterior bundle of the MUCL, located between the anterior and posterior bands, were the most important aspect of the anterior bundle for valgus stability [32]. It was hypothesized that reconstructing just these central fibers

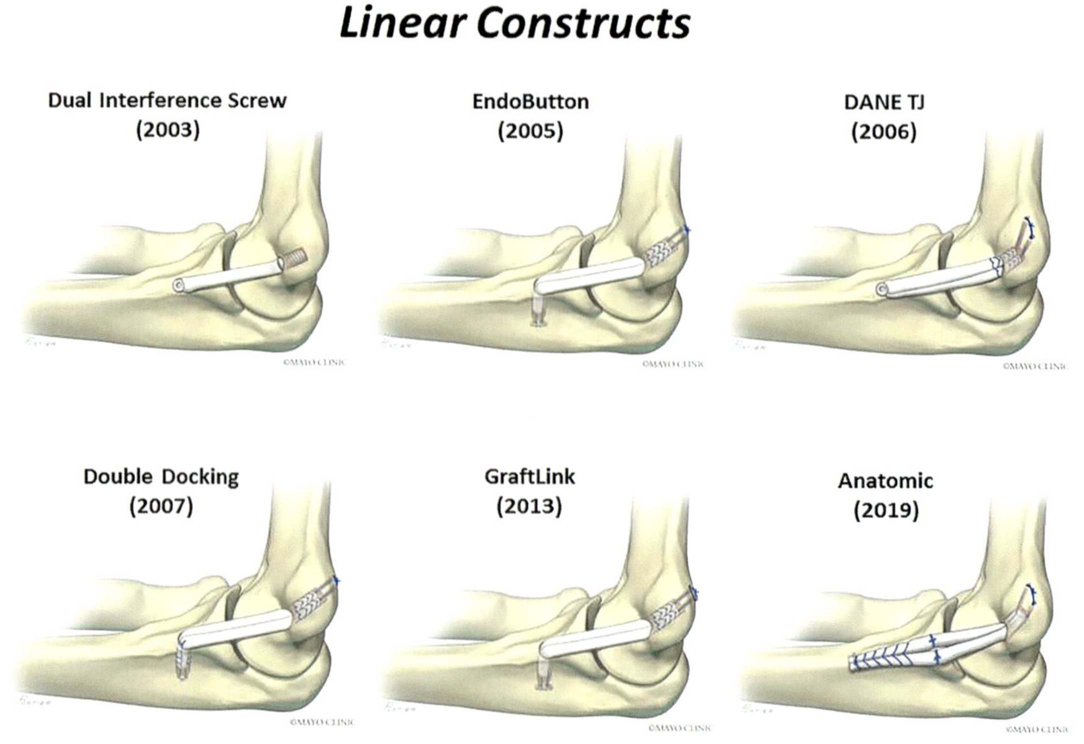

Fig. 15.4 Linear MUCL reconstruction constructs

of the anterior bundle of the MUCL with a linear graft construct would maximize valgus stability while also decreasing the risk of bone bridge fracture and irritation to the ulnar nerve posed by the previous MUCL reconstruction techniques [32]. Many Tommy John techniques utilizing linear constructs were subsequently described, all of which attempted to achieve these theoretical benefits of a linear construct.

Dual Interference Screw Technique (2003)

The first of these linear constructs to be described was the dual interference screw technique, published originally in 2003 [10]. As the name implies, an interference screw is used to fixate the tendon graft on both the ulna and the humerus, thus creating a linear construct. While there is conflicting biomechanical evidence about the structural integrity of the dual interference screw construct [10, 15], the sole clinical study on this technique reported 90% excellent results and just one case of ulnar neuropathy [33].

David Altcheck and Neal ElAttrache Tommy John (DANE TJ) Technique (2006)

Due to the potential of medial epicondyle fractures from drill holes used with interference screws in the humerus [34, 35], Drs. Altchek and ElAttrache published a hybrid linear construct that used docking-style tunnels instead of an interference screw on the humerus [12]. This technique was named the DANE TJ technique and was published in 2006 [12]. The two clinical studies that have evaluated the DANE TJ technique reported 85–86% excellent results with few transient ulnar neuropathies [12, 36].

EndoButton Technique (2005)

Dr. Armstrong proposed a linear construct utilizing EndoButton (Smith & Nephew, Mansfield, MA) ulnar sided fixation and docking-style fixation on the humerus, and then compared this construct to previously described constructs in a biomechanical study [11]. While the biomechanical study found that the EndoButton construct had greater mean peak load to failure than figure of eight or dual interference screw constructs, no clinical data have yet been published.

Double Docking Technique (2007)

In 2007, Dr. Furukawa described another linear construct in which the graft is fixed to both the ulna and humerus through docking constructs [15]. This technique was therefore called the double docking technique [15] and, in a cadaveric study, it was found to have favorable biomechanical properties as compared to other constructs [15]. Like many of the other linear constructs, no clinical data have been reported for the double docking technique.

GraftLink and TightRope Techniques (2013)

Similarly, Dr. Lynch described two linear constructs that have supportive biomechanical data but no clinical results to date. The first technique, called the GraftLink (Arthrex, Naples, FL) technique, utilizes cortical buttons through bicortical drill holes in both the ulna and humerus for graft fixation [17]. The other, called the TightRope (Arthrex, Naples, FL) technique, also utilizes a cortical button through a bicortical drill hole in the ulna but, instead, uses docking-style fixation on the medial epicondyle [37].

Anatomic Technique (2019)

Anatomic studies of MUCL, published after Dr. Jobe first described the Tommy John procedure, have found that the ulnar insertion of the anterior bundle is more extended and distally tapered than was previously thought [38–40]. Because of this finding, Dr. Camp described a unique construct that attempted to more accurately reconstruct the elongated triangular shaped ulnar footprint of the native MUCL anterior bundle [18]. This surgery was therefore called the Anatomic technique. Additionally, it is well known that the graft–bone interface on the humeral side is a common site of failure of MUCL reconstructions that utilize a docking technique. There is concern that this may be related to the high volume of suture in this socket that prevents interdigitation of bone growth into the graft. In an ideal setting, the socket would be drilled to size based on the graft diameter. This would ensure all a tight fit increasing direct graft to bone contact circumferentially with minimal suture to impede healing. To accomplish this goal, the folded end of the graft is fixed into a socket in the medial epicondyle that has been drilled to size. After performing docking-style fixation in the medial epicondyle, the two graft limbs are attached to the ulna proximally with two small all-suture, suture anchors and distally with a single unicortical cortical button. This configuration therefore creates a broad and distally tapered ulnar insertion footprint for the reconstructive graft. It also allows for sequential tensioning of both sides after initial fixation. In a cadaveric study, the Anatomic technique had improved biomechanical parameters compared to the docking technique [18]. No clinical studies have been published on the Anatomic technique to date.

Conclusion

Tommy John surgical techniques have evolved significantly since initially described in 1986 and now refer to a heterogenous group of unique procedures that, broadly speaking, categorize into one of the three groups based on graft configuration: figure of eight, triangular, and linear shaped grafts. Surgical techniques that result in figure of eight and triangular graft constructs have longer clinical track records, while linear constructs are mostly supported by biomechanical data from cadaveric studies thus far. The technical changes that have been implemented over time have been in response to real or perceived limitations of previous iterations of the surgery. The many current techniques vary based on soft tissue management and osseous graft fixation methods. It is critical for elbow surgeons to understand the history of Tommy John surgery, the evolutionary changes that have occurred, and the reasons for these changes to better understand areas of future innovation and improvement.

References

1. Looze CA, Strauss EJ, Jazrawi LM. Ulnar collateral ligament reconstruction past, present, and future. Bull Hosp Jt Dis. 2018;76(1):22–6.
2. Camp CL, Conte S, D'Angelo J, Fealy SA. Epidemiology of ulnar collateral ligament reconstruction in Major and Minor League Baseball pitchers: comprehensive report of 1429 cases. J Shoulder Elb Surg. 2018;27(5):871–8. https://doi.org/10.1016/j.jse.2018.01.024.
3. Camp CL, Conte S, D'Angelo J, Fealy SA. Following ulnar collateral ligament reconstruction, professional baseball position players return to play faster than pitchers, but catchers return less frequently. J Shoulder Elb Surg. 2018;27(6):1078–85. https://doi.org/10.1016/j.jse.2018.01.023.
4. Watson JN, McQueen P, Hutchinson MR. A systematic review of ulnar collateral ligament reconstruction techniques. Am J Sports Med. 2014;42(10):2510–6. https://doi.org/10.1177/0363546513509051.
5. Jobe FW, Stark H, Lombardo SJ. Reconstruction of the ulnar collateral ligament in athletes. J Bone Joint Surg Am. 1986;68(8):1158–63.
6. Andrews JR, Timmerman LA. Outcome of elbow surgery in professional baseball players. Am J Sports Med. 1995;23(4):407–13. https://doi.org/10.1177/036354659502300406.
7. Hechtman KS, Tjin ATEW, Zvijac JE, Uribe JW, Latta LL. Biomechanics of a less invasive procedure for reconstruction of the ulnar collateral ligament of the elbow. Am J Sports Med. 1998;26(5):620–4. https://doi.org/10.1177/03635465980260050401.
8. Thompson WH, Jobe FW, Yocum LA, Pink MM. Ulnar collateral ligament reconstruction in athletes: muscle-splitting approach without transposition of the ulnar nerve. J Shoulder Elb Surg. 2001;10(2):152–7. https://doi.org/10.1067/mse.2001.112881.
9. Rohrbough JT, Altchek DW, Hyman J, Williams RJ 3rd, Botts JD. Medial collateral ligament reconstruction of the elbow using the docking technique. Am J Sports Med. 2002;30(4):541–8. https://doi.org/10.1177/03635465020300041401.
10. Ahmad CS, Lee TQ, ElAttrache NS. Biomechanical evaluation of a new ulnar collateral ligament reconstruction technique with interference screw fixation. Am J Sports Med. 2003;31(3):332–7. https://doi.org/10.1177/03635465030310030201.

11. Armstrong AD, Dunning CD, Ferreira LM, Faber KJ, Johnson JA, King GJ. A biomechanical comparison of four reconstruction techniques for the medial collateral ligament-deficient elbow. J Shoulder Elb Surg. 2005;14(2):207–15.
12. Conway JE. The DANE TJ procedure for elbow medial ulnar collateral ligament insufficiency. Tech Should Elbow Surg. 2006;7(1):36–43.
13. Koh JL, Schafer MF, Keuter G, Hsu JE. Ulnar collateral ligament reconstruction in elite throwing athletes. Arthroscopy. 2006;22(11):1187–91. https://doi.org/10.1016/j.arthro.2006.07.024.
14. Paletta GA Jr, Klepps SJ, Difelice GS, Allen T, Brodt MD, Burns ME, et al. Biomechanical evaluation of 2 techniques for ulnar collateral ligament reconstruction of the elbow. Am J Sports Med. 2006;34(10):1599–603. https://doi.org/10.1177/0363546506289340.
15. Furukawa K, Pichora J, Steinmann S, Faber KJ, Johnson JA, King GJ. Efficacy of interference screw and double-docking methods using palmaris longus and GraftJacket for medial collateral ligament reconstruction of the elbow. J Shoulder Elb Surg. 2007;16(4):449–53. https://doi.org/10.1016/j.jse.2006.09.020.
16. McGraw MA, Kremchek TE, Hooks TR, Papangelou C. Biomechanical evaluation of the docking plus ulnar collateral ligament reconstruction technique compared with the docking technique. Am J Sports Med. 2013;41(2):313–20. https://doi.org/10.1177/0363546512466375.
17. Lynch JL, Pifer MA, Maerz T, Kurdziel MD, Davidson AA, Baker KC, et al. The GraftLink ulnar collateral ligament reconstruction: biomechanical comparison with the docking technique in both kinematics and failure tests. Am J Sports Med. 2013;41(10):2278–87. https://doi.org/10.1177/0363546513498999.
18. Camp CL, Bernard C, Benavitz B, Konicek J, Altchek DW, Dines JS. Reconstruction of the medial ulnar collateral ligament of the elbow: biomechanical comparison of a novel anatomic technique to the docking technique. Orthop J Sports Med. 2019; https://doi.org/10.1177/2325967119857592.
19. Conway JE, Jobe FW, Glousman RE, Pink M. Medial instability of the elbow in throwing athletes. Treatment by repair or reconstruction of the ulnar collateral ligament. J Bone Joint Surg Am. 1992;74(1):67–83.
20. Cain EL Jr, Andrews JR, Dugas JR, Wilk KE, McMichael CS, Walter JC 2nd, et al. Outcome of ulnar collateral ligament reconstruction of the elbow in 1281 athletes: results in 743 athletes with minimum 2-year follow-up. Am J Sports Med. 2010;38(12):2426–34. https://doi.org/10.1177/0363546510378100.
21. Smith GR, Altchek DW, Pagnani MJ, Keeley JR. A muscle-splitting approach to the ulnar collateral ligament of the elbow. Neuroanatomy and operative technique. Am J Sports Med. 1996;24(5):575–80. https://doi.org/10.1177/036354659602400503.
22. Vitale MA, Ahmad CS. The outcome of elbow ulnar collateral ligament reconstruction in overhead athletes: a systematic review. Am J Sports Med. 2008;36(6):1193–205. https://doi.org/10.1177/0363546508319053.
23. Donohue BF, Lubitz MG, Kremchek TE. Elbow ulnar collateral ligament reconstruction using the novel docking plus technique in 324 athletes. Sports Med Open. 2019;5(1):3. https://doi.org/10.1186/s40798-018-0174-8.
24. Dodson CC, Thomas A, Dines JS, Nho SJ, Williams RJ 3rd, Altchek DW. Medial ulnar collateral ligament reconstruction of the elbow in throwing athletes. Am J Sports Med. 2006;34(12):1926–32. https://doi.org/10.1177/0363546506290988.
25. Dines JS, Jones KJ, Kahlenberg C, Rosenbaum A, Osbahr DC, Altchek DW. Elbow ulnar collateral ligament reconstruction in javelin throwers at a minimum 2-year follow-up. Am J Sports Med. 2012;40(1):148–51. https://doi.org/10.1177/0363546511422350.
26. Jones KJ, Dines JS, Rebolledo BJ, Weeks KD, Williams RJ, Dines DM, et al. Operative management of ulnar collateral ligament insufficiency in adolescent athletes. Am J Sports Med. 2014;42(1):117–21. https://doi.org/10.1177/0363546513507695.
27. Erickson BJ, Bach BR Jr, Cohen MS, Bush-Joseph CA, Cole BJ, Verma NN, et al. Ulnar collateral ligament reconstruction: the rush experience. Orthop J Sports Med. 2016;4(1):2325967115626876. https://doi.org/10.1177/2325967115626876.
28. Griffith TB, Ahmad CS, Gorroochurn P, D'Angelo J, Ciccotti MG, Dines JS, et al. Comparison of outcomes based on graft type and tunnel configuration for primary ulnar collateral ligament reconstruction in professional baseball pitchers. Am J Sports Med. 2019;47(5):1103–10. https://doi.org/10.1177/0363546519831705.
29. Bowers AL, Dines JS, Dines DM, Altchek DW. Elbow medial ulnar collateral ligament reconstruction: clinical relevance and the docking technique. J Shoulder Elb Surg. 2010;19(2 Suppl):110–7. https://doi.org/10.1016/j.jse.2010.01.005.
30. Paletta GA Jr, Wright RW. The modified docking procedure for elbow ulnar collateral ligament reconstruction: 2-year follow-up in elite throwers. Am J Sports Med. 2006;34(10):1594–8. https://doi.org/10.1177/0363546506289884.
31. Hechtman KS, Zvijac JE, Wells ME, Botto-van BA. Long-term results of ulnar collateral ligament reconstruction in throwing athletes based on a hybrid technique. Am J Sports Med. 2011;39(2):342–7. https://doi.org/10.1177/0363546510385401.
32. Armstrong AD, Dunning CE, Faber KJ, Johnson JA, King GJ. Single-strand ligament reconstruction of the medial collateral ligament restores valgus elbow stability. J Shoulder Elb Surg. 2002;11(1):65–71. https://doi.org/10.1067/mse.2002.120392.
33. Kodde IF, Rahusen FT, Eygendaal D. Long-term results after ulnar collateral ligament reconstruction of the elbow in European athletes with interference screw technique and triceps fascia autograft. J Shoulder Elb Surg. 2012;21(12):1656–63. https://doi.org/10.1016/j.jse.2012.07.010.

34. Chang ES, Dodson CC, Ciccotti MG. Comparison of surgical techniques for ulnar collateral ligament reconstruction in overhead athletes. J Am Acad Orthop Surg. 2016;24(3):135–49. https://doi.org/10.5435/jaaos-d-14-00323.
35. Jackson TJ, Adamson GJ, Peterson A, Patton J, McGarry MH, Lee TQ. Ulnar collateral ligament reconstruction using bisuspensory fixation: a biomechanical comparison with the docking technique. Am J Sports Med. 2013;41(5):1158–64. https://doi.org/10.1177/0363546513481957.
36. Dines JS, ElAttrache NS, Conway JE, Smith W, Ahmad CS. Clinical outcomes of the DANE TJ technique to treat ulnar collateral ligament insufficiency of the elbow. Am J Sports Med. 2007;35(12):2039–44. https://doi.org/10.1177/0363546507305802.
37. Lynch JL, Maerz T, Kurdziel MD, Davidson AA, Baker KC, Anderson K. Biomechanical evaluation of the TightRope versus traditional docking ulnar collateral ligament reconstruction technique: kinematic and failure testing. Am J Sports Med. 2013;41(5):1165–73. https://doi.org/10.1177/0363546513482567.
38. Dugas JR, Ostrander RV, Cain EL, Kingsley D, Andrews JR. Anatomy of the anterior bundle of the ulnar collateral ligament. J Shoulder Elb Surg. 2007;16(5):657–60. https://doi.org/10.1016/j.jse.2006.11.009.
39. Farrow LD, Mahoney AJ, Stefancin JJ, Taljanovic MS, Sheppard JE, Schickendantz MS. Quantitative analysis of the medial ulnar collateral ligament ulnar footprint and its relationship to the ulnar sublime tubercle. Am J Sports Med. 2011;39(9):1936–41. https://doi.org/10.1177/0363546511406220.
40. Camp CL, Jahandar H, Sinatro AM, Imhauser CW, Altchek DW, Dines JS. Quantitative anatomic analysis of the medial ulnar collateral ligament complex of the elbow. Orthop J Sports Med. 2018;6(3):2325967118762751. https://doi.org/10.1177/2325967118762751.

16 Ulnar Collateral Ligament Reconstruction: Graft Selection and Harvest Technique

James E. Voos and Brandon J. Erickson

Introduction

Ulnar collateral ligament (UCL) reconstruction has proven effective in correcting elbow valgus instability in overhead athletes. Return to the same or higher level of sport has been reported to be as high as 73–90% in the recent literature [1–3]. UCL reconstruction (UCLR) has been described using several well-described methods, including the classic Jobe, modified Jobe, docking, double docking, and other techniques [4–8].

The goal of UCLR is to reproduce the anatomy, tension, and stability of the anterior bundle of the UCL, which is the primary stabilizer of valgus stress to the elbow [2, 4, 9]. Reconstructive options must attempt to resist the tremendous forces generated across the elbow joint during the overhead throwing motion. At end of the late-cocking phase and initiation of the acceleration phase of the throwing cycle, the elbow extends at speeds over 2300° per second generating medial shear forces of nearly 290 N. The valgus load to the elbow at this phase has been documented at 64 N m. This force exceeds the ultimate tensile strength of the native ligament, particularly in the setting of repetitive overhead throwing [10, 11]. The applied load-to-failure moment of the native UCL has been reported by Ahmad et al., Prud'homme et al., and Paletta et al. as 18.8 N m, 20.9 N m, and 30.4 N m, respectively, based on the cyclic loading testing models utilized [12–14]. Hence, every time a pitcher throws, the UCL approaches failure. Supporting structures around the elbow, both bony and soft tissue, help offload the UCL to prevent failure during each pitch.

The selection of an appropriate graft for UCLR, therefore, focuses on obtaining the strongest available graft with the lowest donor site morbidity. The chapter discusses the available graft selection options and harvest techniques utilizing the most current literature.

Graft Selection Options

Ipsilateral or contralateral palmaris longus tendon autograft is the most commonly utilized graft in UCL reconstruction [1–8, 15, 16]. The gracilis tendon is the second most frequently utilized graft. In a series of 100 consecutive overhead throwing athletes, Dodson et al. reported the use of 70 palmaris (59 ipsilateral, 11 contralateral) and 30 gracilis tendons for reconstruction [2]. In the original description of the UCLR procedure by Jobe et al., the donor tendon was the palmaris longus (12 patients), the plantaris (3 patients), and a 3-mm wide and 15-cm long strip of Achilles

J. E. Voos
Department of Orthopaedic Surgery, University Hospitals Cleveland, Cleveland, OH, USA

B. J. Erickson (✉)
Department of Sports Medicine, Rothman Orthopaedic Institute, New York, NY, USA

J. S. Dines et al. (eds.), *Elbow Ulnar Collateral Ligament Injury*,
https://doi.org/10.1007/978-3-030-69567-5_16

tendon (one patient) [4]. Cain et al. reported the largest published series of UCLR to date which included 743 patients [1]. Autograft distribution consisted of 552 palmaris (512 ipsilateral, 40 contralateral), 175 gracilis, and 16 palmaris tendons. Additional autograft sources in the literature include toe extensor tendons and patellar tendon [3].

The authors primarily utilize ipsilateral palmaris tendon autograft in most cases due to ease of harvest in the same surgical field. An exception is in the case of female overhead athletes, such as a javelin thrower, wherein the authors experience the tendon may be smaller than the desired 3 mm. All patients are given the option to utilize palmaris or gracilis tendon autograft based on their desired preference after the procedure has been explained. Allograft tissue is typically only utilized in the revision setting when a reasonable autograft option is not available, although studies have found no significant difference in performance or return to sport (RTS) rates when comparing autograft to allograft [17].

A small percentage of the population has demonstrated an absence of a palmaris tendon. Troha et al. randomly evaluated 200 Caucasian patients for the presence or absence of the palmaris longus tendon [18]. It was absent unilaterally in 3% of patients and bilaterally in 2.5% for a 5.5% total overall absence. Soltani et al. prospectively evaluated 516 patients for the absence of the palmaris tendon based on ethnicity [19]. There was no difference between white (non-Hispanic) and white (Hispanic) patients, with a prevalence of 14.9% and 13.1%, respectively. However, African-American (4.5%) and Asian (2.9%) patients had significantly fewer absences of the palmaris. Furthermore, in patients who only have a palmaris on one side, the authors have occasionally found this palmaris to be less robust, with a shorter tendon length secondary to a low-lying muscle belly. Hence, in these patients the surgeon should be prepared to use a gracilis if needed.

Biomechanical studies have been performed to evaluate the ideal graft choice for UCL reconstruction. In a cadaveric model with a uniaxial load applied to catastrophic failure, Regan et al. reported the palmaris tendon had a load to failure of 358 N compared to 261 N in the native UCL [20]. Paletta et al. reported no difference in load to failure between the intact UCL and a four-strand palmaris reconstruction using the docking technique in a single load-to-failure model without cyclic loading [14].

More recent studies have reported a different result. Armstrong et al. performed cyclic testing of the elbow with incremental increases in load until failure defined as 5-mm elongation [21]. The authors reported the native ligament failed at 142.5 N and the palmaris reconstruction failed at 53 N. The mean number of cycles to failure was 2536 for the intact UCL and 701 for the reconstruction. Using a slightly different loading protocol, Prud'homme et al. reported the native UCL failed at 193.3 N and the palmaris reconstruction failed at 102.7 N [12]. The mean number of cycles to failure was 367 for the intact UCL and 185 for the reconstruction. Larger gracilis and patellar tendon grafts showed no statistical difference in load to failure or number of cycles to failure. The authors concluded there was no biomechanical advantage to a larger graft; therefore, the palmaris is the ideal graft source secondary to its ease of harvest with low morbidity.

Finally, when choosing a graft consideration should be given to future injury risk and ability to RTS at the same or higher level of play. Recent evidence has evaluated outcomes and future injury risk in major league baseball (MLB) and minor league baseball players who underwent UCLR with either a palmaris longus or a hamstring graft [22]. Overall, 195 professional baseball players underwent UCLR with hamstring autograft. This group was compared to matched controls who underwent UCLR with palmaris autograft. No difference in RTS rate or timing of RTS existed between the groups. However, significantly more subsequent injuries to the contralateral lower extremity were seen in the hamstring group versus the palmaris group (25 vs 13, respectively) ($P = 0.040$) while more subsequent injuries to the upper extremity were found in the palmaris group versus the hamstring group (73 vs 55, respectively), although this difference was not significant ($P = 0.052$).

While the ipsilateral palmaris is frequently used as the palmaris graft of choice given its proximity to the operative elbow, when the decision is made to use a hamstring graft, whether to use the ipsilateral or contralateral hamstring is a matter of debate. A recent survey found the majority of MLB team physicians (72.4%) harvest the hamstring from the contralateral (landing) leg [23]. An electromyographic study evaluated hamstring muscle activation in the ipsilateral (drive) versus contralateral (landing) leg in adolescent baseball pitchers during the baseball pitching motion [24]. The study found higher hamstring muscle activity in the drive leg compared to the landing leg, indicating the hamstrings of the drive (ipsilateral) leg are more important during the pitching motion. These results seemed to validate the clinical practice of the MLB team physicians. Finally, a recent study evaluated the outcomes and future injury risk in MLB and minor league baseball players who underwent UCLR with either an ipsilateral or a contralateral hamstring autograft [25]. The study found no difference in RTS rate, performance upon RTS, or subsequent injury rates (hamstring, lower extremity, or upper extremity) between players who underwent UCLR with hamstring autograft from the ipsilateral (drive) or contralateral (landing) leg. Hence, surgeons should counsel patients preoperatively on the risks and benefits of each graft choice for UCLR.

Graft Harvesting Techniques

Palmaris Longus Tendon

The harvesting techniques for the palmaris tendon have been published in recent clinical studies with several small variations [1–5, 7, 8, 26]. It is important in the office and again in the preoperative area to confirm the presence of a palmaris tendon prior to entering the operative suite. The clinical examination to identify the palmaris longus consists of asking the patient to actively oppose the thumb and small finger while slightly flexing the wrist. Both wrists should be checked for the presence/absence of a palmaris longus as the palmaris is often smaller and may be unusable when patients only have a palmaris on one side. If the tendon is present, it can be easily visualized and palpated in the forearm just proximal to the wrist crease (Fig. 16.1). Signing both the surgical site and the palmaris tendon at the level of the wrist is routinely performed by the author (Fig. 16.2). The surgical extremity is positioned using a hand table extension.

A 1-cm incision is made in the distal volar crease of the wrist. Superficial exposure is performed with a dissecting scissor to expose the

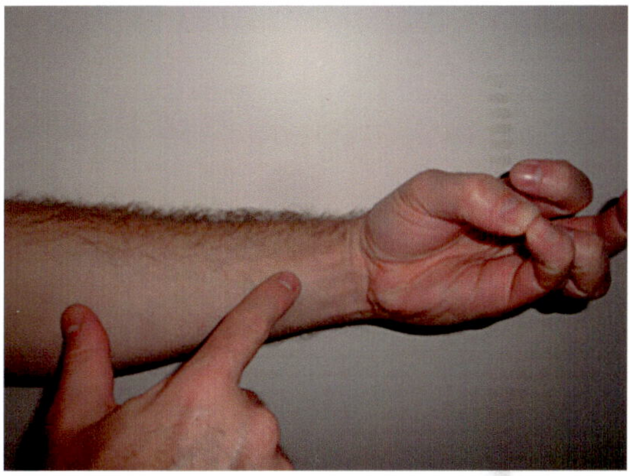

Fig. 16.1 Clinical photograph demonstrating the technique for examining the presence of a palmaris longus tendon. The patient is asked to actively oppose the thumb and small finger while slightly flexing the wrist. If present, the tendon is visualized and palpated just proximal to the wrist crease

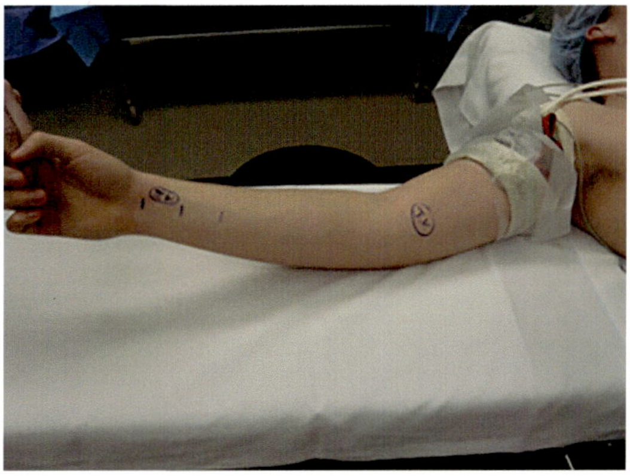

Fig. 16.2 The surgical site and the palmaris tendon harvest site are signed individually in the preoperative holding area to confirm the clinical presence of the tendon

tendon. Caution is exercised to avoid deep dissection to avoid iatrogenic injury to the underlying median nerve. The tendon is delivered from the incision using a right-angle hemostat and tagged with a braided No. 1 or No. 2 suture in a Krackow fashion (Fig. 16.3). This will prep one end of the tendon for later use. The distal end of the tendon is then cut in preparation for harvest. A tendon stripper is then utilized to harvest the tendon (Fig. 16.4). Complete harvest of the tendon is confirmed by visualizing the proximal muscular attachment (Fig. 16.5). Azar et al. have described using two additional small incisions at 7–9-cm intervals along the palmaris to further confirm the ligament has been appropriately identified at the musculotendinous junction before harvest [3] (Fig. 16.6). This step may further decrease the risk of iatrogenic median nerve injury.

After harvest, the tendon is prepared by removing any muscle tissue proximally. The tendon diameter is confirmed using a tendon sizer and is typically 3–3.5 mm in diameter in most cases (Fig. 16.7). The tendon should be at least 10 cm in length and can range up to 20 cm. Most surgical descriptions of UCL reconstruction describe drilling 3–3.5-mm bone tunnels on the ulna; therefore, the graft should accommodate

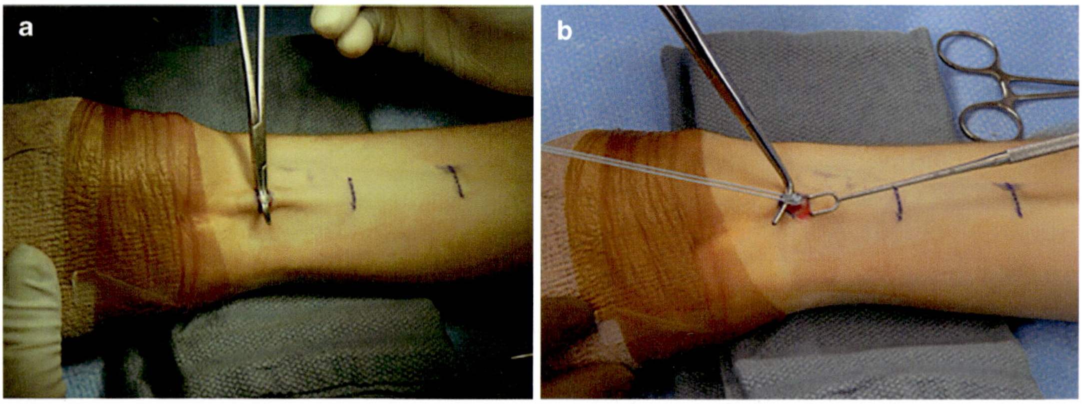

Fig. 16.3 (**a**) The intraoperative image of a right wrist demonstrates delivery of the palmaris tendon through a 1-cm incision in the wrist flexion crease using a curved hemostat. (**b**) The tendon is tagged in a Krackow fashion using a braided suture and its distal attachment is released

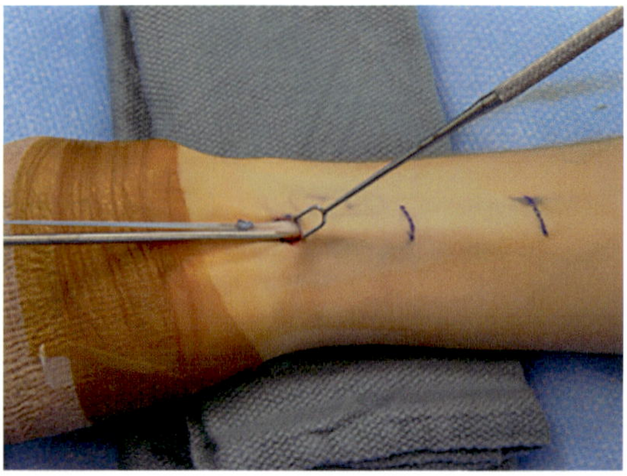

Fig. 16.4 The intraoperative image of a right wrist demonstrates passage of the tendon harvester over the palmaris tendon through a 1-cm incision in the wrist flexion crease

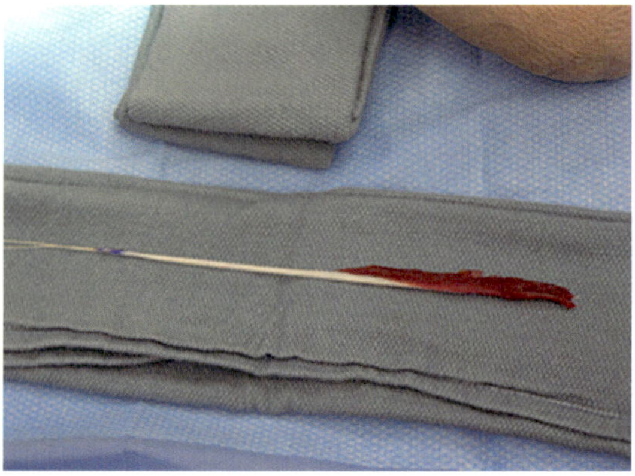

Fig. 16.5 The intraoperative image demonstrates a harvested palmaris tendon with proximal muscle attachments. The tendon is gently debrided of any residual muscle tissue during graft preparation

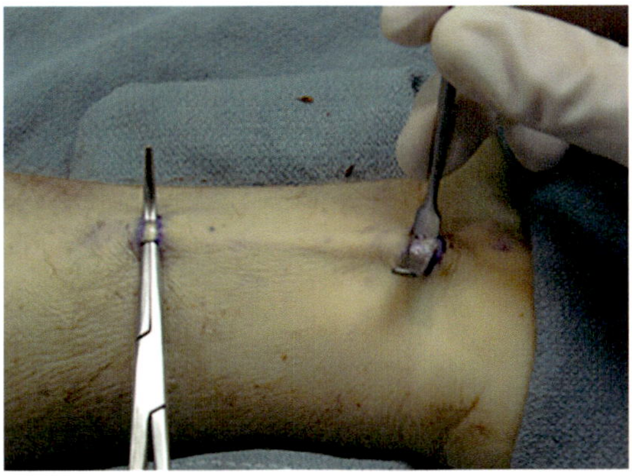

Fig. 16.6 The intraoperative image of a left wrist demonstrates delivery of the palmaris tendon through a 1-cm incision in the wrist flexion crease and a second incision proximal incision confirming identification of the tendon to avoid iatrogenic median nerve injury. (The wrist crease and hand are to the *left* of the image)

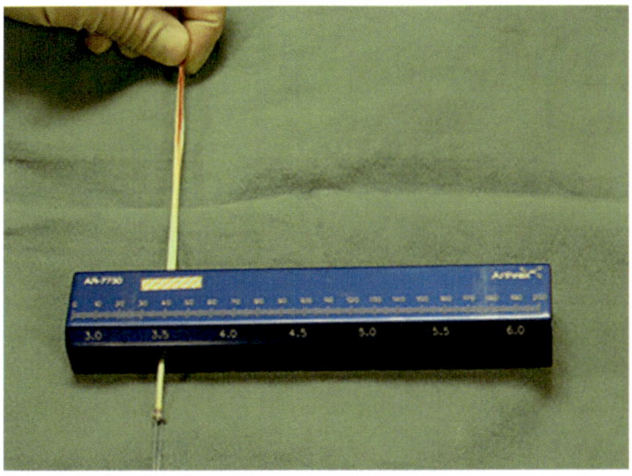

Fig. 16.7 The intraoperative image demonstrates use of a tendon sizer to confirm the palmaris tendon diameter. The tendon is typically 3–3.5 mm in diameter

this [1–3, 5, 8]. The graft is then placed in a moist sponge and protected on the back table.

Gracilis or Semitendinosus Tendon

The gracilis or semitendinosus tendon may be utilized as the primary autograft source for UCLR when the palmaris tendon is absent or in the revision setting when either the palmaris has been previously harvested or a thicker graft is needed because of tunnel issues. In some cases, overhead athletes have elected to use the gracilis as the primary source of autograft secondary to concerns of forearm pain with pitching, although the occurrence of this is quite rare [1, 3]. Harvest of the gracilis from the contralateral leg of the thrower has been reported by Dugas et al. [27]. Contralateral harvest avoids the potential for residual weakness at deep knee flexion angles reported after hamstring harvest that may affect the power generated when pushing off the back leg (ipsilateral) during the throwing cycle [28–30]. The surgeon must consider this when positioning the patient and operative table during the procedure for ease of access to the extremity.

Gracilis and/or semitendinosus tendon harvest is employed most commonly in the setting of anterior cruciate ligament (ACL) reconstruction [28, 31, 32]. The technique for harvest of the tendon for UCLR is quite similar. A gracilis harvest can be performed through a slightly smaller incision due to preservation of the more distal semitendinosus. The gracilis is larger than the palmaris and may require careful trimming of the graft to a diameter of 3–3.5 mm to fit the standard size tunnel or will require the surgeon to upsize the ulnar tunnel to 4.0–4.5 mm.

Harvest of the gracilis is performed using a 2- to 4-cm incision in the anteromedial tibia. The incision is made 1 cm medial to the tibial tubercle and often starts 2 cm distal to the tibial tubercle. The sartorius fascia was identified and incised in line with the fibers taking care to protect the saphenous nerve. Adhesions between the gracilis and semitendinosus tendon or gracilis and gastrocnemius are carefully removed to circumferentially free the tendon (Figs. 16.8 and 16.9). A tendon stripper is then used to harvest the tendon. The knee is flexed during harvest to decrease the risk of saphenous nerve injury and iatrogenic truncation of the tendon [28, 29, 33]. The tendon is often much longer than 10 cm. The proximal muscle is removed from the tendon in a similar fashion as discussed for the palmaris. An alternative "posterior" method of hamstring harvest has been proposed by Prodromos et al. that may allow for easier distinction of the hamstring tendons and improved cosmesis, although this is not used by the authors [32, 34]. The semitendinosus

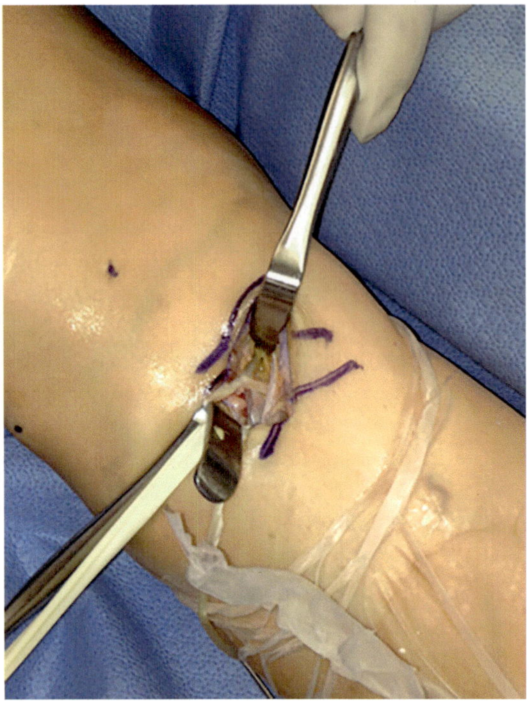

Fig. 16.8 The intraoperative image of a left knee demonstrates the isolated gracilis tendon prior to harvest. The gracilis tendon is then inspected for adhesions to the gastrocnemius, as shown in this image. Adhesions must be freed prior to gracilis harvest to prevent truncation of the tendon

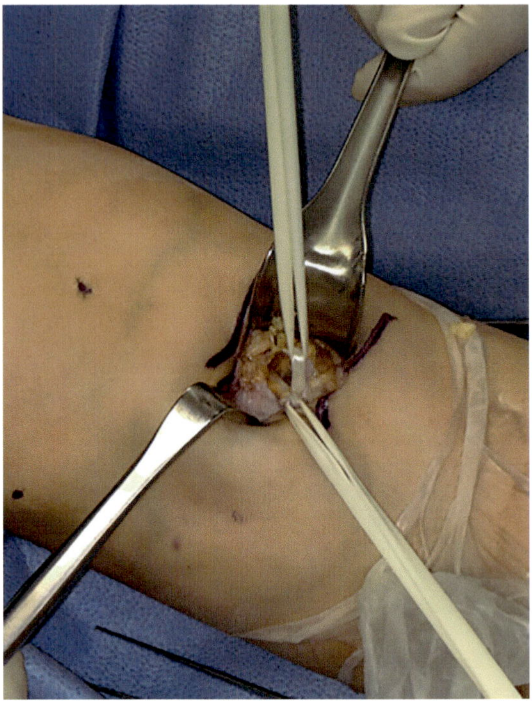

Fig. 16.9 The intraoperative image of a left knee demonstrates the isolated gracilis tendon prior to harvest. Gastrocnemius adhesions have been freed and the tendon is adequately mobilized for harvest

is harvested in a similar manner, ensuring the bands from the semitendinosus to the medial head of the gastrocnemius are released to prevent premature amputation of the tendon.

Complications

Complications of palmaris and hamstring tendon harvest are, fortunately, infrequent. It is important to discuss the potential complications during preoperative planning in order for the patient to make the most informed decision about autograft selection.

A rare, but potentially devastating complication of palmaris tendon harvest is inadvertent transection or harvest of the median nerve [34]. Deep dissection during palmaris tendon harvest should be avoided. The author recommends using an additional proximal incision to confirm the palmaris musculotendinous junction. If the palmaris cannot be clearly identified, an alternative graft choice should be considered.

In the series of UCLRs reported by Azar et al., four (4.4%) patients reported complications related to palmaris harvest. Two patients reported superficial wound infections that resolved with oral antibiotics and two of them reported tightness or tenderness at the harvest site.

Gracilis and semitendinosus tendon harvest complications have primarily been reported in the setting of ACL reconstructions [28–33]. Superficial wound infection, saphenous nerve injury, and loss of knee flexion strength are the most commonly reported complications. The risk of knee flexion weakness may be less when harvesting the gracilis tendon alone [30]. Postoperative sensory disturbance in the saphenous distribution has been reported to be as high as 73% [33]. Sanders et al. reported the saphenous nerve was intimately associated with the gracilis for 4.6 cm in the distal thigh over a segment of the tendon spanning 7.2–11.8 cm proximal to the insertion [33]. This places the nerve at risk when passing the tendon stripper for harvest.

Conclusion

Surgical reconstruction of symptomatic UCL injuries in the overhead athlete has demonstrated high levels of return to play. Graft selection and safe harvest technique are critical steps in UCL reconstruction for a successful outcome. The palmaris longus and gracilis tendon autografts are the most commonly used and accessible options for reconstruction. Complications can be minimized with attention to surgical technique and knowledge of the surrounding neurovascular anatomy.

References

1. Cain EL Jr, Andrews JR, Dugas JR, Wilk KE, McMichael CS, Walter JC 2nd, Riley RS, Arthur ST. Outcome of ulnar collateral ligament reconstruction of the elbow in 1281 athletes: results in 743 athletes with minimum 2-year follow-up. Am J Sports Med. 2010;38(12):2426–34.
2. Dodson CC, Thomas A, Dines JS, Nho SJ, Williams RJ 3rd, Altchek DW. Medial ulnar collateral ligament reconstruction of the elbow in throwing athletes. Am J Sports Med. 2006;34(12):1926–32.
3. Azar FM, Andrews JR, Wilk KE, Groh D. Operative treatment of ulnar collateral ligament injuries of the elbow in athletes. Am J Sports Med. 2000;28(1):16–23.
4. Jobe FW, Stark H, Lombardo SJ. Reconstruction of the ulnar collateral ligament in athletes. J Bone Joint Surg Am. 1986;68:1158–63.
5. Andrews JR, Jost PW, Cain EL. The ulnar collateral ligament procedure revisited: the procedure we use. Sports Health. 2012;4(5):438–41.
6. Smith GR, Altchek DW, Pagnani MJ, Keeley JR. A muscle-splitting approach to the ulnar collateral ligament of the elbow. Neuroanatomy and operative technique. Am J Sports Med. 1996;24(5):575–80.
7. Rohrbough JT, Altchek DW, Hyman J, Williams RJ 3rd, Botts JD. Medial collateral ligament reconstruction of the elbow using the docking technique. Am J Sports Med. 2002;30(4):541–8.
8. Dodson CC, Altchek DW. Ulnar collateral ligament reconstruction revisited: the procedure I use and why. Sports Health. 2012;4(5):433–7.
9. Morrey BF, An KN. Articular and ligamentous contributions to the stability of the elbow joint. Am J Sports Med. 1983;11(5):315–9.
10. Fleisig GS, Escamilla RF. Biomechanics of the elbow in the throwing athlete. Oper Tech Sports Med. 1996;4(2):62–8.
11. Werner SL, Fleisig GS, Dillman CJ, et al. Biomechanics of the elbow during baseball pitching. J Orthop Sports Phys Ther. 1993;17:274–8.
12. Prud'homme J, Budoff JE, Nguyen L, Hipp JA. Biomechanical analysis of medial collateral ligament reconstruction grafts of the elbow. Am J Sports Med. 2008 Apr;36(4):728–32.
13. Ahmad CS, Lee TQ, ElAttrache NS. Biomechanical evaluation of a new ulnar collateral ligament reconstruction technique with interference screw fixation. Am J Sports Med. 2003;31:332–7.
14. Paletta GA Jr, Klepps SJ, Difelice GS, et al. Biomechanical evaluation of 2 techniques for ulnar collateral ligament reconstruction of the elbow. Am J Sports Med. 2006;34:1599–603.
15. Dines JS, Jones KJ, Kahlenberg C, Rosenbaum A, Osbahr DC, Altchek DW. Elbow ulnar collateral ligament reconstruction in javelin throwers at a minimum 2-year follow-up. Am J Sports Med. 2012;40(1):148–51.
16. Argo D, Trenhaile SW, Savoie FH 3rd, Field LD. Operative treatment of ulnar collateral ligament insufficiency of the elbow in female athletes. Am J Sports Med. 2006;34(3):431–7.
17. Cvetanovich GL, Frank RM, Bach BR, Jr., Cohen MS, Bush-Joseph CA, Cole BJ, Romeo AA. Do clinical results and return-to-sport rates after ulnar collateral ligament reconstruction differ based on graft choice and surgical technique? Orthop J Sports Med. 2016;4(11).
18. Troha F, Baibak GJ, Kelleher JC. Frequency of the palmaris longus tendon in North American Caucasians. Ann Plast Surg. 1990;25(6):477–8.
19. Soltani AM, Peric M, Francis CS, Nguyen TT, Chan LS, Ghiassi A, Stevanovic MV, Wong AK. The variation in the absence of the palmaris longus in a multiethnic population of the United States: an epidemiological study. Plast Surg Int. 2012;2012:282959.
20. Regan WD, Korinek SL, Morrey BF, An KN. Biomechanical study of ligaments around the elbow joint. Clin Orthop Relat Res. 1991;271:170–9.
21. Armstrong AD, Dunning CE, Ferreira LM, Faber KJ, Johnson JA, King GJ. A biomechanical comparison of four reconstruction techniques for the medial collateral ligament–deficient elbow. J Shoulder Elb Surg. 2005;14:207–15.
22. Chalmers PN, D'Angelo J, Ma K, Dines JS, Romeo AA. Do outcomes or subsequent injuries differ after ulnar collateral ligament reconstruction with palmaris versus hamstring autograft? Am J Sports Med. 2019;47(6):1473–9.
23. Chalmers PN, Dugas JR, Bach BR Jr., Nicholson GP, Verma NN, Ahmad CS, Romeo AA. Do Major League

Baseball team physicians harvest the semitendinosus from the drive leg or landing leg when performing ulnar collateral ligament reconstruction on elite baseball pitchers? Orthop J Sports Med. 2017;5(7).
24. Zaferiou A, Chalmers PN, Ruby D, Malloy P, Luchetti TJ, Verma NN, Romeo AA. Are the hamstrings from the drive leg or landing leg more active in baseball pitchers? An electromyographic study. J Shoulder Elb Surg. 2017;26(11):2010–6.
25. Chalmers PN, D'Angelo J, Ma K, Ahmad CS, Dines JS, et al. Side of hamstring harvest does not affect performance, return-to-sport rate, or future hamstring injuries after ulnar collateral ligament reconstruction among professional baseball pitchers. Am J Sports Med. 2019;47(5):1111–6.
26. Jones KJ, Osbahr DC, Schrumpf MA, Dines JS, Altchek DW. Ulnar collateral ligament reconstruction in throwing athletes: a review of current concepts. AAOS exhibit selection. J Bone Joint Surg Am. 2012;94(8):e49.
27. Dugas JR, Bilotta J, Watts CD, Crum JA, Fleisig GS, McMichael CS, Cain EL Jr, Andrews JR. Ulnar collateral ligament reconstruction with gracilis tendon in athletes with intraligamentous bony excision: technique and results. Am J Sports Med. 2012;40(7):1578–82.
28. Shelton WR, Fagan BC. Autografts commonly used in anterior cruciate ligament reconstruction. J Am Acad Orthop Surg. 2011;19(5):259–64. Review
29. Prodromos CC, Fu FH, Howell SM, Johnson DH, Lawhorn K. Controversies in soft-tissue anterior cruciate ligament reconstruction: grafts, bundles, tunnels, fixation, and harvest. J Am Acad Orthop Surg. 2008;16(7):376–84.
30. Ardern CL, Webster KE, Taylor NF, Feller JA. Hamstring strength recovery after hamstring tendon harvest for anterior cruciate ligament reconstruction: a comparison between graft types. Arthroscopy. 2010;26(4):462–9.
31. Pagnani MJ, Warner JJ, O'Brien SJ, Warren RF. Anatomic considerations in harvesting the semitendinosus and gracilis tendons and a technique of harvest. Am J Sports Med. 1993;21(4):565–71.
32. Prodromos CC, Han YS, Keller BL, Bolyard RJ. Posterior mini-incision technique for hamstring anterior cruciate ligament reconstruction graft harvest. Arthroscopy. 2005;21(2):130–7.
33. Sanders B, Rolf R, McClelland W, Xerogeanes J. Prevalence of saphenous nerve injury after autogenous hamstring harvest: an anatomic and clinical study of sartorial branch injury. Arthroscopy. 2007;23(9):956–63.
34. Weber RV, Mackinnon SE. Median nerve mistaken for palmaris longus tendon: restoration of function with sensory nerve transfers. Hand (N Y). 2007;2(1):1–4.

17 Primary Repair of Ulnar Collateral Ligament Injuries of the Elbow

Robert S. O'Connell, Felix H. Savoie III, Michael J. O'Brien, and Larry D. Field

Introduction

History

Injuries to the medial ulnar collateral ligament (MUCL) can be devastating in overhead and throwing athletes. Prior to 1986, injury to this ligament was considered to be career-ending. In that year, Dr. Frank Jobe reported on his initial experiences with reconstruction of the MUCL. His first case was a professional pitcher Tommy John, who injured the MUCL in 1974. He had extensive nonoperative management that was unsuccessful in allowing him to return to play (RTP). Unwilling to end his career, he underwent what at that point was considered an experimental surgery to reconstruct the ligament using a palmaris longus autograft. Dr. Jobe gave him a one in a million chance of resuming his career. However, after a long and arduous recovery, he was able to return and pitch successfully for many years. Dr. Jobe continued to perform this operation with increasing success over the years, resulting in a paradigm shift in the treatment and results of injury to the throwing elbow. The surgery now often bears the name "Tommy John" surgery, and the ligament is often called the "Tommy John" ligament by nonmedical personnel.

The "Tommy John" or anterior oblique ligament of the MUCL complex is the primary stabilizer of the elbow to valgus stress [1–8]. When an injury to this ligament in an athlete occurs, conservative management soon after the onset of symptoms may effectively treat the athlete and allow some to return to competition [9, 10]. Podesta et al. showed that the use of platelet-rich plasma (PRP) improves healing rates in conjunction with early bracing and rehabilitation [11]. More recently, Deal et al. treated 23 patients with grade 2 MUCL tears with bracing, physical therapy, and two leukocyte-rich PRP injections and demonstrated a 96% return to play rate [12].

Although often considered, surgical repair of the MUCL in professional athletes failing nonoperative management has produced varying results

Supplementary Information The online version of this chapter (https://doi.org/10.1007/978-3-030-69567-5_17) contains supplementary material, which is available to authorized users.

R. S. O'Connell
Department of Orthopaedic Surgery, Virginia Commonwealth University, Richmond, VA, USA

F. H. Savoie III (✉)
Department of Orthopaedics, Tulane University School of Medicine, New Orleans, LA, USA
e-mail: fsavoie@tulane.edu

M. J. O'Brien
Department of Orthopaedics, Tulane University Medical Center, New Orleans, LA, USA

L. D. Field
Upper Extremity Service and Sports Medicine Program, Mississippi Sports Medicine and Orthopaedic Center, Jackson, MS, USA

J. S. Dines et al. (eds.), *Elbow Ulnar Collateral Ligament Injury*,
https://doi.org/10.1007/978-3-030-69567-5_17

and has not been recommended for professional athletes [13–17]. It remains much more common for professional athletes to show diffuse areas of injury to the MUCL and require grafting. In these patients, treatment with one of the reconstruction procedures pioneered by Jobe and modified by Altchek, Conway, or ElAttrache results in superb recovery and return to play compared to other treatment options [14–16, 18, 19]. Furthermore, most of the published research focuses on male overhand throwers in the professional ranks with regard to MUCL insufficiency. These professional athletes usually present with a ligament that is damaged throughout its entire length, precluding an operative repair and necessitating a reconstruction [15, 16].

Evolution of Repair

Initially, the MUCL graft reconstruction was limited to professional overhead athletes. However, there has seemingly been an exponential increase in the number of patients sustaining these injuries at younger ages [20]. The success of the classic "Tommy John" surgery in professional athletes has led most of these injuries to be managed by the same reconstructive technique. And while the overall rate of elbow injuries in adolescents remains low, the total number continues to rise due to increased participation in organized athletic participation and single-sport specialization with year-round activity [21, 22]. There has been a corresponding increase in MUCL reconstruction in adolescents with one study showing a 22-fold increase between 1994 and 2010 [22, 23]. However, these young athletes and their injuries do not appear to be the same as those sustained by professionals. In fact, one of the issues that led Dr. Jobe to utilize a reconstruction rather than a repair was the "wear and tear" of repetitive microtrauma over many years that resulted in a ligamentous insufficiency rather than a discrete area of injury. Fortunately, in younger athletes, while the injury is still commonly chronic in nature [21], it is often isolated to a single area without degeneration, increasing the chance of success for both nonoperative treatment and direct repair in allowing a return to sport. Unfortunately, there has been little focus on alternative treatment options in these young, nonprofessional athletes who continue to have instability despite conservative treatment and who wish to continue in sports.

Indications and Rationale for Repair

We began seeing these injuries in our younger athletes who wished to continue to compete in the early 1990s. Although we initially treated those requiring surgery with a classic reconstruction, we noticed that unlike their professional counterparts, the ligament in these young athletes appeared almost completely normal except for the area of acute injury. Furthermore, the MUCL is an extraarticular structure and therefore has vascularity that can allow for healing. The proximal MUCL (where most focal tears occur) has been shown to have a consistent dense blood supply compared to the hypovascular distal MUCL [24]. However, another cadaveric study out of the Steadman Phillopon Research Institute has shown equal distribution of vascular endothelial and progenitor cell markers through the proximal and distal MUCL insertions suggesting a well-vascularized ligament throughout its entire course [25]. This likely explains why proximal injuries are more likely to respond to nonoperative management but also supports repair for proximal and distal injuries that fail nonoperative treatment. Rather than extrapolating the data from professional athletes that reconstruction is necessary for all of these patients to return to sports, we developed a protocol of repair. Our indications for repair after failure of nonoperative treatment are listed in Table 17.1.

Using these criteria, our initial study showed that 93% (56 of 60) of these athletes (age range 13–23, avg. 16) returned to play within 6 months (range 4–11.7 months) postoperatively at the same or higher level of competition [26]. Multiple studies have now shown success with MUCL repair, allowing a more rapid return to play with less complications than those reported with the classic reconstruction [13, 27].

Table 17.1 A table comparing indications for repair versus reconstruction of MUCL

Repair	Reconstruction
Failure of nonoperative treatment with partial tears	Failure of nonoperative treatment with partial tears
College level or lower athlete	Professional or semi-professional athlete
No aspirations of professional career	Degenerative/diffuse ligament injury
Focal area of ligament injury on exam, imaging, and inspection	
Healthy mid-substance tissue	
Acute bony avulsion either proximally or distally	
Severe valgus instability after acute injury	

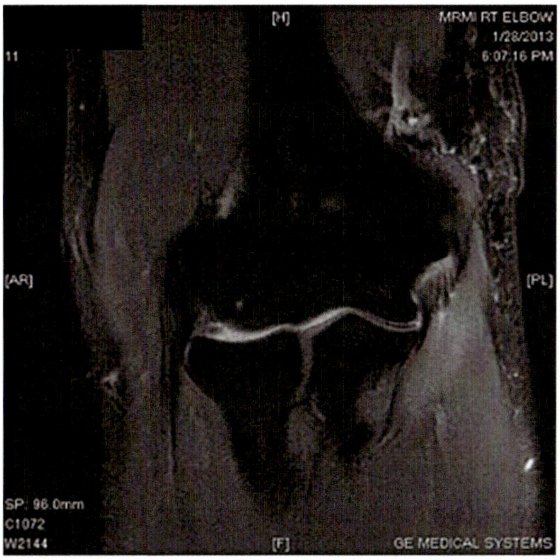

Fig. 17.1 MRA scan of a humeral avulsion of the MUCL amenable to repair

Tulane-MSMOC Protocol

An initial injury to the elbow in a young (nonprofessional) athlete is evaluated by physical examination and radiographs. It is important to evaluate the entire body, beginning with hip range of motion (ROM) and abductor strength, core strength assessment (usually performed by athletic trainer, or physical therapist), scapular position and tracking patterns and the strength of the rotator cuff in addition to the elbow. These athletes may also have inflamed plicas, flexor-pronator inflammation, capitellar osteochondritis dissecans (OCD) and other nonligamentous injuries with or without the MUCL injury.

In the injured elbow, we begin by testing ROM and areas of tenderness. In most cases, the area of injury is easily palpated. Valgus testing is performed at 0°, 30°, 70°, and 90° of flexion, as well as the milking maneuver test, valgus extension overload (VEO) test, and moving valgus stress test. The O'Driscoll moving valgus stress test is the most predictive test available for an injury to the MUCL and is positive if pain is reproduced between 70 and 120 degrees of flexion [28]. If the exam is positive for medial instability, the athlete is initially placed in a hinged brace and started on a comprehensive rehabilitation program. Concurrently, we perform a magnetic resonance imaging (MRI)-arthrogram (MRA). Imaging will often show an area of strain without focal tearing, in which case, nonoperative treatment is continued. In some cases, especially when there was a history of a "pop" in the elbow during throwing, the MRA will show a proximal or distal avulsion with or without a bony fragment. In these young athletes, the rest of the MUCL is usually completely normal and we often recommend repair or continued conservative treatment depending on the patient's desire to return to play (Fig. 17.1).

The decision to repair rather than reconstruct is complex. The ideal candidate is one with a sudden, acute avulsion that is displaced and who shows no other area of injury on history, exam, or imaging. In most cases, however, it is not that straightforward. In patients with more chronic symptoms, the palpation part of the exam becomes more critical in the decision-making process. If the area of major tenderness can be isolated to one area of the ligament (proximal tenderness is more common) and the MRI shows a corresponding area of focal damage, then repair is strongly considered. Furthermore, partial tears on the humeral side that fail to heal with nonoperative treatment are also considered for repair in the nonprofessional athlete (Table 17.1).

In discussing surgery, it is important to stress that the final decision to repair or reconstruct the ligament is made at surgery while directly visualizing the ligament; thus, patient and family are counseled and consent is obtained for both procedures.

Surgical Technique

The patient is placed in the prone position with a tourniquet around the upper arm. A small block or rolled towel is placed under the upper arm for support (Fig. 17.2). An exam under anesthesia is performed to document the ROM and the degree of opening. A diagnostic arthroscopy is performed to confirm the instability and to rule out other pathology.

The shoulder is then internally rotated, and the arm placed on a regular arm board, exposing the medial side of the elbow (Fig. 17.3). The muscle-splitting approach described by Altchek is utilized to expose the MUCL ([18]; Fig. 17.4). The ligament, along with the capsule, is then split along its anterior edge so the undersurface can be completely visualized (Fig. 17.5). At this point, if there are multiple areas of damage to the ligament, a reconstruction with palmaris longus autograft or gracilis allograft can be performed [29]. If the ligament appears to have an isolated area of injury and is otherwise normal, a repair is performed. A bioabsorbable double-loaded suture anchor is placed into the medial epicondyle near the base for proximal avulsions (Fig. 17.6) or directly into the center of the sublime tubercle for

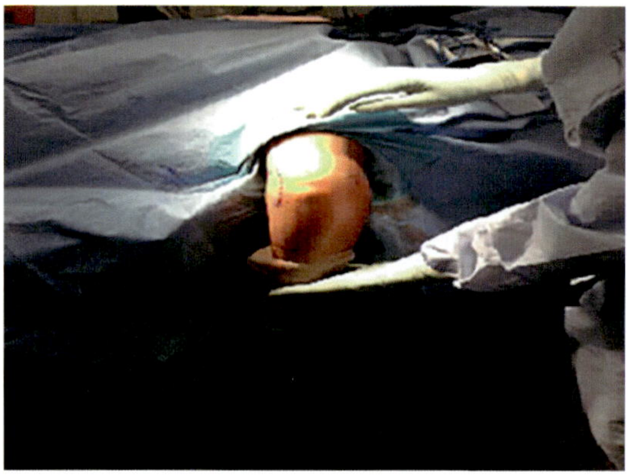

Fig. 17.2 The patient is positioned in the prone position with the elbow elevated on a small rolled towel

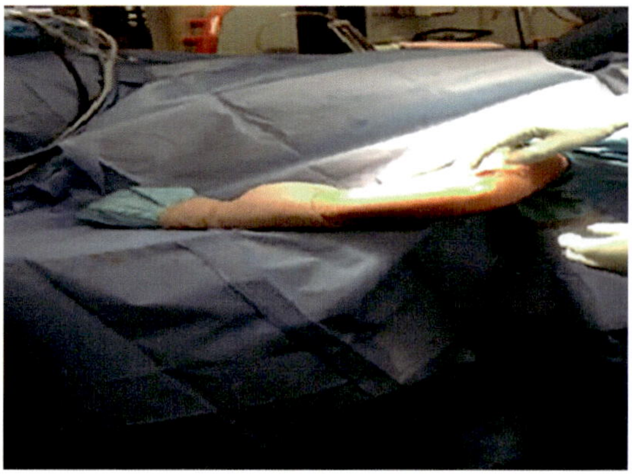

Fig. 17.3 The shoulder is internally rotated which allows the hand to be placed on the arm board, exposing the medial side of the elbow

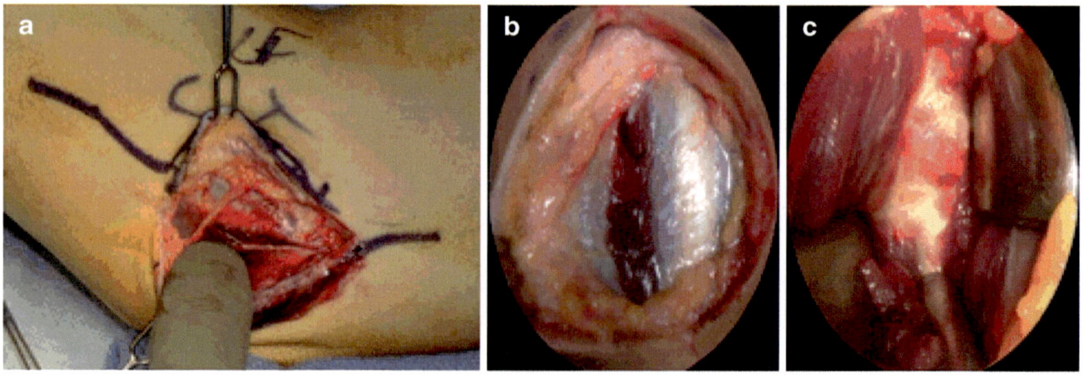

Fig. 17.4 (**a**) The initial medial incision is made and the fascia exposed in preparation to split the fascia. (**b**) The fascia is split to expose the underlying flexor-pronator muscle. (**c**) The muscle is bluntly split, exposing the underlying medial ulnar collateral ligament

distal avulsions. The most reliable way to ensure proper proximal anchor placement is to center the anchor at the base of the epicondyle, ensuring that the ligament will be anatomically reduced to the distal aspect of the epicondyle. The two sets of sutures are then placed in a mattress fashion though the ligament (Fig. 17.7) in order to recreate the normal anatomy and allow the proximal end of the ligament to fold medially onto the distal epicondyle when tensioned (Fig. 17.8a, b).

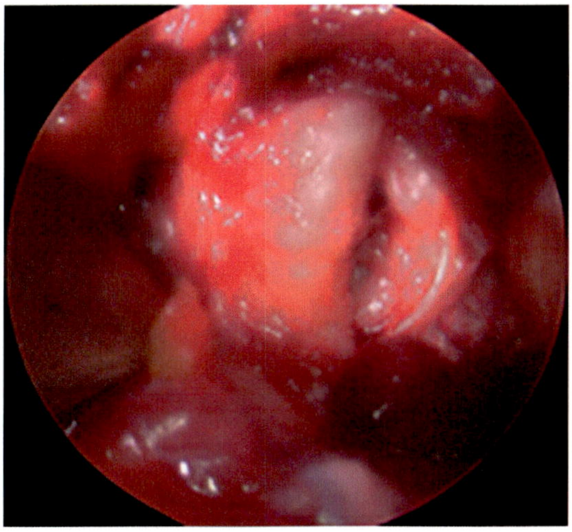

Fig. 17.5 A small incision is made along the anterior aspect of the MUCL, allowing a complete evaluation of both the outer and inner ligament

In special cases, a small part of the flexor-pronator fascia may be harvested and sewn into the ligament to reinforce the native ligament repair, and/or PRP clot may be added to the repair site (Fig. 17.8c).

The elbow is cycled to ensure the ligament is repaired isometrically and the split in the ligament and capsule along the anterior edge is closed with "pants over vest" absorbable suture. The fascia is repaired and the small incision closed with a subcuticular closure.

Post-op Rehabilitation

The patient is placed in a posterior splint for the first week and then switched to a hinged elbow brace. Physical therapy initially focused on leg and core and scapular strengthening is initiated at this time with shoulder and wrist exercises allowed as long as there is no pain in the elbow. We follow the program designed by Wilk, reported most recently by Ellenbecker et al. [30] but allow the milestones to be reached more rapidly with repair compared to reconstruction. It is critical in these early rehab sessions that the brace is worn full time, only removing it for showers. Range of motion is set in a pain-free range, usually 60–90°, and slowly increased in both directions as swelling and pain resolve. In most cases,

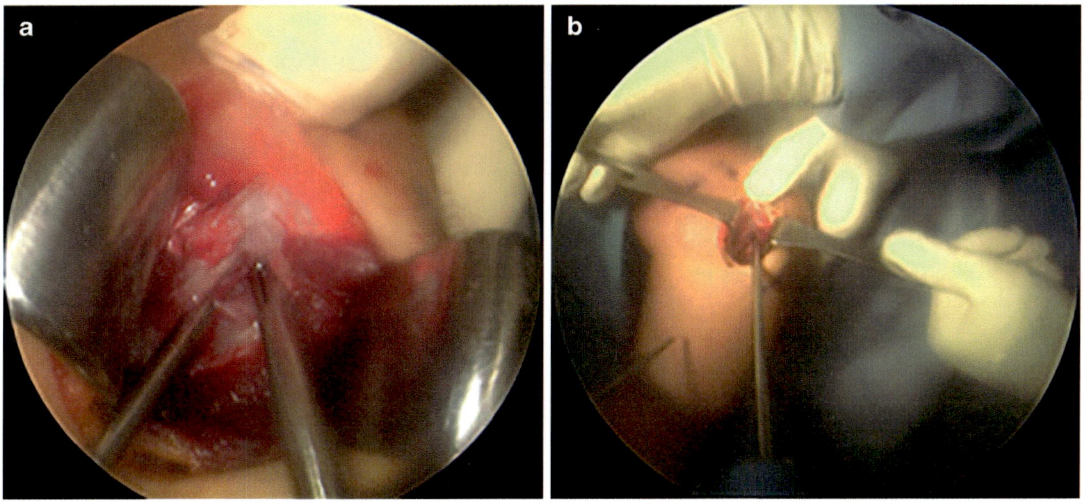

Fig. 17.6 (**a** and **b**) The proximal anchor is placed into the humerus

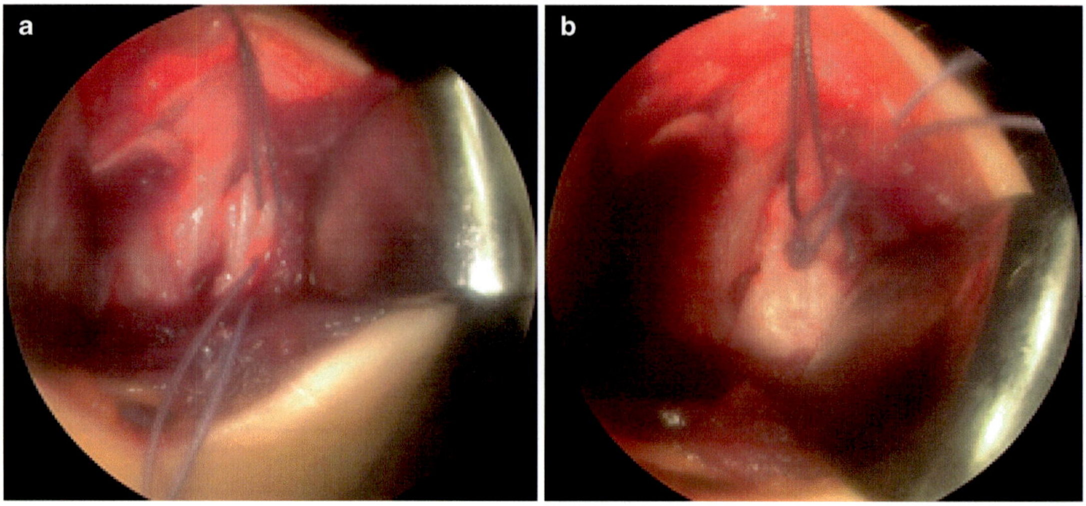

Fig. 17.7 (**a** and **b**) The two sets of sutures are placed through the ligament in horizontal mattress configuration to pull the ligament back to its anatomic position

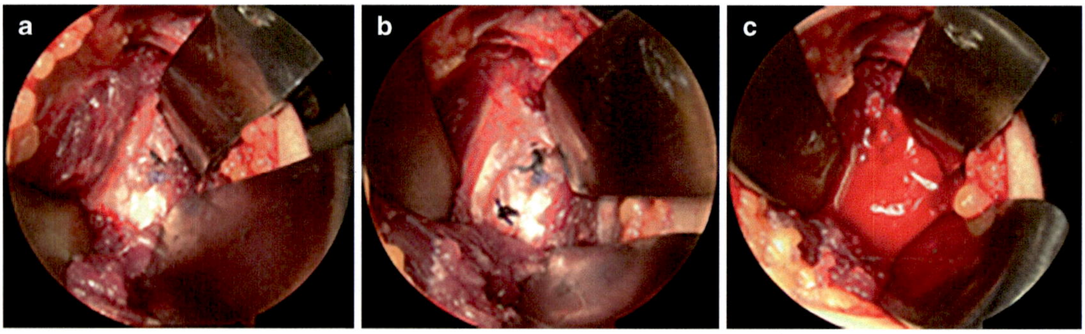

Fig. 17.8 (**a**) Final view of the repaired ligament prior to closure. (**b**) After the ligament is repaired, the split made at the beginning of the case is closed with an absorbable suture. (**c**) In some cases, we now add a clot from PRP to improve the healing of the ligament

by 4 weeks, the brace is allowed to be unlocked. Anywhere from 4 to 6 weeks postoperatively, a more aggressive elbow and wrist rehabilitation is incorporated into the recovery process. Approximately, 6–8 weeks postoperatively, the clinical exam, palpation of the ligament, and a repeat diagnostic ultrasound or MRI should show healing of the ligament and a return to hit and throw program is started in the brace. At this point, many athletes may return to most sports in the brace but are not allowed to do any sports out of the brace. Twelve weeks postoperatively, the program is continued without the brace and the patient may resume sporting activities when the return to play program is completed.

Return to Play

In our initial study, 93% (56 of 60) of these young (age range 13–23, avg. 16) athletes returned to sport within 6 months (range 4–11.7 months) postoperatively at the same or higher level of competition. Forty of the patients had proximal repairs, 11 patients had distal repairs, and 9 patients had both proximal and distal repairs [26]. Fifty-eight of the 60 patients (96%) were able to return to high school or collegiate sports without difficulty, although two patients who continued to play elite level sports 5 years postrepair sustained a late failure requiring reconstruction. Fifty-eight of the 60 patients

(93%) would have the same procedure done again. Fifty-seven of the 60 patients were able to complete their athletic careers without additional surgery.

Functional Outcome

The average postoperative Andrews-Carson Elbow Outcome Score improved from 132 preoperatively to 188 postoperatively ($p < 0.05$), and 93% had good to excellent results [2, 26, 31, 32]. Postoperative means were significantly higher than preoperative means for the subjective, objective, and overall categories of the outcome score for the total population (Table 17.2). Two patients were considered failures according to their functional results and Andrews-Carson rating scale. One patient was a high school baseball player who underwent anchor repair, had a stable exam, excellent core strength, and shoulder mechanics but was still unable to return to throwing. He declined further surgery. The other patient was a freshman college pitcher who was able to play for three more years. However, near the end of his third year of pitching, he developed recurrent symptoms in the elbow. An MRA revealed a new area of injury, however, surgery was declined as he was graduating.

Table 17.2 Andrews and Carson outcome scores

	Preoperative		Postoperative	
	N	%	N	%
Subjective				
Excellent (90–100)	0	0	51	85
Good (80–89)	0	0	5	8
Fair (60–79)	7	12	2	3.5
Poor (60)	53	88	2	3.5
Objective (60)				
Excellent (90–100)	43	72	55	92
Good (80–89)	7	12	2	3.5
Fair (60–79)	5	8	2	3.5
Poor (60)	5	8	1	1
Overall				
Excellent (180–200)	0	0	53	88.3
Good (80–89)	6	10	3	5
Fair (120–159)	42	70	3	5
Poor (120)	12	20	1	1.6

Reoperation

There were three additional surgeries (5%) performed in this repair group, one for arthrofibrosis and two for late failure. One patient was a college baseball player who underwent repair of the MUCL with an anchor and subsequently developed arthrofibrosis and was unable to compete. After conservative treatment for 1 year, he decided that he wanted to play again and returned for arthroscopic treatment with restoration of full ROM. Furthermore, the elbow was stable on exam and MRI. He was able to return to play for two more years.

Two patients were considered to have a successful result but sustained late failure (3.33%). One player completed 2 years of high school athletics and 3 years of college baseball without difficulty. During predraft workouts, he sustained a repeat injury to the MUCL. Repeat surgery with graft reconstruction allowed him to return to college for his senior year. He was drafted and played several years of minor league baseball without elbow complaints. The other patient had a similar history of having a repair at age 14 and returning to high school and junior college baseball without problem. In professional tryouts, he sustained a repeat injury and recently had additional surgery to the elbow, with full recovery and return to baseball.

Complications

Postoperative complications were found in 10% of patients. One patient developed arthrofibrosis necessitating treatment. Three males developed postoperative ulnar nerve symptoms. Two patients had ulnar nerve paresthesias that resolved within 6 weeks postoperatively. Both patients had flexor-pronator mass tears that required repair after the medial collateral ligament (MCL) was addressed. One patient had an ulnar nerve neuropraxia that completely resolved within 8 weeks. This patient had a muscle-splitting approach and we believe that excessive retraction resulted in the neuropraxic injury. None of these patients had preoperative ulnar nerve symptoms and none had an ulnar nerve transposition. A fourth patient had a stitch abscess that resolved with oral antibiotics and removal of the stitch. A fifth patient had a superficial wound infection that required a formal open irrigation and debridement in the office before recovering.

Discussion

The treatment of medial instability of the elbow has classically focused on the elite, high-level male overhead throwing athlete as a result of chronic valgus overloads [14–16, 18, 19]. However, MUCL injuries have also been reported with various injury patterns, including throwing, weight-bearing, extreme torsion, and sudden impact [10, 17, 33, 34]. However, few reports have focused on treating symptomatic instability of the elbow failing conservative treatment with primary repair of the MUCL [13, 26, 27]. In young athletes, repetitive activities such as throwing and gymnastics may produce focal injuries to the MUCL that prevent the continuation of elite level competition. In these athletes, one would expect the ligament to be of better quality and perhaps damaged in only one area. Additionally, if addressed early, the rest of the elbow may be spared the chronic attritional and secondary pathologic changes common in elite throwing athletes, leaving a more biomechanically stable joint amenable to repair and rapid recovery [1, 2, 5, 6, 33, 35, 36]. If the area of injury is localized to the proximal or distal end without midsubstance changes, then repair rather than reconstruction is a viable option. Recent evidence has also shown the excellent vascular supply and favorable healing environment of the MUCL [24, 25]. Repair of the ligament, especially in the absence of secondary pathologic changes allows a more rapid return to sports than the standard reconstruction.

In 1980, Norwood reported on four male patients undergoing primary repair of the ulnar collateral ligament after acute disruption [17]. All patients were able to return to previous activity. In 2002, Salvo et al. reported their results in treating avulsion fractures of the sublime tubercle in throwing athletes. Four of these patients were directly repaired with bioabsorbable anchors with excellent results [37].

More recently, Argo et al. showed excellent overall results in 16 athletes and good results in 2 female athletes who underwent MUCL repair using a variety of techniques. There was only one patient who required graft reconstruction after intraoperative evaluation of the ligament. After surgery, 17 of 18 patients (94%) were able to return to their sport at a mean of 2.5 months [13]. Similarly, in 2008, Richard et al. treated 11 athletes with repair, rather than reconstruction. In their study, 9 of 11 patients (82%) were able to return to sport within 6 months of surgery. While these are small sample sizes, they have similar success as our larger study of 60 patients as discussed above with RTP of 93% at an average of 6 months [26].

Over the last few years, repairs have become more frequent, especially with the addition of ligament augmentation. Recent biomechanical data have shown that MUCL repair with suture tape augmentation can provide similar time-zero failure strength but more resistance to gap formation compared to traditional reconstruction [38]. Similarly, Dugas et al. reported on this technique in 111 overhead athletes with a 92% RTP rate at mean time of 6.7 months [39].

There are a few studies that directly compare MUCL repair with reconstruction; however, most of these focus on elite level throwers. In 1992, Conway et al. reported their results of 14 repairs and 56 reconstructions [15]. In the repair group, 50% were able to return to their previous level of activity prior to injury, while 68% of patients had a similar result in the reconstruction group. The majority of patients were major league professional baseball players (39%). In the repair group, 7 of 14 patients were playing professional baseball with only two (29%) able to return to their same level of play or higher. In the reconstruction group, 20 of 56 patients were playing professional baseball with 13 (65%) able to return to their same or higher level of play. In 2000, Azar et al. reported their results on 59 reconstructions and 8 repairs [14]. In the reconstruction group, 81% of patients were able to return to their previous level of competition or higher. In the repair group, 69% of patients in the repair group were able to return to a similar level of play. However, again all of their patients were male baseball players who played professionally (41%) or in the college ranks (45%).

While there are limited studies evaluating UCL reconstruction in young athletes, we can extrapolate some information from the literature. The RTP rate varies in the literature for reconstruction between 68% and 95% at about 12 months postoperatively [19, 40, 41] in professional athletes. In one of the largest studies by Cain et al. in over 1242 MUCL reconstructions, the RTP rate was 83% at a mean of 11.6 months (range 3–72 months) [41]. Looking specifically at younger athletes, Petty et al. showed a 74% RTP in high-school baseball players at a mean of 11 months after undergoing ligament reconstruction [22]. Similarly, Jones et al. showed an 87% success rate of reconstruction in adolescent athletes with most failures occurring in patients with concomitant injuries to the elbow [42]. These results indicate the reconstruction has similar success rates in adolescents compared to more elite professional athletes. Therefore, the RTP rate for UCL repair tends to be somewhat higher than most studies of reconstruction procedures. It should be emphasized that we believe that this is largely due to patient selection as we are treating elbows that are completely normal other than an isolated ligament injury with excellent healing potential [13–16, 18, 19, 35].

In the very young athlete, long-term outcomes after reconstruction are unknown. The current criteria for success after MUCL reconstruction is one season at the same or higher level of play. The long-term consequences are elusive, but we do know that revision reconstruction has a much lower success rate [11]. In our two patients who had late revision surgery with a graft, there were no technical problems in the reconstruction related to the previous surgery. Indeed, it appeared as though there had been no prior surgical insult. Thus, it would appear that repair when appropriately indicated, can lead to improved results in this younger patient population.

Conclusion

Repair of MUCL remains a viable and most likely underused option in the management of MUCL injuries in these young athletes. Recent literature has shown excellent results and return to play in properly selected athletes [26, 27, 43]. Our current technique involves the use of absorbable anchors with dual suture fixation. Our rehab program has become more aggressive allowing RTP between 3 and 6 months. We recommend primary repair of MUCL for patients participating at the college level of play or younger if the damage is found localized on clinical exam, MRA, and direct inspection. Our conclusion is that select patients can obtain a favorable outcome after repair with a more rapid return to competition when the appropriate patient is selected for primary repair of the MUCL.

References

1. An KN, Morrey BF, Chao EYS. The effect of partial removal of proximal ulna on elbow constraint. Clin Orthop Relat Res. 1986;(209):270–9.
2. Andrews JR, Heggland EJ, Fleisig GS, et al. Relationship of ulnar collateral ligament strain to amount of medial olecranon osteotomy. Am J Sports Med. 2001;29:716–21.
3. Morrey BF, An KN. Articular and ligamentous contributions to the stability of the elbow. Am J Sports Med. 1983;11:315–9.
4. Morrey BF, An KN. Functional anatomy of the ligaments of the elbow. Clin Orthop Relat Res. 1985;(201):84–90.
5. Morrey BF, Tanaka S, An KN. Valgus stability of the elbow. Clin Orthop Relat Res. 1991;(265):187.
6. Regan WD, Korinek SL, Morrey BF, et al. Biomechanical study of ligaments around the elbow joint. Clin Orthop Relat Res. 1991;(271):170–9.
7. Schwab GH, Bennett JB, Woods GW, et al. Biomechanics of elbow instability: the role of the medial collateral ligament. Clin Orthop Relat Res. 1980;(146):42–52.
8. Sojbjerg JO, Ovesen J, Nielsen S. Experimental elbow instability after transaction of the medial collateral ligament. Clin Orthop Relat Res. 1987;(218):186–90.
9. Barnes DA, Tullos HS. An analysis of 100 symptomatic baseball players. Am J Sports Med. 1978;6:62–7.
10. Kenter K, Behr CT, Warren RF, et al. Acute elbow injuries in the national football league. J Shoulder Elb Surg. 2000;9:1–5.

11. Podesta L, Crow SA, Volkmer D, Bert T, Yocum LA. Treatment of partial ulnar collateral ligament tears in the elbow with platelet-rich plasma. Am J Sports Med. 2013;41(7):1689–94. https://doi.org/10.1177/0363546513487979. (PMID:23666850).
12. Deal JB, Smith E, Heard W, et al. Platelet-Rich plasma for primary treatment of partial ulnar collateral ligament tears: MRI correlation with results. Orthop J Sports Med. 2017;5(11) https://doi.org/10.1177/2325967117738238.
13. Argo D, Trenhaile S, Savoie FH, et al. Operative treatment of ulnar collateral ligament insufficiency of the elbow in female athletes. Am J Sports Med. 2006;34(3):431–7.
14. Azar FM, Andrews JR, Wilk KE, et al. Operative treatment of ulnar collateral ligament injuries of the elbow in athletes. Am J Sports Med. 2000;28:16–23.
15. Conway JE, Jobe FW, Glousman RE, et al. Medial instability of the elbow in throwing athletes. J Bone Joint Surg Am. 1992;74:67–83.
16. Jobe FW, Stark H, Lombardo SJ. Reconstruction of the ligament in athletes. J Bone Joint Surg Am. 1986;68:1158–63.
17. Norwood LA, Shook JA, Andrews JR. Acute medial elbow ruptures. Am J Sports Med. 1981;9:16–9.
18. Smith GR, Altechek DW, Pagnani MJ, et al. A muscle-splitting approach to the ulnar collateral ligament of the elbow. Am J Sports Med. 1996;24:575–80.
19. Thompson WH, Jobe FW, Yocum LA, et al. Ulnar collateral ligament reconstruction in athletes: muscle-splitting approach without transposition of the ulnar nerve. J Shoulder Elb Surg. 2001;10:152–7.
20. Olsen SJ, Fleisig GS, Dun S, Loftice J, Andrews JR. Risk factors for shoulder and elbow injuries in adolescent baseball pitchers. Am J Sports Med. 2006;34:905–12.
21. Saper MG, Pierpoint LA, Liu W, et al. Epidemiology of shoulder and elbow injuries among United States high school baseball players: school years 2005–2006 through 2014–2015. Am J Sports Med. 2018;46(1):37–43.
22. Petty DH, Andrews JR, Fleisig GS, Cain EL. Ulnar collateral ligament reconstruction in high school baseball players: clinical results and injury risk factors. Am J Sports Med. 2004;32(5):1158–64.
23. Fleisig GS, Andrews JR. Prevention of elbow injuries in youth baseball pitchers. Sports Health. 2012;4(5):419–24.
24. Buckley PS, Morris ER, Robbins CM, et al. Variations in blood supply from proximal to distal in the ulnar collateral ligament of the elbow: a qualitative descriptive cadaveric study. Am J Sports Med. 2019;47(5):1117–23.
25. Frangiamore SJ, Morris ER, Sibetta AC, et al. Evaluation of endothelial and vascular-derived progenitor cell populations in the proximal and distal UCL of the elbow: a comparative study. Orthop J Sports Med. 2018;6 https://doi.org/10.1177/2325967118777825.
26. Savoie FH III, Trenhaile SW, Roberts J, Field LD, Ramsey LR. Primary repair of ulnar collateral ligament injuries of the elbow in young athletes: a case series of injuries to the proximal and distal ends of the ligament. Am J Sports Med. 2008;36:1066–72. https://doi.org/10.1177/0363546508315201.
27. Richard MJ, Aldridge JMI II, Wiesler ER, Ruch DS. Traumatic valgus instability of the elbow: pathoanatomy and results of direct repair. J Bone Joint Surg Am. 2008;90(11):2416–22. https://doi.org/10.2106/JBJS.G.01448.
28. Field LD, Altchek DW. Evaluation of the arthroscopic valgus instability test of the elbow. Am J Sports Med. 1996;24:177–81.
29. Savoie FHIII, Morgan C, Yaste J, Hurt J, Field LD. Medial ulnar collateral ligament reconstruction using hamstring allograft in overhead throwing athletes. J Bone Joint Surg Am. 2013;95(12):1062–6. https://doi.org/10.2106/JBJS.L.00213.
30. Ellenbecker TS, Wilk KE, Altchek DW, Andrews JR. Current concepts in rehabilitation following ulnar collateral ligament reconstruction. Sports Health. 2009;1(4):301–13. https://doi.org/10.1177/1941738109338553.
31. Andrews JR, Carson WG. Arthroscopy of the elbow. Arthroscopy. 1985;1:97–107.
32. Andrews JR, Timmerman LA. Arthroscopic treatment of posttraumatic elbow pain and stiffness. Am J Sports Med. 1994;22:230–5.
33. Gainor BJ, Piotrowski G, Puhl J, et al. The throw: biomechanics and acute injury. Am J Sports Med. 1980;8:114–8.
34. Mirabello SC, Loeb PE, Andrews JR. The wrist: field evaluation and treatment. Clin Orthop Med. 1992;11:1–25.
35. Fleisig GS, Barrentine SW. Biomechanical aspects of the elbow in sports. Sports Med Arthrosc Rev. 1995;3:149–59.
36. Fleisig GS, Dillman CJ, Escamilla RF, et al. Kinetics of baseball pitching with implications about injury mechanisms. Am J Sports Med. 1995;23:233–9.
37. Salvo JP, Rizio L, Zvijac JE, Uribe JW, Kechtman KS. Avulsion fracture of the ulnar sublime tubercle in overhead throwing athletes. Am J Sports Med. 2002;30(3):426–31.
38. Dugas JR, Walters BL, Beason DP, et al. Biomechanical comparison of ulnar collateral ligament repair with internal bracing versus modified jobe reconstruction. Am J Sports Med. 2016;44(3):735–41.
39. Dugas JR, Looze CA, Capogna B, et al. Ulnar collateral ligament repair with collagen-dipped fibertape augmentation in overhead-throwing athletes. Am J Sports Med. 2019;47(5):1096–102.
40. Dodson CC, Thomas A, Dines JS, et al. Medical ulnar collateral ligament reconstruction of the elbow in throwing athletes. Am J Sports Med. 2006;34(12):1926–32.

41. Cain EL Jr, Andrews JR, Dugas JR, Wilk KE, McMichael CS, Walter JC II, Riley RS, Arthur ST. Outcome of ulnar collateral ligament reconstruction of the elbow in 1281 athletes: results in 743 athletes with minimum 2-year follow-up. Am J Sports Med. 2010;38(12):2426–34. https://doi.org/10.1177/0363546510378100.
42. Jones KJ, Dines JS, Rebolledo BJ, et al. Operative management of ulnar collateral ligament insufficiency in adolescent athletes. Am J Sports Med. 2014;42(1):117–21.
43. Inoue G, Kuwahata Y. Surgical repair of traumatic medial disruption of the elbow in competitive athletes. Br J Sports Med. 1995;29:139–42. https://doi.org/10.1136/bjsm.29.2.139.

Repair and Internal Brace Augmentation of the Medial Ulnar Collateral Ligament

18

Ryan S. Selley, Elizabeth R. Dennis, Eric N. Windsor, James B. Carr II, and Joshua S. Dines

Introduction

The ulnar collateral ligament (UCL) is the primary restraint to valgus stress at the elbow particularly during the late cocking and early acceleration phases of throwing [1–4]. Overhead athletes and pitchers in particular rely heavily on the UCL which is subject to injury with over use. This is especially of concern as younger athletes increasingly engage in single sport specialization, year-round play, and higher ball velocity [5–7]. The UCL is particularly important for baseball pitchers, injury to this ligament was considered career-ending until the advent of the Tommy John or UCL reconstruction procedure in 1974 [8]. UCL reconstruction has undergone several technical modifications since its initial description with higher rates of return to play and low rates of complications [9–14]. However, UCL reconstruction is not without its downsides, rehabilitation takes a period of 12–18 months before return to play [15]. Further, UCL injuries are being reported in younger athletes and as a result being diagnosed earlier in the injury process [16]. Injuries to the UCL can be mild and range from a sprain to partial rupture or in more chronic scenarios, complete deficiency of the ligament [17]. More mild cases of UCL injury can be treated conservatively with rest and therapy; however, a subset of these fail nonoperative management and meet criteria for operative intervention [17]. In these scenarios, orthopedic surgeons have sought other methods of stabilization in the form of UCL repair.

UCL repair has been tried previously with poor outcomes, specifically among pitchers [8, 18]. In an initial reported series on UCL repair in seven professional pitchers, only two returned to playing major league baseball compared with 75% of patients undergoing reconstruction [18]. Another series of patients undergoing either repair or reconstruction noted return to play at previous levels or higher in 63% of the repair group and 81% of the reconstruction groups [19]. Subsequent attempts at repair at this time were less frequently utilized aside from select circumstances in favor of reconstruction secondary to these outcomes.

Despite this, more recent reports of direct suture repair in young athletes with less severe UCL injuries have demonstrated successful outcomes [20, 21]. Savoie et al. reported on a series

R. S. Selley · E. R. Dennis · E. N. Windsor
Department of Orthopaedic Surgery, Hospital for Special Surgery, New York, NY, USA

J. B. Carr II
Sports Medicine Institute, Hospital for Special Surgery, West Palm Beach, FL, USA

J. S. Dines (✉)
Department of Orthopedic Surgery, Sports Medicine and Shoulder Service, Sports Medicine Institute, Hospital for Special Surgery, New York, NY, USA

J. S. Dines et al. (eds.), *Elbow Ulnar Collateral Ligament Injury*,
https://doi.org/10.1007/978-3-030-69567-5_18

of 60 high school and college athletes who underwent direct repair of the UCL with 58 able to return to sports within 6 months of surgery, less than half of the time a typical UCL reconstruction takes to rehabilitate [15, 21]. Dugas et al. have reported similar successful results in UCL repair with augmented techniques using an internal brace [22]. Their cohort of 111 overhead athletes had a 92% return to play rate at a mean of 6.7 months [22]. These results are encouraging and highlight the utility of UCL repair in young overhead athletes as a more favorable option compared to reconstruction allowing safe and faster return to play.

Biomechanics

The UCL is the primary restraint to valgus stress in the elbow during overhead throwing. The anterior band of the UCL is of particular importance and the focus of UCL reconstruction and repair. Several cadaveric studies have analyzed the biomechanics of the internal brace in UCL repair [23–26]. Dugas et al. compared the strength of UCL reconstruction with the modified Jobe technique to UCL repair with internal brace augmentation. They noted significantly less gapping in the repair group compared to the reconstruction group at low cyclic loads; however, they noted no difference in time-zero failure strength with respect to maximum torque, torsional stiffness, and gap formation [24]. In a similar study with slight modification, Bodendorfer et al. compared the UCL reconstruction docking technique to repair with internal brace and noted no significant difference between groups in terms of load-to-failure, gapping, or valgus opening angle during cyclic loading at time zero [23]. Contrarily, Urch et al. compared UCL repair and reconstruction with a three-strand technique with results that favor reconstruction in terms of load-to-failure testing for yield torque, yield angle, and ultimate torque. They did, however, note that the repair state restored valgus laxity to native values at all degrees of elbow flexion [26]. Lastly, Jones et al. compared UCL reconstruction and repair under cyclic fatigue mechanics. They observed that after 10, 100, and 500 flexion extension cycles and applied valgus stress, the repair group demonstrated significantly less gap formation than the reconstruction group [25]. The above results suggest that UCL repair is similar in time-zero strength to the native UCL state as well as the reconstructed states, and in some circumstances maybe more durable than UCL reconstruction.

UCL Repair Indications

Correct indications for UCL surgical intervention are crucial to obtaining a successful outcome. The authors of this chapter categorize patients into three different categories: reconstruction, repair, and repair + internal brace. The first determination is if a patient would benefit from a reconstruction versus repair. Candidates for repair are young, overhead athletes with partial UCL tears refractory to conservative management and those with proximal or distal avulsions. Other considerations include level of competition, desired timing for return to sport and concomitant injuries. MRI evaluation is helpful in determining quality of tissue prior to intra-operative evaluation and with setting patient expectations with regard to repair or reconstruction on the day of surgery. Intra-operative determinants are the last factor, these include gross assessment of the UCL tissue quality, contraindications to repair include poor quality, large bony avulsions or ossification within the ligament that once excised render the ligament incompetent. Lastly, when considering whether or not to augment with an internal brace, the authors assess the quality of potential repair; if it is felt that the tissue is adequate for repair but would benefit from additional stability, then an internal brace is added as a supplement (Fig. 18.1). There is little evidence to guide decision-making in this regard and is largely left to expert opinion.

Surgical Technique

Several surgical techniques for UCL repair have been described, these include direct suture repair, repair with bone tunnels or repair with

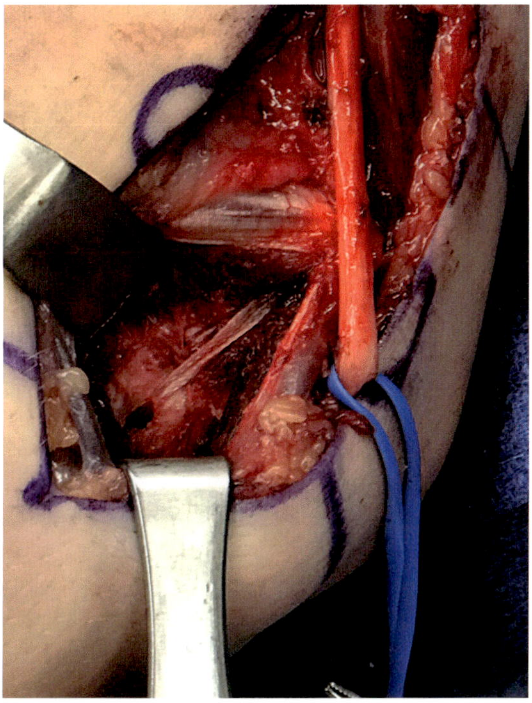

Fig. 18.1 When it is felt that the native tissue is adequate for repair but would benefit from additional stability, an internal brace is added to the repair construct

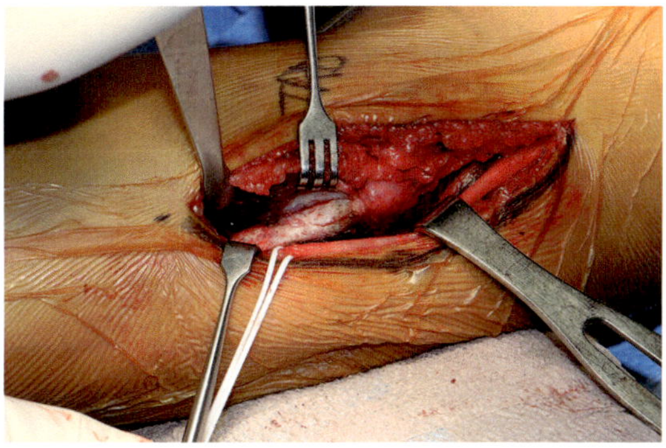

Fig. 18.2 The UCL is visualized through the FCU dissection and a subperiosteal dissection is performed anteriorly and distally

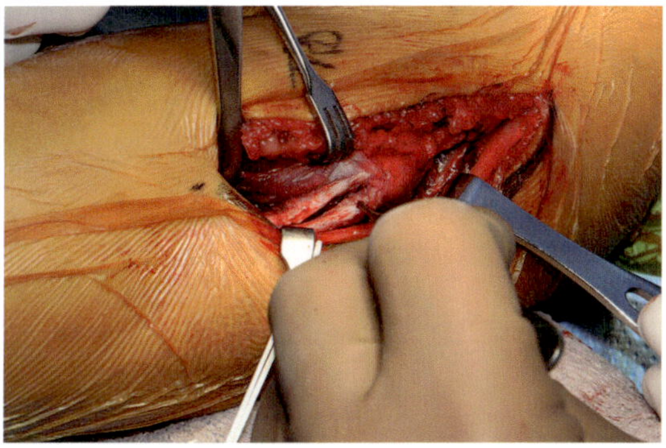

Fig. 18.3 The native ligament is analyzed for tear location and whether its integrity is amenable to repair. Any attenuated or friable tissue is sharply debrided leaving the healthy ligamentous tissue intact

suture anchors [18, 20, 21, 27]. We present our preferred technique for UCL repair. The patient is positioned supine on the operating table with the operative extremity on a hand table. Prior to prep and drape, an exam under anesthesia is performed documenting range of motion throughout all elbow arcs of motion, blocks to extension in particular are noted. Next the operative extremity is prepped and draped along with the contralateral leg should the need for a hamstring autograft arise if UCL reconstruction is required. The arm is exsanguinated and a tourniquet is raised to 250 mmHg. A medial-based incision is made extending from the medial epicondyle toward the sublime tubercle with sharp dissection carried down through skin and subcutaneous tissue to the level of fascia. A muscle splitting approach in the flexor carpi ulnaris (FCU) is utilized. The ulnar nerve is not exposed unless preoperative subluxation or symptoms necessitates transposition. After mobilization of the FCU, the UCL is visible and subperiosteal dissection is performed anteriorly and distally with a combination of scalpel and soft tissue elevator (Fig. 18.2). At this point, the ligament is analyzed for location of tear and if it would be amenable to repair. Any attenuated or friable tissue is sharply debrided leaving healthy ligamentous tissue intact (Fig. 18.3). In the case of partial tears, the tear is completed and the free end is whip stitched using suture tape in a Krakow fashion. Next a hole for the 3.5 mm swivel lock (Arthrex, Naples, FL, USA) is drilled at the side of injury (insertion of the UCL on the medial epicondyle or sublime tubercle) (Fig. 18.4a). The hole is tapped (Fig. 18.4b), and the anchor is loaded with the free suture end that is attached to the UCL; if it is deemed that the repair would benefit from an internal brace (Arthrex, Naples,

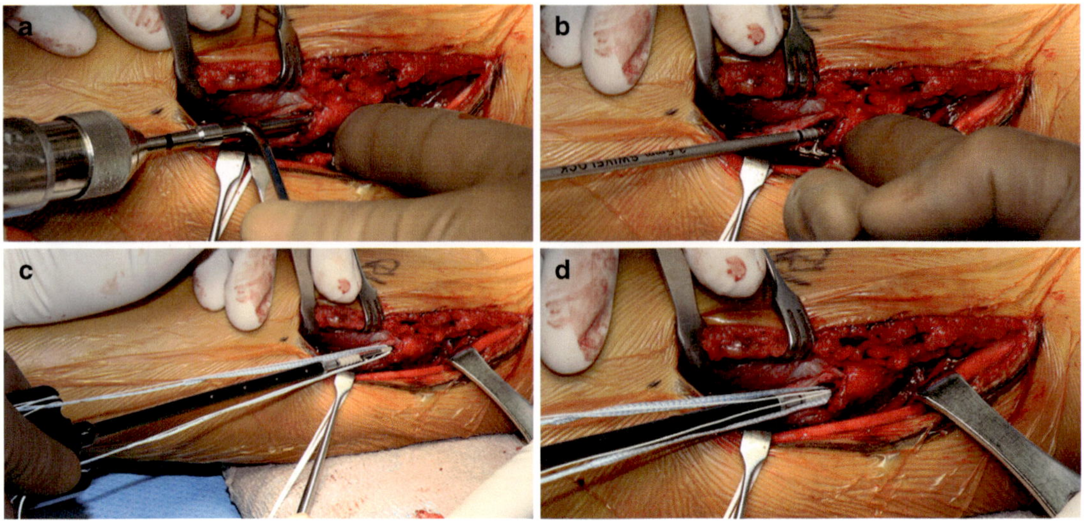

Fig. 18.4 (**a**) The insertion site for a 3.5 mm swivel lock (Arthrex, Naples, FL, USA) is drilled at the origin of the native UCL. (**b**) The drill hole is tapped. (**c**), An internal brace (Arthrex, Naples, FL, USA) is loaded into the anchor. (**d**) The loaded anchor is inserted with the elbow in 30 degrees of flexion and slight varus force

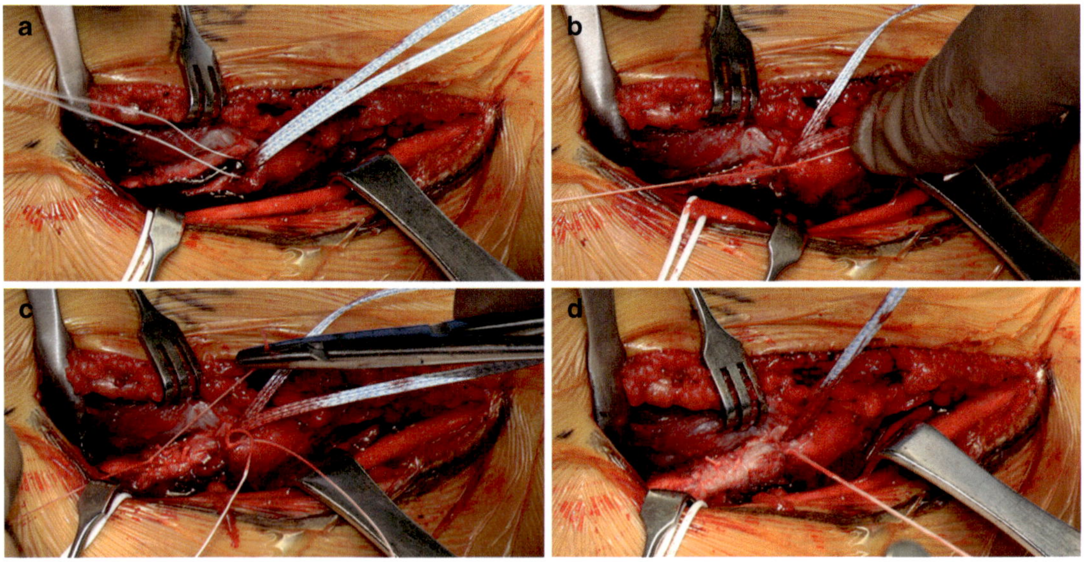

Fig. 18.5 (**a**–**d**) The free suture loaded through the anchor is used to repair the underlying native ligament

FL, USA), then this is loaded into the anchor as well (Fig. 18.4c). The anchor is then inserted with the elbow in 30 degrees of flexion and slight varus force (Fig. 18.4d). The free suture loaded through the anchor is used to repair the underlying native ligament (Fig. 18.5a–d). Next, in the case of internal brace use, the opposite site for anchor placement is prepared in a similar fashion and a second 3.5 mm swivel lock is loaded on the other end of the internal brace (Fig. 18.6a). Prior to fixation, the elbow is taken through a range of motion to ensure that no over constraint has occurred and the remaining half of the internal brace is secured with the ulnohumeral joint

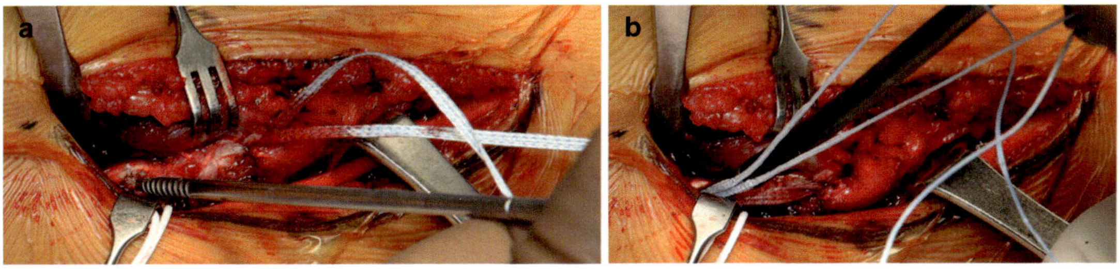

Fig. 18.6 (**a**) The distal site for the internal brace insertion prepared in a similar fashion. (**b**) The internal brace is loaded into a second 3.5 mm swivel lock and secured at the distal insertion site. Prior to final fixation, the elbow is taken through a range of motion to ensure that the construct is not over-constrained. The distal end of the internal brace is secured with the ulnohumeral joint reduced in relative extension

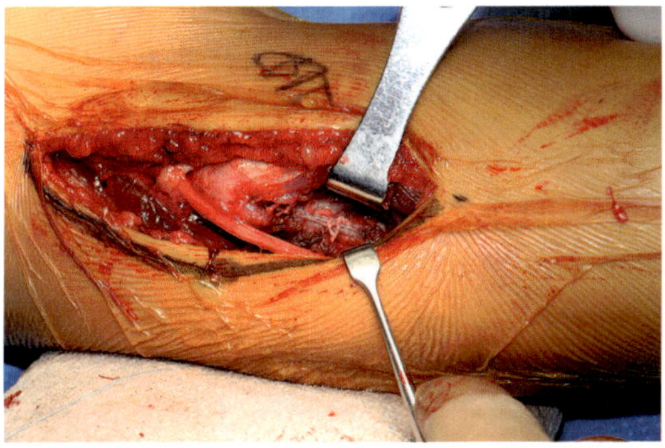

Fig. 18.7 The final UCL repair construct augmented with the internal brace

reduced in relative extension (Fig. 18.6b). The elbow is then taken through range of motion to ensure that there are no impediments to motion and the ends of the suture are cut. The final construct can be seen in Fig. 18.7. Next, the wound is copiously irrigated and closed in a layered fashion. The patient is placed in a soft dressing and a brace is placed locked in 90 degrees of flexion.

Patients who undergo UCL repair with internal brace augmentation undergo an accelerated rehabilitation schedule when compared to the traditional UCL reconstruction protocol with most athletes returning to throwing in competition at 6 month postoperatively. The two main complications that have been reported include ulnar nerve symptoms either related to compression or subluxation and heterotopic bone formation [22].

Outcomes

Historically, outcomes of UCL repair demonstrated poor results and low return to play rates. The initial reports by Norwood et al. in 1981 in four players noted that only two players were able to return to sport [27]. In 1992, Conway et al. reported on their experience with UCL repair and reconstruction, of the 14 patients who underwent direct repair, 7 were able to return to the same level of play [18]. Of these 14, however, 7 were professional athletes and only of 2 of the 7 were able to return to the Major League Baseball (MLB) [18]. Due to these poor results, UCL reconstruction was considered the gold standard for return to sport in overhead throwing athletes and minimal consideration was given to UCL repair. Recent investigations, however, have demonstrated promising results. Argo et al. published a series of 18 female athletes undergoing UCL repair with 17 returning to their respective sports [20]. Subsequently, Savoie et al. published their experience with a direct UCL repair in 60 overhead athletes with a mean age of 17.2 years; they noted that 93% of athletes demonstrated good to excellent outcomes and a 97% rate of return to play at an average of 6 months postoperatively [21]. Dugas et al. most recently published a series about 111 patient who underwent UCL repair with internal brace augmentation. They noted a 92% rate of return to sport at an average of 6.7 months from surgery. Further, they noted improvements in Kerlan-Jobe Orthopaedic Clinic (KJOC) scores in all patients with a mean score of 88.2, and significantly more improvement from year 1 to year 2 postoperatively (86.2 vs. 91.1). These results demonstrate that UCL repair maybe a superior option in appropriately indicated patients with UCL injuries.

Conclusion

UCL injuries are a heterogeneous group of pathology with a multitude of treatment options. Our knowledge of how to treat these injuries has expanded greatly over the past several decades. When specifically considering UCL repair, recent studies with modern techniques in appropriately indicated patients demonstrate excellent outcomes with faster return to play compared to a UCL reconstruction cohort.

References

1. Morrey BF, An KN. Articular and ligamentous contributions to the stability of the elbow joint. Am J Sports Med. 1983;11:315–9.
2. Regan WD, Korinek SL, Morrey BF, An KN. Biomechanical study of ligaments around the elbow joint. Clin Orthop Relat Res. 1991;(271):170–9.
3. Fleisig GS, Andrews JR, Dillman CJ, Escamilla RF. Kinetics of baseball pitching with implications about injury mechanisms. Am J Sports Med. 1995;23:233–9.
4. Fleisig GS, Kingsley DS, Loftice JW, et al. Kinetic comparison among the fastball, curveball, change-up, and slider in collegiate baseball pitchers. Am J Sports Med. 2006;34:423–30.
5. Feeley BT, Agel J, LaPrade RF. When is it too early for single sport specialization? Am J Sports Med. 2016;44:234–41.
6. Bruce JR, Andrews JR. Ulnar collateral ligament injuries in the throwing athlete. J Am Acad Orthop Surg. 2014;22:315–25.
7. Whiteside D, Martini DN, Lepley AS, Zernicke RF, Goulet GC. Predictors of ulnar collateral ligament reconstruction in Major League Baseball pitchers. Am J Sports Med. 2016;44:2202–9.
8. Jobe FW, Stark H, Lombardo SJ. Reconstruction of the ulnar collateral ligament in athletes. J Bone Joint Surg Am. 1986;68:1158–63.
9. Dodson CC, Thomas A, Dines JS, Nho SJ, Williams RJ 3rd, Altchek DW. Medial ulnar collateral ligament reconstruction of the elbow in throwing athletes. Am J Sports Med. 2006;34:1926–32.
10. Paletta GA Jr, Wright RW. The modified docking procedure for elbow ulnar collateral ligament reconstruction: 2-year follow-up in elite throwers. Am J Sports Med. 2006;34:1594–8.
11. Koh JL, Schafer MF, Keuter G, Hsu JE. Ulnar collateral ligament reconstruction in elite throwing athletes. Arthroscopy. 2006;22:1187–91.
12. Dines JS, ElAttrache NS, Conway JE, Smith W, Ahmad CS. Clinical outcomes of the DANE TJ technique to treat ulnar collateral ligament insufficiency of the elbow. Am J Sports Med. 2007;35:2039–44.
13. Bowers AL, Dines JS, Dines DM, Altchek DW. Elbow medial ulnar collateral ligament reconstruction: clinical relevance and the docking technique. J Shoulder Elb Surg. 2010;19:110–7.
14. Cain EL Jr, Andrews JR, Dugas JR, et al. Outcome of ulnar collateral ligament reconstruction of the elbow in 1281 athletes: results in 743 athletes with minimum 2-year follow-up. Am J Sports Med. 2010;38:2426–34.
15. Makhni EC, Lee RW, Morrow ZS, Gualtieri AP, Gorroochurn P, Ahmad CS. Performance, return to competition, and Reinjury after Tommy John surgery in Major League Baseball pitchers: a review of 147 cases. Am J Sports Med. 2014;42:1323–32.
16. Erickson BJ, Nwachukwu BU, Rosas S, et al. Trends in medial ulnar collateral ligament reconstruction in the United States: a retrospective review of a large private-payer database from 2007 to 2011. Am J Sports Med. 2015;43:1770–4.
17. Zaremski JL, McClelland J, Vincent HK, Horodyski M. Trends in sports-related elbow ulnar collateral ligament injuries. Orthop J Sports Med. 2017;5:2325967117731296.
18. Conway JE, Jobe FW, Glousman RE, Pink M. Medial instability of the elbow in throwing athletes. Treatment by repair or reconstruction of the ulnar collateral ligament. J Bone Joint Surg Am. 1992;74:67–83.
19. Azar FM, Andrews JR, Wilk KE, Groh D. Operative treatment of ulnar collateral ligament injuries of the elbow in athletes. Am J Sports Med. 2000;28:16–23.
20. Argo D, Trenhaile SW, Savoie FH 3rd, Field LD. Operative treatment of ulnar collateral ligament insufficiency of the elbow in female athletes. Am J Sports Med. 2006;34:431–7.
21. Savoie FH 3rd, Trenhaile SW, Roberts J, Field LD, Ramsey JR. Primary repair of ulnar collateral ligament injuries of the elbow in young athletes: a case series of injuries to the proximal and distal ends of the ligament. Am J Sports Med. 2008;36:1066–72.
22. Dugas JR, Looze CA, Capogna B, et al. Ulnar collateral ligament repair with collagen-dipped FiberTape augmentation in overhead-throwing athletes. Am J Sports Med. 2019;47:1096–102.
23. Bodendorfer BM, Looney AM, Lipkin SL, et al. Biomechanical comparison of ulnar collateral ligament reconstruction with the docking technique versus repair with internal bracing. Am J Sports Med. 2018;46:3495–501.

24. Dugas JR, Walters BL, Beason DP, Fleisig GS, Chronister JE. Biomechanical comparison of ulnar collateral ligament repair with internal bracing versus modified Jobe reconstruction. Am J Sports Med. 2016;44:735–41.
25. Jones CM, Beason DP, Dugas JR. Ulnar collateral ligament reconstruction versus repair with internal bracing: comparison of cyclic fatigue mechanics. Orthop J Sports Med. 2018;6:2325967118755991.
26. Urch E, Limpisvasti O, ElAttrache NS, et al. Biomechanical evaluation of a modified internal brace construct for the treatment of ulnar collateral ligament injuries. Orthop J Sports Med. 2019;7:2325967119874135.
27. Norwood LA, Shook JA, Andrews JR. Acute medial elbow ruptures. Am J Sports Med. 1981;9:16–9.

The Role of Arthroscopy in Athletes with Ulnar Collateral Ligament Injuries

19

Curtis Bush and John E. Conway

Introduction

Medial elbow pain is common in the overhead throwing athlete. The diagnosis of medial ulnar collateral ligament (MUCL) injuries is mostly based on a history of medial elbow pain, physical exam findings, and imaging studies. The repeated valgus load that causes MUCL attenuation or rupture might also cause ulnar nerve symptoms, posterior impingement, formation of posteromedial osteophytes , formation of loose bodies, stress fractures of the ulna, lateral plica syndrome, trochlea chondromalacia, and less commonly capitellar osteochondritis dissecans (OCD) lesions. Operative treatment of acute MUCL tears may involve open repair [1] or graft reconstruction, whereas operative treatment of chronic MUCL insufficiency involves open graft reconstruction. Failure to address associated conditions may compromise outcomes of reconstruction. With direct visualization afforded by arthroscopy, the diagnosis and treatment of concomitant pathology may be accomplished at the time of MUCL reconstruction, making elbow arthroscopy a useful adjuvant in the evaluation and treatment of elbow pain in the overhead athlete. The objective of this chapter is to review the indications and techniques of elbow arthroscopy in athletes with MUCL insufficiency.

C. Bush (✉)
Texas Orthopedic Associates, Fort Worth, TX, USA
e-mail: curtisbush@texashealth.org

J. E. Conway
TCU Baseball, Texas Orthopedic Associates, LLP, Fort Worth, TX, USA

Diagnostic Arthroscopy

The diagnosis of ulnar collateral ligament (UCL) injury is based on clinical history, physical examination, and diagnostic tests including stress radiographs, ultrasound, and magnetic resonance imaging (MRI) arthrography . The physical exam for valgus instability can be difficult and is often unreliable [2]. Furthermore, Timmerman and Andrews found little difference between the clinical exam and exam under anesthesia, with neither particularly accurate in evaluating the stability of the ulnohumeral articulation. In Dr. Frank Jobe's landmark description of MUCL reconstruction for valgus instability, arthroscopy was not a routine element of the reconstructive procedure. Timmerman and Andrews, however, found that arthroscopic exam was most helpful in detecting instability in cases with equivocal clinical findings. Altchek's modification of the Jobe reconstruction (the "docking technique") included routine arthroscopy to improve the diagnosis and treatment of concomitant intraarticular pathology [3]. In a later publication by the same authors, arthroscopy was no longer routine but

J. S. Dines et al. (eds.), *Elbow Ulnar Collateral Ligament Injury*,
https://doi.org/10.1007/978-3-030-69567-5_19

instead reserved for patients with preoperative exam findings of extension overload [4]. Although it was once considered to be an effective diagnostic tool in the evaluation of MUCL instability, that role has diminished significantly due to limited capacity to evaluate the appearance and function of the MUCL arthroscopically [4, 5] .

Timmerman and Andrews showed that only the anterior 20–30%, approximately 2–3 mm, of the anterior bundle of the UCL could be adequately visualized with the arthroscope through the anterolateral portal. Meanwhile, the posterior 30–50% of the posterior bundle could be visualized through the posterolateral portal [6]. Visualization was only slightly improved with a 70° scope, which offers a wider field of view around the corner of the ulna. Longitudinal cuts made by the researchers could not be visualized, which suggests that naturally occurring tears likewise may be missed. Following a transverse cut, only the most anterior aspect of the defect (2 mm) could be visualized. Based on these findings, the arthroscopic appearance of a normal ligament does not necessarily preclude the possibility of MUCL tear [6, 7].

Early limitations with the arthroscopic exam of the MUCL led to the development of the arthroscopic "stress test," designed to evaluate the dynamic function of the ligament. The arthroscopic "stress test" [2] places a valgus stress across the ulnohumeral joint in 70° of flexion with the scope in the anterolateral portal (Fig. 19.1). Field et al. showed that opening of the medial ulnohumeral joint 1–2 mm required complete release of anterior bundle. By also releasing the posterior bands and/or placing the forearm in full pronation, one might see a greater ulnohumeral opening, but only after having released the anterior band [8]. Posterior bundle tears with/without partial anterior bundle tears did not create any discernible instability arthroscopically. Based on the findings in this study, the arthroscopic stress test has very limited ability to detect partial tears of the UCL, though the limitations of the test may simply reflect our inability to recreate in vivo forces of throwing. The stress test has not proven to be a particularly reliable test and rarely alters the diagnosis or treatment of MUCL insufficiency [4, 5]. The diagnosis of MUCL insufficiency is usually decided before heading to the operating room, based mostly on history, physical exam, and MRI findings [4, 5]. In a limited number of cases, one might find that an arthroscopic exam is helpful in choosing between ligament repair and reconstruction. With that said, isolated repairs are less

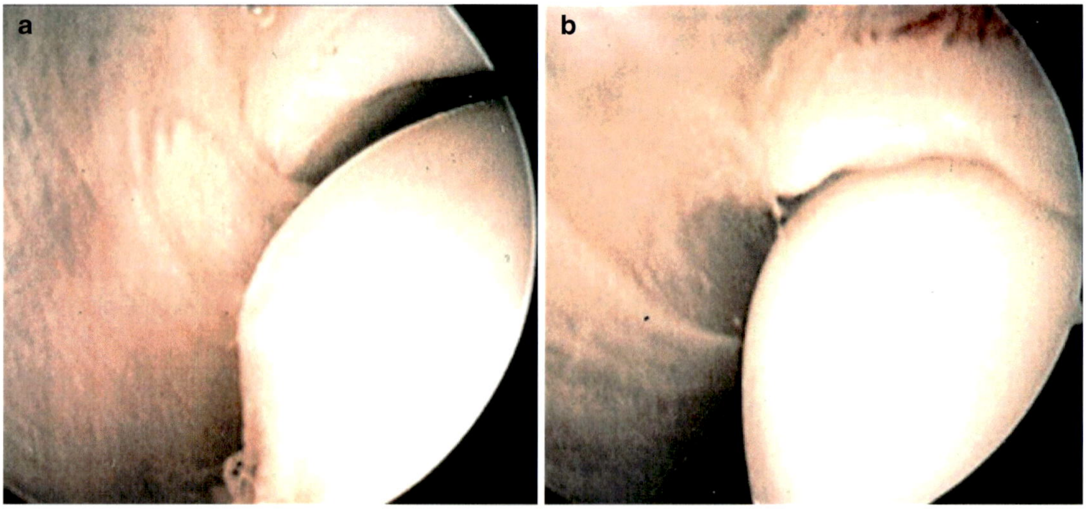

Fig. 19.1 (**a**) Arthroscopic valgus stress test without stress. (**b**) Arthroscopic view showing opening of the ulnohumeral ligament consistent with UCL insufficiency

commonly performed compared to full reconstructions based on historically inferior outcomes. Chap. 17 covers this in more detail [5, 9].

Though elbow arthroscopy has limitations as it relates directly to the treatment of MUCL tears, it has substantial utility in the diagnosis and treatment of the intraarticular pathology that often accompanies chronic MUCL insufficiency. The repeated valgus load of the pitching motion that causes MUCL attenuation or rupture might also cause ulnar nerve symptoms, lateral plica syndrome, posterior impingement, trochlea chondromalacia, formation of posteromedial osteophytes, formation of loose bodies, stress fractures of the ulna, and less commonly capitellar OCD lesions. Concurrent treatment of these conditions is important to the success of MUCL reconstruction surgery. Fortunately, awareness of the prevalence and presentation of MUCL injuries in the overhead throwing athlete has improved in the sports medicine community, and with better awareness and improved imaging techniques fewer chronic sequelae of MUCL insufficiency seem to accumulate. Nevertheless, elbow arthroscopy remains an indispensable skill set when treating the overhead throwing athlete.

Posterior Impingement

Chronic MUCL insufficiency in the overhead throwing athlete can result in valgus extension overload, which may then develop into posterior impingement. Posterior impingement is a broad term subcategorized into posterolateral impingement, posterior impingement, and posteromedial impingement. Arthroscopy has an essential role in the management of each.

Posterolateral Impingement

Posterolateral impingement can present with lateral gutter pain with throwing, palpation, moving valgus stress test, flexion, and extension. These are also findings associated with an olecranon stress fracture or loose body; therefore, one must also consider them among the differential diagnoses. The underlying cause of posterolateral impingement is not well known, though it is generally believed that valgus laxity occurring with MUCL insufficiency leads to reduced resistance to valgus loading, increases in radiocapitellar contact pressures and perhaps symptomatic entrapment of the plica. The posterolateral type impingement may involve the lateral gutter plica or radiocapitellar plica (meniscus). Kim et al. found that 58% of symptomatic patients complained of clicking or catching, and 25% complained of swelling [10]. Exam findings include lateral gutter pain with palpation, moving valgus stress test, flexion, extension, and the flexion–pronation test. The flexion–pronation test, described by Antuna and O'Driscoll, is a provocative test in which the pronated elbow is passively flexed from an extended position. One might find reproducible, painful snapping of plica over the radial head elicited with this maneuver, usually between 90° and 110° of flexion [11]. Akagi and Nakamura demonstrated in a patient with plica impingement that with <90° of flexion the synovial fold is in the joint and that it slips distally over the radial head with flexion >100° [12]. Kim et al. [10] reported that 25% of symptomatic patients had a positive flexion–pronation test. MRI is helpful in making the diagnosis of posterolateral impingement and might reveal thickened or nodular plicae. There are limited data correlating plica size and symptoms, though thickness ≥3 mm and nodularity are suggestive of plica syndrome. Kim et al. [10] reported that 9 of 12 patients had an abnormally thickened plica.

Arthroscopic findings in a patient with symptomatic lateral gutter plica include frayed margins, hypertrophy, capillary infiltration with hyperemia, and lateral ulnar chondromalacia. Arthroscopic findings of radiocapitellar plica syndrome are similar but with anterolateral radial head chondromalacia—from snapping back and forth over the radial head—as opposed to the lateral ulna (Fig. 19.2). Kim et al. [10] found that all patients

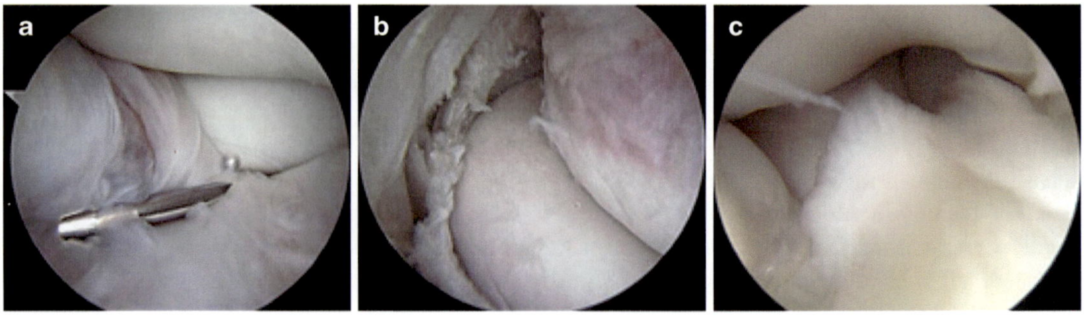

Fig. 19.2 (**a**) Arthroscopic view of radiocapitellar plica. (**b**) Chondral damage evident secondary to abrasion of plica against capitellum. (**c**) Lateral gutter plica

demonstrated a thickened, hypertrophic synovial plica and eight (67%) patients had associated synovitis and inflammation of the adjacent capsular tissue. Seven (58%) patients demonstrated chondromalacia with visible articular chondral changes, most commonly involving the capitellum and posterolateral distal humerus (five patients), followed by the radial head (two patients).

For the majority of cases, the scope is best placed in the posterolateral portal and instruments in the direct posterior radiocapitellar portal. The author's preferred method of plica resection is to place the scope in the posterolateral portal and shaver through the direct posterolateral portal or midradiocapitellar portal. The scope may also be placed in the direct posterolateral portal and shaver through the midradiocapitellar portal. Care should be taken to preserve the anconeus muscle fascia. We might suggest using minishavers because they remove less fascia and allow better access to the ulnohumeral joint, radiocapitellar joint, and the lateral margin of the radial head.

Outcomes of arthroscopic treatment of posterolateral impingement are generally good. Antuna and O'Driscoll reported on 14 patients with posterolateral impingement in which 54% had a positive flexion–pronation test, 93% had chondromalacia visualized arthroscopically, and 86% excellent outcomes following arthroscopic excision. Kim et al. [10] reported on 12 patients in which 25% had a positive flexion–pronation test, 58% had chondromalacia, and 92% excellent result with arthroscopic resection [11].

Posteromedial Impingement

Posteromedial impingement is the most common diagnosis (51%) for which arthroscopic elbow surgery is performed in athletes [13]. Andrews and Timmerman noted that posterior extension injury was the most common diagnosis associated with MUCL injuries [14]. In their group of baseball players treated with elbow arthroscopy for posteromedial impingement, MUCL injuries were initially underestimated. Among the patients requiring a second surgery, 25% required MUCL reconstruction.

Posteromedial impingement may develop as a course of chronic valgus extension overload. Overload is caused by the combination of medial elbow tension, lateral compression, and valgus extension. Wilson and Andrews describe a wedging effect of the olecranon into the olecranon fossa, with abutment of the medial outer rim of the olecranon and inner rim of the olecranon fossa of the humerus [15]. MUCL insufficiency that increases valgus laxity alters both the contact pressure and area on the posteromedial olecranon and partially explains the development of posteromedial olecranon osteophyte formation [16]. The impingement appears to occur during late acceleration, ball release, and early follow-through phases of throwing. Physical exam findings may include pain in extension and valgus stress. Crepitance and/or loss of elbow extension may also be seen. In the throwing athlete, posteromedial impingement should focus the physician's attention toward instability. Imaging evaluation of posteromedial impingement may include CT and/or MRI. Ko et al. [17] found that the most common imaging manifestations of posteromedial impingement were joint space narrowing, subchondral sclerosis, and osteophyte formation. The authors concluded that CT is superior to MRI in detecting joint space narrowing, medial olecranon subluxation, and loose bodies, whereas bone marrow edema and associated soft tissue injuries were more readily visualized on MRI. Conway et al. reported that over 50% of their patients undergoing UCL reconstruction or repair had posteromedial osteophytes.

Posterior medial gutter synovitis may occur in isolation or along with other posterolateral pathology. This condition usually resolves without surgery. In the senior author's experience, this condition may respond to injections and is rarely treated with synovectomy.

Direct Posterior Impingement

Repetitive hyperextension of the elbow may also cause a discrete form of posterior impingement. This injury pattern is seen in softball players and seen in other repetitive hyperextension activities where pain occurs in extension. Radiographic findings include osteophyte/reactive lesions of the olecranon tip and thickening of the bone bridge between the coronoid and olecranon fossae. UCL tears are usually not present in association with this process. Primary osteoarthritis (OA) may develop predominately in the posterior elbow creating posterior impingement, though this is seen almost exclusively in males between the fourth and sixth decades [18].

Trochlear Chondromalacia

MUCL insufficiency that increases valgus laxity leads to an increase in total contact pressure on the PM trochlea while decreasing the overall contact area and shifting it medially [19]. Trochlear chondromalacia may be detected on high-resolution, high-field, thin-section MRI with intraarticular contrast on sagittal and axial sequences, appearing as subchondral edema signal, insufficiency stress patterns, osteochondral collapse, and/or marginal exostosis. When confirmed arthroscopically, these lesions may only require debridement and/or chondroplasty (Fig. 19.3). Formal microfracture is rarely necessary. To improve visualization and protect the ulnar nerve during this procedure, one might consider maintaining the elbow at 45–90° of elbow flexion, using a curved retractor, a 2.7-mm microshaver, and briefly increasing the fluid pressure manually. Here we stress the importance of leaving the posteromedial capsule intact, which is facilitated by the use of the smaller shaver and momentarily increasing fluid pressure.

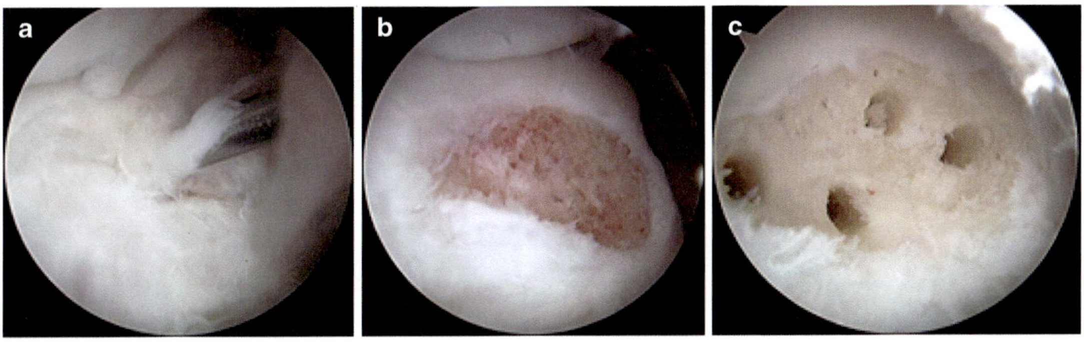

Fig. 19.3 (**a**) Trochlear chondral lesion. (**b**) Trochlear chondral lesion delineated after debridement. (**c**) Microfracture of the lesion

Olecranon Exostosis and Fragmentation

Repetitive stress on the posteromedial olecranon may cause stress reactions, stress fractures of the posteromedial tip or transversely through the more proximal process, and exostosis formation/fragmentation. Olecranon exostosis formation was found in 24% of asymptomatic professional baseball pitchers and in 50% of players aged 30–35 years [20]. Exostoses and fragmentation may be detected on preoperative imaging. Conventional X-ray view may underestimate the actual fragment size. The senior author presented a radiographic technique using an anteroposterior (AP) view of the elbow with the patient seated, the shoulder abducted 90°, externally rotated 40°, and elbow flexed 140° [20]. This X-ray view may provide a more accurate estimate of the size and location of medial olecranon exostoses.

The objective of arthroscopic treatment is to remove loose fragments and restore the normal shape of the olecranon. The posterior impingement view, described earlier and depicted in Fig. 19.4, helps define the size of the posterior medial exostosis to be removed. Excessive olecranon resection can negatively affect the results of elbow surgery [14] and one should avoid resecting more than 3 mm of the normal posterior medial margin. Kamineni et al. showed in a biomechanical model that 3 mm incremental olecranon resection created stepwise valgus angulation and that resection greater than 3 mm may jeopardize MUCL function due to added strain on the ligament [19]. These findings challenged the rationale of removing any amount of normal bone. An adequate resection may be facilitated by using two to three working portals and moving the scope, instruments, and retractors between them as needed. The two primary portals are the posterior central and posterolateral portals, and a good accessory portal is the high posterolateral portal (Fig. 19.5). Resection may be performed using sharpened miniosteotomes and small bone cutting shavers (used with a retractor). We recommend using retractors to protect the ulnar nerve and switching portals as often as needed for visibility and access. We recommend against using suction or burrs due to the tendency to over-resect. We might also recommend clearing all bone fragments and debris after resection and closing the deep layer of all posterolateral portals. As shown in Table 19.1, the outcomes in terms of return to play following olecranon resection are generally good.

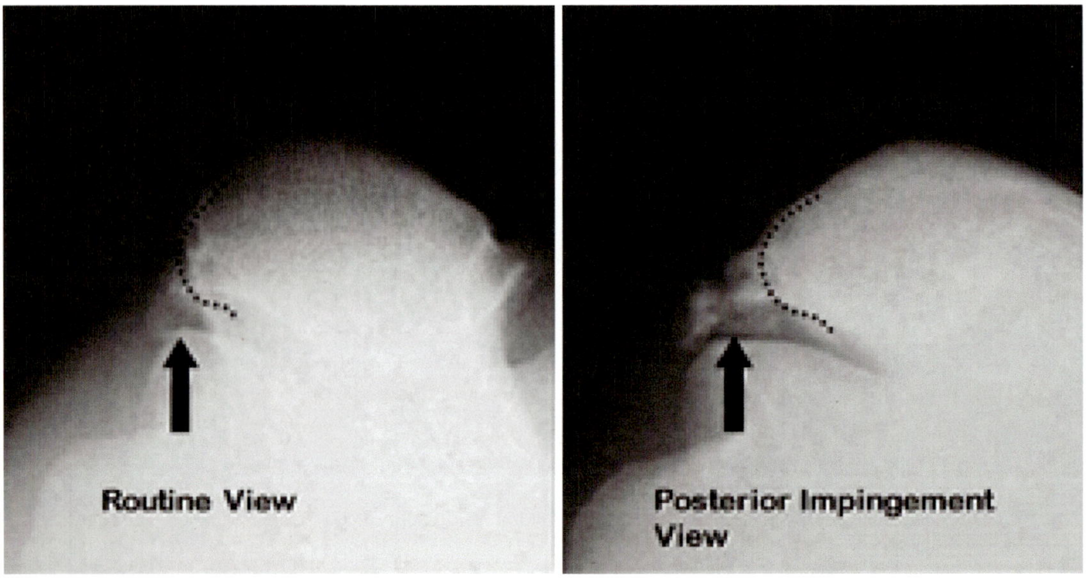

Fig. 19.4 Posterior impingement view defining posterior medial exostosis

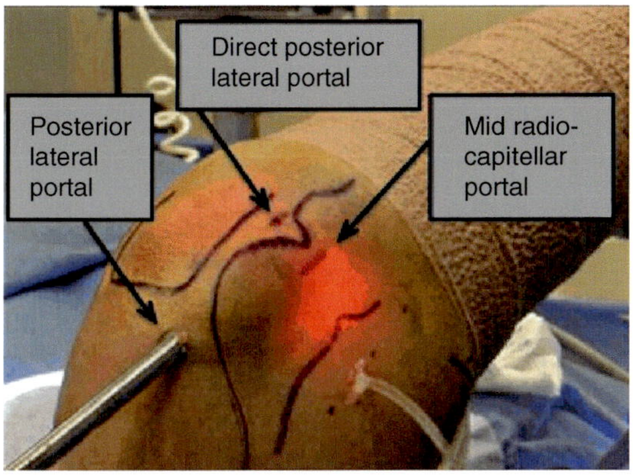

Fig. 19.5 Posterior portals most commonly used to remove posterior medial exostosis

Table 19.1 Outcomes in terms of return to play following olecranon resection

Rossenwasser *AANA* 1991	83%
Rossenwasser *AANA* 1991	74%
Ward *JHSurg* 1993	78%
Andrews *AJSM* 1995	73%
Fideler *JSES* 1997	74%
Hepler *Arthroscopy* 1998	95%
Reedy *Arthroscopy* 2000	85%
Cohen *Arthroscopy* 2011	77%

Loose Bodies

Loose bodies may cause painful mechanical symptoms and produce crepitus, tenderness, and motion loss. Radiographs routinely underestimate the presence/quantity of loose bodies [21, 22]. Loose bodies may appear anterior, posterior, lateral, and rarely medial (Fig. 19.6). Treatment usually involves simple fragment removal unless the fragment is needed for OCD repair.

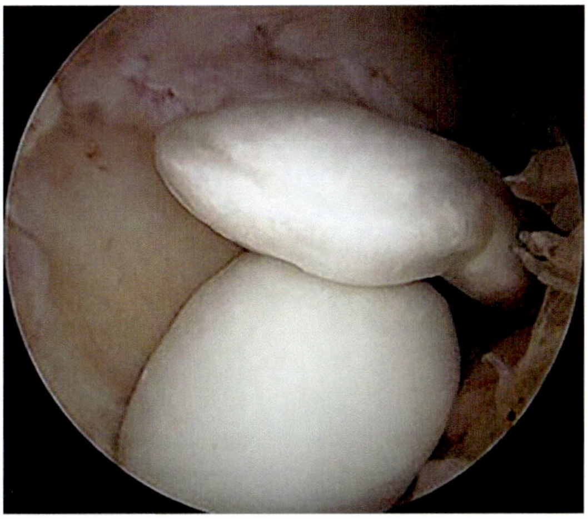

Fig. 19.6 Multiple loose bodies in lateral gutter

Capitellar Osteochondritis Dissecans

Capitellar osteochondritis dissecans lesions are rarely seen in association with UCL injury, however, the treating physician must be prepared to manage such lesions if they occur. With larger OCD lesions, it may be best to treat the OCD first and stage the UCL reconstruction at a later time. The diagnosis and treatment of OCD of the capitellum is a lengthy discussion to itself and is beyond the scope of this chapter.

Surgical Technique

Elbow arthroscopy can be quite technically demanding and each physician may have his or her own learning curve. As it is with other disciplines in orthopedics, it is important in elbow arthroscopy that the treating surgeon understand his/her learning curve and commit only to procedures that fall under that curve. It is very helpful to be familiar and comfortable using multiple patient positions, including the supine cross body, supine suspended, lateral decubitus, and prone positions. It is particularly important to be comfortable with elbow arthroscopy in the supine position when an arthroscopic procedure is called upon in conjunction with MUCL reconstruction. We recommend this position in order to avoid the need to reposition and redrape during surgery. When arthroscopy is indicated with UCL reconstruction, we recommend performing the arthroscopic portion of the procedure before the open portion. Associated arthroscopic procedures are usually simple and relatively short, for example, plica excision, loose body removal, chondroplasty. There are circumstances in which it might be best to perform the open procedure prior to arthroscopy. For instance, when performing contracture release surgery or other complex arthroscopic procedures in combination with ulnar nerve neurolysis, it is probably best to perform the nerve surgery before the arthroscopic procedure.

Portal placement is an essential step toward successful elbow arthroscopy. The standard portals used are the high (proximal) anterior medial, high anterior lateral, posterior central, posterior lateral, and posterior direct radiocapitellar. Accessory portals might include a high posterior lateral and midradiocapitellar portal. The first arthroscopic portal is usually anterior, unless one expects to perform the entire procedure through posterior portals.

The initial anterior portal may be made either medial or lateral, and there is debate on this subject [23, 24]. Surgeon preference and patient diagnosis may determine which is most suitable. The three commonly described anteromedial portals are the standard anteromedial, proximal anteromedial, and midanteromedial portals. The standard anteromedial portal offers excellent visualization of the anterolateral elbow joint, but is probably most commonly used for capsular retractors. As described by Andrews and Carson, it is located 2 cm anterior and 2 cm distal to the prominence of the medial epicondyle. The median nerve-to-sheath distance averages between 6 and 14 mm for this portal [25]. The high or proximal, anteromedial portal is described as 2 cm proximal to the prominence of the medial epicondyle and just anterior to the medial intermuscular septum [26]. Some have described it as much as 2 cm anterior to the septum [24]. This portal provides visual access to the lateral joint structures, though perhaps less visualization of superior capsular structures, the lateral capitellum, and the radiocapitellar joint space in comparison to the standard anteromedial portal [25]. The midanteromedial portal is a modification of the proximal anteromedial portal and is located 1 cm proximal and 1 cm anterior to the prominence of the medial epicondyle [27].

The distal anterolateral portal is less commonly used than the other lateral portals due to safety concerns and is typically reserved for retraction. It is located 3 cm distal and 1 cm anterior to the prominence of the lateral epicondyle. The midanterolateral portal is most useful for visualizing the medial elbow structures and debridement of the anterior radiocapitellar joint surfaces. It is located 1 cm anterior to the prominence of the lateral epicondyle and just proximal to the anterior margin of the radiocapitellar joint space. The high or proximal, anterolateral portal is thought to provide the most extensive evaluation of the joint, especially when viewing the radiocapitellar joint [25, 28]. It is located 1–2 cm proximal to the prominence of the lateral epicondyle.

The posterior portals are relatively safer than the anterior portals. The posterior central portal is commonly the initial posterior portal and provides visualization of the olecranon fossa, olecranon tip, posterior trochlea, and the medial recess. It is typically located 2–4 cm proximal to the olecranon tip and midway between the medial and lateral condyles. The posterolateral portal can provide a view of the olecranon fossa, olecranon tip, and posterior and central trochlea, medial recess, lateral recess, and the posterior radiocapitellar joint. It is located 3 cm proximal to the olecranon and through the lateral border of the triceps tendon. The direct posterolateral portal may also be known as the midlateral portal, the dorsal lateral portal, or the soft spot portal. This portal typically provides the best view of the radiocapitellar joint. It is located at the center of the triangle defined by the prominence of the lateral epicondyle, prominence of the olecranon, and the radial head. The lateral radiocapitellar portal is a difficult portal to create and use due to limited space. It is useful in the management of capitellar OCD lesions and radiocapitellar chondral injuries. It is located at the radiocapitellar joint line where an 18-gauge needle may be used to localize the appropriate portal position.

Elbow arthroscopy requires specialized instrumentation. We recommend the availability of a minishaver system, curved 3.2 mm retractors, sharpened miniosteotomes, sharpened minicurettes (3–0, 4–0), and beaver blades.

Rehabilitation Considerations

When one or multiple arthroscopic procedures described earlier are performed in conjunction with MUCL reconstruction, the risk of postoperative stiffness increases. Motion recovery should be the first priority for therapists. At the time of surgery, we might recommend thoroughly irrigating the joint and extending the elbow to evacuate any hemarthrosis before final ligament fixation. Postoperatively, we do not recommend shortening the immobilization period unless microfracture is performed, in which case we recommend limiting motion or continuous passive motion (CPM) to 10–50° of motion for the first 10 days, then 40–100° for 10 days.

Conclusion

The throwing motion places extreme stresses across the elbow, which may result in medial, lateral, and posterior pathology. Clearly, the focus of this chapter is on the medial-based pathology, namely UCL insufficiency. However, failure to treat radiocapitellar changes and/or posterior impingement may result in suboptimal outcomes. For this reason, thorough understanding of elbow biomechanics as it relates to the throwing athlete and a mastery of elbow arthroscopy are critical to success when treating the throwing athlete.

References

1. Dugas JR, Looze CA, Capogna B, Walters BL, Jones CM, Rothermich MA, Fleisig GS, Aune KT, Drogosz M, Wilk K, Emblom BA, Cain EL. Ulnar collateral ligament repair with collagen-dipped FiberTape augmentation in overhead-throwing athletes. Am J Sports Med. 2019;47:1096–102.
2. Timmerman LA, Andrews JR. Undersurface tear of the ulnar collateral ligament in baseball players. Am J Sports Med. 1994;22(1):33–6. 64
3. Rohrbough JT, Altchek DW, Hman J, Williams RJ III, Botts JD. Medial collateral ligament reconstruction of the elbow using the docking technique. Am J Sports Med. 2002;30:541–8.
4. Bowers AL, Dines JS, Dines DM, et al. Elbow medial ulnar collateral ligament reconstruction: clinical relevance and the docking technique. J Shoulder Elb Surg. 2010;19:110–7. 10
5. Cain EL, Andrews JR, Dugas JR, Wilk KE, McMichael C, Walter JC, Riley R, Arthur ST. Outcome of ulnar collateral ligament reconstruction of the elbow in 1281 athletes: results in 743 athletes with minimum 2-year follow-up. Am J Sports Med. 2010;38:2426–34. 73
6. Timmerman LA, Andrews JR. Histology and arthroscopic anatomy of the ulnar collateral ligament of the elbow. Am J Sports Med. 1994;22(5):667–73. 63
7. Timmerman LA, Schwartz ML, Andrews JR. Preoperative evaluation of the ulnar collateral ligament by magnetic resonance imaging and computed tomography arthrography. Am J Sports Med. 1994;22(1):26–32. 65
8. Field LD, Altchek DW. Evaluation of the arthroscopic valgus instability test of the elbow. Am J Sports Med. 1996;24(2):177–81. 21
9. Azar FM, Andrews JR, Wilk KE. Operative treatment of ulnar collateral ligament injuries in the elbow in athlete. Am J Sports Med. 2000;28:16–23. 74
10. Kim DH, Gambardella RA, Elattrache NS, Yocum LA, Jobe FW. Arthroscopic treatment of posterolateral elbow impingement from lateral synovial plicae in throwing athletes and golfers. Am J Sports Med. 2006;34(3):438–44.
11. Antuna SA, O'Driscoll SW. Snapping plicae associated with radiocapitellar chondromalacia. Arthroscopy. 2001;17(5):491–5.
12. Akagi M, Nakamura T. Snapping elbow caused by the synovial in the radiohumeral joint. J Shoulder Elb Surg. 1998;7(4):427–9.
13. Reddy AS, Kvitne RS, Yocum LA, Elattrache NS, Glousman RE, Jobe FW. Arthroscopy of the elbow: a long-term clinical review. Arthroscopy. 2000;16(6):588–94. 54
14. Andrews JR, Timmerman LA. Outcome of elbow surgery in professional baseball players. Am J Sports Med. 1995;23:407–13.

15. Wilson FD, Andrews JR, Blackburn T, Mccluskey G. Valgus extension overload in the pitching elbow. Am J Sports Med. 1983;11(2):83–8.
16. Ahmad C, Park MC, Elattrache NS. Elbow medial ulnar collateral ligament insufficiency alters posteromedial olecranon contact. Am J Sports Med. 2004;32(7):1607–12. 90
17. Ko CC, Tai MH, Lin CH, Tzeng WS, Chen JH, Shu G, Wu CD, Chen CKH. Posteromedial olecranon impingement of the pitching elbow: additional finding provided by CT. Eur J Radiol. 2016;85:211–7.
18. Morrey BF. Primary degenerative arthritis of the elbow: treatment by ulnohumeral arthroplasty. J Bone Joint Surg. 1992;74A:410–3.
19. Kamineni S, Elattrache N, Odriscoll S, Ahmad C, Hirohara H, Peale P, An K, Morrey BF. Medial collateral ligament strain with partial posteromedial olecranon resection: a biomechanical study. J Bone Joint Surg Am. 2004;86(11):2424–30. 91
20. Conway J. Olecranon exostosis in throwers. Presentation at American orthopedic society of sports medicine annual meeting. 2000.
21. Ogilvie-Harris DJ, Schemitsch E. Arthroscopy of the elbow for removal of loose bodies. Arthroscopy. 1993;9:5–8.
22. Ward WG, Belhobek GH, Anderson TE. Arthroscopic elbow finding: correlation with preoperative radiographic studies. Arthroscopy. 1992;8:498–502.
23. Abboud J, Ricchetti E, Tjoumakaris F, et al. Elbow arthroscopy basic setup and portal placement. J Am Acad Orthop Surg. 2006;14:312–8.
24. O'Driscoll S, Morrey BF. Arthroscopy of the elbow: diagnostic and therapeutic benefits and hazards. J Bone Joint Surg Am. 1992;74A:84–94.
25. Stothers K, Day B, Regan W. Arthroscopy of the elbow: anatomy, portal sites, and a description of the proximal lateral portal. Arthroscopy. 1995;11(4):449–57.
26. Poehling GG, Whipple TL, Sisco L, Goldman B. Elbow arthroscopy, a new technique. Arthroscopy. 1989;5:222–81.
27. Lindenfeld TN. Medial approach in elbow arthroscopy. Am J Sports Med. 1990;18:413–7.
28. Verhaar J, van-Mameren H, Brandsma A. Risks of neurovascular injury in elbow arthroscopy: starting anteromedially or anterolaterally? Arthroscopy. 1991;7:287–90.

Biomechanics of Reconstruction Constructs

20

Melissa A. Wright and Anand M. Murthi

Introduction

Ulnar collateral ligament (UCL) injuries in overhead athletes are common because the motion of throwing subjects the elbow to high valgus stresses during every pitch. It has been estimated that the UCL receives forces of up to 3100°/s and valgus stresses of up to 64 N m [1, 2]. Until the 1970s, this injury was career ending because non-operative management yielded poor results and no surgical treatments were available. In 1974, Jobe performed the first UCL reconstruction on major league pitcher Tommy John, and the procedure bears the pitcher's name. The first published series in UCL reconstruction was subsequently published by Jobe in 1986 [3]. This original Jobe technique of reflecting the flexor–pronator muscles prior to autograft ligament reconstruction yielded excellent results with 63% return to play [3]. Newly available technologies and surgical approaches have contributed to the improvements in this technique with a focus on minimizing muscle disruption. In this chapter, we review the original technique and newer techniques that have evolved. We also review the biomechanical data available on various procedures.

M. A. Wright
Department of Orthopaedics, MedStar Union Memorial Hospital, Baltimore, MD, USA

A. M. Murthi (✉)
Shoulder and Elbow Surgery, MedStar Union Memorial Hospital/Georgetown University School of Medicine, Baltimore, MD, USA
e-mail: Anand.m.murthi@medstar.net

Jobe Technique

The goal of the classic Jobe technique was to restore elbow stability using a reconstruction to restore the anterior band of the UCL [3]. The procedure involved a takedown of the flexor–pronator mass and submuscular ulnar nerve transposition. The entire flexor–pronator musculature was reflected off the medial condyle and proximal ulna to provide an uncompromised view of the surgical reconstruction site. The primary goal was to reconstruct the anterior band of the UCL. A palmaris longus graft was then woven through 3.2 mm bone tunnels at the sublime tubercle of the ulna and medial epicondyle of the distal humerus in a figure of eight fashion (Fig. 20.1). This procedure was later modified by Smith et al. by using a muscle-splitting approach, thus avoiding the morbidity associated with the takedown of the flexor–pronator mass [4]. This became known as the modified Jobe technique and is one of the popular techniques available today.

In 2002, Mullen et al. [5] evaluated the Jobe procedure in the laboratory by comparing it to the intact state using 14 cadaveric elbows. The specimens were fixed on a load frame, and a 50-N

J. S. Dines et al. (eds.), *Elbow Ulnar Collateral Ligament Injury*,
https://doi.org/10.1007/978-3-030-69567-5_20

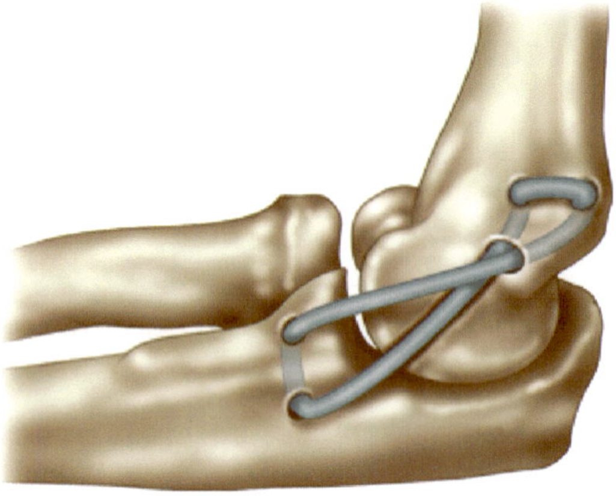

Fig. 20.1 Jobe technique. Bone tunnels are placed at the sublime tubercle and medial humeral epicondyle. A palmaris longus graft is weaved in a figure of eight fashion and tied with sutures

force was used to elevate the forearm, creating a 5-N-m moment on the medial side of the elbow. Displacement was measured at 30° intervals from 30° to 120° of elbow flexion. The UCL was then transected and the specimen was tested. Finally, the elbows were reconstructed using the traditional Jobe technique and tested in the same fashion. The investigators found that sectioning the anterior bundle of the UCL increased displacement from 140% to 150% during the range of motion. When the UCL was reconstructed with the Jobe technique, displacement ranged from 98 to 112% during range of motion compared to the intact state. These differences were statistically significant. This basic biomechanical study gives mechanical credibility to the Jobe reconstruction method.

Ciccotti et al. also looked at the biomechanics of the Jobe technique compared to the native UCL and the docking technique [6]. In this study of 10 cadaveric specimens, the authors potted the elbows and mounted them on a custom elbow loading system. The investigators then subjected the elbows to a valgus load of 5 N m for 6–8 s and then offloaded them. They performed each loading test five times at 30° intervals from 30° to 110° of elbow flexion. Once this was done, the elbows were placed at 90° of flexion to simulate the throwing position and then loaded to failure. Results from this study showed that the maximal elongation of the anterior band of the native UCL did not change with elbow flexion; however, the valgus laxity decreased with increasing flexion angles. The same result was observed in elbows reconstructed with the Jobe technique and the docking technique, and no differences were observed compared to the intact state. In terms of load to failure, the native UCL was stronger than both reconstructions by almost 80%. Modes of failure of the native UCL were 50% ulnar avulsion, 5% humeral avulsion, and 45% midsubstance tear, whereas the Jobe technique showed 70% ulnar tunnel fracture, 20% midsubstance tear, and 10% suture pullout, and for the docking technique, there were 40% ulnar tunnel fracture, 40% suture pullout, 10% midsubstance tear, and 10% humeral tunnel fracture.

Docking Technique

Rohrbough et al. described the docking technique in 1996 [7]. In this technique, the authors placed ulnar tunnels similarly to what is used in the traditional Jobe technique, but they replaced the humeral tunnels with a single bony tunnel with two converging exit suture holes. The graft is secured using sutures over a bone bridge. This technique was designed to improve graft tensioning while minimizing the number or bone tunnels in the humerus [7, 8]. Care must be taken to measure and cut the graft to fit snugly into the humeral socket to prevent graft slippage and loosening. Cohen et al. tested the load to failure of 10 elbow pairs to determine the optimal position for tensioning the UCL docking reconstruction [9]. The load to failure of the native ligament was significantly higher than in the reconstructed ligament tensioned at either position, but there was no significant difference in load to failure between the reconstruction tensioned at 30° or 90° of flexion. Valgus laxity (degrees per Newton-meter) when the reconstruction was tensioned at 30° was more similar to the native ligament than when tensioned at 90°, but difference in valgus laxity between all three states was not statistically significant. Fixation is generally recommended at 30° of flexion. A case series of the docking technique by Bowers et al. looking at 21 throwers, 5 of which were professional and 11 were college players, showed 19 (90%) of 21 excellent results and 2 of 21 good results with no complications [8].

In a biomechanical study, Armstrong et al. [10] compared the docking technique to figure of eight, Endobutton, and interference screw techniques. The investigators tested 20 cadaveric elbows by potting them and placing them on a custom jig (Fig. 20.2). A cyclic load of 20 N was applied for 200 cycles. The load was then increased by 10 N increments until ligament failure occurred or a gap formation greater than 5 mm was seen. A palmaris tendon graft was used for the reconstruction in all four of the different reconstruction states. The investigators found that the intact elbow failed at 142.5 ± 39.4 N, whereas all other reconstruction techniques failed at much lower loads. The docking technique failed at 53.0 ± 9.5 N and the Endobutton group failed at 52.5 ± 10.4 N. Interference screw and figure-eight reconstructions were the weakest, failing at 41.0 ± 16.0 N and 33.3 ± 7.1 N, respectively. Moreover, the docking and Endobutton techniques failed at a much higher number of cycles than the interference screw and figures of eight groups. No intrasubstance failures were reported. The primary mode of failure was tendon pullout from the tendon–suture interface in the docking, figure of eight, and Endobutton techniques. In the interference screw cohort, failure occurred via dissociation of the tendon from the tendon–screw interface.

Hurbanek et al. proposed the addition of an interference screw to the docking technique [11]. They used nine matched cadaveric elbows and compared the traditional docking technique to docking with the addition of a 4.75-mm bioabsorbable screw. The investigators found a statistically significant difference in valgus instability of the elbow between the intact and docking alone groups. There was no difference in laxity of the UCL between the intact and the docking + interference screw groups. The most common mode of failure in both groups was suture pulling out of the tendon. The stiffness of the interference screw construct was higher than in the traditional docking group (14.7 N/mm vs. 9.9 N/mm; $p = 0.044$). The authors concluded that the addition of a bioabsorbable interference screw might enhance fixation strength.

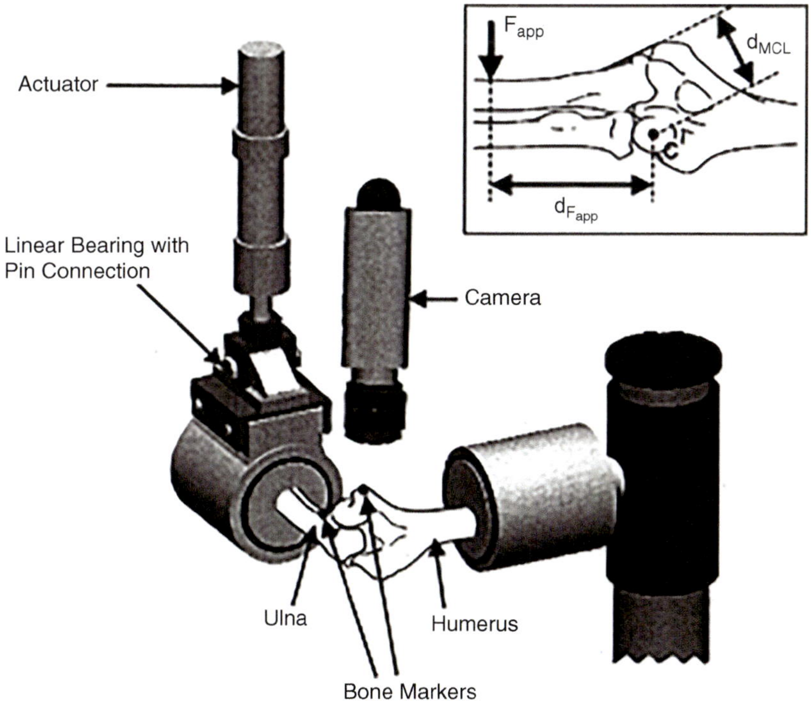

Fig. 20.2 Test setup. (Reprinted from [9], with permission from Elsevier)

Bernas et al. examined the time-zero biomechanical properties of the docking technique in an attempt to better define safe rehabilitation [12]. They used eight cadaveric elbows and measured strain on their UCL reconstruction in three settings: passive range of motion, 22.2 N isometric flexion and extension contractions, and 3.34 N-m varus and valgus torques at 90° of flexion. They found that strain increased by 7% (>3% considered unsafe) with flexion beyond 50°. Isometric contractions were performed at 90° and also caused unsafe levels of strain; the strain, however, was not increased beyond the level seen with simple flexion to 90°. Valgus stress increased the strain significantly. The authors concluded that motion from 0° to 50° is safe following UCL reconstruction with a docking technique and that isometric strengthening may be safe as long as it is performed in the 0–50 degree zone. Valgus stress should be avoided.

Suture Anchor Technique

In the early 1990s, the advent of new suture anchor technology led to their use in reconstruction of the UCL [13]. Suture anchors were thought to obviate the need for bone tunnels and therefore to prevent complications such as bone bridge fracture and screw pullout. In all UCL reconstructions, preventing sublime tubercle and/or medial condyle fracture and protecting the ulnar nerve are paramount for a good outcome. These issues stimulated new, safer techniques that continue to provide strong constructs. In 1998, Hechtman et al. [14] described a technique using suture anchors as the primary form of fixation of the UCL graft. In this procedure, the investigators identified the origin of the anterior bundle at the anteroinferior border of the medial epicondyle and created an anteroposterior trough just distal to it, large enough to accommodate a palmaris longus graft. Two anchors were placed on the medial and lateral borders of the anterior bundle origin. Next, the insertion of the anterior bundle was identified on the sublime tubercle, where a vertical trough was made. Two anchors were placed at the anterior and posterior borders of the anterior bundle insertion. The center of the graft was fixed to the epicondyle with a 2-0 suture. The free limbs were passed under the ulnar anchor sutures and tied back to the epicondyle with the arm at 45° of flexion (Fig. 20.3).

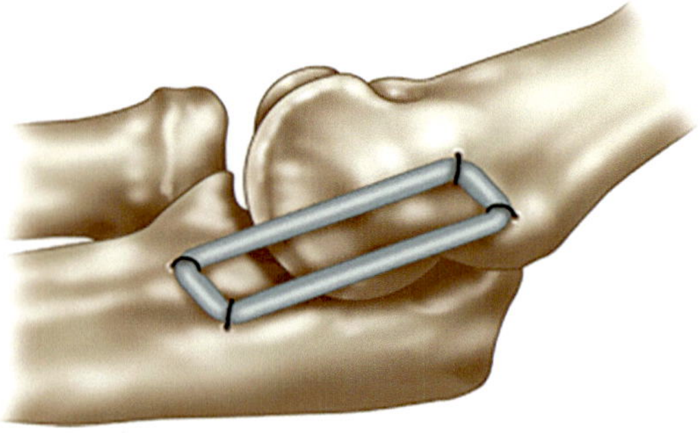

Fig. 20.3 Suture anchor technique. Suture anchors are placed at the sublime tubercle and medial epicondyle. A palmaris longus graft is secured to the anchors and tied to itself with sutures

Hechtman et al. [14] compared this new reconstruction technique with the classic Jobe technique using 31 cadaveric elbows. Length measurements were collected throughout the range of motion arc. Specimens were then taken through the same range of motion and strain measurements were similarly calculated. The investigators found that toward extension, strain increased in the anterior band of the normal and anchor groups, but were decreased in the tunnel group. Moreover, the posterior band was lax in the normal and anchor groups, but tight in the tunnel group. No significant difference in maximal valgus load to failure versus intact was found between the two groups, with 76.3% in the tunnel group and 63.5% in the anchor group. Primary mode of failure in the intact group was a tear in the anterior bundle, and no tears were seen in the posterior bundle. Of the tears in the intact group, 68% occurred at the ligament–bone interface and 32% were intrasubstance. In the Jobe technique group, 65% of failures occurred by suture slippage, 14% by humeral fracture, 14% by ulnar fracture, and 7% by intraligamentous failure. In the anchor group, 53% of samples failed from suture slippage, 18% by suture failure, 6% by intraligament failure, 12% by ulnar bone fracture, and 12% by anchor pullout. The authors concluded that although there was no difference in resistance to valgus stress, suture anchor fixation was more anatomic. However, it is important to note that in this study, fixation strength in the suture anchor group was significantly lower than in the intact ligament, plus this technique creates an onlay reconstruction versus the intraosseous bone tunnel/docking techniques which may create an issue with bony healing. These may be some reasons why this procedure showed a dismal 30% clinical failure rate in clinical studies [13, 15].

Interference Screw Technique

To avoid ulnar tunnel complications, avoid muscle dissection, and decrease the risk of nerve injury, Ahmad et al. described an interference screw technique in which both the ulnar and humeral sides of the graft are fixed with interference screws [16]. This technique was described in a cadaveric study in which the investigators created 5 mm bone tunnels at the isometric anatomic insertion sites on the sublime tubercle and medial epicondyle. The ulnar tunnel was drilled at a 45° angle to the long axis of the ulna to a depth of 20 mm, and the humeral tunnel was placed 5 mm distal to the anterior tip of the epicondyle directed to exit at the superior aspect of the epicondyle. An ipsilateral palmaris longus tendon graft was used. Fixation was achieved with five 15 mm interference screws. The elbows were mounted on a custom frame and loaded with a valgus load of 3 N m at 15° intervals from 0 to 120° of elbow flexion.

When compared to the intact state, the reconstructed state had lower stiffness (42.81 ± 11.6 N/mm vs. 20.28 ± 12.5 N/mm; $p < 0.05$), but there was no difference in ultimate moment (34.29 ± 6.9 N/m vs. 30.55 ± 19.24 N/m). No differences were seen in valgus stability of the elbow. The authors concluded that this technique returned elbow kinematics to near normal and achieved failure strength comparable to that of the native elbow. The investigators did not compare their technique to other established reconstruction techniques.

McAdams et al. [17] used a bioabsorbable interference screw technique and compared it to the docking technique. In this study, 16 elbows were mounted on a custom jig and a cyclic valgus load was applied to the intact state and to the reconstructed specimens. The investigators looked at the valgus angle that was created after 1, 10, 100, and 1000 cycles. They found that the valgus angle was significantly greater in the docking technique group than in the intact and interference screw groups at 1, 10, and 100 cycles. No difference between the groups was seen after 1000 cycles. The authors concluded that a bioabsorbable interference screw technique can better restore the native elbow biomechanics at early cyclic loading.

Subsequent studies comparing interference screw fixation techniques with other techniques suggest that interference screw fixation may have lower load to failure than other techniques [10, 18]. Interference screw fixation was compared with the traditional Jobe technique in a study by Large et al. [18]. Using 10 matched cadaveric elbows, the investigators looked at differences between the two reconstruction techniques under valgus load at four different flexion angles. The investigators showed that elbows reconstructed via the Jobe technique reproduced the overall stiffness of the intact UCL at all angles tested. Interference screw stiffness was lower than the intact state at almost all tested degrees of flexion. In terms of load to failure, the elbows reconstructed with the Jobe technique failed at 22.7 N m absorbing 1.59 N m of energy, whereas the interference screws failed at 13.4 N m absorbing only 0.97 N m of energy (=0.0045). The bone tunnels in the Jobe technique failed 40% of the time, whereas 70% of the interference screw constructs failed by graft slippage. The authors concluded that the traditional Jobe technique appears to be superior to interference screw fixation. The study by Armstrong et al. previously discussed also suggested that interference screw fixation is inferior to the docking technique and endobutton technique [10].

High-Strength Suture Tape Augmentation

High-strength suture tape augmentation with the InternalBrace (Arthrex) has become a widespread concept for reinforcing various ligament reconstructions and repairs throughout the body, including the UCL [3, 4]. A suture tape, often collagen coated, is fixed in the orientation of a reconstructed or repaired ligament to reduce the stress on the ligament above a certain threshold of strain and provide improved biomechanical stability. UCL repair, once abandoned due to poor clinical outcomes, has seen a resurgence in recent years with the advent of the high-strength suture tape augmentation technology. Dugas et al. performed a biomechanical study on 18 cadaver elbows and found no difference in ultimate torque failure, rotational stiffness, or gap formation between UCL repair in conjunction with high-strength suture tape augmentation and the modified Jobe reconstruction technique [19]. At repetitive low loads, there was actually less gap formation in the repair with suture tape augmentation. Bodendorfer et al. followed up this study with a biomechanical analysis comparing UCL repair with suture tape augmentation to UCL reconstruction with the docking technique [20]. They similarly found similar biomechanical properties between the two techniques in terms of ultimate failure, valgus opening, and gap formation. Small studies have demonstrated high rates of return to play (92% at 6 months) in patients undergoing UCL repair with suture tape augmentation, adding clinical relevance to the biomechanical data [21].

Given the success of suture tape augmentation in improving the biomechanics of UCL repair, Bernholt et al. compared the biomechanical performance of the docking UCL reconstruction with and without high-strength suture tape augmentation [22]. They found that mean stiffness and mean ultimate failure torque in the UCL reconstruction with suture tape augmentation were equivalent to the native UCL, whereas stiffness and ultimate failure torque were lower in the standard reconstruction with docking technique group. Mean ulnohumeral gapping was not different among the standard reconstruction, the reconstruction with suture tape augmentation, and the native UCL. The most common modes of failure in the reconstruction with suture tape augmentation specimens were ulnar tunnel fracture (58%), followed by graft failure (42%). In the standard docking reconstruction, graft failure was by far the most common mode of failure (75%). These findings demonstrate that suture tape augmentation of UCL reconstruction increases the stiffness and ultimate failure torque of the construct relative to reconstruction alone. Whether these improved biomechanical properties translate into clinical outcomes remains to be seen.

Other Novel Techniques

A new technique for UCL reconstruction using an adjustable cortical fixation device (ACL TightRope, Arthrex) has been described in which a cortical button and tensioning sutures are used to fix the graft on the ulnar side through a single tunnel. This technique places the graft directly against the ulnar bone with just one tunnel, without the risks of an interference screw. Lynch et al. performed a biomechanical study comparing the adjustable cortical fixation device to a traditional docking technique [23]. There were no differences in joint kinematics between 15° and 75° of flexion, but at 90° the novel device had significantly higher angular displacement. The adjustable cortical fixation device also had inferior failure torque compared to the intact elbow, whereas the docking technique did not differ from the intact elbow in terms of failure torque.

Another new technique for UCL reconstruction is using two linked adjustable cortical fixation devices (GraftLink, Arthrex), which fixes the graft with cortical buttons and self-reinforcing tensioning sutures on both the humeral and ulnar sides. Lynch et al. compared this dual linked cortical fixation device reconstruction technique to the traditional docking technique and found no difference in joint kinematics between the native state and either reconstruction techniques [24]. Although the dual cortical fixation device was less stiff, there was no difference in torque at failure between the docking technique and the dual linked cortical fixation device. As new techniques are described for UCL reconstruction, it is important to rigorously compare their biomechanical properties to those of established clinically successful techniques.

Anatomic Considerations

Regardless of the reconstruction technique that is chosen, a biomechanically sound reconstruction starts with an accurate understanding of the anatomy that is being recreated. Early anatomic studies of the UCL found its insertion on the sublime tubercle to be a relatively small area approximately 5.5 mm distal to the articular surface [25]. However, more recent studies have described a long insertion, extending beyond the sublime tubercle, as far as 24.5 mm distal to the articular surface [26], calling into question the traditional ulnar tunnel placement 5 mm from the joint line in UCL reconstruction. Erickson et al. studied the biomechanics of this broader UCL footprint and found that the distal and middle thirds contributed little to elbow stability [27]. There were no differences in gap resistance at 5 N-m of valgus load between specimens that were intact, those with the distal third of the insertion removed, and those with the distal and middle thirds removed. When the proximal third of the ligament was sectioned, the ligament failed in half of the specimens. Although the UCL insertion may be broader than initially thought, the proximal portion of the insertion is most critical to the biomechanical properties of the ligament. Despite this, however, Dutton et al. did not find differences in valgus stability and ultimate torque failure when they performed UCL reconstruction at various positions along this UCL insertion footprint [28]. They reconstructed the UCL on 18 cadaveric specimens using a standard docking technique. They placed the ulnar tunnel at 5, 10, or 15 mm from the joint line and found no differences in valgus rotation under a 3-N-m stress and no differences in ultimate torque failure. While the most proximal portion of the UCL insertion may be the greatest contributor to stability, reconstruction done up to 15 mm from the joint line appears to provide equivalent biomechanical stability to the elbow and could be useful in revision settings or in the setting of challenging anatomic variations.

Conclusions

Numerous procedures exist for reconstruction of the UCL in overhead-throwing athletes looking to return to a high level of sport. Biomechanical studies show that these reconstruction techniques fall short from restoring native stability to the elbow under valgus load. The classic Jobe and docking techniques appear to come closest to replicating the strength of the native UCL than other techniques. However, there is potential for bone tunnel fracture when using the Jobe technique. Bone tunnel fracture appears to be less common with the docking technique, but failure can occur at the suture. Conclusive biomechanical data are not yet available on the newer techniques. Results with interference screw fixation are equivocal in the studies reviewed. The suture anchor and adjustable cortical fixation device techniques have shown some positive results in the laboratory. Reinforcement of reconstruction or repair techniques with a high-strength suture augmentation technique may provide a biomechanical profile more similar to the native ligament, but further studies are needed.

References

1. Feltner ME, Dapena J. Dynamics of the shoulder and elbow joints of the throwing arm of the baseball pitch. Int J Sports Biomech. 1989;5:420–50.
2. Fleisig GS, Andrews JR, Dillman CJ, Escamilla RF. Kinetics of baseball pitching with implications about injury mechanisms. Am J Sports Med. 1995;23:233–9.
3. Jobe FW, Stark H, Lombardo SJ. Reconstruction of the ulnar collateral ligament in athletes. J Bone Joint Surg Am. 1986;68:1158–63.
4. Smith GR, Altchek DW, Pagnani MJ, Keeley JR. A muscle-splitting approach to the ulnar collateral ligament of the elbow. Neuroanatomy and operative technique. Am J Sports Med. 1996;24:575–80.
5. Mullen DJ, Goradia VK, Parks BG, Matthews LS. A biomechanical study of stability of the elbow to valgus stress before and after reconstruction of the medial collateral ligament. J Shoulder Elb Surg. 2002;11:259–64.
6. Ciccotti MG, Siegler S, Kuri JA, Thinnes JH, Murphy DJ. Comparison of the biomechanical profile of the

intact ulnar collateral ligament with the modified Jobe and the docking reconstructed elbow: an in vitro study. Am J Sports Med. 2009;37:974–81.
7. Rohrbough JT, Altchek DW, Hyman J, Williams RJ III, Botts JD. Medial collateral ligament reconstruction of the elbow using the docking technique. Am J Sports Med. 2002;30:541–8.
8. Bowers AL, Dines JS, Dines DM, Altchek DW. Elbow medial ulnar collateral ligament reconstruction: clinical relevance and the docking technique. J Shoulder Elb Surg. 2010;19:110–7.
9. Cohen SB, Woods DP, Siegler S, Dodson CC, Namani R, Ciccotti MG. Biomechanical comparison of graft fixation at 30 degrees and 90 degrees of elbow flexion for ulnar collateral ligament reconstruction by the docking technique. J Shoulder Elb Surg. 2015;24(2):265–72.
10. Armstrong AD, Dunning CE, Ferreira LM, Faber KJ, Johnson JA, King GJ. A biomechanical comparison of four reconstruction techniques for the medial collateral ligament-deficient elbow. J Shoulder Elb Surg. 2005;14:207–15.
11. Hurbanek JG, Anderson K, Crabtree S, Karnes GJ. Biomechanical comparison of the docking technique with and without humeral bioabsorbable interference screw fixation. Am J Sports Med. 2009;37:526–33.
12. Bernas GA, Ruberte Thiele RA, Kinnaman KA, Hughes RE, Miller BS, Carpenter JE. Defining safe rehabilitation for ulnar collateral ligament reconstruction of the elbow: a biomechanical study. Am J Sports Med. 2009;37(12):2392–400.
13. Langer P, Fadale P, Hulstyn M. Evolution of the treatment options of ulnar collateral ligament injuries of the elbow. Br J Sports Med. 2006;40:499–506.
14. Hechtman KS, Tjin ATE, Zvijac JE, Uribe JW, Latta LL. Biomechanics of a less invasive procedure for reconstruction of the ulnar collateral ligament of the elbow. Am J Sports Med. 1998;26:620–4.
15. Williams RJ III, Urquhart ER, Altchek DW. Medial collateral ligament tears in the throwing athlete. Instr Course Lect. 2004;53:579–86.
16. Ahmad CS, Lee TQ, Elattrache NS. Biomechanical evaluation of a new ulnar collateral ligament reconstruction technique with interference screw fixation. Am J Sports Med. 2003;31:332–7.
17. McAdams TR, Lee AT, Centeno J, Giori NJ, Lindsey DP. Two ulnar collateral ligament reconstruction methods: the docking technique versus bioabsorbable interference screw fixation – a biomechanical evaluation with cyclic loading. J Shoulder Elb Surg. 2007;16:224–8.
18. Large TM, Coley ER, Peindl RD, Fleischli JE. A biomechanical comparison of 2 ulnar collateral ligament reconstruction techniques. Arthroscopy. 2007;23:141–50.
19. Dugas JR, Walters BL, Beason DP, Fleisig GS, Chronister JE. Biomechanical comparison of ulnar collateral ligament repair with internal bracing versus modified Jobe reconstruction. Am J Sports Med. 2016;44(3):735–41.
20. Bodendorfer BM, Looney AM, Lipkin SL, et al. Biomechanical comparison of ulnar collateral ligament reconstruction with the docking technique versus repair with internal bracing. Am J Sports Med. 2018;46(14):3495–501.
21. Walters BL, Cain EL, Emblom BA, Frantz JT, Dugas JR. Ulnar collateral ligament repair with internal brace augmentation: a novel UCL repair technique in the young adolescent athlete. Orthop J Sports Med. 2016;4:1.
22. Bernholt DL, Lake SP, Castile RM, Papangelou C, Hauck O, Smith MV. Biomechanical comparison of docking ulnar collateral ligament reconstruction with and without an internal brace. J Shoulder Elb Surg. 2019;28(11):2247–52.
23. Lynch JL, Maerz T, Kurdziel MD, Davidson AA, Baker KC, Anderson K. Biomechanical evaluation of the TightRope versus traditional docking ulnar collateral ligament reconstruction technique: kinematic and failure testing. Am J Sports Med. 2013;41(5):1165–73.
24. Lynch JL, Pifer MA, Maerz T, et al. The GraftLink ulnar collateral ligament reconstruction: biomechanical comparison with the docking technique in both kinematics and failure tests. Am J Sports Med. 2013;41(10):2278–87.
25. Dugas JR, Ostrander RV, Cain EL, Kingsley D, Andrews JR. Anatomy of the anterior bundle of the ulnar collateral ligament. J Shoulder Elb Surg. 2007;16(5):657–60.
26. Farrow LD, Mahoney AJ, Stefancin JJ, Taljanovic MS, Sheppard JE, Schickendantz MS. Quantitative analysis of the medial ulnar collateral ligament ulnar footprint and its relationship to the ulnar sublime tubercle. Am J Sports Med. 2011;39(9):1936–41.
27. Erickson BJ, Fu M, Meyers K, et al. The middle and distal aspects of the ulnar footprint of the medial ulnar collateral ligament of the elbow do not provide significant resistance to valgus stress: a biomechanical study. Orthop J Sports Med. 2019;7(2):2325967118825294.
28. Dutton PH, Banffy MB, Nelson TJ, Metzger MF. Anatomic and biomechanical evaluation of ulnar tunnel position in medial ulnar collateral ligament reconstruction. Am J Sports Med. 2019;47(14):3491–7.

Figure of 8 Technique and Outcomes

21

Tony Wanich, Joseph H. Choi, and Lewis A. Yocum

Introduction

The figure of 8 technique developed by Dr. Frank Jobe was the first described technique for ulnar collateral ligament (UCL) reconstruction [1]. It was this technique that was first performed on Tommy John whose name has become synonymous with this procedure. While the originally described technique has undergone several evolutions and modifications, the fundamental basis of the reconstruction remains the same.

The figure of 8 reconstruction takes its name from the configuration of the reconstructed ligament which loops through drill holes in the ulna and humerus to create a figure of 8. Dr. Jobe's original technique for UCL reconstruction utilized release of the flexor-pronator mass during the surgical approach. Additionally, the ulnar nerve was mobilized to further aid in visualization. While the initial reconstruction performed by Dr. Jobe did not include transposition of the ulnar nerve, all other cases in his initial report had routine ulnar nerve transposition as part of the procedure. The figure of 8 reconstruction involves creation of two drill holes in the ulna and three drill holes in the humerus. The ulnar drill holes were placed anterior and posterior to the sublime tubercle, while the drill holes in the humerus were located at the UCL insertion on the medial epicondyle with exit holes placed on the posterior aspect of the distal humerus within the ulnar groove.

Due to the high rate of complications, the original technique as described by Dr. Jobe has been subsequently modified. In his original report, Dr. Jobe reported a 31% incidence of ulnar nerve problems following surgery. His subsequent report involving a larger series of patients still demonstrated a 21% incidence of ulnar nerve problems [2]. This high rate of ulnar nerve issues prompted the first significant evolution in this technique, namely the muscle splitting approach.

Dr. Jobe first described the muscle splitting approach as a way to reduce ulnar nerve complications. Smith et al. mapped out the neuroanatomy of the ulnar nerve during a muscle splitting approach, helping to establish a safe zone [3].

The modified Jobe technique is the senior author's preferred method for reconstruction of the UCL [4]. The primary modification involves the use of the muscle splitting approach, which

Supplementary Information The online version of this chapter (https://doi.org/10.1007/978-3-030-69567-5_21) contains supplementary material, which is available to authorized users.

T. Wanich (✉)
High Mountain Orthopedics, Wayne, NJ, USA
e-mail: drwanich@highmountainorthopedics.com

J. H. Choi
Orthopaedic Surgery, Seton Hall Orthopedics, Paterson, NJ, USA

L. A. Yocum
Kerlan-Jobe Orthopaedic Clinic, Los Angeles, CA, USA

J. S. Dines et al. (eds.), *Elbow Ulnar Collateral Ligament Injury*,
https://doi.org/10.1007/978-3-030-69567-5_21

obviates the need for routine ulnar nerve transposition and changes the humeral tunnel placement from the posterosuperior aspect of the medial epicondyle to the anterosuperior aspect.

Modified Jobe Technique

The procedure is begun with the patient placed supine with the arm abducted on an arm board or hand table. Following induction of general anesthesia, the elbow is tested for range of motion, carrying angle and instability, while palpating the ulnar nerve to make sure it is posterior to the medial epicondyle and to rule out subluxation.

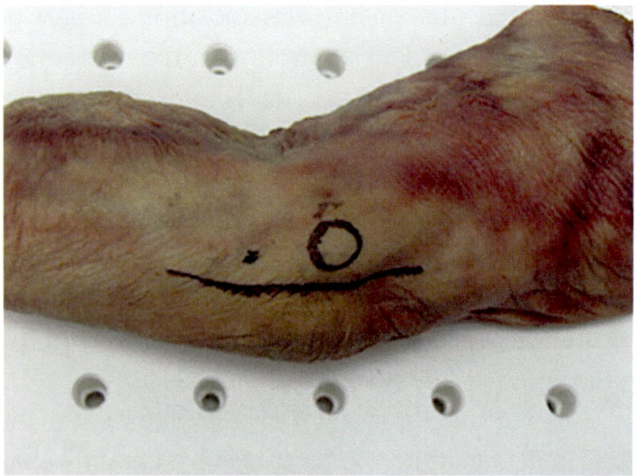

Fig. 21.1 Medial view of the arm with the medial epicondyle, sublime tubercle, and course of the ulnar nerve outlined

A marking pen is used to outline the medial epicondyle, the sublime tubercle, and the course of the ulnar nerve (Fig. 21.1). Following inflation of a nonsterile tourniquet to 250 mmHg, a 10-cm incision is made, centered over the medial epicondyle and just posterior to the sublime tubercle. After hemostasis is achieved by cauterizing superficial vessels, blunt dissection is carefully performed in order to visualize and protect the medial antebrachial cutaneous nerve and its branches. The medial antebrachial cutaneous nerve and its branches have been shown to cross the surgical incision at an average of 3.1 cm distal to the medial epicondyle (Fig. 21.2) [5]. Once the nerve is identified, it is mobilized, protected, and retracted with a vessel loop.

The fascia overlying the flexor-pronator musculature is subsequently visualized (Fig. 21.3). The incision for the muscle split is through the posterior one-third of the common flexor-pronator mass within the anterior fibers of the flexor carpi ulnaris muscle. This is demarcated by a dense raphe in the fascia overlying the flexor carpi ulnaris and palmaris longus muscles superficially and the flexor carpi ulnaris and flexor digitorum superficialis muscles deeper within the internervous plane, as defined by Smith et al. [3].

An incision is made in line with the fibers of the fascial raphe of the flexor carpi ulnaris muscle extending from the medial epicondyle to approximately 1 cm distal to the sublime tubercle. The fascial raphe is more readily identified at

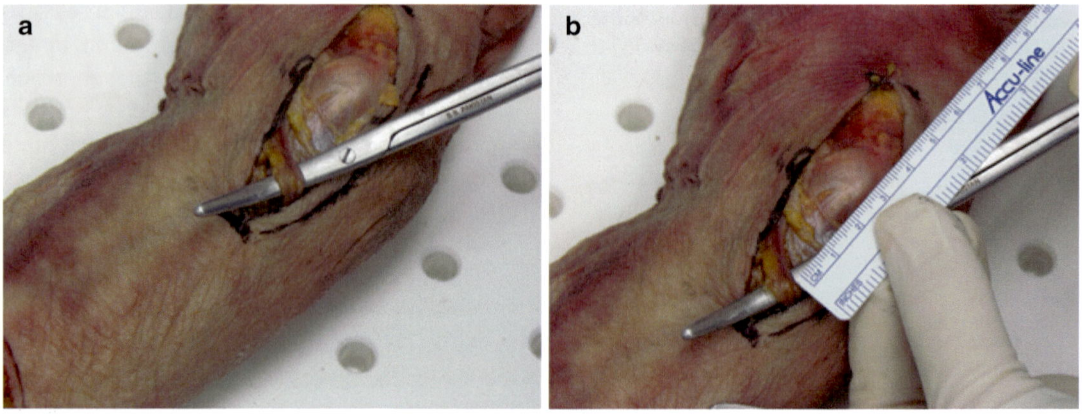

Fig. 21.2 (**a**) Medial antebrachial cutaneous nerve identified. (**b**) Medial antebrachial cutaneous nerve and branches have been shown to cross the incision at approximately 3.1 cm distal to the medial epicondyle

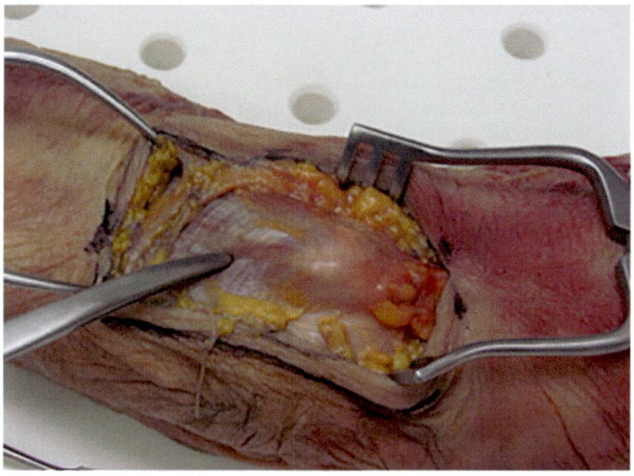

Fig. 21.3 Fascia overlying the flexor-pronator musculature

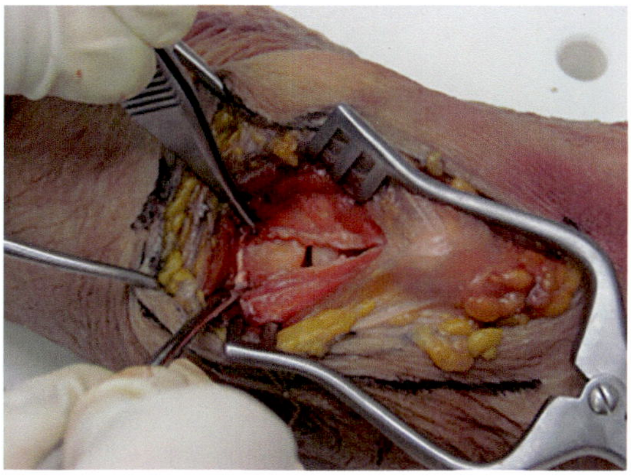

Fig. 21.5 The ulnohumeral articulation visualized via an incision through the UCL and capsule

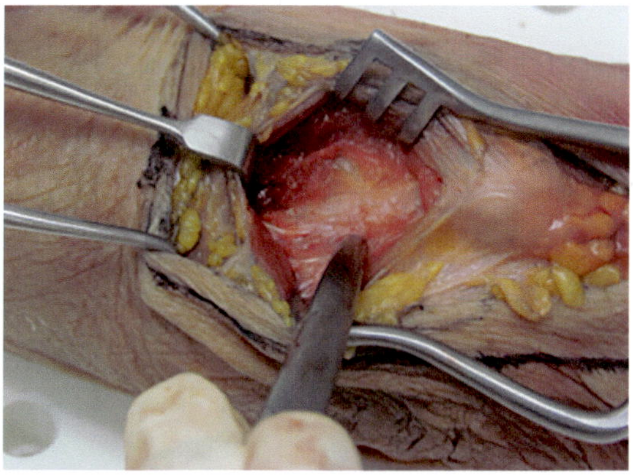

Fig. 21.4 The UCL and capsule

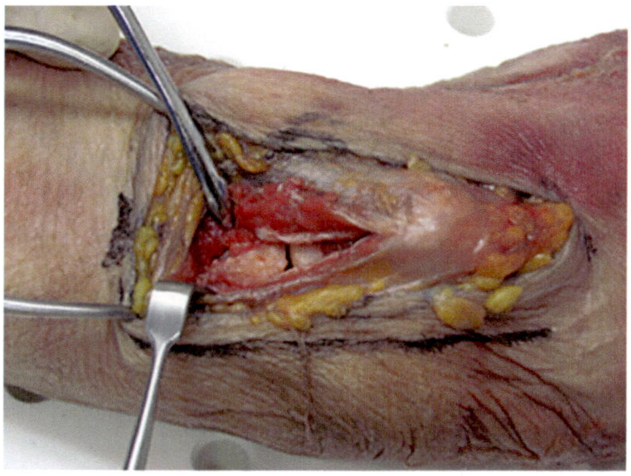

Fig. 21.6 Anterior and posterior portions of the split UCL elevated allowing visualization of the UCL attachments on the sublime tubercle and medial epicondyle

the distal portion of the incision as the flexor-pronator musculature separates and becomes more easily defined. In cases where the fascial raphe is not visualized, the incision is made in the anterior aspect of the flexor carpi ulnaris.

During the incision, the ulnar nerve is identified by palpation and protected to ensure the dissection does not extend too far posteriorly. The underlying muscle is then split and elevated with a blunt periosteal elevator down to the level of the UCL and capsule (Fig. 21.4). Once the UCL is visualized, a longitudinal incision is made through the UCL and capsule to expose the underlying ulnohumeral articulation (Fig. 21.5). A valgus stress test is performed to confirm instability and insufficiency of the ligament. The anterior and posterior portions of the split UCL are elevated to allow visualization of the attachments of the UCL on the sublime tubercle and the medial epicondyle and are then tagged with a 0 Vicryl stitch (Fig. 21.6).

To expose the anterosuperior aspect of the medial epicondyle, an L-shaped incision is made with a short vertical limb anterior and parallel to the intermuscular septum and a transverse limb in line with the fibers of the flexor-pronator fascia (Fig. 21.7). A blunt periosteal elevator is used to elevate the musculature to expose the anterosuperior aspect of the medial epicondyle. Following the exposure of the sublime tubercle and medial epicondyle, the tunnels can then be created.

The ulnar tunnels are made first using a 3.5-mm drill to create two convergent holes anterior

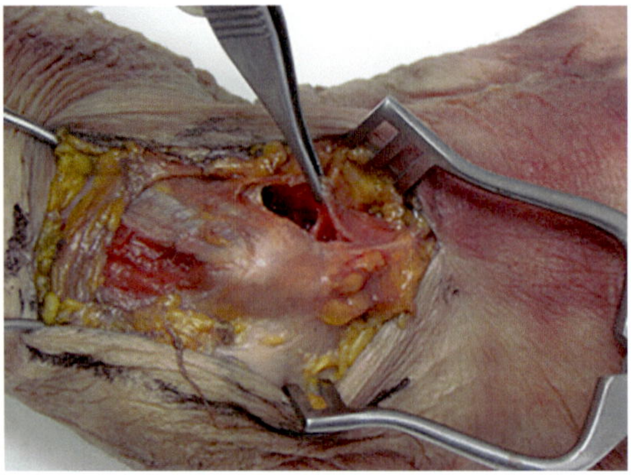

Fig. 21.7 Exposure of the anterosuperior aspect of the medial epicondyle

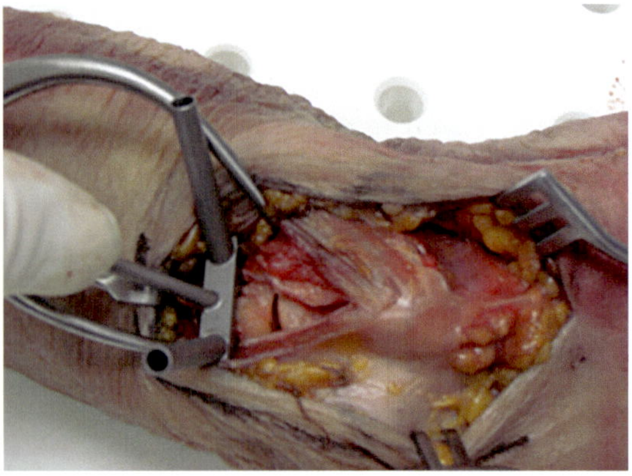

Fig. 21.8 Two convergent ulnar tunnels being created anterior and posterior to the sublime tubercle. Note the posterior hole is slightly proximal with respect to the anterior hole

and posterior to the sublime tubercle, with the posterior hole placed slightly more proximal (Fig. 21.8). It is important to monitor the orientation of drilling to prevent penetration into the ulnohumeral joint, given the proximity of the joint to the bony tunnels. The tunnels are connected with a small curette leaving a 0.5–1 cm bone bridge between the holes.

The insertion of the UCL on the anterior aspect of the medial epicondyle is noted and a 3.5-mm drill is aimed proximally to create a single tunnel directed anterior to the medial intermuscular septum, taking care not to penetrate the superior cortex of the medial epicondyle (Fig. 21.9). The hole is subsequently enlarged

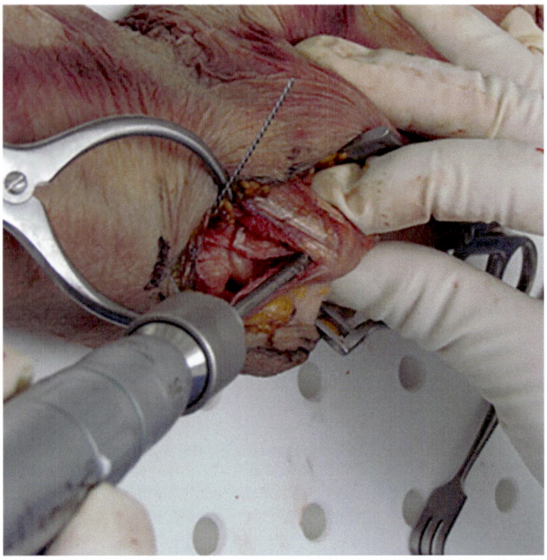

Fig. 21.9 At the native insertion of the UCL on the medial epicondyle, a single tunnel is created directed anterior and medial to the intermuscular septum

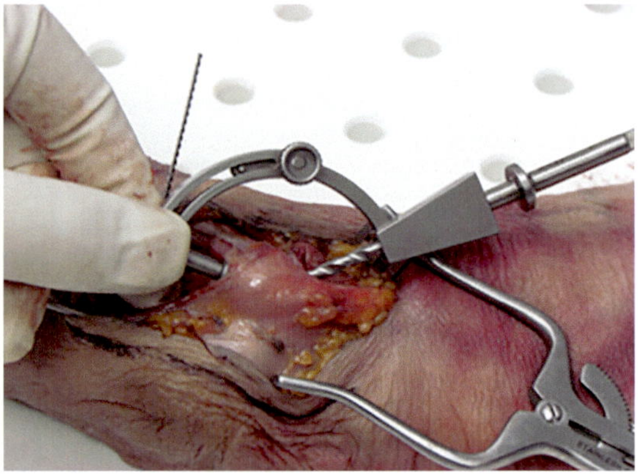

Fig. 21.10 Drill guide used for creating two converging tunnels on the anterosuperior medial epicondyle

with a 4.5-mm drill. A hemostat or curette is inserted into the tunnel to serve as a guide for the creation of the two converging tunnels on the anterosuperior medial epicondyle (Fig. 21.10). The first anterior proximal tunnel is placed slightly anterior to the epicondylar attachment of the intermuscular septum, with the second tunnel placed 1 cm anterior to the first (Fig. 21.11) [6]. The converging humeral tunnels are drilled with a 3.2-mm bit from proximal to distal aiming toward the hemostat placed in the main humeral

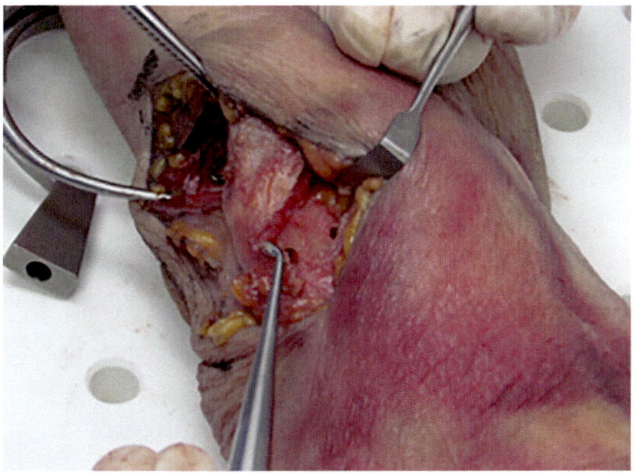

Fig. 21.11 Two converging tunnels on the anterosuperior medial epicondyle. The anterior proximal tunnel is placed slightly anterior to the epicondylar attachment of the intermuscular septum and the second tunnel is 1 cm anterior to the first

tunnel, taking care to ensure a bony bridge of at least 5 mm separates them.

After the tunnels are drilled, the tourniquet is released and the wound is irrigated and hemostasis is achieved prior to graft harvesting. There are a number of potential donor sites for graft harvesting including the palmaris longus, gracilis, toe extensor, plantaris, and the Achilles tendon [4, 7]. The authors' preference is to use the ipsilateral palmaris tendon. It is important during the preoperative assessment to ensure the patient has a palmaris longus. If the palmaris is absent as is the case in 20% of the population, the authors' preferred secondary graft is the contralateral gracilis.

If the palmaris tendon is used, its insertion is palpated at the wrist crease and a 1–2-cm transverse incision is made. Once the tendon is exposed, a hemostat is used to isolate and grasp the tendon while making sure the median nerve is protected. Additional incisions are made every 8 cm along the length of the palmaris until the musculotendinous junction is identified. The use of the hemostat is continued in order to isolate the tendon and protect the nerve. A number 1 Ethibond suture is used to create a locking stitch at the distal end of the tendon prior to releasing its distal insertion. Once the distal end is secured, the proximal end is subsequently released. The graft should be 15–20 cm in length and 5 mm in diameter.

During graft passage, the arm is held between 30 and 40° of flexion with a varus force applied for graft tensioning. A 22-gauge wire is folded in half and twisted on itself to serve as a suture passer to facilitate graft passage through the tunnels. The graft end that is tagged is first passed through the ulnar tunnels from anterior to posterior, along with a suture loop leaving the looped end posteriorly. The tagged end is then pulled through the distal humeral tunnel exiting the anteromedial hole. As the graft is subsequently passed through the anterolateral hole, another suture loop is passed with the looped end, exiting the distal humeral tunnel along with the tagged end of the graft. Once again, the tagged end is then passed through the ulnar tunnel, this time from the posterior to anterior using the suture loop. The free end of the graft is then whipstitched with a number 1 Ethibond suture and passed through the distal humeral hole with the previously passed suture loop.

Tension is applied to the graft while the arm is placed under varus stress and the ulnohumeral joint is visualized to assess adequacy of the reconstruction (Fig. 21.12). A free needle is used to secure the distal end of the graft to the native UCL and the proximal end to the medial intermuscular septum. A 0 Vicryl suture is used to suture the graft to itself to further tighten the construct and minimize the chance of graft slippage. The remnants of the original UCL are sutured over the graft for additional strength. After hemostasis is obtained, the fascia overlying

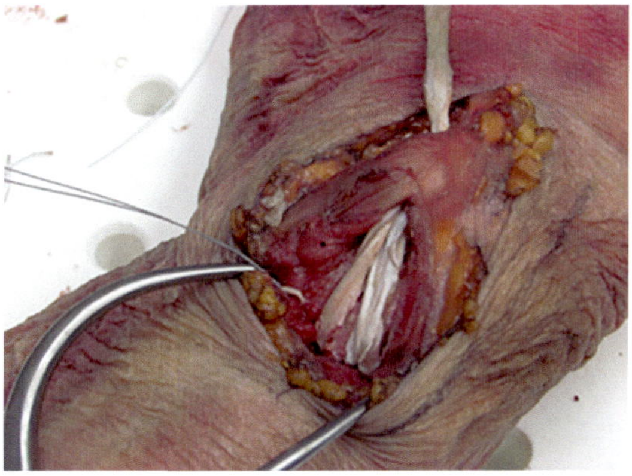

Fig. 21.12 Tension applied to the graft to assess adequacy of the reconstruction

the flexor carpi ulnaris is reapproximated followed by a subcutaneous and subcuticular closure [8]. The elbow is immobilized in a posterior splint with side slabs, to prevent rotation, at 90° of flexion and neutral rotation for 7–10 days.

American Sports Medicine Institute (ASMI) Modification

Dr. Andrews has published the largest series of UCL reconstructions utilizing his modifications to the original Jobe technique [9]. The primary modification involves anterior elevation and retraction of the flexor-pronator mass without release during the surgical approach. In addition, this approach necessitates routine transposition of the ulnar nerve, which is done subcutaneously versus submuscularly as described by Dr. Jobe [1]. The drill holes are placed in the same position as Dr. Jobe's original technique with the proximal humeral tunnels exiting the posterior cortex.

Postoperative Rehabilitation

0–10 days:

- Splint is worn for 7–10 days with the elbow in 90° flexion.
- No valgus stress to the elbow.
- Wrist circles.
- Ball/putty squeeze.

10–14 days:

- Full active forearm pronation and supination range of motion.
- Full active wrist radial and ulnar deviation range of motion. Gentle stretching of wrist and fingers is okay.
- Active and active assistive wrist flexion and extension range of motion exercises.
- Instruct a family member/caregiver in active and active assistive exercises for the shoulder.

2–4 weeks (bracing is optional at the surgeons' discretion):

- Active range of motion (ROM) 30–100° in week 2.
- Advance to 15–110° in week 3.
- Advance to 10–120° in week 4.
- Two weeks postoperation, begin a lower extremity conditioning (bike, no running for first 2 months) and core stabilization program after incision is closed (starting earlier, you run the risk of getting perspiration in or on the wound, increasing the risk of infection).
- Avoid forced full extension or flexion for the first month.
- Continue range of motion for forearm, wrist, and shoulder as needed.
- Scapular stabilizing exercises.
- Week 4 shoulder/wrist/elbow isometrics.

4–6 weeks:

- Should have full motion.
- Light rotator cuff strengthening avoiding valgus stress.
- In week 5, begin light resistance exercises including 1 lb wrist curls, extension/pronation/supination, elbow flexion, and extension.
- Begin active assistive range of motion (AAROM) to full flexion, but *do not force flexion.*
- Continue exercises in phase I.

6–8 weeks:

- Athlete should obtain full range of motion at elbow, wrist, forearm, and shoulder joints.
- Progressive elbow strengthening exercises.
- Progressive shoulder internal/external rotation strengthening.
- Add throwers ten program.

2–4 months:

- Continue active, resistive exercises for the entire extremity, including the rotator cuff.
- Continue lower body and trunk conditioning program.
- Continue joint mobilization as needed.
- Maintain full elbow range of motion.

4.5–5 months:

- If there is no swelling and the athlete has full, pain-free elbow range of motion, the athlete may start the throwing program and/or agilities specific to their sport in weeks 18–20.

Table 21.1 UCL figure of 8 reconstruction outcomes

Author	Flexor-pronator mass approach	Number of patients	Ulnar nerve transposition	Percent excellent results on Conway scale (%)	Rate of ulnar nerve complications (%)
Jobe et al. [1]	Detached	16	Submuscular	63	31
Conway et al. [2]	Detached	71	Submuscular	68	21
Andrews and Timmerman [9]	Elevated and retracted	12	Subcutaneous	78	11
Azar et al. [7]	Elevated and retracted	78	Subcutaneous	81	I
Thompson et al. [4]	Split	83	Not performed	82	5
Cain et al. [12]	Elevated and retracted	743	Subcutaneous	83	7
Petty et al. [13]	Elevated and retracted	27	Subcutaneous	74	16

5–12 months:

- Initiation and progression of an interval throwing program with pitching from a mound at 70% of maximum ability by month 8 or 9.

12 months:

- If the athlete has full, pain-free elbow and shoulder range of motion with full strength, the athlete may begin throwing in competition.

Outcomes

In his original series, Dr. Jobe reported 63% of patients returned to play at the same level with an overall complication rate of 31% [1]. As the figure of 8 technique has evolved, so have the outcomes with regard to lower complications and improved rate of return to play. Using a modified Jobe technique, the senior author demonstrated 82% excellent results based on the modified Conway scale with a 5% rate of transient ulnar nerve symptoms [4]. When those with prior surgery were excluded, the rate of excellent results jumped to 92%. Other authors have demonstrated similar findings as outlined in Table 21.1 below as adapted from Jones et al. and Vitale et al. [10–13].

The modified Jobe technique and the docking technique are the two most common techniques for UCL reconstruction with a trend toward increased use of the docking technique in recent studies, although outcomes have been similar between both groups [14]. In a single surgeon study of 25 patients, there was no difference in KJOC scores, need for additional surgery, or return to play between the modified Jobe and docking technique at 7-year follow-up [15].

References

1. Jobe FW, Stark H, Lombardo SJ. Reconstruction of the ulnar collateral ligament in athletes. J Bone Joint Surg Am. 1986;68(8):1158–63.
2. Conway JE, Jobe FW, Glousman RE, Pink M. Medial instability of the elbow in throwing athletes. Treatment by repair or reconstruction of the ulnar collateral ligament. J Bone Joint Surg Am. 1992;74(1):67–83.
3. Smith GR, Altchek DW, Pagnani MJ, Keeley JR. A muscle-splitting approach to the ulnar collateral ligament of the elbow. Neuroanatomy and operative technique. Am J Sports Med. 1996;24(5):575–80.
4. Thompson WH, Jobe FW, Yocum LA, Pink MM. Ulnar collateral ligament reconstruction in athletes: muscle-splitting approach without transposition of the ulnar nerve. J Shoulder Elb Surg. 2001;10(2):152–7.
5. Lowe JB 3rd, Maggi SP, Mackinnon SE. The position of crossing branches of the medial antebrachial cutaneous nerve during cubital tunnel surgery in humans. Plast Reconstr Surg. 2004;114(3):692–6.
6. Greiwe RM, Bjerke-Kroll B, Ahmad CS. Medial collateral ligament reconstruction. Oper Tech Orthop. 2009;19(4):243–50.
7. Azar FM, Andrews JR, Wilk KE, Groh D. Operative treatment of ulnar collateral ligament injuries of the elbow in athletes. Am J Sports Med. 2000;28(1):16–23.

8. Olsen SJ 2nd, et al. Risk factors for shoulder and elbow injuries in adolescent baseball pitchers. Am J Sports Med. 2006;34(6):905–12.
9. Andrews JR, Timmerman LA. Outcome of elbow surgery in professional baseball players. Am J Sports Med. 1995;23(4):407–13.
10. Jones KJ, Osbahr DC, Schrumpf MA, Dines JS, Altchek DW. Ulnar collateral ligament reconstruction in throwing athletes: a review of current concepts. AAOS exhibit selection. J Bone Joint Surg Am. 2012;94(8):e49.
11. Vitale MA, Ahmad CS. The outcome of elbow ulnar collateral ligament reconstruction in overhead athletes: a systematic review. Am J Sports Med. 2008;36(6):1193–205.
12. Cain EL Jr, Andrews JR, Dugas JR, Wilk KE, McMichael CS, Walter JC 2nd, et al. Outcome of ulnar collateral ligament reconstruction of the elbow in 1281 athletes: results in 743 athletes with minimum 2-year follow-up. Am J Sports Med. 2010;38(12):2426–34.
13. Petty DH, Andrews JR, Fleisig GS, Cain EL. Ulnar collateral ligament reconstruction in high school baseball players: clinical results and injury risk factors. Am J Sports Med. 2004;32(5):1158–64.
14. Griffith TB, Ahmad CS, Gorroochurn P, D'Angelo J, Ciccotti MG, Dines JS, Altchek DW, Camp CL. Comparison of outcomes based on graft type and tunnel configuration for primary ulnar collateral ligament reconstruction in professional baseball pitchers. Am J Sports Med. 2019;47(5):1103–10. https://doi.org/10.1177/0363546519831705. Epub 2019 Mar 21. PMID: 30896975.
15. Arner JW, Chang ES, Bayer S, Bradley JP. Direct comparison of modified jobe and docking ulnar collateral ligament reconstruction at midterm follow-up. Am J Sports Med. 2019;47(1):144–50. https://doi.org/10.1177/0363546518812421. Epub 2018 Nov 30. PMID: 30500269

Ulnar Collateral Ligament Reconstruction: Docking Technique

22

Joshua S. Dines, Alexandra D. Berger, Jonathan S. Yu, Brittany Dowling, and David W. Altchek

Introduction

Prior to Jobe's description of a reconstruction technique for ulnar collateral ligament (UCL) insufficiency, the injury was career ending [1]. Despite successful results in about 70% of cases, concerns with elevation of the flexor-pronator mass, ulnar nerve complications, and relatively large bone tunnels in the medial epicondyle of the humerus led to modifications to Jobe's technique. One of the most novel modifications was the "docking technique" [2]. Differences included (1) arthroscopic evaluation and management, when indicated, of concomitant intra-articular pathology, (2) maintenance of the ulnar nerve in situ unless symptoms specifically indicate transposition, (3) use of a muscle-splitting approach through the flexor mass, and (4) "docking" of the graft into a humeral socket. Ulnar preparation remained the same as the originally described Jobe. These modifications facilitated improved graft tensioning while minimizing the number of large tunnels drilled in the relatively small medial epicondyle. The intraoperative morbidity was minimized by the muscle-splitting approach and the reservation of ulnar nerve transposition only when indicated based on preoperative exam. This is our preferred technique for UCL reconstruction.

Supplementary Information The online version of this chapter (https://doi.org/10.1007/978-3-030-69567-5_22) contains supplementary material, which is available to authorized users.

J. S. Dines (✉)
Sports Medicine and Shoulder Service, Sports Medicine Institute, Hospital for Special Surgery, New York, NY, USA

A. D. Berger
University of Miami, Jupiter, FL, USA

J. S. Yu
Hospital for Special Surgery, New York, NY, USA

B. Dowling
Sports Performance Center, Midwest Orthopaedics at Rush, Chicago, IL, USA

D. W. Altchek
Sports Medicine and Shoulder Service, Hospital for Special Surgery, New York, NY, USA

Preoperative Considerations

History

Athletes with injury to their UCL will complain of medial-sided elbow pain. With regard to baseball players, the pain typically occurs during the late cocking and early acceleration phases of throwing. Occasionally, the injury will be acute as evidenced by a pop while throwing, but more commonly it is a chronic or acute-on-chronic scenario. In these cases, the athletes may report decreased pitch velocity or control, and they may find it difficult to warm up. It is important to ask about ulnar nerve symptoms, as these are commonly associated with UCL tears. Transient

J. S. Dines et al. (eds.), *Elbow Ulnar Collateral Ligament Injury*, https://doi.org/10.1007/978-3-030-69567-5_22

ulnar paresthesias that occur during throwing are likely due to the valgus instability. These typically resolve after reconstruction of the ligament. More persistent sensory symptoms, or motor symptoms, indicate intrinsic pathology to the nerve. These cases require transposition at the time of UCL reconstruction. Mechanical symptoms such as catching or locking may be due to posteromedial olecranon osteophytes and/or loose bodies. It is important to realize that all medial-sided elbow pain is not UCL insufficiency. A thorough differential diagnosis includes: flexor-pronator tendonosis, ulnar neuritis, stress fractures of the olecranon or ulna, and posteromedial osteophytes.

Physical Examination

A thorough physical exam of an athlete with elbow pain begins with an assessment of the proximal components of the kinetic chain, including the shoulder, scapula, core, and lower extremities, as injuries to these areas can lead to changes in throwing biomechanics and subsequent elbow injury. The medial and lateral recesses should be performed to detect the presence of an effusion. Patients will often have tenderness along the course of the ligament. Focal tenderness in the area of the flexor-pronator mass or various bony landmarks, including the posterior olecranon or radial head, may signify associated pathology. A positive compression test or positive Tinel's sign at the cubital tunnel may suggest the presence of ulnar neuropathy.

UCL competency is assessed with several specific physical examination maneuvers. The valgus stress test is performed with the elbow flexed at 30° and the forearm pronated. A valgus stress is applied to detect any widening at the ulnohumeral joint. Even in the absence of frank instability, some patients will complain of pain with this maneuver. The moving valgus stress test, as described by O'Driscoll, is extremely sensitive for UCL tears [3]. The patient is seated upright with the arm placed in the abducted and externally rotated position to simulate the throwing position. A valgus stress is applied to the elbow, which is ranged quickly from full flexion to extension. The maneuver is designed to simulate the valgus forces experienced during the overhead throw. In a positive test, a patient complains of pain from 70 to 120° of flexion arc. Despite O'Driscoll's reporting 100% sensitivity, in our experience, even in patients with UCL tears, this test is often dependent on when the player last threw. Occasionally, players with UCL insufficiency who have been resting for weeks can have a negative moving valgus stress test, whereas those with tears that threw within the few days prior to being examined will almost always have a positive test.

Imaging

Imaging evaluation includes standard anteroposterior (AP) and lateral radiographs of the elbow. With chronic valgus loading of the UCL, varying degrees of ligamentous ossification may be observed. At our institution, we routinely use noncontrast magnetic resonance imaging (MRI) to diagnose UCL pathology (Fig. 22.1). It can also help identify other signs of valgus extension overload. Reported sensitivity for noncontrast

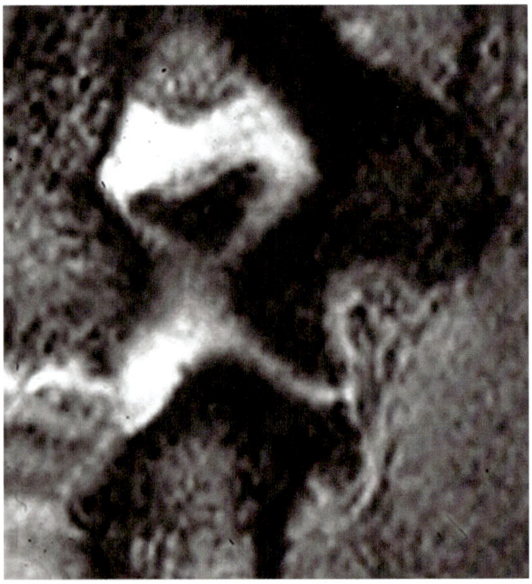

Fig. 22.1 Coronal MRI showing a complete tear of the UCL

MRI approaches 75% and specificity has been reported to be 100% for UCL tears.

Indications and Contraindications

We reserve ligament reconstruction for athletes with medial-sided elbow pain consistent with UCL insufficiency who have failed conservative treatment. Additionally, they must be willing to be compliant with the year-long rehabilitation process typically required after reconstruction.

In contrast to the original description of the docking technique, in which elbow arthroscopy was routinely performed in all elbows prior to UCL reconstruction, we only perform arthroscopy on patients with preoperative physical exam or imaging findings consistent with valgus extension overload.

Ulnar nerve transposition is indicated for athletes with motor changes due to ulnar nerve pathology or persistent sensory deficits. We prefer to use an anterior subcutaneous ulnar nerve transposition technique.

Preoperatively, we identify the source of our graft for ligament reconstruction. Gracilis or palmaris grafts are our preferred choices.

UCL reconstruction is contraindicated in patients unwilling to go through the prolonged postoperative rehabilitation course. Additionally, if the athlete does not have the opportunity to play baseball again, the surgery is likely unnecessary. An example of this would be the high school athlete who is not talented enough to play in college. Clearly, active infection is a contraindication.

Surgical Technique

Anesthesia and Positioning

The procedure is performed under regional anesthesia with the patient supine and the injured arm on an arm board. We apply a nonsterile tourniquet to the upper arm, and the arm is prepped and draped sterilely. If arthroscopy is indicated, the arm is placed in a Spyder arm holder, and the arthroscopy is performed with the patient supine.

Surgical Landmarks/Incisions

At this point, the previously determined graft is harvested. If the Palmaris longus tendon is to be used, we make a small transverse incision just proximal to the wrist flexor crease. A no. 1 braided, nonabsorbable suture is placed in a Krackow fashion in the tendon prior to utilizing a tendon stripper to harvest the graft. We then exsanguinate the arm and inflate the tourniquet. A medial incision starting 1 cm proximal to the medial epicondyle extending distally over the UCL to a point about 2 cm past the sublime tubercle is made (Fig. 22.2).

A muscle-splitting approach through the posterior third of the common flexor mass within the anterior fibers of the flexor carpi ulnaris is used. A submuscular dissection is used to expose the anterior bundle of the ligament. The joint is exposed by incising the native ligament in line with its fibers (Fig. 22.3). UCL laxity can be confirmed by joint surface separation of 3 mm or more with the application of a valgus stress. We place a 2–0 Vicryl suture on each side of the ligament to be used for repair later in the case.

Next, we turn our attention to the creation of the ulnar tunnel. Burr holes are made anteriorly and posteriorly on the sublime tubercle using a 3.5-mm burr taking care to maintain at least a 1-cm bone bridge between the holes. The tunnel is created by connecting the holes with a curved

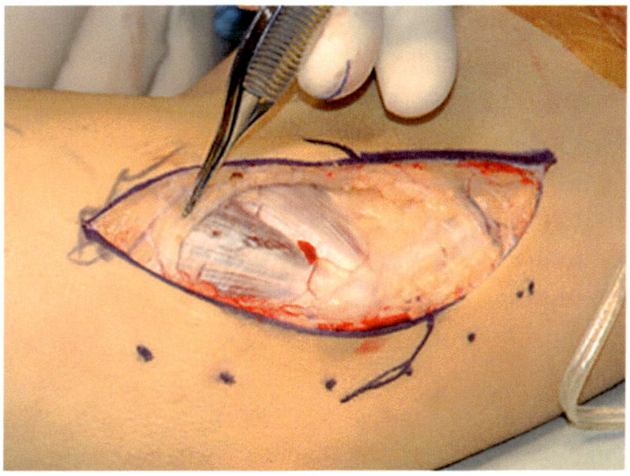

Fig. 22.2 Medially based incision beginning just proximal to the medial epicondyle and extending distally past the sublime tubercle

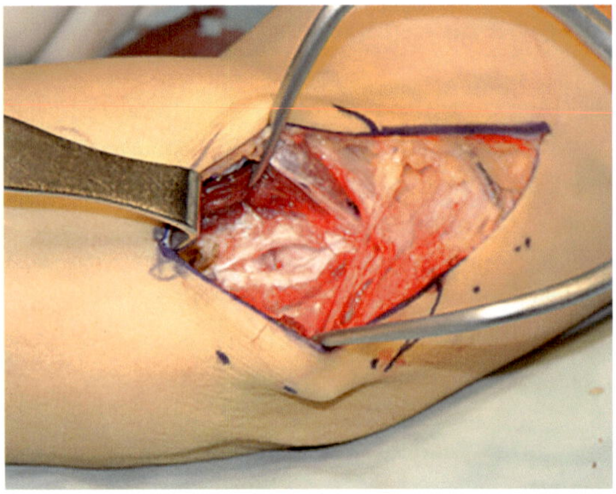

Fig. 22.3 Native ligament exposed through a muscle-splitting approach, which is then incised in line with its fibers

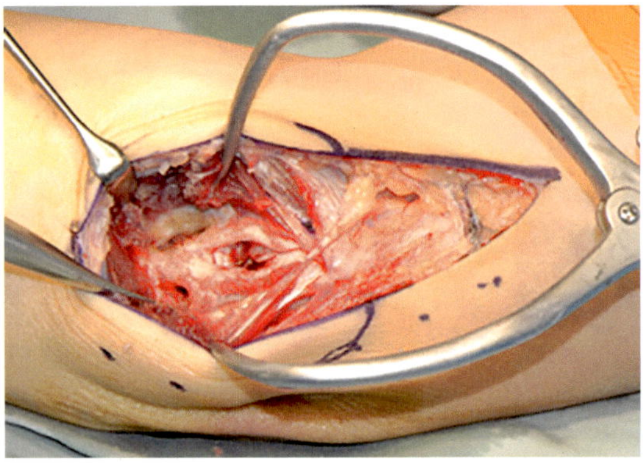

Fig. 22.4 Ulnar tunnel created in the sublime tubercle

curette (Fig. 22.4). A shuttling suture is placed through the tunnel and clamped for later use. If at any time during the approach or drilling of burr holes, the ulnar nerve cannot be safely protected, it should be transposed.

On the humeral side, a 4-mm burr is used to create the humeral tunnel in the origin of the UCL on the anterior-distal aspect of the medial epicondyle (Fig. 22.5). Care should be taken to avoid being too shallow in the epicondyle, leaving only a thin roof of bone over the graft. The tunnel is drilled longitudinally along the axis of the medial epicondyle to a depth of 15 mm. Two connecting puncture holes are made with a dental burr. These exit punctures should be located about 10 mm apart on the anterior surface of the epicondyle. Shuttling sutures are then brought

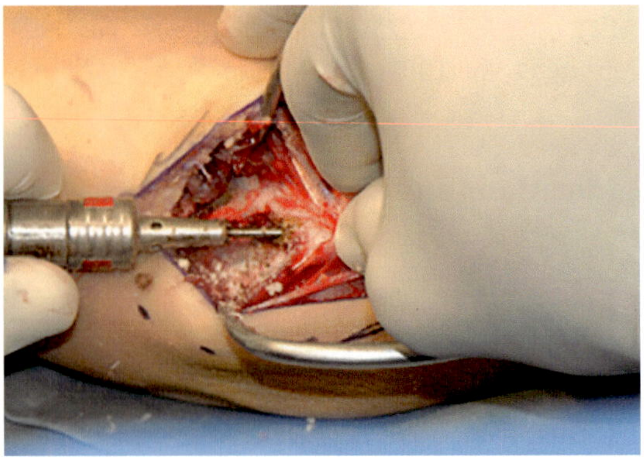

Fig. 22.5 Humeral socket drilled to a depth of about 15 mm in the medial epicondyle

through the humeral tunnel out of each exit puncture and clamped for later use.

The graft is shuttled through the ulnar tunnel. The native ligament is repaired using the previously placed sutures while the elbow is flexed 30° with the forearm supinated while a varus stress is applied. The posterior limb of graft is then shuttled into the medial epicondylar tunnel, and the grasping suture is pulled through the inferior exit portal. Application of tension through the grasping suture keeps this limb of graft "docked" in the humeral tunnel. The elbow is again reduced with a varus force and the forearm supinated for cycling and tensioning of the graft. The anterior graft limb is then positioned next to the humeral tunnel to estimate the needed length (Fig. 22.6). A nonabsorbable suture is passed in a Krackow fashion for the estimated length to be positioned in the tunnel. With tension maintained on the posterior limb, and the elbow reduced with varus and supination, the anterior limb suture is shuttled through the tunnel and out the superior exit portal. Tension on the Krackow docks the anterior limb adjacent to the posterior within the humeral tunnel. Final graft tensioning is verified, and the grasping sutures are tied over a bone bridge (Fig. 22.7).

The tourniquet is deflated, and hemostasis is achieved. The fascia of the muscle splitting approach is reapproximated. The wound is closed in layers, and the patient is placed in a posterior splint with the elbow flexed about 50° and the forearm supinated to reduce the joint.

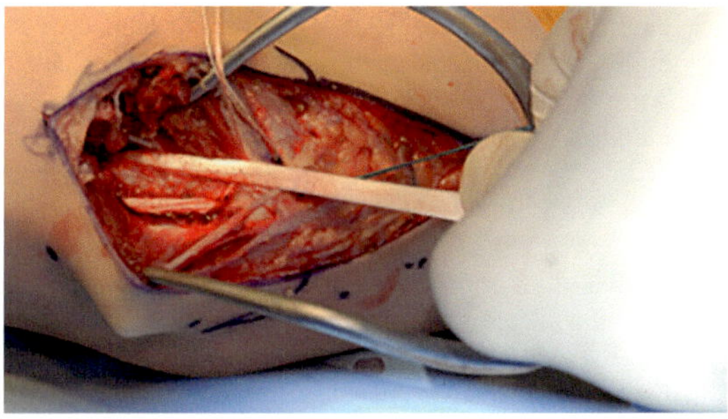

Fig. 22.6 With posterior limb of graft docked, the amount of graft needed for anterior limb is estimated

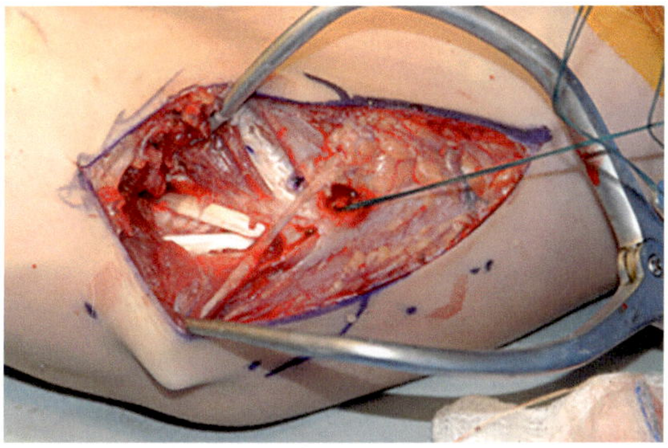

Fig. 22.7 Final graft configuration

Postoperative Protocol

Patients are switched to a hinged elbow brace at 1 week postoperatively. Because the anterior and posterior bands of the reconstructed ligament are not isometric, bracing is used to prevent excessive strain on the graft at extremes of range of motion. Motion is allowed from 60 to 100° and it is advanced by about 15° per week. The goal is a full range of motion by 6–8 weeks after surgery at which point the use of the brace is discontinued. Physical therapy is instituted to work on rotator cuff, forearm, core, and lower extremity strengthening. Any residual loss of elbow motion is addressed. Most baseball players start an interval throwing program at about 4 months after surgery and progress to throwing off a mound at about 8 months. Return to competitive pitching is allowed about 12 months after surgery.

Results

Rohrborough reported the results of Altchek's first 36 patients treated with the docking technique. In this series, 92% (33/36) of patients returned to a preinjury level of play for at least 1 year, and all 22 professional or collegiate athletes returned to or exceeded prior competition levels [2]. A larger, more recent follow-up study by the same group reconfirmed these data with excellent outcomes in 90% (90/100) [4]. There were three (3%) postoperative complications, including two patients who required ulnar nerve transposition for ulnar nerve symptoms and one patient who required arthroscopic lysis of adhesions.

Several groups have modified the docking technique by using multiple-stranded grafts to increase the amount of collagen incorporated in the reconstruction [5–7]. Koh and Bowers both reported on the results using a three-strand construct modification of the docking technique, with excellent outcomes in 85% and 90% of patients, respectively [5, 7]. Paletta and Wright used a four-strand construct modification of the docking technique in elite baseball players [6]. Their results showed that 92% of the athletes return to the same or higher level of play. Two postoperative complications occurred including one transient ulnar nerve neurapraxia and an ulnar tunnel stress fracture. Donohue et al. reported on results for a 4-strand "docking plus" technique with a return to play rate of 91% [8].

A systematic review by Vitale et al. in 2008 illustrated that the docking technique with a muscle-splitting approach and decreased handling of the ulnar nerve resulted in improved outcomes and reduced complications compared to other UCL reconstruction techniques [9]. A separate review by Watson et al. in 2014 showed that the docking technique compared to the Jobe technique resulted in a significantly higher return to play rate, 90% and 67% respectively, and lower complication rates, 6% and 29% respectively [10].

More recently in 2019, Arner et al. compared the docking technique to the modified Jobe technique and found no statistically significant differences in return to play, KJOC scores, or rates for subsequent surgeries [11]. These results were similar to an outcomes comparison in 2019 by Griffith et al. in professional baseball players. Their results demonstrated that return to play rates were similar for docking and modified Jobe techniques (80% vs 82%) while rates for subsequent surgery (10% vs 15%) and revision surgery (3% vs 6%) were slightly lower for the docking technique [12].

A recent survey of 159 American Shoulder and Elbow Surgeons revealed that 66% of the group preferred the docking technique as their method for UCL reconstruction [13].

References

1. Jobe FW, Stark H, Lombardo SJ. Reconstruction of the ulnar collateral ligament in athletes. J Bone Joint Surg Am. 1986;68:1158–63.
2. Rohrbough JT, Altchek DW, Hyman J, Williams RJ III, Botts JD. Medial collateral ligament reconstruction of the elbow using the docking technique. Am J Sports Med. 2002;30:541.
3. O'Driscoll S, Lawton R, Smith A. The moving valgus stress test for medial collateral ligament tears of the elbow. Am J Sports Med. 2005;33(2):231–9.
4. Dodson CC, Thomas A, Dines JS, Nho SJ, Williams RJ III, Altchek DW. Medial ulnar collateral ligament reconstruction of the elbow in throwing athletes. Am J Sports Med. 2006;34(12):1926–32.
5. Koh JL, Schafer MF, Keuter G, Hsu JE. Ulnar collateral ligament reconstruction in elite throwing athletes. Arthroscopy. 2006;22(11):1187–91.
6. Paletta GA, Wright RW. The modified docking procedure for elbow ulnar collateral ligament reconstruction. Am J Sports Med. 2006;34(10):1594–8.
7. Bowers A, Dines J, Dines D, Altchek DW. Elbow medial ulnar collateral ligament reconstruction: clinical relevance and the docking technique. J Shoulder Elb Surg. 2010;19(2S):110–7.
8. Donohue BF, Lubitz MG, Kremchek TE. Elbow ulnar collateral ligament reconstruction using the novel docking plus technique in 324 athletes. Sports Med Open. 2019;5(3):1–9.
9. Vitale MA, Ahmad CS. The outcome of elbow ulnar collateral ligament reconstruction in overhead athletes: a systematic review. Am J Sports Med. 2008;36(6):1193–2005.
10. Watson JN, McQueen P, Hutchinson MR. A systematic review of ulnar collateral ligament reconstruction techniques. Am J Sports Med. 2014;42(10):2510–6.
11. Arner JW, Chang ES, Bayer S, Bradley JP. Direct comparison of modified Jobe and docking ulnar collateral ligament reconstruction at midterm follow-up. Am J Sports Med. 2019;47(1):144–50.
12. Griffith TB, Ahmad CS, Gorroochurn P, D'Angelo J, Ciccotti MG, Dines JS, Altchek DW, Camp CL. Comparison of outcomes based on graft type and tunnel configuration for primary ulnar collateral ligament reconstruction in professional baseball pitchers. Am J Sports Med. 2019;47(5):1103–10.
13. Hurwit DJ, Garcia GH, Liu J, Altchek DW, Romeo A, Dines J. Management of ulnar collateral ligament injury in throwing athletes: a survey of the American Shoulder and Elbow Surgeons. J Shoulder Elb Surg. 2017;26(11):2023–8.

23 Ulnar Collateral Ligament Reconstruction: American Sports Medicine Institute Technique and Outcomes

Marcus A. Rothermich and Jeffrey R. Dugas

Introduction

Over the past several decades, injuries to the medial ulnar collateral ligament (UCL) of the elbow have become increasingly more common in overhead athletes. First described in javelin throwers in 1946, these injuries have gained more attention in the late twentieth century and early twenty-first century in baseball players [1]. Biomechanical literature has demonstrated that the chronic and repetitive valgus stress placed on the medial structures of the elbow during the throwing motion contribute to the high incidence of UCL injuries in overhead athletes [2, 3]. In recent years, these injuries have been shown to occur with an increasingly higher incidence in younger athletes, leading to the recognition of an epidemic of medial elbow injuries primarily in youth baseball players [4, 5]. This health crisis in young athletes has accelerated the research regarding the optimal treatment techniques for these injuries as well as opportunities for prevention of UCL injuries.

The surgical treatment of UCL injuries has evolved since the initial UCL reconstruction procedure was performed on Tommy John by Dr. Frank Jobe in 1974 [6]. Since that time, a variety of modifications to this original surgical technique have emerged [7–14]. These include the modified Jobe technique, the docking technique, the DANE TJ technique, the American Sports Medicine Institute (ASMI) technique, and primary repair of the ligament. Although these procedures are all variants of the original Jobe technique, each has demonstrated successful outcomes in restoring medial elbow stability and allowing athletes to return to play at high levels [15–21].

In the treatment of a patient with medial elbow pain, a complete clinical evaluation including the history of the elbow injury, the physical examination, and appropriate imaging is critical in making an accurate diagnosis of injury to the UCL. Following the confirmation of this diagnosis, a discussion of conservative and surgical treatment options is necessary before the decision is made to proceed with operative management. After surgery, the post-operative rehabilitation of the elbow is an important component of a successful outcome and eventual return to play. Although patient outcomes are excellent with UCL reconstruction and particularly with the ASMI modification of the Jobe technique, prevention of these injuries in young athletes is a priority for the sports medicine

M. A. Rothermich
Department of Orthopaedic Surgery, Andrews Sports Medicine and Orthopaedic Center, Birmingham, AL, USA

J. R. Dugas (✉)
Andrews Sports Medicine and Orthopaedic Center, Birmingham, AL, USA
e-mail: Jeff.dugas@andrewssm.com

J. S. Dines et al. (eds.), *Elbow Ulnar Collateral Ligament Injury*, https://doi.org/10.1007/978-3-030-69567-5_23

community. Continued education of modern guidelines for pitching counts and recommended throwing technique is critical for players, parents, and coaches in youth baseball to decelerate the epidemic of UCL injuries.

Clinical Evaluation

History

The clinical evaluation of medial elbow pain in an overhead athlete typically begins with a thorough discussion of the history of symptoms. It is important to differentiate between an acute traumatic injury and a more chronic, insidious development of elbow pain. Some pitchers can isolate which phase of the throwing cycle causes the onset of pain, and this information can be valuable to the examining clinician. Classically, pain in the late cocking and early acceleration phase of throwing is consistent with UCL injury as this phase generates the highest torque and valgus stress across the medial elbow [22–27]. Many pitchers cannot describe an acute injury or traumatic event that causes the pain, but instead describe a decrease in throwing accuracy or velocity. This decrease in performance is typically associated with structural damage to the medial elbow, and often is the key piece of history described by the patient during the clinical evaluation.

In addition to the description of the pain onset, a qualitative discussion of the nature and location of the pain is an important component of the clinical history. Pain in the medial elbow isolated on the medial epicondyle and distal to the epicondyle is most concerning for UCL injury. It is also critical to note any paresthesia symptoms radiating down the upper extremity, as this is often an indicator of concomitant ulnar nerve pathology. This plays an important role in the treatment plan, as ulnar nerve symptoms may necessitate an ulnar nerve transposition to be performed at the time of UCL reconstruction.

A final element of a thorough history is a discussion with the patient and the family regarding both previous injuries to that extremity and the future goals of the patient. An understanding of where the athlete is at on the career timeline can be valuable in recognizing potential motivating factors regarding treatment decisions. A high school athlete seeking a college scholarship often has different ambitions than a recreational player or a player nearing retirement from the sport. This comprehensive history involving the nature and timeline of the injury, the location and quality of the pain, and the psychosocial factors related to the patient and the family are all contributory elements toward a thorough understanding of the clinical scenario.

Physical Examination

After the thorough history has been obtained, the next step in the clinical evaluation of the patient with medial elbow pain is the physical examination. A general inspection of the elbow consists of evaluating for an effusion, medial ecchymosis, and a resting flexion contracture. Additionally, testing the range of motion compared to the contralateral extremity is helpful in assessing for a dynamic flexion contracture of the dominant arm [28–30]. This range of motion testing can also serve to detect general ligamentous laxity. Importantly, pain at the medial elbow with resisted wrist flexion typically indicates pathology of the flexor-pronator muscle mass, originating over the medial elbow and often associated with UCL injuries. Pain in the posteromedial olecranon fossa with terminal extension is often indicative of concomitant valgus extension overload which is also often seen in the setting of UCL pathology.

Following inspection and range of motion testing, palpation of the medial elbow from the medial epicondyle to the sublime tubercle is critical in the evaluation for UCL injury. Ideally, this palpation occurs with the elbow in 50–70° of flexion to best expose the UCL from underneath the flexor-pronator muscle mass [9]. Pain over the medial epicondyle or within 1–2 cm distal to the epicondyle is often associated with UCL pathology [30]. Stability testing is performed with the forearm in pronation and a valgus force applied to the elbow flexed to approximately 30°,

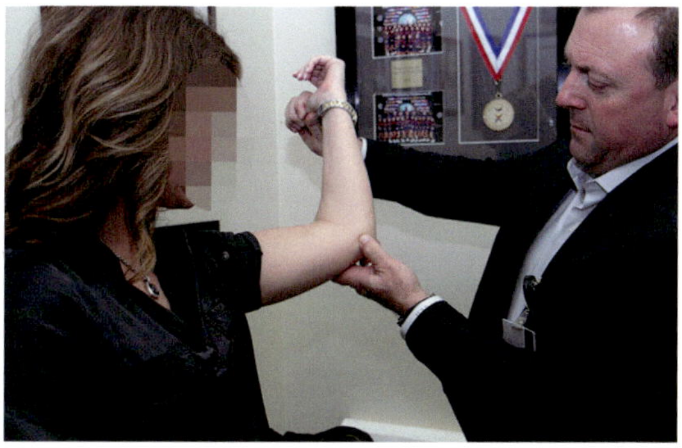

Fig. 23.1 Milking maneuver

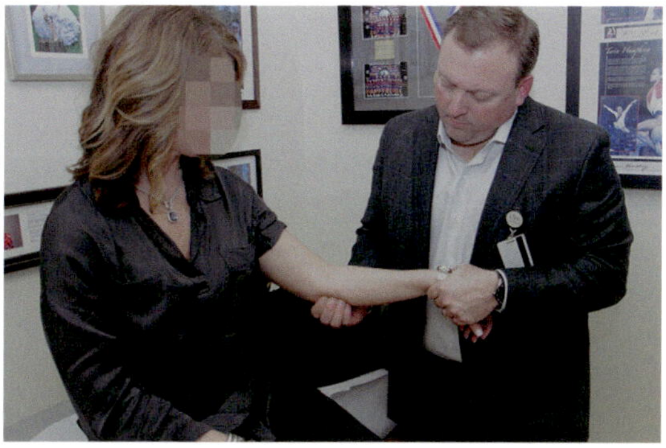

Fig. 23.2 Moving valgus stress test

which isolates the anterior bundle of the UCL [7, 9]. The diagnosis of instability is often subjective and this valgus stress testing is used only to support the diagnosis of UCL injury [31].

The final element of the physical examination of the elbow is the provocative maneuver testing to assess for UCL damage. A common provocative test is the "milking maneuver" which places a valgus stress on the medial elbow by pulling on the supinated thumb with the shoulder in external rotation [32]. The elbow is brought through a range of motion with palpation of the UCL distal to the medial epicondyle, and pain elicited with this maneuver indicates a positive test (Fig. 23.1). Additionally, the "moving valgus stress test" applies a valgus stress to the elbow as the upper extremity is brought through a throwing motion [33]. With the shoulder in 90° abduction, the elbow is hyperflexed to 120° and then quickly and smoothly extended to 30° with a constant valgus force applied to the elbow (Fig. 23.2). This reproduces the late cocking and early acceleration phases of the pitching cycle, and pain caused by this test is also indicative of UCL injury.

Imaging

During the clinical evaluation of patients with medial elbow pain, routine radiographs are typically taken to evaluate for avulsion fractures, loose bodies, or osteophytes in the elbow [34]. The standard 5-view series includes an anterior-posterior (AP), lateral, axial, and internal and external oblique views. For most patients with normal radiographs and clinical suspicion for UCL pathology, magnetic resonance imaging (MRI) is subsequently performed to evaluate the status of the UCL.

MRI arthrography continues to be the gold standard for the diagnosis of partial and complete UCL tears in symptomatic patients. The literature has demonstrated a definitive improvement in the diagnostic accuracy of MRI arthrography [35, 36]. While non-contrast MRI demonstrated a 57% sensitivity and 100% specificity for diagnosing UCL tears, MRI with an intra-articular dye injection improved the sensitivity to 92% while maintaining a 100% specificity for accurate diagnosis [35, 36]. Complete tears often demonstrate dye extravasation into the surrounding soft tissues, whereas partial undersurface tears typically demonstrate a "T-sign" which indicates an undersurface tear with dye pooling around the intact superficial layer of the distal UCL (Fig. 23.3). The combination of routine radiographs and advanced imaging can complement the comprehensive history and physical examination to provide a complete clinical evaluation of the patient with medial elbow pain.

Treatment

Conservative

After the diagnosis of UCL injury has been made, the next step in the counseling of the patient is a

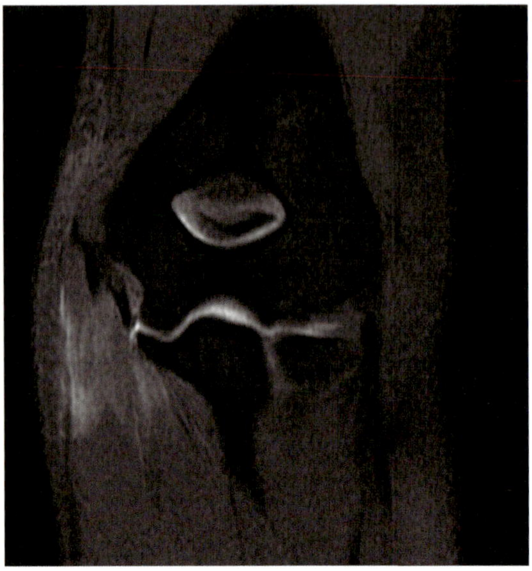

Fig. 23.3 MRI arthrogram with T-sign

thorough discussion of treatment options. This conversation should include a variety of conservative as well as surgical treatment modalities. A critical element of the diagnosis of the UCL injury is the differentiation between a partial tear and a complete tear of the ligament. This classification is often made after the physical examination and evaluation of the MRI arthrogram of the elbow.

For overhead athletes with partial tears, conservative management is an appropriate initial treatment algorithm. This typically involves a period of "active rest" in which inflammation is controlled and overhead throwing is restricted for at least 2–6 weeks following the diagnosis [37, 38]. An active rest period includes range of motion exercises, strengthening of the flexor-pronator musculature (typically consisting of a high-repetition, low-weight program), core exercises, and potentially bracing in the setting of an unstable elbow or bony avulsions in pediatric patients.

In addition to a period of active rest, some patients elect to proceed with platelet-rich plasma injections during the conservative management of UCL injuries. PRP refers to autologous blood that is centrifuged to isolate a platelet concentration higher than baseline levels, which includes a significantly higher growth factor concentration. The goal of PRP injections is to increase the return to play rate in patients with UCL injuries that are refractory to traditional conservative management. Ideally, a successful PRP injection in addition to a supervised throwing program could avoid the need for surgical intervention and decrease the total recovery time for these patients. At ASMI, adult partial UCL tears are often treated with ultrasound-guided PRP injections in competitive overhead athletes [39–42].

Following a period of active rest with or without a PRP injection, the patient is progressed to a plyometric program with rhythmic stabilization drills to improve muscular balance. An advanced interval-throwing program is then initiated and the player is progressed toward a gradual return to play.

Conservative management of overhead athletes with partial UCL tears has traditionally been met with mixed results. Rettig and colleagues initially reported a 42% return to play rate with non-operative management of partial UCL tears at an average of 24.5 weeks [38]. More recent literature including PRP injections in appropriate candidates has been more encouraging. Dines and colleagues recently reported a 73% rate of good to excellent outcomes following PRP injections in high-level players who had failed a traditional conservative treatment course, with a mean time of return to play at 12 weeks [42]. For overhead athletes with continued pain following conservative management of partial UCL tears and for patients with complete tears, operative intervention is the most appropriate next step of the treatment algorithm.

Operative

Several operative techniques are available for treatment of UCL tears in overhead athletes. For patients with partial tears and high-quality native tissue, there has been recent renewed interest in a primary repair of the ligament [14, 43]. UCL repair with internal brace augmentation has had encouraging early results in appropriately selected patients [14]. For patients with complete tears and poor-quality native tissue, UCL reconstruction is still the gold standard of surgical treatment. Following the initial UCL reconstruction procedure by Dr. Frank Jobe in 1974, there have been several modifications to the original technique [6–14]. Dr. James Andrews developed the ASMI modification of the Jobe technique by retracting the flexor-pronator muscle mass medially rather than releasing it, as well as performing a subcutaneous ulnar nerve transposition as opposed to submuscular. This modification remains the primary technique for UCL reconstructions performed at ASMI.

The patient is brought to the operating room and placed supine with the operative upper extremity on an arm board. If the contralateral gracilis tendon is to be harvested due to the lack of a palmaris longus tendon, the contralateral leg is prepped and draped as well. Examination under anesthesia is performed, and the shoulder is externally rotated with the elbow in 30° of flexion. A half stack of towels is placed under the elbow, and full stack is placed under the wrist. A tourniquet is set at 250 mmHg and is inflated after exsanguination with an Esmarch bandage.

A 10-cm incision is made just posterior to the medial epicondyle, with one third of the incision proximal to the medial epicondyle and two thirds distal to the epicondyle (Fig. 23.4). After sharp dissection through the skin, subcutaneous skin flaps are developed and the medial antebrachial cutaneous nerve is identified superficial to the fascia (on average 3 cm distal to the medial epicondyle) and is protected with a vessel loop (Fig. 23.5) [44]. The ulnar nerve is then identified in the cubital tunnel posterior to the medial epicondyle and is carefully dissected from the medial intermuscular septum proximally to the first muscular branch of the flexor carpi ulnaris distally. This nerve is also protected with a vessel loop. A strip of the medial intermuscular septum is then released proximally and is carefully dissected. This remains attached distally and will be used following UCL reconstruction to form a soft tissue sling keeping the ulnar nerve transposed anterior to the medial epicondyle.

The muscle belly of the flexor-pronator mass is then elevated with a 15-blade scalpel, exposing the anterior bundle of the UCL. The ligament is evaluated from its origin on the medial epicondyle to its insertion on the sublime tubercle. Following this inspection, the anterior bundle of the native UCL is splint longitudinally in line with its fibers. If any bony ossicles are present within the substance of the ligament, these are removed to expose the intra-articular space of the elbow joint. If any loose bodies or osteophytes are present, these can be removed under direct visualization.

Following this preparation of the elbow joint, graft harvest is then performed. If the palmaris longus is present, this is the gold standard graft for UCL reconstruction. Interestingly, the absence of a palmaris longus tendon in 3–15% of the population has been linked to ethnic trends [45, 46]. Non-Hispanic whites are most commonly missing the tendon, with the reliable presence of the palmaris longus most common in patients of Asian descent. Three transverse incisions are used to harvest the palmaris longus ten-

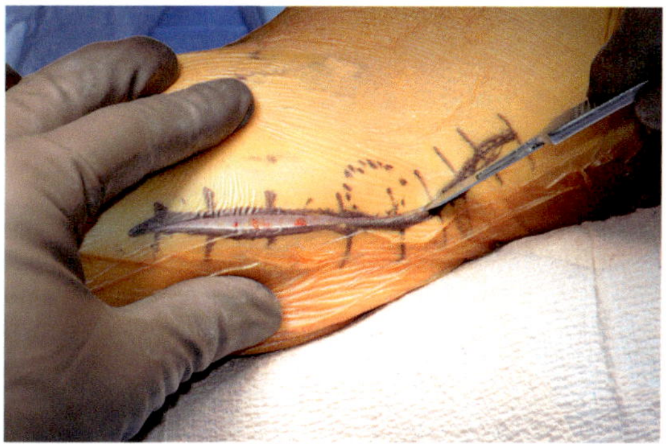

Fig. 23.4 UCL reconstruction incision

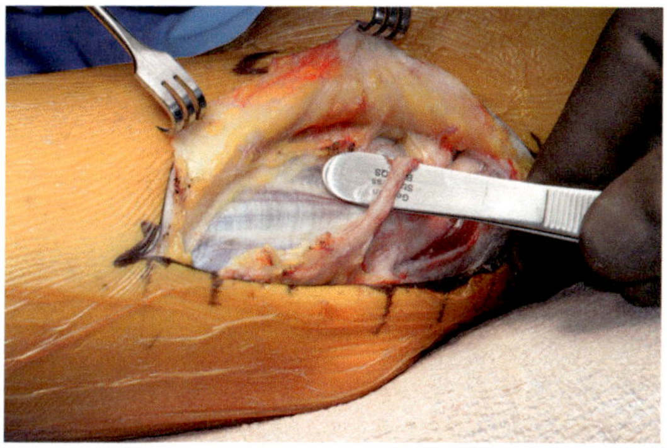

Fig. 23.5 Medial antebrachial cutaneous nerve

don, and are often marked pre-operatively by having the patient flex the wrist while opposing the thumb to the small finger. Starting with the most distal incision at the proximal wrist crease, and second small incision is made 2 cm proximal to the first. The critical element of transecting the palmaris longus tendon from the most distal incision is ensuring that the median nerve or flexor carpi radialis tendon is not harvested. Following transection of the palmaris longus tendon, the tendon is then pulled out through the second, more proximal incision. A locking whipstitch is placed on the distal end of the tendon with a #0 Ticron suture and traction is placed on the tendon to identify the musculotendinous junction. A third small incision is then made at the junction of the proximal third and distal two thirds of the forearm. The tendon is removed from the third small incision with a hemostat. The tendon is then transected at the proximal aspect of the tendon for a minimum graft length of 13 cm. Excess muscle is cleaned from the tendon and the free end of the tendon is also whipstitched. This graft is then placed in a moist sponge on the back table until the elbow is ready for graft passage.

If the palmaris longus is absent or of insufficient length, the contralateral gracilis is then harvested [17]. In the contralateral leg, an oblique incision is made over the pes anserine tendons with full-thickness skin flaps, and the sartorial fascia is identified and incised. The sartorial fascia is then reflected and the gracilis tendon is identified. This is freed from the undersurface of the sartorial fascia with a hemostat. The tendon is freed from soft-tissue adhesions to prevent transection. An open tendon stripper is used to harvest the tendon by passing it in line with the trajectory of the gracilis tendon with the knee in a flexed and externally rotated ("figure-4") position. Following proximal harvest at the musculotendinous junction, the tendon is transected at the conjoined insertion of the gracilis and semitendinosis tendons distally. Excess muscle is then removed from the tendon with the end of a metallic ruler and both ends are whipstitched with #2 Vicryl suture with a minimum length of 13 cm. The prepared graft is then placed in a moist sponge on the back table until the elbow is ready for graft passage.

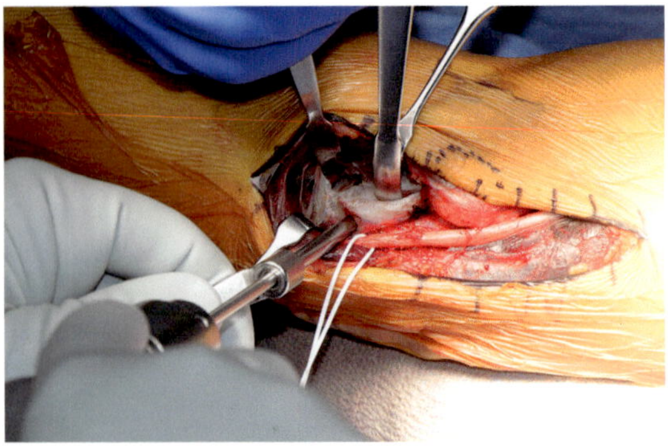

Fig. 23.6 Sublime tubercle tunnel drilling

Following graft preparation, bone tunnels are drilled to prepare the elbow for graft passage. The distal bone tunnel on the sublime tubercle is typically drilled first, often approximately 10 mm from the articular surface of the ulna. For a palmaris longus graft, a 3.6-mm drill bit is used, whereas a 4-mm drill bit is used for a gracilis graft. The first drill hole is started posteriorly on the sublime tubercle and is aimed anteriorly and laterally (Fig. 23.6). After a unicortical drill hole is made, a hemostat is placed into the drill hole and a second tunnel is drilled 1 cm anterior to the first drill hole and is directed posteriorly until the hemostat is contacted. Angled curettes are passed through the tunnel and the tunnel is irrigated to remove bony debris. A curved Hewson suture passer is used to pass the graft through the ulnar tunnel that has been created.

The tunnel drilled about the medial epicondyle of the humerus is lambda-shaped, and begins with a drill hole from the UCL origin on the anteroinferior aspect of the medial epicondyle. This is aimed proximally and exits the posterosuperior medial epicondyle as far lateral as possible (Fig. 23.7) [24]. Again, a hemostat is placed in first drill hole and a second tunnel is drilled 1 cm from the posterosuperior exit point of the first drill hole (Fig. 23.8). When the hemostat is again contacted with the drill bit, the tunnels are cleared with a curette and irrigated. The graft is then passed through the medial epicondyle with the Hewson suture passer in a figure-8 fashion.

Following passage of the graft in a figure-8 fashion, the arm is placed in 15–20° of flexion and a varus force is placed on the elbow to close

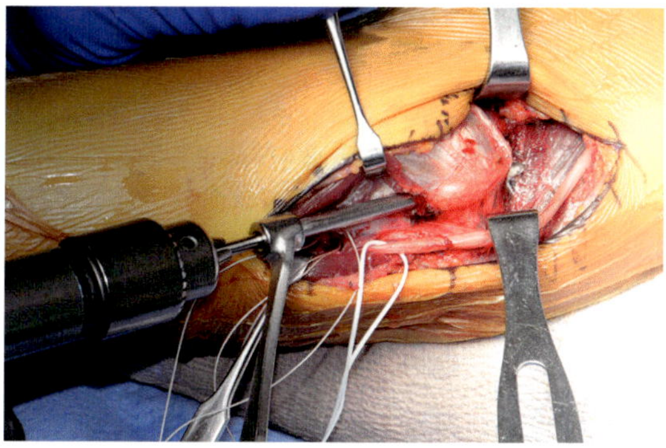

Fig. 23.7 Medial epicondyle tunnel drilling1

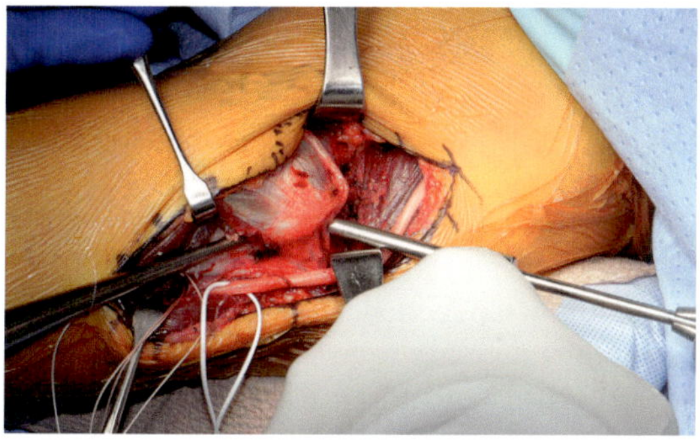

Fig. 23.8 Medial epicondyle tunnel drilling2

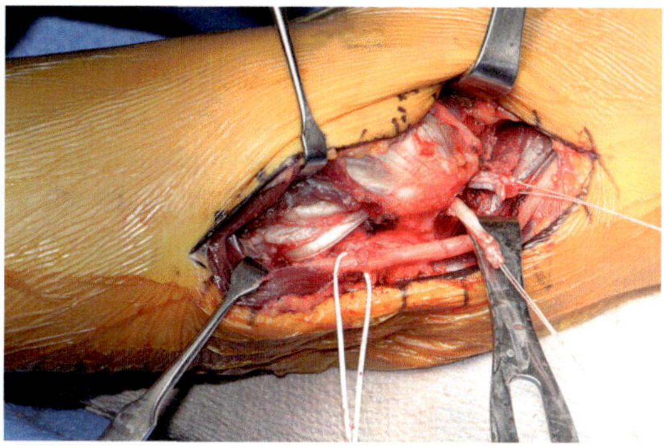

Fig. 23.9 Graft passage

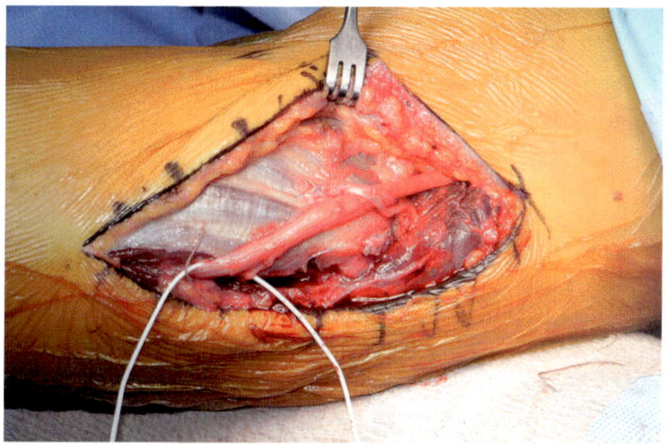

Fig. 23.10 Subcutaneous ulnar nerve transposition

down the medial joint line (Fig. 23.9). With this tension on the graft, the two limbs of the graft are sewn together between the two proximal drill holes on the medial epicondyle with #0 Ticron suture. Excess graft is removed and the native ligament is closed with #0 Ticron suture. Finally, the graft is sewn to the native ligament with the same #0 Ticron suture.

After securing the graft and completing the UCL reconstruction, the ulnar nerve is transposed anteriorly to the medial epicondyle and loosely secured with the slip of soft tissue from the medial intermuscular septum with 3-0 Ticron sutures (Fig. 23.10). Following the ulnar nerve transposition, the elbow is taken through a range of motion to ensure that the ulnar nerve is not compressed. The cubital tunnel is then closed with #0 Vicryl suture and an antipropagation stitch is placed in the most distal aspect of the flexor carpi ulnaris fascial split.

At this point, the tourniquet is let down and the bipolar electrocautery is used to achieve hemostasis. A drain is placed and the wound is thoroughly irrigated and closed with a 2-0 Vicryl and running 3-0 subcuticular Prolene with an escape stitch. The upper extremity is cleaned and steri-strips, sterile dressings, and a posterior splint are applied at 90° flexion with the wrist in neutral position.

Rehabilitation

The rehabilitation following UCL reconstruction is a critical component for the overhead athlete to safely return to play. A detailed protocol has been designed by Dr. Kevin Wilk and is utilized on patients at ASMI following surgery [47]. This program has been broken into four phases: an immediate post-operative phase, an intermediate phase, an advanced strengthening phase, and a return to play phase.

The immediate post-operative phase includes the first 3 weeks following UCL reconstruction, and focuses on controlling the post-operative inflammation of the elbow, protecting the reconstruction, and limiting the muscle atrophy that occurs in the elbow following surgery. A posterior elbow splint is typically applied at the time of surgery and is discontinued after the first week. During week 1, gripping exercises and shoulder isometrics without shoulder external rotation are begun. After the splint is removed, a hinged elbow brace is applied during week 2 and elbow range of motion is allowed from 30° to 105° with wrist range of motion exercises and elbow extension isometrics. During week 3, passive elbow range of motion is advanced from 15° to 115° with the initiation of active wrist, elbow, and shoulder range of motion.

The intermediate phase includes weeks 4–8 and focuses on gradually progressing the elbow to full range of motion while improving strength. The brace is unlocked from 0° to 125° during week 4 and one-pound weights are used during wrist, elbow, shoulder, and scapular strengthening exercises. During week 5, the brace is discontinued and full active range of motion at the elbow is allowed. Activity is gradually increased and during week 6 the Advanced Throwers Ten Program is initiated, a collection of activities designed to improve strength and endurance of the operative upper extremity. These activities continue during week 7.

The advanced strengthening phase, which includes weeks 8–14, consists primarily of core strengthening, plyometrics, eccentric elbow exercises, and isotonic forearm strengthening. During week 10 the plyometrics program progresses from two-handed chest passes near the body to soccer and side throws. If the progression of the rehabilitation continues without significant pain, the conclusion of the advanced strengthening phase in week 14 includes bench presses, lat pulldowns, and an interval hitting program.

The final phase of the UCL reconstruction rehabilitation program at ASMI includes an eventual return to competitive throwing. From week 15 to week 32, power and endurance training continues to progress. The interval throwing program begins during week 16 with an important stretching program to be performed before and after the long toss. For most overhead athletes, this program allows for a gradual return to competitive throwing at the conclusion of the ASMI rehabilitation protocol.

Outcomes

With the advancement of our understanding of UCL injuries through biomechanical studies and progressive rehabilitation protocols, the outcomes following UCL surgery continue to be highly satisfactory. Several large-scale studies have demonstrated consistently high return to play rates for players in both short-term and long-term follow-up periods [4, 15, 48, 50]. Also, recent literature has shown similar outcome data regardless of both surgical technique and graft used in elite baseball players.

The largest cohort of short-term outcomes was published in 2010 and reported outcomes on 1281 patients at ASMI following UCL reconstruction by Dr. Andrews [4]. This minimum 2-year follow-up data demonstrated a return to play rate at the same or higher level of 83% in these patients. The cohort began throwing at an average of 4.4 months and returned to competition at an average of 11.6 months following the UCL rehabilitation protocol. The outcomes were not significantly different regardless of graft choice or previous injury. In addition to a high return to play rate, there was a low complication rate in these patients. From this cohort, 53 patients (4.2%) had subsequent arthroscopic olecranon osteophyte debridement and only nine patients (0.7%) had a recurrent UCL tear with revision UCL reconstruction.

These encouraging short-term outcomes were supported by later long-term outcome data on the same patient cohort [15]. A total of 313 baseball players with minimum 10-year follow-up data demonstrated an identical 83% return to play rate. The nature of the longer follow-up period allowed for a greater retrospective evaluation of player performance following surgery. Career longevity in this cohort was an average of 3.6 years following surgery, and 86% retired for reasons other than the elbow. Following retirement in these patients, 93% were satisfied overall with the outcome of the UCL reconstruction experience and 98% of patients had the ability to throw recreationally.

A recent study supported the excellent return to play outcomes seen from the short-term and long-term cohort at ASMI. A large cohort of 566 professional baseball pitchers with a minimum 2-year follow-up demonstrated an overall return to play rate of 79.9% at an average of 14.5 months [51]. These players were treated at several different high-volume centers, and a variety of surgical techniques and graft types were utilized with no significant differences in outcomes for the different techniques or grafts.

Prevention

Although the treatment and rehabilitation following UCL reconstruction has yielded generally favorable outcomes and high return to play rates in elite overhead athletes, the incidence of UCL injuries in youth baseball players continues to rise annually. There have been several factors described to explain the high rates of injury in young overhead athletes. Biomechanical analysis has demonstrated that the elbow experiences 64 N•m of torque during the pitching motion [52–55]. This varies for different types of pitches thrown, with the curveball causing greater torque than the fastball or changeup. Several environmental factors have been identified that also contribute to the rise of elbow injuries in youth baseball. The increasing emphasis on playing for travel teams and participating in elite showcases, as well as the growth in the number of indoor facilities in northern states, have made year-round play much more prevalent in recent years for young athletes.

At ASMI, the incidence of surgical UCL injuries in Division-I collegiate baseball players has been studied recently in a large-scale national injury registry [56]. With 99.0% of Division-I baseball programs participating, the data have demonstrated a consistently high incidence of surgical UCL injuries in Division-I baseball. Over 200 surgeries have been reported annually for the 2017–2018 and 2018–2019 college baseball seasons, with a surgical rate of 0.77 surgeries on the UCL per Division-I program during that time [57]. The average age over that time was 19.9 years old, indicating that these injuries are happening predominantly on underclassmen. With a primary UCL surgery at a young age, these players are often set up for potential recurrent problems in the future if they continue to play in the major leagues for another decade or more following surgery. Clearly, the high incidence of UCL surgery at a young age is a major concern for young players and their parents, coaches, scouts, and collegiate and professional baseball organizations.

With the increasing incidence of UCL injuries in young players, an emphasis has been placed on the development of guidelines for youth baseball organizations to help prevent the continued acceleration of the injury rate. Recommendations for prevention include avoiding pitching when fatigued, observing a 4-month period of rest during the calendar year, following the current age-appropriate pitch count regulations, pitching no more than 100 innings per calendar year and not playing on multiple teams with overlapping seasons, and using appropriate pitching mechanics. By following these guidelines, a young overhead athlete has the best chance to avoid a surgical UCL injury early in the career timeline.

Complications

Although recent outcome data have shown continued improvement in return to play rates in high-level athletes, complications following surgery do still unfortunately occur. For a player who has undergone surgical intervention and progressed through the exhaustive rehabilitation program, a recurrent injury to the medial elbow is a devastating complication. Thankfully, the rate of recurrent UCL injuries continues to be low in baseball players. When a recurrent tear occurs, a difficult treatment decision is encountered by the athlete to proceed with conservative treatment or a secondary operative intervention. For revision UCL procedures, both revision UCL reconstruction and the modern UCL repair with internal brace augmentation are both viable treatment options.

Revision UCL Reconstruction

With the consistent increase in the incidence of primary UCL reconstruction and the declining age at the time of this procedure in overhead athletes, the rate of revision UCL reconstruction in this population is also expected to rise over time in the future. The national Division-I UCL Injury Registry at ASMI has demonstrated an average revision rate of 2.6% of UCL surgeries performed in collegiate baseball players from 2017 to 2019 [57]. In professional players, recent data have shown a 4.9% revision rate in players from the minor and major leagues [50]. Outcome data have demonstrated an average time of revision to be 47 months following primary UCL reconstruction [58]. In this cohort of professional baseball players, 76.6% of players returned to play at any level, whereas only 55.3% were able to return to the same level of play. The career length in the patients following the revision procedure in one study ranged from 2.6 to 3.2 years following surgery [50]. Although revising the previously drilled bone tunnels with secondary graft choices in the revision setting is technically challenging, revision UCL reconstruction remains an option for high-level overhead athletes.

UCL Repair with Internal Brace Augmentation

There has been a renewed interest in UCL repair for treating both primary UCL injuries as well as in the revision setting. The recent modification of the repair procedure includes the addition of a collagen-coated FiberTape (Arthrex) to augment the repair [14]. This augmentation serves as an additional backstop to the valgus stress applied to the medial elbow during the pitching motion, and the biologic addition of the collagen helps in healing of the repair. Although this procedure is ideal in young patients with high-quality native UCL tissue, there has been interest in UCL repair as an option in high-level baseball players with a recurrent tear in a reconstructed UCL. Early outcome data following UCL repair have been encouraging. In 111 patients who underwent UCL repair with internal brace augmentation at ASMI with a minimum 2-year follow-up, a return to play rate of 92% was seen at the same or higher level of competition at an average 6.7 months following surgery [14]. Although these data are based on patients who underwent a primary UCL repair of the native ligament, the surgical technique avoiding the drilling of bone tunnels and the accelerated rehabilitation protocol is an interesting and attractive option for consideration in high-level throwers who have sustained a recurrent UCL tear of a reconstructed ligament. Certainly, the outcome data following UCL repair in the revision setting will be an area of increased interest in the future.

Conclusion

In overhead athletes with medial elbow pain, UCL injuries continue to be a major cause of morbidity and loss of playing time. In these patients, a thorough clinical evaluation including a detailed history of the injury, a complete physical examination, and appropriate imaging is critical to determine the nature of the pathology. For patients with damage to the UCL who have failed conservative treatment, UCL reconstruction remains an excellent surgical option. At ASMI, the modified surgical technique and specific rehabilitation protocol have consistently yielded satisfactory outcomes and a high return to play rate for these players. While complications including recurrent UCL tear remain low, revision UCL reconstruction and primary UCL repair with internal brace augmentation are surgical treatment options. Research related to the outcomes following the recently modified UCL repair technique is ongoing, but early outcome data are encouraging. Although the treatment and rehabilitation protocols typically yield satisfactory outcomes, the incidence of elbow injuries in young athletes continues to rise. Prevention of these injuries through an awareness of common causes and adherence to current playing guidelines is a primary goal for the future of youth baseball.

References

1. Waris W. Elbow injuries of javelin-throwers. Acta Chir Scand. 1946;93(6):563–75.
2. Fleisig GS, Andrews JR, Dillman CJ, Escamilla RF. Kinetics of baseball pitching with implications about injury mechanisms. Am J Sports Med. 1995;23(2):233–9.
3. Werner SL, Fleisig GS, Dillman CJ, Andrews JR. Biomechanics of the elbow during baseball pitching. J Orthop Sports Phys Ther. 1993;17:274–8.
4. Cain EL, Andrews JR, Dugas JR, Wilk KE, McMichael CS, Walter JC, et al. Outcome of ulnar collateral ligament reconstruction of the elbow in 1281 athletes. Am J Sports Med. 2010;38(12):2426–34.
5. Fleisig GS, Andrews JR. Prevention of elbow injuries in youth baseball pitchers. Sports Health. 2012;1(4):314–20.3 Andrews JR, Jost PW, Cain EL. The ulnar collateral ligament procedure revisited-the procedure we use. Sports Health. 2012;4:438–41.
6. Jobe FW, Stark H, Lombardo SJ. Reconstruction of the ulnar collateral ligament in athletes. J Bone Joint Surg Am. 1986;68(8):1158–64.
7. Yocum LA, Wanich T. Ulnar collateral ligament reconstruction. In: Dines J, Altchek DW, Andrews JR, ElAttrache NS, editors. Sports medicine of baseball. Philadelphia: Lippincott Williams & Wilkins; 2012. p. 231–43.
8. Safran M, Ahmad CS, Elattrache NS. Ulnar collateral ligament of the elbow. Arthroscopy. 2005;21(11):1381–95.
9. Cain EL, Dugas JR, Wolf RS, Andrews JR. Elbow injuries in throwing athletes-a current concepts review. Am J Sports Med. 2003;31:621–35.
10. Ahmad CS, ElAttrache NS. Elbow valgus instability in throwing athlete. J Am Acad Orthop Surg. 2006;14:693–700.
11. Thompson WH, Jobe FW, Yocum LA, Pink MM. Ulnar collateral ligament reconstruction in athletes-muscle-splitting approach without transposition of the ulnar nerve. J Shoulder Elb Surg. 2001;10:152–7.
12. Savoie FH, Trenhaile SW, Roberts J, Field LD, Ramsey JR. Primary repair of ulnar collateral ligament injuries of the elbow in young athletes-a case series of injuries to the proximal and distal ends of the ligament. Am J Sports Med. 2008;36(6):1066–72.
13. Rohrbough JT, Altchek DW, Hyman J, Williams RJ III, Botts JD. Medial collateral ligament reconstruction of the elbow using the docking technique. Am J Sports Med. 2002;30:541–8.
14. Dugas JR, Looze CA, Capogna B, Walters BL, Jones CM, Rothermich MA, et al. Ulnar collateral ligament repair with collage-dipped FiberTape augmentation in overhead athletes. Am J Sports Med. 2019;47(5):1096–102.
15. Osbahr DC, Cain EL, Raines BT, Fortenbaugh D, Dugas JR, Andrews JR. Long-term outcomes after ulnar collateral ligament reconstruction in competitive baseball players- follow-up with minimum of 10 years. American Academy of Orthopaedic Surgeons Annual Meeting. 2013 March 11–15; Chicago, IL.
16. Azar FM, Andrews JR, Wilk KE, Groh D. Operative treatment of ulnar collateral ligament injuries of the elbow in athletes. Am J Sports Med. 2000;28:16–23.
17. Dugas JR, Bilotta J, Watts CD, Crum JA, Fleisig GS, McMichael CS, et al. Ulnar collateral ligament reconstruction with gracilis tendon in athletes with intraligamentous bony excision. Am J Sports Med. 2012;20(7):1578–82.
18. Bennett GE. Shoulder and elbow lesions of the professional baseball pitcher. JAMA. 1941;117(7):4.
19. King JW, Brelsford HJ, Tullos HS. Analysis of the pitching arm of the professional baseball pitcher. Clin Orthop. 1969;67:116–23.
20. Norwood LA, Shook JA, Andrews JR. Acute medial elbow ruptures. Am J Sports Med. 1981;9(1):16–9.
21. Andrews JR, Jost PW, Cain EL. The ulnar collateral ligament procedure revisited- the procedure we use. Sports Health. 2012;4:438–41.
22. Dugas JR, Cain EL. Ulnar nerve injury in the throwing athlete. In: ElAttrache NS, Harner CD, Mirzayan R, Sekiya JK, editors. Surgical techniques in sports medicine. Philadelphia: Lippincott Williams & Wilkins; 2007. p. 299–305.
23. Conway JE, Jobe FW, Glousan RE, Pink M. Medial instability of the elbow in throwing athletes-treatment by repair or reconstruction of the ulnar collateral ligament. J Bone Joint Surg Am. 1992;74:67–83.
24. Dugas JR, Ostrander RV, Cain EL, Kingsley D, Andrews JR. Anatomy of the anterior bundle of the ulnar collateral ligament. J Shoulder Elb Surg. 2007;16:657–60.
25. Vitale MA, Ahmad CS. The outcome of elbow ulnar collateral ligament reconstruction in overhead athletes-a systematic review. Am J Sports Med. 2008;36(6):1193–205.
26. Dugas JR, Bullens-Borrow A. Instability and arthroscopy. In: Johnson DL, Mair SD, editors. Clinical sports medicine. Philadelphia: Mosby Elsevier; 2006. p. 341–51.
27. Wilson FD, Andrews JR, Blackburn TA, McCluskey G. Valgus extension overload in the pitching elbow. Am J Sports Med. 1983;11:83–8.
28. Azar FM. History and examination of the thrower's elbow. Sports Med Arthroscopy Rev. 2003;11(1):10–4.

29. Dugas JR, Weiland AJ. Vascular pathology in the throwing athlete. Hand Clin. 2000;16:477–85.
30. Lee ML, Rosenwasser MP. Chronic elbow instability. Orthop Clin North Am. 1999;30:81–9.
31. Rijke AM, Goitz HT, McCue FC, Andrews JR, Berr SS. Stress radiography of the medial elbow ligaments. Radiology. 1994;19(1):213–6.
32. Veltri DM, Field LD, Deutsch A, Altcher A, Potter H. The milking maneuver-a new test to evaluate the MCL of the elbow in the throwing athlete. J Shoulder Elb Surg. 1995;4(1):4A.
33. O'Driscoll SWM, Lawton RL, Smith AM. The "moving valgus stress test" for medial collateral ligament tears of the elbow. Am J Sports Med. 2005;33(2):231–9.
34. Salvo JP, Rizio L, Zvijac JE, Uribe JW, Hechtman KS. Avulsion fracture of the ulnar sublime tubercle in overhead throwing athletes. Am J Sports Med. 2002;30(3):426–31.
35. Schwartz ML, AL-Zahrani S, Morwessel RM, Andrews JR. Ulnar collateral ligament injury in the throwing athlete-evaluation with saline-enhanced MR arthrography. Radiology. 1995;197(1):297–9.
36. Timmerman LA, Schwartz ML, Andrews JR. Preoperative evaluation of the ulnar collateral ligament by magnetic resonance imaging and computed tomography arthrography. Evaluation in 25 baseball players with surgical confirmation. Am J Sports Med. 1994;22(1):26–31.
37. Miller CD, Savoie FH III. Valgus extension injuries of the elbow in the throwing athlete. J Am Acad Orthop Surg. 1994;2:261–9.
38. Rettig AC, Sherrill C, Snead DS, Mendler C, Mieling P. Nonoperative treatment of ulnar collateral ligament injuries in throwing athletes. Am J Sports Med. 2001;21:15–7.
39. Chen FS, Rokito AS, Jobe FW. Medial elbow problems in the overhead-throwing athlete. J Am Acad Orthop Surg. 2001;9:99–113.
40. Lee KS, Rosas HG, Craig JG. Musculoskeletal ultrasound: elbow imaging and procedures. Semin Musculoskelet Radiol. 2010;14(4):449–60.
41. Sasaki J, Takahara M, Ogino T, Kashiwa H, Ishigaki D, Kanauchi Y. Ultrasonographic assessment of the ulnar collateral ligament and medial elbow laxity in college baseball players. J Bone Joint Surg Am. 2002;84-A(4):525–31.
42. Dines JS, Williams PN, ElAttrache N, Conte S, Tomczyk T, Osbahr DC, et al. Platelet-rich plasma can be used to successfully treat elbow ulnar collateral ligament insufficiency in high-level throwers. Am J Orthop. 2016 Jul-Aug;45(5):296–300.
43. Timmerman LA, Andrews JR. Undersurface tear of the ulnar collateral ligament in baseball players. A newly recognized lesion. Am J Sports Med. 1994;22(1):33–6.
44. Lowe JB, Maggi SP, Mackinnon SE. The position of crossing branches of the medial antebrachial cutaneous nerve during cubital tunnel surgery in humans. Plast Reconstr Surg. 2004;114(3):692–6.
45. Soltani AM, Peric M, Francis CS, Nguyen TT, Chan LS, Ghiassi A, et al. The variation in the absence of the palmaris longus in a multiethnic population of the United States: an epidemiological study. Plast Surg Int. 2012;31:Article ID 282959.
46. Sebastin SJ, Puhaindran ME, Lim AYT, Lim IJ, Bee WH. The prevalence of absence of the palmaris longus-a study in a Chinese population and a review of the literature. J Hand Surg Br. 2005;30(5):525–7.
47. Ellenbecker TS, Wilk KE, Altchek DW, Andrews JR. Current concepts in rehabilitation following ulnar collateral ligament reconstruction. Sports Health. 2009;1(4):301–13.
48. Andrews JR, Timmerman LA. Outcome of elbow surgery in professional baseball players. Am J Sports Med. 1994;23:407–13.
49. Petty DH, Andrews JR, Fleisig GS, Cain EL. Ulnar collateral ligament reconstruction in high school baseball players-clinical results and injury risk factors. Am J Sports Med. 2004;32(5):1158–64.
50. Glogovac G, Grawe BM. Outcomes with a focus on return to play for revision ulnar collateral ligament surgery among elite-level baseball players. Am J Sports Med. 2019;47(11):2759–63.
51. Griffith TB, Ahmad CS, Gorroochum P, D'Angelo J, Ciccotti MG, Dines JS, et al. Comparison of outcomes based on graft type and tunnel configuration for primary ulnar collateral ligament reconstruction in professional baseball players. Am J Sports Med. 2019;47(5):1103–10.
52. Olsen SJ, Fleisig GS, Dun S, Loftice J, Andrews JR. Risk factors for shoulder and elbow injuries in adolescent baseball pitchers. Am J Sports Med. 2006;34(6):905–12.
53. Fleisig GS, Kingsley DS, Loftice JW, Dinnen KP, Ranganathan R, Dun S, et al. Kinetic comparison among the fastball, curveball, change-up, and slider in collegiate baseball pitchers. Am J Sports Med. 2006;34(3):423–30.
54. Escamilla RF, Barrentine SW, Fleisig GS, Zheng N, Takada Y, Kingsley D, et al. Pitching biomechanics as a pitcher approaches muscular fatigue during a simulated baseball game. Am J Sports Med. 2007;35(1):23–33.
55. Lyman S, Fleisig GS, Andrews JR, Osinski ED. Effect of pitch type, pitch count, and pitching mechanics on risk of elbow and shoulder pain in youth baseball pitchers. Am J Sports Med. 2002;30(4):463–8.
56. Rothermich MA, Conte SA, Aune KT, Fleisig GS, Cain EL, Dugas JR. Incidence of elbow ulnar collateral ligament surgery in collegiate baseball players. Orthop J Sports Med. 2018;6(4):2325967118764657.
57. Rothermich MA, Conte SA, Hart KM, Fleisig GS, Cain EL, Dugas JR. Incidence of UCL surgery in collegiate baseball players. American Orthopaedic Society for Sports Medicine Annual Meeting. 2019 July 11–14; Boston, MA.
58. Camp CL, Desai V, Conte S, Ahmad CS, Ciccotti M, Dines JS, et al. Revision ulnar collateral ligament reconstruction in professional baseball: current trends, surgical techniques, and outcomes. Orthop J Sports Med. 2019;7(8):2325967119864104.

Ulnar Collateral Ligament Reconstruction: Alternative Surgical Techniques

24

Brandon A. Simonetta, Benjamin C. Service, Neal S. ElAttrache, and Daryl C. Osbahr

Introduction

The number of UCL reconstructions performed annually has rapidly increased in recent years, especially in throwing athletes [1]. By subjecting the elbow to massive valgus force during competition, throwing athletes are at risk for injury to the ulnar collateral ligament (UCL) of the elbow [2]. While a trial of nonsurgical treatment is recommended as the initial treatment for UCL injury, many of these athletes need surgical reconstruction of the UCL to return to their preinjury level of performance. The modern surgical management of UCL injuries in throwing athletes was based upon the initial method described by Jobe et al. [3]. While the fundamental goals of reconstruction of the UCL still focus on returning the athlete to the sport, the evolution of UCL reconstruction has led to research regarding almost every step of the surgery.

Research has quantified the magnitude of the forces on the elbow during the throwing motion; the late cocking and acceleration phases can result in valgus moments that near 290 N [2]. The primary restraint to valgus forces on the elbow, as seen during the overhead throwing motion, is the anterior bundle of the UCL [4]. Due to these high forces, the reconstructed ligament must achieve strength near that of the native UCL. Innovation regarding UCL reconstruction has focused on three aspects of the surgery: the type of approach, humeral graft fixation, and ulnar graft fixation. Multiple techniques have been investigated regarding the biomechanical effects of varied graft fixation methods that differ from bone tunnel figure-of-eight graft passage as initially described by Dr. Frank Jobe.

Modifications of the figure-of-eight technique have been developed to facilitate anatomic reconstruction and strength comparable to the native UCL. Furthermore, surgical techniques have also been developed to facilitate graft fixation in an expeditious and secure manner. The spectrum of humeral graft fixation has included the figure-of-eight technique, docking technique [5], interference screw fixation [6], suture anchor fixation [7], and cortical suspensory fixation [8]. Graft fixation options for the ulna have included tunnel utilization, interference screw fixation [9], and cortical suspensory fixation [8].

The most common UCL surgical techniques have been the figure-of-eight and the docking technique [10, 11]; however, other alternative techniques have been proposed to improve out-

B. A. Simonetta (✉)
Department of Orthopedic Surgery, Orlando Health Orthopedic Institute, Orlando, FL, USA

B. C. Service · D. C. Osbahr
Orlando Health Orthopedic Institute, Orlando, FL, USA

N. S. ElAttrache
Kerlan-Jobe Orthopaedic Clinic, Los Angeles, CA, USA

J. S. Dines et al. (eds.), *Elbow Ulnar Collateral Ligament Injury*, https://doi.org/10.1007/978-3-030-69567-5_24

comes and decrease the risk for complications, such as bone tunnel fracture and failure of fixation. Two of the most common alternative techniques include interference screw and cortical suspensory fixation of the tendinous graft. The main benefits of these alternative fixation methods have been to facilitate ease of technique and limit complications, but a relative paucity of clinical outcomes data exists for these newer fixation methods compared to the figure-of-eight and docking techniques. The literature on these techniques has mostly focused on surgical methods and biomechanical assessments. Nonetheless, the concepts behind these UCL reconstruction techniques are important to consider, as we optimize surgical outcomes relating to UCL injuries in the future .

UCL Reconstruction: Biomechanical Assessment

Biomechanical studies have compared the various UCL reconstruction techniques with the native ligament. Additionally, the integrity of various graft constructs has been compared to established techniques. These studies have attempted to quantify the strength of the reconstruction options and the kinematics to optimize outcomes.

Much of the literature has focused on load to failure due to the considerable forces during the throwing motion [12]. Paletta et al. compared the valgus moment measured to failure of the native ligament in comparison to reconstructed ligaments using the figure-of-eight and docking techniques [13]. The native UCL had a maximal valgus moment to failure of 18.8 N m. In comparison to the figure-of-eight technique (8.9 N m), the docking technique had a significantly greater maximal valgus moment to failure (14.3 N m, $p = 0.0148$). The docking technique was not statistically different from the native UCL valgus moment to failure. The location of failure was most common at the suture–tendon interface for the figure-of-eight reconstructions; the docking technique failed most commonly due to suture failure. For both types of reconstructions, bone tunnel fracture was the second most common reason for the loss of graft integrity. The strain of each reconstruction type was also assessed at 3 N m, with the docking technique having significantly less strain compared to the figure-of-eight technique ($p = 0.378$). While research has shown excellent Conway scale outcomes with the use of the figure-of-eight technique, the greater maximal valgus moment to failure and decrease strain with the docking technique has led to further research on this method over the past decade .

In a study by Armstrong et al., a biomechanical evaluation of the native ligament was compared to four reconstruction methods [14]. The four methods of UCL reconstruction included: (1) figure-of-eight technique, (2) docking technique as described by Rohrbough [5], (3) ulnar metal interference screw fixation with humeral docking technique (DANE TJ), and (4) ulnar cortical suspensory fixation with humeral docking technique. The peak load was measured to failure with the elbow flexed 90°; the increasing load was applied in a cyclic manner until 5 mm of joint displacement occurred. For the native anterior bundle of the UCL, the peak load to failure was 142.5 N. All of the reconstruction techniques had a peak load to failure significantly less than the native ligament ($p = 0.001$). The docking technique had a significantly greater peak load to failure in comparison to both the figure-of-eight and interference screw reconstructions. The cortical suspensory technique was found to have a significantly greater load to failure in comparison to the figure-of-eight technique .

Additionally, both the docking (701 cycles) and suspensory (703 cycles) reconstructions endured a significantly greater number of cycles before failure in comparison to the figure-of-eight technique (333). The failure of the graft occurred at the suture–tendon interface with UCL reconstructions using the figure-of-eight, docking, and suspensory fixation methods. Grafts with interference screw fixation failed at the screw–tendon interface; two grafts actually tore during interference screw insertion and required subsequent revision with another graft to complete the biomechanical analysis.

Jackson et al. tested the load to failure in cadaver elbows using a single-bundle graft construct [8]. UCL reconstruction with bisuspensory cortical fixation was compared to the docking technique as described by Rohrbough [5]. Suspensory fixation of the proximal ends of the graft was achieved with the Arthrex ACL Tightrope RT (Arthrex, Naples, FL). The ultimate torque to failure was 25.1 N m for the docking technique and 26.5 N m for the bisuspensory fixation; these were not significantly different ($p = 0.78$). The failure occurred at the suture–tendon interface in six of six (100%) of the cadaver elbows reconstructed with bisuspensory fixation and in five of six (83%) of the elbows reconstructed using the docking technique, with the remaining failure occurring as an ulnar bone bridge fracture. For both reconstruction types, valgus laxity was similar to the elbow with a native UCL from 0 to 120° of elbow range of motion .

Reconstruction of the UCL using interference screw fixation was evaluated by Ahmad et al. [6]. In their study, the native ligament was compared with UCL reconstruction using interference screw fixation for both humeral and ulnar graft fixation. A doubled palmaris longus graft was used and tensioned at 60°. The data demonstrated an ultimate valgus moment for intact elbows (34.0 N m) that was not significantly different from the reconstructed elbows (30.6 N m). Graft failure was most commonly due to the graft rupture (60%) followed by ulnar tunnel fracture (20%). The biomechanical stability of this technique and ease of interference screw insertion in the ulna have encouraged research regarding interference screw fixation in conjunction with the docking technique (DANE TJ technique).

In summary, none of the classic UCL reconstruction methods have been found to consistently match the native UCL in terms of the biomechanical load to failure. Generally, the evidence supports the docking technique over the figure-of-eight techniques in regard to strength. The data are less clear in delineating the biomechanical advantages when using the docking method in conjunction with interference screws, suture anchors, or cortical suspensory devices. More recent studies suggest that UCL repair with internal brace augmentation may be superior to all types of reconstruction in appropriate patients, which is discussed in a separate chapter.

Results of biomechanical studies are valuable but must be subsequently supported by clinical data, especially as these time zero biomechanical studies do not account for the biomechanics of the reconstruction techniques when the graft has reached final maturation. No single biomechanical study can support the supremacy of one type of reconstruction technique; surgeon experience and clinical research must also be used to guide which reconstruction is best for each patient. We will now discuss three of these alternative UCL reconstruction techniques that may provide successful outcomes and minimize complications in both the primary and revision surgical settings.

Surgical Approach

The patient is placed in the supine position in the surgical theater, with a hand table to support the upper extremity. A tourniquet is applied to the upper arm outside of the sterile field. After a standard sterile preparation, the patient is draped in a normal fashion. Appropriate antibiotics are given for surgical prophylaxis prior to incision. The tourniquet is typically inflated to approximately 100–125 mmHg above the systolic blood pressure to control bleeding in the surgical field. Adjusted to the patient's size, an approximately 8 cm incision is made to allow for visualization of the medial epicondyle and the proximal–medial ulna in the region of the sublime tubercle. The medial antebrachial cutaneous nerve and branches are identified and protected.

Deep dissection is then performed to expose the ulnar collateral ligament. Two surgical approaches are typically used in modern-day UCL reconstruction surgery: flexor-pronator split and flexor-pronator elevation. The flexor-pronator split approach is performed at the anterior margin of the flexor carpi ulnaris, which targets the internervous plane between the flexor digitorum superficialis and the flexor carpi ulnaris. The flexor-pronator split approach does not require exposure in the region of the ulnar nerve or subsequent ulnar nerve transposition. The flexor-pronator elevation approach is performed more posteriorly between the humeral and ulnar heads of the flexor carpi ulnaris in the plane on the ulnar nerve; therefore, this approach requires an obligatory ulnar nerve transposition.

In both alternative UCL reconstruction techniques, routine subcutaneous ulnar nerve transposition is not necessary but may be performed depending upon the desired approach. However, ulnar nerve transposition may be considered if the patient has evidence of ulnar subluxation on physical exam, documented ulnar nerve conduction pathology, or sensory paresthesias in the ulnar nerve distribution.

Retraction of the flexor-pronator muscle group will allow visualization of the UCL. Confirmatory findings of an avulsion fracture, calcifications within the ligament, pathologic ligamentous laxity, and/or ligament disruption are then evaluated. Based on patient factors and surgeon preference, the palmaris or gracilis tendon grafts are harvested in the usual manner.

Surgical Technique: DANE TJ UCL Reconstruction

Potential advantages of interference screw fixation in the ulna have led to its use in conjunction with the docking technique for humeral fixation. This combination of two concepts is referred to the DANE TJ technique, in acknowledgment of innovation by Dr. David Altchek, Dr. Neal ElAttrache, and the first professional baseball player, Tommy John, to have a UCL reconstruction [9]. Some surgeons have even subsequently suggested utilizing interference screws for both ulnar and humeral fixation.

The ulna is prepared by identifying the sublime tubercle for interference screw placement. The bone tunnel should be angled toward the lateral aspect of the ulna, just distal to the region of the supinator crest, with a depth of 15 mm (Fig. 24.1). To prevent iatrogenic injury to the articular surface, the ulnar joint surface and the bone tunnel should be separated by 3–4 mm of subchondral bone. The diameter of the tunnel is usually equal to the diameter of the folded end of the stitched tendon graft .

Preparation of the humeral tunnel for the docking technique begins with the identification of the humeral insertion of the UCL on the inferior medial epicondyle. Drilling of the docking tunnel is performed in a distal-to-proximal direction with a 4.5 mm diameter drill bit. Two exit tunnels are drilled using a 2.7 mm drill bit with the distal aspect of each tunnel meeting in the 4.5 mm tunnel. The distal tunnel size is checked to ensure proper graft docking; if needed, the tunnel size can be increased to allow for the passage of the graft. A bone bridge of at least 5 mm between the 2.7 mm drill holes is needed to prevent fracture of the bone during knot tying.

Ulnar graft fixation is then performed (Fig. 24.2). The folded end of the graft is secured in the ulnar tunnel with a biotenodesis screw (Arthrex Inc., Naples, FL) that approximates the diameter of the tunnel. A smaller screw may be needed with a thicker autograft.

Humeral graft tensioning and fixation are then performed (Fig. 24.3). With the ulnohu-

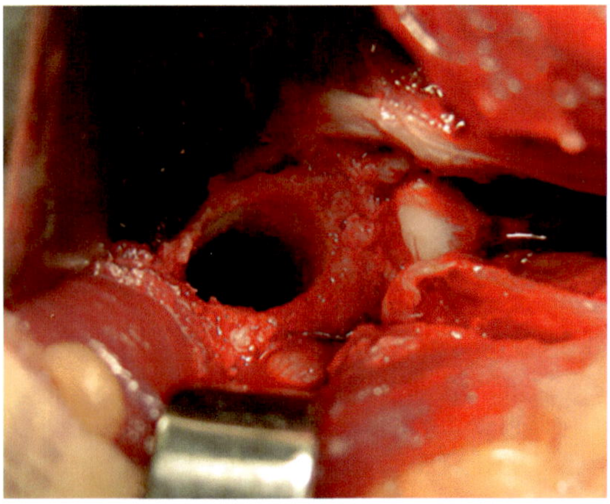

Fig. 24.1 Ulnar socket drilled in sublime tubercle. Note the preservation of bone bridge between socket and articular cartilage

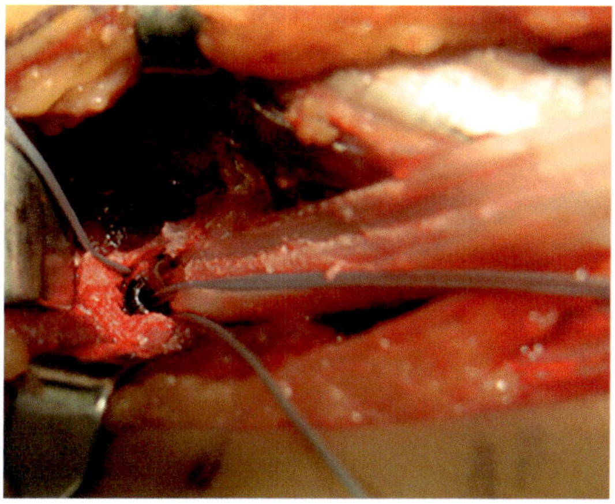

Fig. 24.2 The folded end of the graft is secured in the ulnar socket with an interference screw

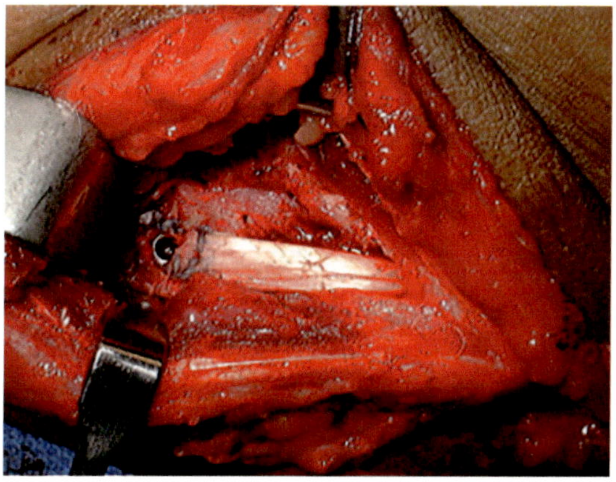

Fig. 24.3 Humeral graft tensioning and fixation is performed

meral joint appropriately positioned in a reduced position, the two ends of the graft are measured for proper tensioning in relation to the medial epicondyle. After removing the excess tendon, the two ends of the graft are prepared with a locking stitch using a nonabsorbable suture (Number 2 Fiberwire, Arthrex Inc., Naples, FL). The respective stitch for each end of the graft is then passed through one of the humeral tunnels, and the graft is seated in its ideal position. The native UCL is repaired before tensioning the graft. The suture ends are then tied over the bony bridge of the medial epicondyle with the ulnohumeral joint in a reduced position .

Surgical Technique: Cortical Suspensory UCL Reconstruction [8]

Cortical suspensory fixation in UCL reconstruction has been adapted from the anterior cruciate reconstruction literature. In both primary UCL reconstruction and in revision cases, cortical suspensory fixation can offer an alternative graft fixation method, especially in patients with bony defects that limit fixation options at the anatomic insertions of the UCL. Either proximal or distal suspensory fixation can be used in conjunction with established techniques such as the docking technique or interference screw fixation. For patients in whom both proximal and distal suspensory fixation is additionally desired, a cortical bisuspensory technique can be used [8] .

After a muscle splitting approach and identification of an incompetent UCL anterior bundle, sharp dissection is used to identify the proximal and distal insertions of the native ligament. The humeral tunnel is prepared using a 3.2 mm spade tip pin, which is placed at the inferior medial epicondyle. The pin is left in place and over-drilled with a 4.5 mm cannulated drill to create a 15 mm bone tunnel. The cortical suspensory implant (Arthrex ACL Tightrope RT, Arthrex, Naples, FL) is passed through the bone tunnel so that the implant is secured and seated on the proximal and slightly anterior cortex of the medial column of the distal humerus. The graft is passed through the looped end of the suspension suture and folded across the loop to create a doubled graft. This humeral graft fixation technique can be used with multiple fixation options for the ulna including interference screw fixation and cortical suspensory fixation.

The ulnar tunnel at the sublime tubercle is identified to locate the desired location for tunnel placement of the distal suspensory fixation. The 3.2 mm spade-tip pin is used to guide the cortical suspensory button placement; after initial perpendicular bony penetration, the pin is directed 30° posteriorly and 30° distally. The pin is left in place to allow the 4.5 mm cannulated drill to create a bone tunnel measuring about 30 mm. The cortical suspensory implant is then passed through the tunnels and seated on the lateral ulnar cortex, with the tightrope loop resting outside of the bone tunnel. The graft is then passed through the looped end of the suspension suture and folded across the loop to create a doubled graft. The cinching suture is ready for graft seating and tensioning. Ulnar fixation with the suspensory technique can be used with various fixation options proximally, including bone tunnels, suture anchors, interference screw fixation, the docking technique, and suspensory fixation. Prior to fixation of any UCL reconstruction, the native UCL is then repaired.

In cases of bisuspensory fixation, graft tensioning and fixation have been proposed to be performed in the following fashion. The folded graft should measure approximately the same diameter as the drill bit diameter and be at least 15 cm in length. The graft should be passed through the tightrope loop of the proximal and distal suspensory fixation devices, with the graft divided into thirds at each loop location. Position the central third of the graft between the two tightrope loops; this will allow later end-to-end suturing after seating the folded graft in each tunnel. The humeral cinching suture is used to seat the proximal end of the graft by pulling in-line with graft seating. Next, the cinching suture of the ulnar suspensory implant is pulled to seat the ulnar portion of the graft, with up to 20 mm of the distal graft within the ulnar tunnel. The tensioning of the distal end of the graft within the ulna should be performed with the ulnohumeral joint reduced anatomically while maintaining a varus force at 30° of flexion. With the central third of the graft well tensioned, the proximal and distal ends of the graft should have adequate length to cross the joint line for secure fixation to each other utilizing figure-of-eight nonabsorbable sutures (Number 2 Fiberwire, Arthrex Inc., Naples, FL).

Surgical Technique: Anatomic UCL Reconstruction [15]

Recent studies on the anatomy of the UCL have demonstrated that the ulnar insertional footprint is more broad and tapered distally than previously thought [16, 17]. As a result, Camp et al. [15] developed a novel anatomic UCL reconstruction technique based on this new anatomic understanding.

After a standard approach, a 4.0 mm socket with a 15 mm depth and 2 small (2 mm) perforating tunnels are drilled into the humerus in the same manner as the docking technique. Two shuttle sutures are then used to pass an all-suture adjustable suspensory loop (Arthrex, Inc., Naples, FL) from the smaller 2 mm tunnels out through the 4 mm socket. A palmaris graft is then folded in half and the suspensory loop is assembled around the center of the graft. The loop is then tensioned until the graft is 10 mm into the humeral socket.

Focus is then shifted to the ulnar fixation. Two 1.3 mm all-suture anchors (FiberTak, Arthrex) are placed just distal to the joint line at the anterior and posterior footprints of the native ligament (approximately 5 mm apart). These are set aside for future use. A 2-0 absorbable suture is then used to repair the native capsule and ligament if amenable. This suture is placed prior to passing the graft, but is tied afterward. A closed-loop number 0 nonabsorbable suture is then used to suture together the two distal limbs of the graft using a whipstitch technique. The excess graft is excised. The loop suture is then cut to create two free ends, which are then loaded onto an intramedullary cortical suspensory button (Arthrex, Inc., Naples FL).

The sutures from the two anchors are now passed around each limb of the graft, with the more anterior anchor being passed around the anterior limb and the posterior anchor around the posterior limb. The graft is then tensioned and cycled. The arm is put into 30 degrees of flexion and a varus load is applied. While maintaining this position and force, the sutures from the anchors are tied around each limb of the graft, securing it to the proximal aspect of the UCL footprint on the ulna.

For the distal ulnar fixation, a 3.2 mm, unicortical hole is drilled at the apex of the UCL footprint. The suspensory button is inserted into the intramedullary canal and deployed. The sutures are tensioned in order to reduce the graft to the

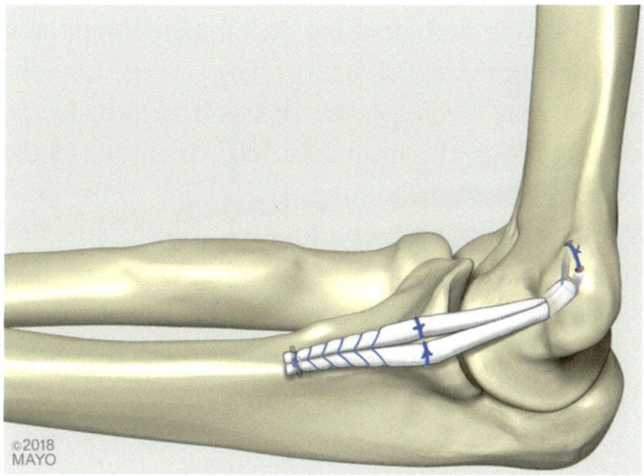

Fig. 24.4 Anatomic UCL reconstruction technique

ulna. Sutures are tied over the top of the graft, creating a closed-loop construct. The suspensory loop on the humeral side is again tensioned, and the suture ends are tied over the bone bridge to create a closed-loop construct. Finally, the sutures that were originally passed through the capsule and ligament for repair are tied in order to ensure that the graft remains extra-articular (Fig. 24.4).

Surgical Closure and Postoperative Care

The wound is then closed in layers, beginning with the flexor-pronator mass fascia, and ending with the skin. Release of the tourniquet should be performed prior to skin closure to ensure proper hemostasis. Standard dressings are applied, and a long arm splint is applied with a neutral forearm position and the elbow flexed slightly less than 90°.

The splint should be removed after 7–10 days to allow for assessment of the wound and to initiate an early gentle range of motion of the elbow, shoulder, and wrist. After splint removal, a hinged elbow brace can be used, but there is no consensus regarding the guidelines for utilization. In one literature review of UCL reconstruction, hinged elbow braces were used in only 139 of 351 (40%) patients [11]. Gentle strengthening of the forearm muscles can begin in the first postoperative month. However, valgus stresses on the graft should be avoided until after the second postoperative month, and throwing activities should not begin until at least 4 months after the reconstruction.

The postoperative rehabilitation program recommended for each reconstruction technique has many similarities; however, there is a paucity of literature describing differences in rehabilitative principles according to surgical technique. The study by Cain utilizing a figure-of-eight technique reviewed 1281 patients that were treated postoperatively with a 4-phase rehabilitation protocol as described by Wilk et al. [18]. They advocated for use of a hinged elbow brace. Full range of motion was ideally reached by 6 weeks while protecting the UCL reconstruction from valgus stress. Strengthening exercises were initiated at week 3 and were advanced at week 9. Throwing programs were typically started at week 16, and return to competition around 12 months after surgery.

Discussion

UCL reconstruction is a complex surgical procedure that is being performed with increasing frequency [10]. The surgical technique has evolved from the initial figure-of-eight technique with the goal of improving the biomechanical properties and to facilitate the ease of reconstruction. Based on the literature, the most common techniques for UCL reconstruction are the figure-of-eight and the docking techniques [10, 11]. The docking technique was an initial modification of the figure-of-eight technique that improved both the ultimate load to failure [13] and aimed to preserve some of the bone integrity through minimization of bone tunnel size. As a result of these improvements, there has been a trend toward increased use of the docking technique over the figure-of-eight technique. However, a recent single surgeon cohort study by Arner et al. [19] found that the modified Jobe and docking techniques are equivalent in regards to return to play, Kerlan-Jobe Orthopaedic Clinic scores, and the need for subsequent surgery. This suggests that the previous predilection for the docking technique based mostly on biomechanical studies may not be clinically significant. More recent advancements have focused on continued biomechanical and surgical improvements as well as focusing on creating a more anatomic reconstruction.

Cadaveric studies focusing on anatomy have demonstrated that the central fibers of the anterior and posterior bands of the anterior bundle of the UCL are the most isometric division during elbow motion [20]. As opposed to the tunnels converging around the sublime tubercle on the ulnar side, single-bundle reconstruction of these central fibers can be achieved with interference screw fixation as described by Ahmad [6] that can be reconstructed in a doubled graft technique using the DANE TJ technique [9], or can be recreated utilizing cortical suspensory fixation. More recent studies have suggested that the ulnar insertion of the UCL is more elongated and tapered distally than previously depicted [16, 17]. This was the focus of a novel anatomic reconstruction technique described by Camp et al. [15].

DANE TJ UCL Reconstruction

In terms of the interference screw fixation, the DANE TJ technique allows the surgeon to use familiar concepts to facilitate a solid UCL reconstruction and has also shown good clinical outcomes. The risk of bone tunnel fracture has inspired much of the research regarding UCL reconstruction. The DANE TJ technique avoids the use of ulnar bone tunnels, which eliminates the risk of ulnar bone tunnel fracture. This avoidance of bone tunnels has led to failures of the UCL reconstructions in new locations. Biomechanical studies suggest the suture–tendon interface was a frequent location for graft failure in the figure-of-eight, docking, and cortical suspensory techniques [8, 14]. The suture–tendon interface does not exist with interference screw fixation; however, failure with interference screw fixation was associated with graft rupture, ulnar tunnel fracture, and graft damage during insertion [6, 14]. Despite this limitation, graft damage during screw insertion is uncommonly reported with routine use of modern interference screw designs and materials.

The humeral docking technique component helps minimize the use of large bone tunnels, which may decrease the risk of fracture. In the docking site, the graft has 360° exposure to the bone for biologic healing. Tensioning of the graft is also facilitated by pulling the sutures attached to the ends of the graft in-line through the smaller bone tunnels; secure fixation is easily achieved when tying these suture ends over the bony bridge. As reported with figure-of-eight and cortical suspensory techniques, biomechanical studies of the docking technique have also suggested that the suture–tendon interface was the most frequent location for graft failure [8, 14]. Although some advocates, therefore, suggest the utilization of interference screw fixation on the humeral side, suture–tendon interface failure has not been commonly reported in the clinical setting .

The ulnar fixation of the DANE TJ technique uses the interference screw placed at the sublime tubercle. This allows for anatomic reconstruction of the anterior bundle of the UCL using a familiar technique to many orthopedic surgeons. Biomechanically, interference screw fixation has been shown to offer a similar valgus moment to failure as the native UCL [6]. The avoidance of bone tunnels not only helps facilitate the surgery, but also allows for a doubled reconstruction of the anterior bundle in its anatomic location. However, the interference screw itself does limit the amount of bone within the tunnel available for bone–tendon healing. While offering excellent frictional fixation of the graft in a secure manner, the interference screw pressure may form an avascular zone that limits the biologic incorporation. Additionally, the interference screw may have difficulty achieving stable fixation in revision cases with significant bone loss at the sublime tubercle .

In a clinical case series, Dines et al. described the outcomes of the DANE TJ technique in 22 patients [9]. With a mean follow-up duration of 35 months, their hybrid technique had an 86% excellent outcome on the modified Conway scale. For the 20 athletes that participated in baseball, 17 (85%) had an excellent result. These results are similar to other large series by Cain and Andrews [10]. Additionally, 3 of the 22 patients had revision UCL reconstruction; 2 of the 3 revision patients had an excellent result. Postsurgical ulnar nerve pathology was observed in only one revision patient who had prior UCL reconstruction and ulnar nerve transposition. Outcomes for the DANE TJ hybrid technique support its similarity to prior data regarding primary UCL reconstruction. For revision UCL reconstruction, the DANE TJ method offers an alternative technique to the traditional docking or figure-of-eight methods.

Cortical Suspensory UCL Reconstruction

The suspensory fixation technique is a relatively new type of fixation for use in UCL reconstruction. Humeral or ulnar graft fixation with suspensory fixation can aid graft tensioning by allowing graft tensioning in-line with graft seating, similar to the DANE TJ technique. By suspending the graft in the bone tunnel, a greater exposure of the graft to the bone may allow for better healing at the bone–tendon junction. Additionally, the avoidance of aperture fixation can be helpful in revision situations with bone loss at the sublime tubercle or the inferior medial epicondyle .

Despite the benefits of suspensory fixation, some limitations may exist in relation to this technology. When utilizing cortical suspensory fixation on one side (i.e., either ulnar or humeral), graft slippage may theoretically occur through the endobutton fixation. When performing a bisuspensory technique, graft slippage may also occur; however, the reconstruction also relies on suture–tendon interface fixation that may also be a source of failure. Despite these potential limitations, biomechanical studies have supported a solid fixation mechanism when utilizing the cortical suspensory technique in the setting of clinical success being reported when using this technology in other surgical procedures, including ACL reconstruction. In recent years, studies have found cortical suspensory fixation for UCL reconstruction to have both good clinical outcomes [21] and biomechanics that are comparable to the docking technique [22]. Further research is warranted to directly compare clinical outcomes of cortical suspensory device fixation to other UCL reconstruction fixation techniques.

Anatomic UCL Reconstruction

This novel UCL reconstruction technique developed by Camp et al. [15] has promising initial biomechanical results. In their cadaveric study, this technique was found to have superior strength and resistance to valgus torque when compared with the docking technique. They also found that reconstructions using this new anatomic technique performed similar to native UCL specimens from prior biomechanical studies. By providing a more anatomic reconstruction, Camp et al. hypothesized that this technique more accurately recreates normal joint kinematics. This increased initial strength may allow for earlier initiation of throwing programs and ultimately quicker return to play.

Due to the relatively recent publication of this novel anatomic technique, there is limited information available beyond the previously discussed study. Future research on this novel technique is warranted based on these early results. More biomechanical studies comparing the anatomic technique to the docking and modified Jobe techniques would be beneficial to ensure reproducibility. Clinical trials with patient-oriented outcomes will truly reveal if this technique proves to be practically superior to the current, well-established reconstruction techniques.

Conclusion

The clinical outcomes of UCL reconstruction have been best studied regarding the figure-of-eight technique and the docking technique. Driven by the nature of these injuries during athletic performance, studies have emphasized the return to the presurgical level of sport as a holistic evaluation of the athlete's outcome after UCL reconstruction [23]. Additionally, complications and revision surgery have also been examined.

For athletes with an incompetent UCL, the alternative UCL reconstruction techniques have been shown to have a solid biomechanical profile and excellent outcomes on par with other UCL reconstruction techniques. Additionally, it can be agreed that some of these techniques allow for a more anatomic reconstruction and help facilitate the ease of graft tensioning and graft fixation using familiar implants. A novel anatomic reconstruction technique seems to be the first technique to show improved biomechanical properties in comparison to the docking technique. More research on its biomechanics and eventually its clinical outcomes is warranted. With the significant increase in UCL reconstructions being performed each year, these alternative techniques will certainly continue to amass attention within the orthopedic sports medicine literature.

References

1. Mahure SA, et al. Disproportionate trends in ulnar collateral ligament reconstruction: projections through 2025 and a literature review. J Shoulder Elb Surg. 2016;25(6):1005–12.
2. Werner SL, et al. Biomechanics of the elbow during baseball pitching. J Orthop Sports Phys Ther. 1993;17(6):274–8.
3. Jobe FW, Stark H, Lombardo SJ. Reconstruction of the ulnar collateral ligament in athletes. J Bone Joint Surg Am. 1986;68(8):1158–63.
4. Callaway GH, et al. Biomechanical evaluation of the medial collateral ligament of the elbow. J Bone Joint Surg Am. 1997;79(8):1223–31.
5. Rohrbough JT, et al. Medial collateral ligament reconstruction of the elbow using the docking technique. Am J Sports Med. 2002;30(4):541–8.
6. Ahmad CS, Lee TQ, ElAttrache NS. Biomechanical evaluation of a new ulnar collateral ligament reconstruction technique with interference screw fixation. Am J Sports Med. 2003;31(3):332–7.
7. Hechtman KS, et al. Long-term results of ulnar collateral ligament reconstruction in throwing athletes based on a hybrid technique. Am J Sports Med. 2011;39(2):342–7.
8. Jackson TJ, et al. Ulnar collateral ligament reconstruction using bisuspensory fixation: a biomechanical comparison with the docking technique. Am J Sports Med. 2013;41(5):1158–64.
9. Dines JS, et al. Clinical outcomes of the DANE TJ technique to treat ulnar collateral ligament insufficiency of the elbow. Am J Sports Med. 2007;35(12):2039–44.
10. Cain EL Jr, et al. Outcome of ulnar collateral ligament reconstruction of the elbow in 1281 athletes: results in 743 athletes with minimum 2-year follow-up. Am J Sports Med. 2010;38(12):2426–34.
11. Vitale MA, Ahmad CS. The outcome of elbow ulnar collateral ligament reconstruction in overhead athletes: a systematic review. Am J Sports Med. 2008;36(6):1193–205.
12. Fleisig GS, et al. Biomechanics of overhand throwing with implications for injuries. Sports Med. 1996;21(6):421–37.
13. Paletta GA Jr, et al. Biomechanical evaluation of 2 techniques for ulnar collateral ligament reconstruction of the elbow. Am J Sports Med. 2006;34(10):1599–603.
14. Armstrong AD, et al. A biomechanical comparison of four reconstruction techniques for the medial collateral ligament-deficient elbow. J Shoulder Elb Surg. 2005;14(2):207–15.
15. Camp, et al. Reconstruction of the medial ulnar collateral ligament of the elbow: biomechanical comparison of a novel anatomic technique to the docking technique. Orthop J Sports Med. 2019;7(7)
16. Dugas JR, Ostrander RV, Cain EL, Kingsley D, Andrews JR. Anatomy of the anterior bundle of the ulnar collateral ligament. J Shoulder Elbow Surg. 2007;16(5):657–60.
17. Farrow LD, Mahoney AJ, Stefancin JJ, Taljanovic MS, Sheppard JE, Schickendantz MS. Quantitative analysis of the medial ulnar collateral ligament ulnar footprint and its relationship to the ulnar sublime tubercle. Am J Sports Med. 2011;39(9):1936–41.
18. Wilk KE, Arrigo C, Andrews JR. Rehabilitation of the elbow in the throwing athlete. J Orthop Sports Phys Ther. 1993;17(6):305–17.
19. Arner JW, Chang ES, Bayer S, Bradley JP. Direct comparison of modified Jobe and docking ulnar collateral ligament reconstruction at midterm follow-up. Am J Sports Med. 2019;47(1):144–50.
20. Ochi N, et al. Anatomic relation between the medial collateral ligament of the elbow and the humero-ulnar joint axis. J Shoulder Elb Surg. 1999;8(1):6–10.
21. Lynch, et al. Biomechanical evaluation of the TightRope versus traditional docking ulnar collateral ligament reconstruction technique: kinematic and failure testing. Am J Sports Med. 2013;41(5):1165–73.
22. Myeroff C, Brock JL, Huffman GR. Ulnar collateral ligament reconstruction in athletes using a cortical button suspension technique. J Shoulder Elb Surg. 2018;27(8):1366–72.
23. Conway JE, et al. Medial instability of the elbow in throwing athletes. Treatment by repair or reconstruction of the ulnar collateral ligament. J Bone Joint Surg Am. 1992;74(1):67–83.

Combined Flexor-Pronator Mass and Ulnar Collateral Ligament Injuries

25

Alexander Christ, Joshua S. Dines, Christopher Chin, and David W. Altchek

Introduction

Valgus moments of the elbow are primarily resisted by the anterior bundle of the ulnar collateral ligament (UCL). When the UCL becomes attenuated or fails in the overhead throwing athlete, tendinosis and/or tears in the flexor-pronator mass can also occur, which may affect the athlete's ability to throw and return to competition. A subgroup of athletes with both UCL and flexor-pronator mass injuries was first described by Conway et al. and later shown to have inferior outcomes when compared to athletes with UCL injury alone [1, 2]. The most prominent risk factor for combined injury is age greater than 30 years, with prior steroid injection possibly playing a role.

The importance of the flexor-pronator mass as a dynamic valgus stabilizer in the elbow has been demonstrated in cadaveric, in vivo, and clinical outcomes studies. Through cadaveric dissection, Davidson et al. demonstrated that the flexor carpi ulnaris primarily and the flexor digitorum superficialis secondarily are in line with the UCL anatomically and able to provide resistance to valgus stress [3]. Park and Ahmad similarly demonstrated in UCL-deficient, cadaveric models that contraction of flexor carpi ulnaris and flexor digitorum superficialis provided the most correction of valgus angle when compared to elbows with an intact UCL [4]. Electromyography has also shown that pitchers with valgus instability have decreased flexor-pronator mass activity during the throwing motion, further confirming the action of the flexor-pronator mass as a dynamic stabilizer against valgus stress [5, 6].

Clinical outcomes based on the surgical approach underscore the importance of the flexor-pronator mass as a valgus stabilizer as well. Multiple groups have described a muscle-splitting approach that limits dissection through the flexor-pronator mass [7, 8]. This approach is now widely used and may generate improved clinical outcomes when compared to the original approach described by Jobe, where the flexor-pronator mass was detached and mobilized off of the medial epicondyle for visualization of the UCL.

Diagnosis

Diagnosis of combined UCL–flexor-pronator mass injuries requires a thorough physical exam and imaging studies. Patients present with history and physical exam findings consistent with val-

A. Christ
Hospital for Special Surgery, New York, NY, USA

J. S. Dines (✉)
Department of Orthopedic Surgery, Sports Medicine and Shoulder Service, Sports Medicine Institute, Hospital for Special Surgery, New York, NY, USA

C. Chin · D. W. Altchek
Sports Medicine and Shoulder Service, Hospital for Special Surgery, New York, NY, USA

J. S. Dines et al. (eds.), *Elbow Ulnar Collateral Ligament Injury*,
https://doi.org/10.1007/978-3-030-69567-5_25

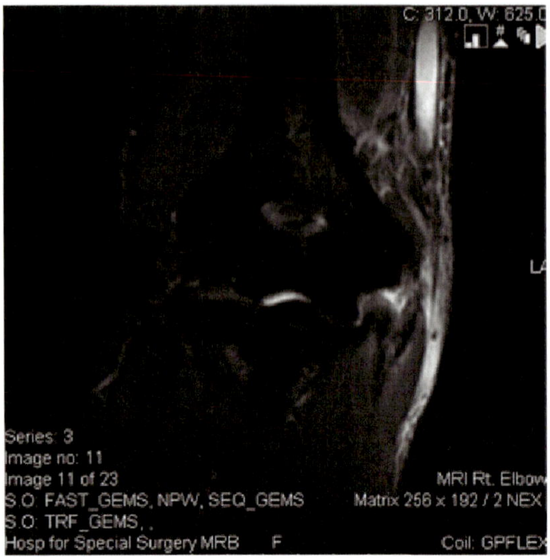

Fig. 25.1 Coronal plane MR image highlighting combined UCL tear and flexor-pronator tear

gus instability of the elbow including medial elbow pain, inability to throw secondary to pain, weakness, and pain reproduced upon resisted wrist flexion and forearm pronation. In the only published study examining the characteristics of patients with combined injuries, all patients described chronic elbow pain and instability, and half of the patients described acute-on-chronic medial elbow pain. In that same series, preoperative MRI reliably diagnosed pathologic changes in the flexor-pronator mass as well as the UCL. Therefore, preoperative MRI is indicated in all cases to assess both the extent of UCL injury and the integrity of the flexor-pronator mass (Fig. 25.1).

Operative Treatment

In cases of mild-to-moderate tendinosis, the tissue can be debrided through the same muscle splitting approach or through a separate anterior flexor-pronator incision, based on surgeon preference.

If a severe tendinosis, a partial tear, or a complete tear of the flexor-pronator mass in the setting of a concomitant UCL tear is seen, a flexor-pronator elevating approach is used. The UCL is reconstructed using the surgeon's preferred technique. After completion of the ligament reconstruction, the flexor-pronator tendon pathology is addressed. Degenerated, torn tissue can be debrided and repaired back to the medial epicondyle using a suture repair with No. 1 Ethibond through 1.5 mm transosseous tunnels. The suture limbs extending from the medial epicondyle from the UCL reconstruction are then used in the repair as well. If there is more extensive tearing or debrided tendon, additional 1.5 mm transosseous tunnels can be made at the native origin of the flexor-pronator mass on the anterosuperior aspect of the medial epicondyle of the humerus to aid in the repair [2]. If indicated, an ulnar nerve transposition can be performed after the repair of the flexor-pronator mass. The fascia of the flexor-pronator mass should then be repaired, followed by the closure of the surgical wound in layers. The elbow is then placed in a plaster splint in 45° of flexion with the forearm in a supinated position.

Rehabilitation

The postoperative protocol for patients is the same, regardless of isolated UCL reconstruction versus combined UCL reconstruction and flexor-pronator mass debridement or repair. The arm is kept in a splint for 1 week, after which the sutures are removed and the elbow is managed in a hinged brace for 3 weeks. Motion in the brace is allowed from 45 to 90° of flexion, which is advanced slowly over 5 weeks. Formal physical therapy without the brace is initiated at 6 weeks with rotator cuff and forearm exercises, taking care not to overload the flexor-pronator mass. Patients start an interval throwing program at around 4 months and are not allowed to pitch competitively until at least 9 months to a year after surgery.

Outcomes and Complications

Conway et al. were the first to describe these combined injuries in throwing athletes [1]. In their series, 9 of 70 throwers (12.8%) had such pathology. After surgical treatment, seven of the nine (78%) returned to their previous level of play. More recently, Osbahr and colleagues looked at a subgroup of patients undergoing UCL reconstruction that underwent concomitant flexor-pronator repair. Eight of 187 patients had such an injury, and only one of eight returned to their previous level of play [2]. Five of the eight had poor outcomes. Clearly, these results are inferior to those reported with isolated UCL reconstruction. It is important to recognize that these were all professional baseball players, and therefore, return to the previous level of play was difficult, but these numbers are in stark contrast to the 90% or greater return to the previous level of play for players with isolated UCL injuries that undergo reconstructive surgery [9, 10]. Interestingly, one reason for the better results in the Conway series may be due to the fact that they were using the historical flexor-pronator take-down approach, as opposed to the muscle splitting approach . Our present treatment algorithm is to use this same approach for combined pathology, which may result in improved outcomes in the future.

The main complication seen in patients with combined UCL and flexor-pronator mass injuries is reoperation. In the Osbahr series, three of eight patients underwent reoperation for flexor-pronator mass tear postoperatively. Two had flexor-pronator mass debridements that subsequently tore, while the third was initially treated for a full tear and retore his flexor-pronator mass. Only one of these three returned to major league baseball. Due to the high reoperation rate in that series using the flexor-splitting approach, the authors suggest using the flexor-pronator mass take-down approach for all combined injuries, as it allows for better visualization and assessment of the flexor-pronator mass and minimizes dissection of the musculature.

References

1. Conway JE, Jobe FW, Glousman RE, Pink M. Medial instability of the elbow in throwing athletes. Treatment by repair or reconstruction of the ulnar collateral ligament. J Bone Joint Surg Am. 1992;74(1):67–83.
2. Osbahr DC, Swaminathan SS, Allen AA, Dines JS, Coleman SH, Altchek DW. Combined flexor-pronator mass and ulnar collateral ligament injuries in the elbows of older baseball players. Am J Sports Med. 2010;38(4):733–9.
3. Davidson PA, Pink M, Perry J, Jobe FW. Functional anatomy of the flexor pronator muscle group in relation to the medial collateral ligament of the elbow. Am J Sports Med. 1995;23(2):245–50.
4. Park MC, Ahmad CS. Dynamic contributions of the flexor-pronator mass to elbow valgus stability. J Bone Joint Surg Am. 2004;86-A(10):2268–74.
5. Glousman RE, Barron J, Jobe FW, Perry J, Pink M. An electromyographic analysis of the elbow in normal and injured pitchers with medial collateral ligament insufficiency. Am J Sports Med. 1992;20(3):311–7.
6. Hamilton CD, Glousman RE, Jobe FW, Brault J, Pink M, Perry J. Dynamic stability of the elbow: electromyographic analysis of the flexor pronator group and the extensor group in pitchers with valgus instability. J Shoulder Elb Surg. 1996;5(5):347–54.
7. Smith GR, Altchek DW, Pagnani MJ, Keeley JR. A muscle-splitting approach to the ulnar collateral ligament of the elbow. Neuroanatomy and operative technique. Am J Sports Med. 1996;24(5):575–80.
8. Thompson WH, Jobe FW, Yocum LA, Pink MM. Ulnar collateral ligament reconstruction in athletes: muscle-splitting approach without transposition of the ulnar nerve. J Shoulder Elb Surg. 2001;10(2):152–7.
9. Rohrbough JT, Altchek DW, Hyman J, Williams RJ 3rd, Botts JD. Medial collateral ligament reconstruction of the elbow using the docking technique. Am J Sports Med. 2002;30(4):541–8.
10. Vitale MA, Ahmad CS. The outcome of elbow ulnar collateral ligament reconstruction in overhead athletes: a systematic review. Am J Sports Med. 2008;36(6):1193–205.

Ulnar Nerve Issues in Throwing Athletes

26

Michael E. Angeline, Albert O. Gee, Joshua S. Dines, and David W. Altchek

Introduction

The ulnar collateral ligament (UCL) reconstruction surgery has evolved over time since it was first performed by Dr. Jobe in 1974 [1]. The original technique described a submuscular ulnar nerve transposition that was performed in each case [2]. Since that time, further iterations have utilized a subcutaneous transposition, while others have moved away from an obligatory transposition of the nerve, performing it only selectively when indicated [3–11]. This progression has shown improved outcomes of UCL reconstruction surgery, particularly in regard to postoperative ulnar nerve complications that have lessened with newer techniques.

M. E. Angeline (✉)
Mercy Health System, Janesville, WI, USA
e-mail: mangeline@mhemail.org

A. O. Gee
Orthopaedics and Sports Medicine, University of Washington Medical Center, Seattle, WA, USA

J. S. Dines
Department of Orthopedic Surgery, Sports Medicine and Shoulder Service, Sports Medicine Institute, Hospital for Special Surgery, New York, NY, USA

D. W. Altchek
Sports Medicine and Shoulder Service, Hospital for Special Surgery, New York, NY, USA

History

When Dr. Frank Jobe performed his landmark operation to reconstruct the UCL of the elbow [2], he used a surgical approach that released the flexor-pronator musculature off the medial humeral epicondyle, dissected out and mobilized the ulnar nerve prior to UCL reconstruction, and performed a submuscular ulnar nerve transposition at the completion of the procedure (Figs. 26.1 and 26.2).

In the original series of 16 elite throwing athletes, Jobe reported a significant complication rate of 31%, which was mostly postoperative ulnar nerve dysfunction [2]. Of the five patients who had ulnar nerve symptoms after reconstruction, two required additional surgery for ulnar nerve neurolysis. Despite this complication rate, this procedure was considered a success as 63% of these athletes were able to return to their previous level of the overhead sport.

In a follow-up series, which included the original series described by Jobe, Conway and colleagues evaluated 71 athletes that underwent either UCL repair or reconstruction with palmaris longus autograft (14 repairs, 56 reconstructions) using the same original technique that included submuscular ulnar nerve transposition [12]. Follow-up ranged from 2 to 15 years and the authors found a return to the previous competition level rate of 68% at an average of 1 year after surgery. Again, complications mostly involved

J. S. Dines et al. (eds.), *Elbow Ulnar Collateral Ligament Injury*,
https://doi.org/10.1007/978-3-030-69567-5_26

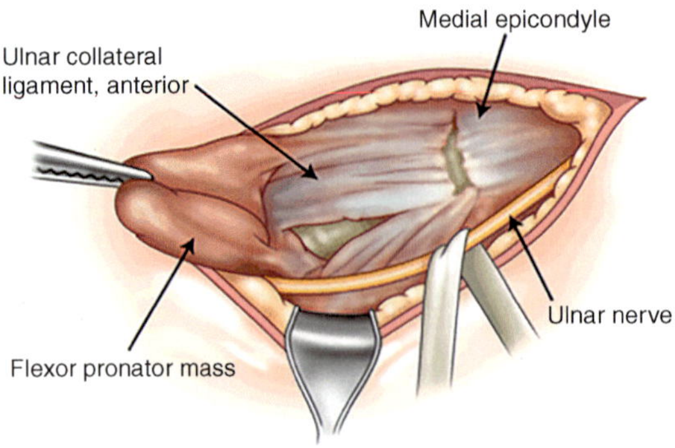

Fig. 26.1 Illustration of the original approach to the anterior band of the ulnar collateral ligament as described by Jobe [2]. This technique called for a detachment of the flexor-pronator mass from the medial epicondyle in order to expose the UCL and also for the purpose of submuscular ulnar nerve transposition

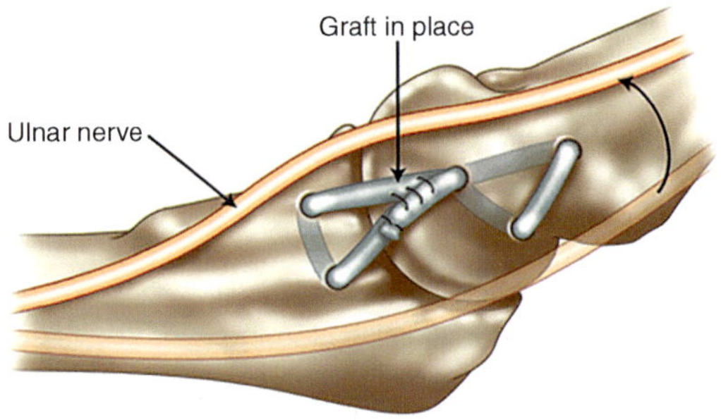

Fig. 26.2 Illustration of the UCL reconstruction graft in a figure-of-eight configuration from the original Jobe technique [2]. Also diagrammed is the transposition of the ulnar nerve

ulnar nerve problems postoperatively and were reported in 15 patients (21%) of which nine required further decompression surgery. At the final follow-up, five patients continued to have ulnar nerve paresthesias and one patient had notable muscle wasting.

Surgical Modifications

In light of the high rate of postoperative ulnar nerve complications, Jobe's original technique was modified in an effort to limit the extent of dissection and detachment of the flexor-pronator mass and minimize handling of the ulnar nerve.

The Hospital for Special Surgery (HSS) Technique

Smith et al. [13] were the first to describe a muscle-splitting approach in place of elevating the entire flexor-pronator mass in a study conducted at HSS. They described a safe zone in the posterior one-third of the common flexor muscle bundle to expose the UCL. The authors performed a cadaveric study, in which they plotted points of innervation of the flexor-pronator from branches of the median and ulnar nerve and identified a watershed area between the two nerve distributions that defined the muscle-split (Fig. 26.3).

In their initial series of 22 patients who underwent UCL surgery (6 traditional reconstructions, 5 had augmented repairs, and 11 primary repairs with suture-anchors) through this approach, they noted no clinical evidence of neuropathy of either the ulnar or median nerve at 1 year after surgery [13].

Using this muscle splitting approach, Rohrbough et al. [7] described a series of 36 patients who underwent UCL reconstruction using a newly described humeral bone tunnel configuration, decreasing the number of drill holes from three to a single tunnel, which was termed the “docking technique” (Fig. 26.4). In their series, ulnar nerve transposition was only performed if the patient had a history of chronic nerve symptoms preoperatively and characteristic findings on physical examination. A total of two patients underwent a subcutaneous ulnar nerve transposition, which was stabilized with a fascial sling. One patient had ulnar nerve paresthesias that resolved within 3 weeks after surgery. Overall, 33 of 36 patients returned to their preinjury level of activity or higher at a mean follow-up of 3.3 years.

In a more recent follow-up of UCL reconstructions performed using this same docking technique, Dodson et al. [9] found ongoing excellent results in 90% of the 100 patients in this series. A total of 22 patients underwent subcutaneous ulnar nerve transposition using an intermuscular septal sling [14]. This resulted in a

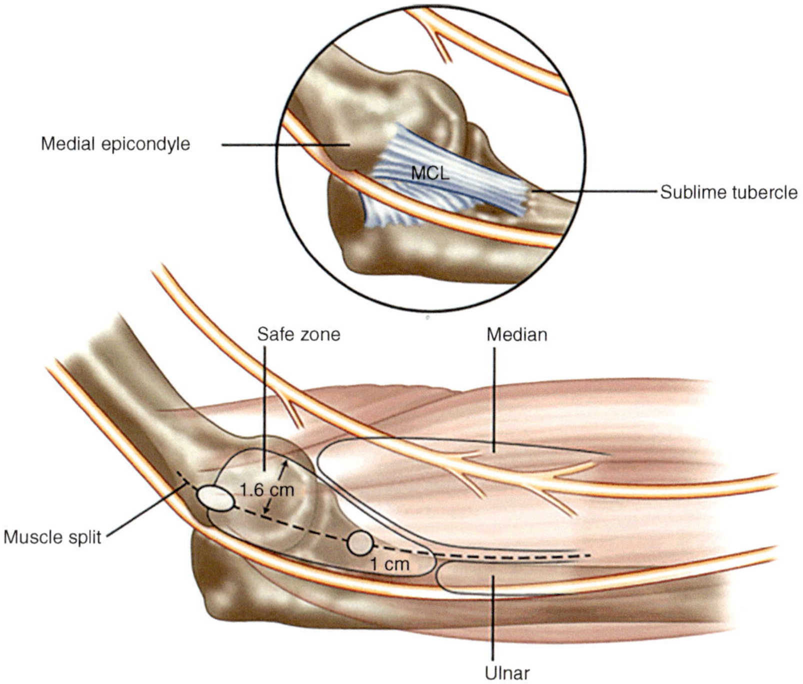

Fig. 26.3 A diagram of the "safe zone" for a muscle-split approach and the relationship of this split to the underlying UCL [13]

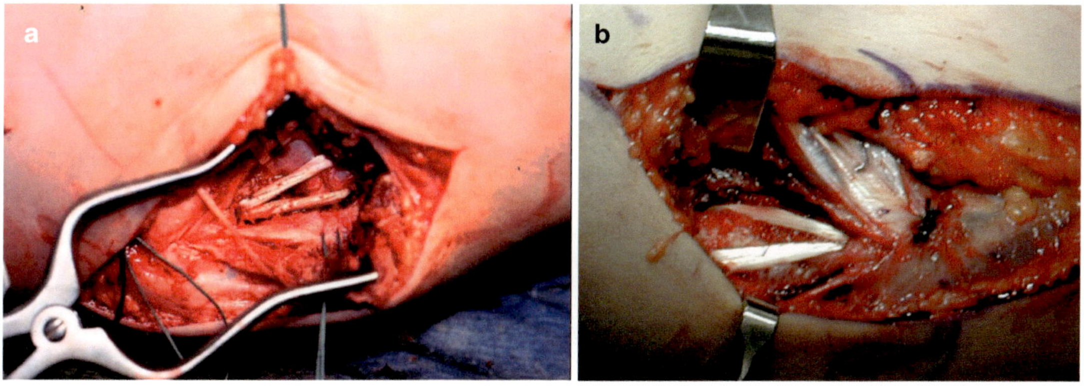

Fig. 26.4 (**a**) Clinical photo of the docking technique using a double-stranded palmaris longus graft. (**b**) Diagram of the docking technique illustrating the graft configuration and docking of both free ends into a single humeral tunnel with a bone bridge to secure and tension the graft [9]

2% complication rate as related to the ulnar nerve. These two patients had no preoperative nerve symptoms, and both had complete resolution of their symptoms after subsequent ulnar nerve transposition and had excellent results at final follow-up.

American Sports Medicine Institute (ASMI) Technique

During this same time period, another group of surgeons at the ASMI developed an alternate modification of Jobe's original surgical technique that was first published by Azar et al. [5]. They performed UCL surgery using a technique in which they retracted the flexor carpi ulnaris (FCU) anteriorly without detaching the muscle of the humeral epicondyle. Routine ulnar nerve transposition was performed in each case; however, they performed a subcutaneous ulnar nerve transposition in their technique using slings developed from the underlying fascia of the flexor-pronator musculature (Fig. 26.5). In their series of 91 throwing athletes who underwent UCL surgery (13 direct repairs and 78 reconstructions), they reported one case of transient ulnar nerve symptoms and found that 9 out of 10 patients who had preoperative ulnar nerve neuritis had resolution postoperatively. In this series, 79% of the throwing athletes who underwent reconstruction returned to their preinjury level or higher, while only 63% of direct repair patients were able to return to the same level of throwing activity.

In a follow-up to this original series, Cain et al. [15] evaluated a series of 1281 athletes (942 patients had a minimum 2-year follow-up) who underwent UCL surgery using this same surgical technique of FCU retraction anteriorly without detachment and subcutaneous ulnar nerve transposition in each case. The vast majority of these patients was overhead-throwing athletes and underwent autograft reconstruction, primarily using palmaris longus. They reported a return to preinjury or higher level of competition in 83% of patients.

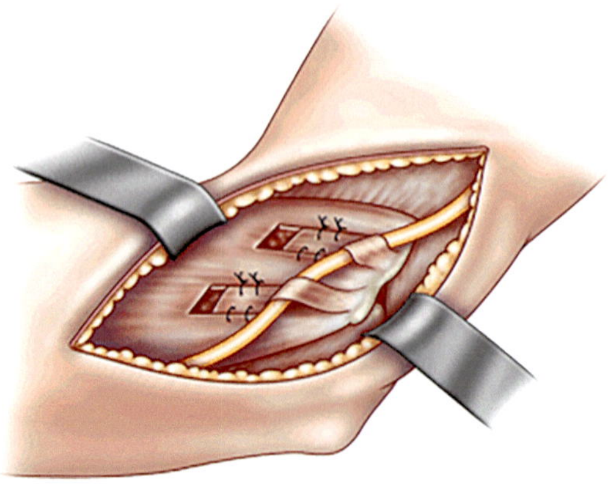

Fig. 26.5 Illustration of the subcutaneous ulnar nerve transposition which is secured using two fascial slings that have been elevated from the flexor-pronator mass [5]

Again, the most common postoperative complication was ulnar nerve related. They reported a total of 121 patients (16%) with neuropraxia of the nerve, of which the vast majority (99 out of 121) completely resolved at 6 weeks. Only one patient had the motor and sensory deficits, which required further operative intervention. They noted that postoperative ulnar nerve dysfunction did not affect the rate of return to previous level of competition.

In this large series, the authors noted that their ulnar nerve complication rate was 20% in the early part of their data collection period (these were all transient neuropraxias). In response, they modified their ulnar nerve transposition technique, where instead of two fascial slings as described originally, they now utilize either one sling of fascia from the flexor mass or a single strip of the medial intermuscular septum that remains attached to the medial epicondyle of the humerus. This resulted in a decrease in the rate of postoperative ulnar nerve symptoms [6].

In a hybrid technique that was published by Thompson, Jobe, and colleagues [11], the authors utilized the muscle splitting approach to the UCL as described by Smith et al. [13] (HSS technique) but utilized the original tunnel and graft configuration from Jobe's original technique [2]. In addition, the ulnar nerve was left alone and no transpositions were performed, even in patients who presented with signs of preoperative ulnar nerve irritation. In their series of 83 patients, they noted a 5% ulnar nerve complication rate postoperatively, and all resolved without further surgery. Interestingly, 21% of athletes had ulnar nerve symptoms preoperatively, but none of these patients had ulnar nerve transposition, and at final follow-up, there were no instances of residual ulnar neuropathy. The authors postulated that minimizing the exposure and handling of the nerve were responsible for the lower rate of complications after surgery and that even those athletes who had preoperative symptoms had resolution after UCL reconstruction without neurolysis and transposition of the ulnar nerve. They attributed this to a traction neuropraxia due to valgus instability that resolved after UCL reconstruction, and therefore, the nerve symptoms would be expected to resolve as well.

Ulnar Nerve Dysfunction in Throwing Athletes

Ulnar nerve problems are common in the throwing athlete and the second most common entrapment neuropathy in the upper extremity [16]. The anatomy of the ulnar nerve and the course in which it travels through the upper extremity make it susceptible to injury, especially when the elbow is loaded in the extremes that come with throwing sports such as baseball pitching [15].

Ulnar Nerve Anatomy and Sites of Compression

Starting proximally, a common potential site of compression is at the arcade of Struthers. This is located approximately 8 cm proximal to the medial epicondyle and represents a deep fascial band in the arm, which attaches the medial head of the triceps to the medial intermuscular septum. This arcade has been reported in 70% of individuals and is a common compression site of the ulnar nerve that can result in persistent ulnar nerve dysfunction despite appropriate ulnar nerve decompression and transposition at the cubital tunnel [16–18]. Especially in throwing athletes, the medial head of the triceps can become hypertrophic in this region and be more likely to cause nerve compression at the arcade as well as more distally as the nerve travels down toward the medial epicondyle.

More distally, the nerve comes around the elbow posterior to the medial epicondyle and enters the cubital tunnel. The tunnel floor is made up of the medial olecranon, posteromedial elbow capsule, and ulnar collateral ligament; the cubital tunnel retinaculum (arcuate ligament) makes up the roof of the tunnel. Osteophyte formation at the medial epicondyle or the olecranon can be sites of nerve compression and thickening of the overlying arcuate ligament or an accessory anconeus epitrochlearis muscle (the arcuate ligament is believed to be the normal remnant of the epitrochlearis muscle, but the muscle can be persistent in some individuals) can also cause stenosis of the cubital tunnel leading to neuropathy.

As the nerve exits the tunnel and passes between the two heads of the FCU muscle origin, the aponeurosis of the muscle here can also be a site of compression as well as bone spurs that can develop at the sublime tubercle where the UCL inserts on the ulna.

Additionally, the ulnar nerve can be hypermobile and subluxate and/or dislocate anteriorly around the edge of the medial epicondyle. Asymptomatic subluxation of the nerve has been documented in 16% of individuals [19]. In the throwing athlete with repetitive subluxations of the nerve with flexion extension of the elbow, the chronic friction that develops as a result of this phenomenon can lead to inflammation and nerve symptoms [20].

The throwing motion itself has been shown to increase tension within the ulnar nerve at the elbow. Aoki et al. [15] showed in a biomechanical study in cadaveric specimens that the average maximal strain on the ulnar nerve during the overhead-throwing motion was over 13% at the cubital tunnel. They noted that this value approached the elastic limit of the nerve and postulated that this stretch had the potential to limit the blood flow to the nerve. With repetitive stretch, a part of the pathophysiology leading to ulnar neuritis may be related to deficiencies in perfusion to the nerve as well. These studies were done with the UCL intact, and other authors have noted that it is possible to have ulnar nerve dysfunction independent of the continuity of the ligament [17, 21]. With this concept in mind, a more recent cadaveric biomechanical study by Mihata et al. [22] investigated the effect of UCL insufficiency on ulnar nerve elongation in the simulated throwing position. Overall, the authors found that there was a significant positive correlation between elbow valgus laxity and ulnar nerve strain when the UCL was torn but not when it was intact. In the setting of increased valgus laxity due to UCL insufficiency, the results of this study suggest that there is increased an elongation of the ulnar nerve that could exacerbate cubital tunnel syndrome during the throwing motion.

Evaluation of the Ulnar Nerve in the Throwing Elbow

The throwing athlete will present similarly to those patients with ulnar nerve problems in general. Symptoms include numbness, tingling, or burning sensation in an ulnar distribution in the forearm or hand, which are common complaints early in the disease process. Late findings may include weakness or atrophy of the hand intrinsic musculature. Medial elbow pain is also a common presenting symptom and pitchers may report heaviness or clumsiness of the hand and fingers after throwing several innings. In patients with subluxation of the nerve at the elbow, they may note a snapping or popping sensation with flexion-extension or during throwing motion at the medial elbow.

Physical examination should include a thorough assessment of the cervical spine for evidence of radiculopathy or cervical disk disease. At the elbow, often there will be a positive Tinel's sign at the cubital tunnel and the nerve itself may be tender to palpation. The ulnar nerve should also be palpated with flexion and extension of the elbow to determine whether it is subluxation or dislocating out of the condylar groove. The elbow flexion test can be performed, which is a provocative test in which the elbow is flexed with forearm supination and wrist extension for several minutes. If ulnar nerve paresthesias worsen with this position, the test is positive. Sensation changes are often noted in the ring and small finger of the hand, and two-point discrimination can be checked and compared with the contralateral hand to assess the degree of neuropathy. Motor findings are rare in the early phase of compression neuropathy, but intrinsic weakness can be subtle and detected before forearm extrinsic weakness such as grip strength.

Routine plain X-rays of the elbow should be performed to assess for degenerative arthritis or bone spurs that may cause compression as well as any previous fracture or deformity and the possibility of heterotopic ossification in the soft tissues. Magnetic resonance imaging (MRI) can be useful in ruling out space-occupying mass lesions, bone spurs, the presence of an anomalous anconeus epitrochlearis muscle, and the UCL can be evaluated simultaneously.

Electrodiagnostic testing can confirm the diagnosis and the location of the compression. It may also identify a secondary compression location ("double crush" phenomenon) and also give an assessment of the severity of neuropathy. Although helpful, these tests have been shown to possess a 10% false negative rate and should not be solely relied on to make a determination of ulnar neuropathy at the elbow [20].

Treatment

Initially, the focus should be on nonoperative treatment and avoidance of inciting activities [23]. The overhead athlete should be advised to rest until the nerve symptoms resolve. Ice, padding of the cubital tunnel to avoid any pressure on this area, and gentle physical therapy (including posterior capsular stretching exercises at the shoulder) are instituted for the first 4–6 weeks. Nonsteroidal anti-inflammatory medications may be helpful and splinting, especially at night, should be considered depending on the severity of nerve symptoms. When the athlete attempts to return to sport, throwing mechanics may need to be evaluated for potential improvements in technique. Once the symptoms have resolved, a strengthening program should be instituted with a focus on dynamic elbow stabilizers and an interval throwing program can be initiated. If symptoms persist despite conservative treatment, then surgical options should be discussed with the patient.

The surgical options include in situ decompression of the nerve without transposition, and either subcutaneous or submuscular anterior transposition. Historically, medial epicondylectomy has been described but is not recommended especially in the throwing athlete as the resection of the epicondyle has the potential to disrupt the flexor-pronator origin and affect muscle strength which is crucial for dynamic elbow stabilization [20]. In situ decompression is also not recommended in the throwing athlete as it does not address the potential tension that occurs within the nerve with throwing motion and will have a poor chance of alleviating neuropathy without an anterior translation of the nerve.

The subcutaneous transposition requires less soft-tissue dissection and leaves the flexor-pronator mass origin in its normal state and may allow for a quicker recovery after surgery. However, the nerve is brought superficial where it remains at risk for trauma, hypersensitivity at the skin, and is believed to be more susceptible to kinking. The submuscular transposition on the other hand violates a portion of the flexor-pronator mass, involves more dissection, and potentially results in a longer recovery. The nerve is better protected within a soft tissue envelope and has a more direct course to the forearm, and is less prone to kinking or ongoing traction stresses on the nerve.

Although well-designed studies are lacking comparing subcutaneous versus submuscular transposition, both techniques have had favorable outcomes. Rettig et al. performed subcutaneous nerve transposition in 20 athletes and reported 19 returned to previous athletic competition at 12 weeks after surgery. Aoki et al. [24], in a small series of adolescent baseball players, reported five out of six returned to the previous level of play 5 months after subcutaneous ulnar nerve transposition. The submuscular transposition also showed a reasonable return to throwing in a study by Del Pizzo [25] in 15 throwers. A more recent cohort study by Erickson et al. [26] examined the performance and rate of return to sport (RTS) among professional baseball players after ulnar nerve decompression/transposition. From 2010 to 2016, 52 players were found to have undergone isolated ulnar nerve decompression/transpositions. Overall, 92% of the surgical procedures involved anterior subcutaneous transpositions and it was noted that 62% were successfully able to RTS.

The surgeon must always consider the competency of the UCL in the setting of ulnar nerve irritation in the throwing elbow. If the ligament is torn, then the decision to reconstruct the ligament is already made; however, even in the setting of microinstability of the UCL, strong consideration should be given to concomitant UCL reconstruction to prevent ongoing valgus instability and persistent elbow problems. However, the management of the ulnar nerve when performing a UCL reconstruction still remains controversial. An epidemiological study by Hodgins et al. [27] identified all UCL reconstructions performed in New York State from 2002 to 2011 using the New York Statewide Planning and Research Cooperative System (SPARCS) database. Overall, the number of UCL reconstructions performed per year increased at a rate of 193% during the study period. Additionally, the frequency of concomitant ulnar nerve procedures was found to significantly increase by 400%. This disproportionate increase in ulnar nerve procedures was also noted in a systematic review of UCL reconstruction of the elbow by Erickson et al. [28]. Of the 2019 patients included within the study, 69.9% of the patients underwent concomitant ulnar nerve transposition at the time of UCL reconstruction despite only 18.0% of the patients having preoperative ulnar nerve symptoms. This disproportionate increase in ulnar nerve procedures contradicts the Rush experience [29]. Of the 187 patients undergoing UCL reconstruction from 2004 to 2014, only 41.8% underwent subcutaneous ulnar nerve transposition with all patients having some form of preoperative ulnar nerve symptoms. This concept of reserving ulnar nerve transposition for only those patients with preoperative symptoms was mirrored in a recent survey of Major League Baseball (MLB) team orthopedic surgeons [30]. Thirty orthopedic surgeons with a mean experience of 9.37 years as a team physician responded to the survey and it was noted that 93.3% of the surgeons do not routinely transpose the ulnar nerve in pitchers with no preoperative ulnar nerve symptoms or examination findings at the time of UCL reconstruction. While there is no literature to date strongly supporting a recommendation for the management of the ulnar nerve in the setting of UCL reconstruction, the practitioner must be aware of the potential nerve-related complications. A

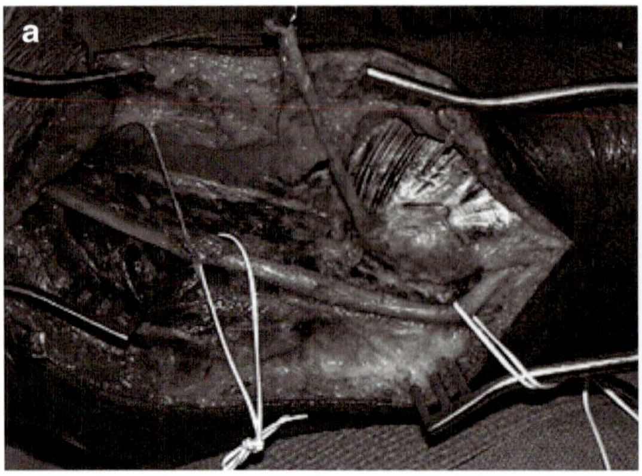

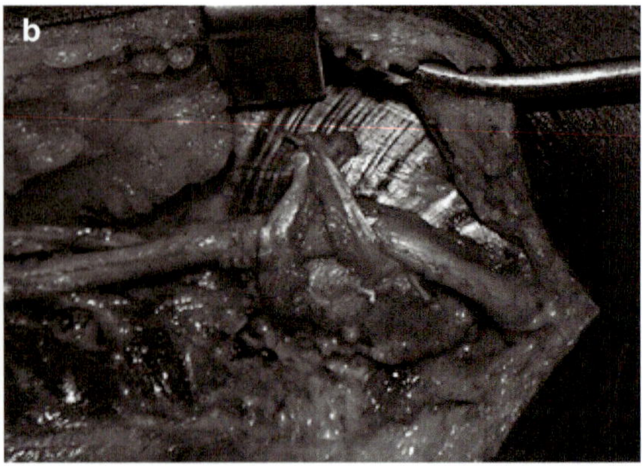

Fig. 26.6 (**a**) Clinical photo of ulnar nerve transposition. The intermuscular fascial sling that has been dissected from the intermuscular attachment and remains attached to the medial epicondyle is visualized, and the ulnar nerve has been dissected and tagged with two vessel loops [14]. (**b**) Clinical photo of a subcutaneous ulnar nerve transposition. The intermuscular fascial V-sling has been sutured to the fascial overlying the flexor-pronator mass to prevent the nerve from falling back behind the medial epicondyle. (From [14], reprinted with permission from Elsevier limited)

systematic review by Clain et al. [31] noted that concomitant ulnar nerve transposition was associated with a higher rate of ulnar neuropathy (16.1%) compared with the group without ulnar nerve transposition (3.9%). Subgroup analysis further revealed that submuscular transposition was associated with a significantly higher rate of reoperation (12.7%) compared with those undergoing subcutaneous transposition (0%).

Authors' Preferred Technique for Ulnar Nerve Transposition

Our preference for UCL reconstruction is to perform a docking technique with a double-stranded ipsilateral palmaris longus through a muscle splitting approach [7]. We will examine the elbow preoperatively as described previously for signs and symptoms of ulnar neuritis and will only transpose the nerve in those situations.

When ulnar nerve transposition is performed, we use a subcutaneous technique as previously described by Tan et al. [14]. The nerve is identified proximal to the cubital tunnel and posterior to the medial intermuscular septum. It is dissected out from proximal to distal and freeing it up completely from the arcade of Struthers to the two heads of the FCU. Once the nerve is adequately dissected, it is protected throughout the remainder of the UCL reconstruction procedure. Once the reconstruction portion of the procedure has been completed, we transpose the ulnar nerve anterior to the medial epicondyle and then hold it there with a band of the intermuscular septum. This is performed by dividing and dissecting out a longitudinal strip of the medial intermuscular septum starting approximately 8 cm proximal to the medial epicondyle. This strip of septum is taken distally until it is attached only to the medial epicondyle. This is then fashioned into an inverted V and sutured onto the fascia overlying the flexor-pronator musculature or subcutaneous tissue to prevent the nerve from subluxation back behind the epicondyle (Fig. 26.6).

Conclusion

The trend with time has been toward performing fewer obligatory ulnar nerve transpositions as part of UCL surgery and only moving the nerve when there are significant preoperative ulnar nerve symptoms [32, 33]. At the same time, as the surgical approach evolved away from a flexor-pronator muscle group detachment and toward a muscle splitting approach, the technique for nerve transposition has gone consistently to a subcutaneous placement of the nerve. These modifications have led to improvements in postoperative outcomes and a low rate of complications involving the ulnar nerve.

The surgeon must be cognizant of the fact that the ulnar nerve is in extremely close proximity throughout the entire UCL reconstruction procedure and that great care must be given to protect it from injury. However, with sound technique utilizing either surgical approach (HSS or ASMI) or prudent handling of the ulnar nerve, successful outcomes can be achieved in a high percentage of cases with minimal postoperative complications.

References

1. Langer P. Evolution of the treatment options of ulnar collateral ligament injuries of the elbow. Brit J Sports Med. 2006;40(6):499–506. https://doi.org/10.1136/bjsm.2005.025072.
2. Jobe FW, Stark H, Lombardo SJ. Reconstruction of the ulnar collateral ligament in athletes. J Bone Joint Surg Am. 1986;68(8):1158–63.
3. Koh JL, Schafer MF, Keuter G, Hsu JE. Ulnar collateral ligament reconstruction in elite throwing athletes. Arthroscopy. 2006;22(11):1187–91. https://doi.org/10.1016/j.arthro.2006.07.024.
4. Bowers AL, Dines JS, Dines DM, Altchek DW. Elbow medial ulnar collateral ligament reconstruction: clinical relevance and the docking technique. J Shoulder Elb Surg. 2010;19:110–7. https://doi.org/10.1016/j.jse.2010.01.005.
5. Azar FM, Andrews JR, Wilk KE, Groh D. Operative treatment of ulnar collateral ligament injuries of the elbow in athletes. Am J Sports Med. 2000;28(1):16–23.
6. Cain EL, Andrews JR, Dugas JR, et al. Outcome of ulnar collateral ligament reconstruction of the elbow in 1281 athletes: results in 743 athletes with minimum 2-year follow-up. Am J Sports Med. 2010;38(12):2426–34. https://doi.org/10.1177/0363546510378100.
7. Rohrbough JT, Altchek DW, Hyman J, Williams RJ, Botts JD. Medial collateral ligament reconstruction of the elbow using the docking technique. Am J Sports Med. 2002;30(4):541–8.
8. Hyman J, Breazeale NM, Altchek DW. Valgus instability of the elbow in athletes. Clin Sports Med. 2001;20(1):25–45. - viii.
9. Dodson CC, Thomas A, Dines JS, Nho SJ, Williams RJ, Altchek DW. Medial ulnar collateral ligament reconstruction of the elbow in throwing athletes. Am J Sports Med. 2006;34(12):1926–32. https://doi.org/10.1177/0363546506290988.
10. Petty DH. Ulnar collateral ligament reconstruction in high school baseball players: clinical results and injury risk factors. Am J Sports Med. 2004;32(5):1158–64. https://doi.org/10.1177/0363546503262166.
11. Thompson W. Ulnar collateral ligament reconstruction in athletes: muscle-splitting approach without transposition of the ulnar nerve. J Shoulder Elb Surg. 2001;10(2):152–7. https://doi.org/10.1067/mse.2001.112881.
12. Conway JE, Jobe FW, Glousman RE, Pink M. Medial instability of the elbow in throwing athletes. Treatment by repair or reconstruction of the ulnar collateral ligament. J Bone Joint Surg Am. 1992;74(1):67–83.
13. Smith GR, Altchek DW, Pagnani MJ, Keeley JR. A muscle-splitting approach to the ulnar collateral ligament of the elbow. Neuroanatomy and operative technique. Am J Sports Med. 1996;24(5):575–80.
14. Tan V, Pope J, Daluiski A, Capo JT, Weiland AJ. The V-sling: a modified medial intermuscular septal sling for anterior transposition of the ulnar nerve. J Hand Surg Am. 2004;29(2):325–7. https://doi.org/10.1016/j.jhsa.2003.11.011.
15. Aoki M, Takasaki H, Muraki T, Uchiyama E, Murakami G, Yamashita T. Strain on the ulnar nerve at the elbow and wrist during throwing motion. J Bone Joint Surg Am. 2005;87(11):2508–14.
16. Bencardino JT, Rosenberg ZS. Entrapment neuropathies of the shoulder and elbow in the athlete. Clin Sports Med. 2006;25(3):465–87. https://doi.org/10.1016/j.csm.2006.03.005.
17. Keefe DT, Lintner DM. Nerve injuries in the throwing elbow. Clin Sports Med. 2004;23(4):723–42. https://doi.org/10.1016/j.csm.2004.04.012.
18. Glousman RE. Ulnar nerve problems in the athlete's elbow. Clin Sports Med. 1990;9(2):365–77.
19. Childress HM. Recurrent ulnar-nerve dislocation at the elbow. Clin Orthop Relat Res. 1975;108:168–73.
20. Zemel NP. Ulnar neuropathy with and without elbow instability. Hand Clin. 2000;16(3):487–95. -x.
21. Treihaft MM. Neurologic injuries in baseball players. Semin Neurol. 2000;20(2):187–93. https://doi.org/10.1055/s-2000-9827.
22. Mihata T, Akeda M, Künzler M, McGarry MH, Neo M, Lee TQ. Ulnar collateral ligament insufficiency affects cubital tunnel syndrome during throwing motion: a cadaveric biomechanical study. J Shoulder Elb Surg. 2019;28(9):1758–63. https://doi.org/10.1016/j.jse.2019.02.009.
23. Cain EL, Dugas JR, Wolf RS, Andrews JR. Elbow injuries in throwing athletes: a current concepts review. Am J Sports Med. 2003;31(4):621–35.
24. Aoki M, Kanaya K, Aiki H, Wada T, Yamashita T, Ogiwara N. Cubital tunnel syndrome in adolescent baseball players: a report of six cases with 3- to 5-year follow-up. Arthroscopy. 2005;21(6):758. https://doi.org/10.1016/j.arthro.2005.03.030.
25. Del Pizzo W, Jobe FW, Norwood L. Ulnar nerve entrapment syndrome in baseball players. Am J Sports Med. 1977;5(5):182–5.

26. Erickson BJ, Chalmers PN, D'Angelo J, Ma K, Romeo AA. Performance and return to sport after ulnar nerve decompression/transposition among professional baseball players. Am J Sports Med. 2019;47(5):1124–9. https://doi.org/10.1177/0363546519829159.
27. Hodgins JL, Vitale M, Arons RR, Ahmad CS. Epidemiology of medial ulnar collateral ligament reconstruction: a 10-year study in New York state. Am J Sports Med. 2016;44(3):729–34. https://doi.org/10.1177/0363546515622407.
28. Erickson BJ, Chalmers PN, Bush-Joseph CA, Verma NN, Romeo AA. Ulnar collateral ligament reconstruction of the elbow: a systematic review of the literature. Orthop J Sports Med. 2015;3(12):2325967115618914. https://doi.org/10.1177/2325967115618914.
29. Erickson BJ, Bach BR Jr, Cohen MS, Bush-Joseph CA, Cole BJ, Verma NN, Nicholson GP, Romeo AA. Ulnar collateral ligament reconstruction: the rush experience. Orthop J Sports Med. 2016;4(1):2325967115626876. https://doi.org/10.1177/2325967115626876.
30. Erickson BJ, Harris JD, Fillingham YA, Cvetanovich GL, Bush-Joseph CA, Bach BR Jr, Romeo AA, Verma NN. Treatment of ulnar collateral ligament injuries and superior labral tears by major league baseball team physicians. Arthroscopy. 2016;32(7):1271–6. https://doi.org/10.1016/j.arthro.2016.01.034.
31. Clain JB, Vitale MA, Ahmad CS, Ruchelsman DE. Ulnar nerve complications after ulnar collateral ligament reconstruction of the elbow: a systematic review. Am J Sports Med. 2019;47(5):1263–9. https://doi.org/10.1177/0363546518765139.
32. Vitale MA, Ahmad CS. The outcome of elbow Ulnar collateral ligament reconstruction in overhead athletes: a systematic review. Am J Sports Med. 2008;36(6):1193–205. https://doi.org/10.1177/0363546508319053.
33. Purcell DB, Matava MJ, Wright RW. Ulnar collateral ligament reconstruction. Clin Orthop Relat Res. 2007;455:72–7. https://doi.org/10.1097/BLO.0b013e31802eb447.

Revision Ulnar Collateral Ligament Reconstruction

27

Terrence S. Daley-Lindo, Andrew J. Rosenbaum, Michael A. Flaherty, Christopher Chin, Neal S. ElAttrache, Joshua S. Dines, and Daryl C. Osbahr

Introduction

Repetitive overloading associated with the throwing motion can cause microscopic tears in the UCL with subsequent ligament attenuation and failure [1, 2]. Surgical reconstruction of the UCL has been found to be effective in correcting valgus elbow instability allowing most overhead athletes (83%) to return to the previous or higher level of competition in less than 1 year [3]. Retears of the reconstructed ligament are uncommon, with a large series investigating complications by Andrews et al. reporting a 2% retear rate [4]. The small retear rate may be due to the higher tensile strength of the grafts used in reconstruction (357 N for palmaris longus tendon [5], 837 N for gracilis tendon [6]) compared to the native UCL (260 N). The high strength of the graft used may expose poor cortical bone, poor quality of soft tissue, and technique as the cause for poor outcome.

The actual rate of retear may be higher than the reported 2%, as it is possible that some patients are unable or unwilling to undergo a second long rehab period required after reconstruction and thus do not seek revision surgery. Given the low retear rate in primary reconstruction as well as the limited indications for reconstruction, revision procedures are infrequently performed. However, with the trend toward an increasing number of high school overhead throwing athletes having primary reconstructions, and subsequently more professional athletes, the number of revision procedures will continue to increase [7]. This chapter explores failed UCL reconstruction, evaluation for revision, treatment options, techniques, and outcomes following revision surgery.

Suboptimal Outcomes and Complications After Primary Reconstruction

The original UCL reconstruction technique had a >30% complication rate [8]. Complications are

T. S. Daley-Lindo (✉)
Department of Orthopedics, Orlando Health, Orlando, FL, USA

A. J. Rosenbaum
Orthopaedic Surgery, The Bone and Joint Center, Albany Medical Center, Albany, NY, USA

M. A. Flaherty
The Bone and Joint Center, Capital Region Orthopaedics Group, Albany, NY, USA

C. Chin
Sports Medicine and Shoulder Service, Hospital for Special Surgery, New York, NY, USA

N. S. ElAttrache
Kerlan-Jobe Orthopaedic Clinic, Los Angeles, CA, USA

J. S. Dines
Department of Orthopedic Surgery, Sports Medicine and Shoulder Service, Sports Medicine Institute, Hospital for Special Surgery, New York, NY, USA

D. C. Osbahr
Orlando Health Orthopedic Institute, Orlando, FL, USA

J. S. Dines et al. (eds.), *Elbow Ulnar Collateral Ligament Injury*, https://doi.org/10.1007/978-3-030-69567-5_27

now estimated to occur at a reported rate ranging from 3 to 25% [9]. Ulnar neuropathies, sensory nerve paresthesias, fixation loss, and graft site complications including infection, tightness, and tenderness, have been described.

Although excellent results are seen in primary reconstruction, suboptimal outcomes do occur, with prior elbow surgery a major risk factor [10]. Conway et al. reported that patients who underwent elbow surgery prior to UCL reconstruction had a significantly decreased chance of returning to their previous level of sports participation [11]. The previous surgeries included arthroscopic loose body removal, diagnostic arthroscopy, osteophyte debridement, ulnar nerve transposition, and prior UCL repair. Of the patients having undergone a prior elbow surgery, only 33% had an excellent outcome. The specific outcomes of the two patients who underwent revision UCL reconstruction were not discussed.

In technique-related complications, considerations include the approach to the flexor pronator mass (e.g., detachment vs. muscle-splitting technique), type of humeral tunnels (e.g., posterior, anterior), graft fixation technique (e.g., figure-of-8, docking technique), type of graft used, indications and technique for ulnar nerve transposition, performance of diagnostic arthroscopy, and if any additional procedures are to be performed at the time of reconstruction. In a meta-analysis performed by Vitale and Ahmad, these factors were evaluated in eight studies describing 493 patients [12]. Better outcomes were observed with the muscle-splitting approach, as compared to detachment of the flexor-pronator mass; with avoidance of obligatory ulnar nerve transposition; and when the docking or modified docking technique was used instead of a figure-of-8 technique.

In a large case series by Cain et al., 55 of 942 patients who underwent UCL reconstruction required 62 subsequent elbow surgeries, ranging from 6 months to 7 years after reconstruction [3]. Although arthroscopic debridement of an olecranon osteophyte was the most common reason for a second procedure (53 of the 55 patients), 1% of the patients required revision surgery. Additionally, four patients required open reduction and internal fixation of avulsion fractures of the medial epicondyle at the tunnel site.

Indications for Revision Surgery for Failed UCL Reconstruction

The decision to revise a failed UCL reconstruction is dependent on several factors, including the history, physical examination findings, and most importantly, patient expectations. Because revision surgery is generally associated with inferior outcomes and more complications, suboptimal results are not uncommon and patients must understand that they may not return to their pre-injury level of play, the primary measure of success with regard to UCL reconstruction [13, 14].

Patients with a torn UCL graft may complain of medial elbow pain, stiffness, or ulnar nerve symptoms, which are similar findings to those observed with a primary tear. They may describe an acute event that caused their recurrent UCL pain, or present with a more insidious onset of symptoms. Of the 15 patients studied by Dines et al. who underwent revision UCL surgery, seven identified an acute event, while the remainder had a more chronic history of medial elbow pain [15]. The average time from initial reconstruction to revision surgery was 36 months (range, 12–76 months).

Preoperative Evaluation and Considerations for UCL Reconstruction

Physical examination must include inspection, palpation, and determination of elbow range of motion. Palpation about the medial elbow and previous incision will show the position of the ulnar nerve and pinpoint area of tenderness (ulnar vs. humeral failure). Valgus stress testing and a moving valgus test should also be performed in all patients. Range of motion about the elbow should also be evaluated for osteophyte formation or loose bodies which may have recurred or been untreated previously. Preoperative radiographs and magnetic resonance imaging can aid in diag-

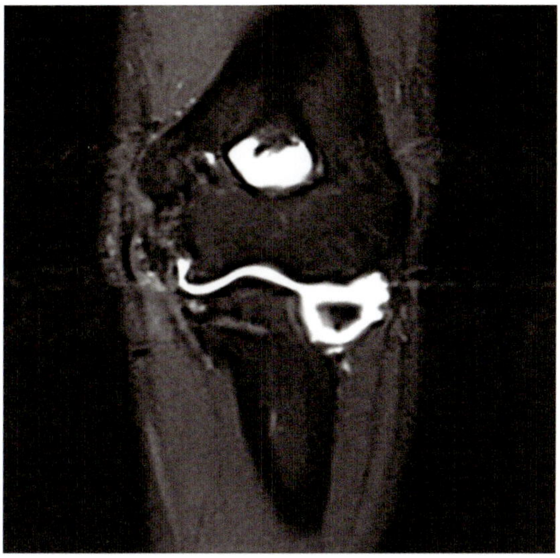

Fig. 27.1 Coronal magnetic resonance image showing retear of UCL status post figure-of-8 technique

nosis and clinical decision-making (Fig. 27.1). Anteroposterior (AP), lateral oblique, reverse axial (cubital tunnel view), and bilateral valgus stress radiographs of the elbow are obtained to evaluate for arthritic changes, bony UCL avulsion, ligamentous calcification, and/or posteromedial osteophytes [16]. Magnetic resonance imaging (MRI) is currently the modality of choice in detecting UCL tears. However, in the setting of prior UCL reconstruction Wear et al. showed 24% of patients had continued intermediate signal on T1 or T2 MRI [17]. Postoperative MRI of the UCL can also show thickening of the graft due to double-bundle technique, which can be confused with changes in the common flexor [18]. MR arthrogram interrogation of the reconstructed UCL has been found to have increased sensitivity in detecting partial tears [18]. Along with prior operative records from the primary reconstruction, thin slice computed tomography (CT) scan with sagittal, coronal, and 3D reconstructions should be obtained prior to all revisions to better evaluate prior tunnels, including size and location, to better plan revision reconstruction. Knowledge of the surgical technique used is important as it is difficult to perform a docking procedure on a patient who had a previous Jobe procedure. Type and size graft used is also important to plan for tunnel size and possible bone loss. The position of the ulnar nerve and previous transposition must be reviewed as well as other intraoperative findings, complications, and additional procedures performed. Revision surgery must be individually tailored to each patient based on the previous operation, and clinical evaluation and imaging.

When possible, previous incisions should be used. A careful dissection is imperative, as the medial antebrachial cutaneous and ulnar nerves may be encased in scar tissue, especially if prior ulnar nerve transposition was performed. Different techniques have been described for revision UCL surgery, including direct repair, the modified Jobe [10], DANE TJ (David Altcheck, Neal ElAttrache, Tommy John) [15], docking [9], and suspension button [8] fixation techniques.

Principles of Revision Surgery for Failed UCL Reconstruction

The technique and type of graft the surgeon feels most comfortable with should be utilized, and options include ipsilateral or contralateral palmaris autograft, contralateral gracilis autograft, and allograft. If bone tunnels are larger, the surgeon may consider utilizing gracilis autograft to allow for a larger graft. Although there are studies recommending the utilization of allograft in primary UCL reconstruction, the authors do not prefer utilizing allograft for both primary and revision UCL reconstruction [19]. However, certain situations such as bone loss, previous technique, and ulnar nerve position may dictate specific treatment options and make revision more challenging. The surgeon must have contingency plans for all potential sources of graft fixation failure. Ulnar and humeral bone tunnel quality and the presence of ulnar cortical bone loss are one such example and one of the most important factors that can influence which reconstruction technique to use. The surgeon must be prepared to deal with bone loss at the time of surgery, and the authors recommend having options for bone grafting from both autograft sites and allograft sources. If bone stock is a major concern when reviewing the imaging or at the time of surgery, the authors must be prepared to consider bone grafting with a staged reconstruction; in the author's experience; however, this is very rarely necessary.

Ulnar Bone Loss

The DANE TJ is useful when faced with ulnar bone loss (see Chap. 19 for details regarding the DANE procedure). It is a hybrid procedure combining a proximal docking technique with interference screw fixation on the ulna [20]. By fixing the UCL to a single tunnel distally, the ligament's native anatomy is more closely restored, as anatomical studies have shown the UCL to have a narrow insertion on the ulna's sublime tubercle. Because multiple drill holes in the ulna are unnecessary, the DANE TJ is effective in cases of insufficient bone stock on the sublime tubercle. This technique also decreases the risk of ulna bone bridge fracture. Excellent outcomes have been reported in 86% of patients undergoing reconstruction with the DANE TJ technique [21].

Lee et al. [8] assessed the applicability of suspension button fixation in the setting of ulnar cortical bone loss. In this cadaveric study, a guidewire was drilled through the center of the ulnar footprint of the ligament into the lateral ulnar cortex. The guidewire should be angled at about 30° in the coronal and sagittal planes to protect the posterior interosseous nerve. A cannulated reamer is used to drill the sockets after which the graft is shuttled into the ulna. Several suspensory buttons exist, which can be used for fixation (Fig. 27.2). While there are no reports of clinical outcomes using this technique, the investigators found elbow kinematics with the suspension button reconstruction to be comparable to those of the UCL in its intact state, and failure testing identified comparable fixation loads as compared to historical controls, even with the presence of ulnar cortical bone loss.

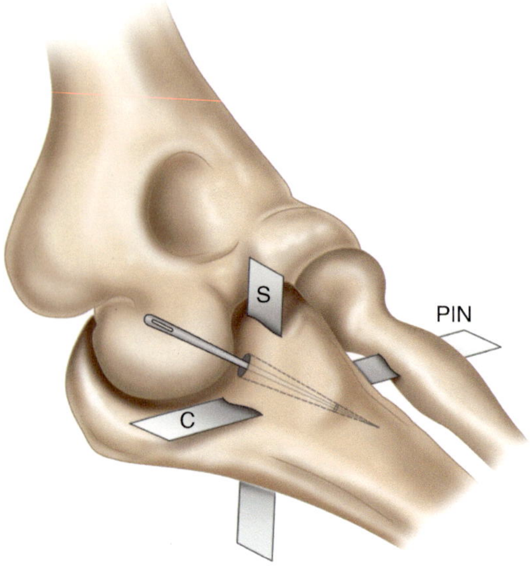

Fig. 27.2 Guidewire angled 30° in the coronal and sagittal plane to avoid posterior interosseous nerve [8]

Humeral Bone Loss

Humeral bone loss presents a much more complicated clinical scenario for the treating surgeon. No good options exist to secure the graft into a fractured or insufficient medial epicondyle (Fig. 27.3). If, after counseling the patient about the prolonged recovery course and less-than-ideal clinical outcomes, patients wish to proceed, a staged procedure can be used. Bone grafting of the humeral tunnels should be done at the index procedure. After incorporation of the bone graft is confirmed by computed tomography (CT) scan, the revision UCL reconstruction can be carried out.

Additional procedures may be performed at the time of revision surgery. In the Dines et al. case series examining revision UCL surgery, four patients underwent concomitant revision ulnar nerve transposition, and one underwent ulnar nerve transposition for the first time. Open posteromedial osteophyte resection, flexor muscle repair, and transposition of the medial antebrachial cutaneous nerve may also be necessary.

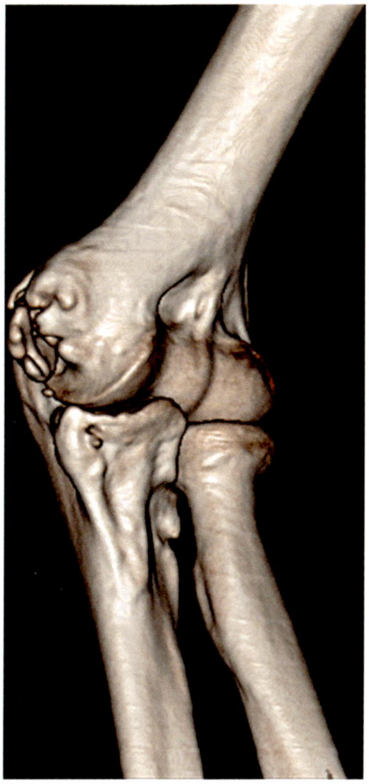

Fig. 27.3 Fractured humeral socket after UCL reconstruction

Outcomes Following Revision Surgery for Failed UCL Reconstruction

The paucity of data on functional outcomes following revision UCL surgery makes it challenging to establish objective guidelines and recommendations for return to competition [4, 21, 22]. Of the 15 patients in the Dines et al. series, only five (33%) were able to return to their previous level of competition for at least 1 year. Andrews presented similar data in a presentation titled "Complications of Failed Medial UCL Reconstructions and Evaluation of Revision Surgery" [4]. Of the seven patients who underwent revision surgery in this series, only two returned to their previous level of play or higher (<30%) [4]. Although these outcomes are worse than those seen after primary reconstruction (83%), given the complexity of revision surgery and the technical difficulties of revision UCL surgery, it is not surprising [3].

Dines et al. reported a 40% complication rate in their revision series, a higher rate than that seen after primary surgery (3–25%) [3, 10]. Although six players developed postoperative complications, most were effectively treated conservatively with physical therapy and anti-inflammatory medications. The patients conservatively managed for stiffness, transient ulnar neuritis, and medial epicondylitis were all able to return to their previous level of play, having excellent outcomes following revision surgery. There was one patient with stiffness requiring an arthroscopic lysis of adhesions and excision of an olecranon spur. This patient was ultimately classified as having a poor outcome. A rerupture of the revised UCL occurred at 15 months post-revision in another patient. At the time of retear, the patient had returned to his previous level of play for 3 months. He retired from baseball after this, and was considered to have had a poor outcome.

Some studies suggest that one in nine Major League Baseball (MLB) pitchers require UCL reconstruction, making them a unique and excellent cohort to follow in regard to UCL injuries [3, 12]. Dines et al. found a 75% rate of return to preinjury competition for MLB pitchers who underwent revision UCL surgery. However, they did not discuss whether these players returned to their preinjury pitching workload [15]. Jones et al. sought to determine the functional outcomes of MLB players after revision UCL reconstruction by evaluating pitching workload (appearances for relief pitchers, games started/innings pitched for starters; earned run average, strike outs per nine innings, walks per nine innings) [22]. In their case series, 78% (14/18) of pitchers were able to return to MLB play within two full seasons. Relief pitchers were able to resume 50% of their preinjury workload, while starting pitchers reached only 35% of their preinjury workload. Based on these findings, the authors believe starting pitchers to be at higher risk for suboptimal outcomes in the revision setting, and that they may benefit from transition to a relief role [22].

A study performed by Camp et al. [23] using the MLB Health and Injury Tracking System, identified 47 MLB and minor league pitchers who underwent revision UCL reconstruction from 2010 to 2014. Of these pitchers, 76.6% (35/47) were able to return to play at any level and 55.3% (26/47) were able to return to play at the same level. The previously reported levels of return to play are noted to be much lower than this study. It was noted that major league players had a significantly higher rate of return to play (73.1%) compared to minor league players (39.5%). There was no significant difference found in the career length, time to return to play or return to same level of play between major and minor league pitchers.

Summary

Primary reconstruction of the UCL can be accomplished via many proven techniques, with an 83% rate of return to previous or higher level of competition in less than 1 year [4]. However, complications and poor outcomes are at times observed, albeit infrequently. Rerupture is a rare complication estimated to occur in 2% of patients but may be vastly underreported. Little is known about optimal treatment for rerupture and the outcomes following revision UCL surgery. In the setting of intact bone tunnels, many of the techniques used for primary reconstruction can be used for revision surgery. When ulnar cortical bone loss is present, options become more limited, with the DANE TJ and endobutton techniques showing good results. Cadaveric studies have also shown a suspension button construct to be an effective treatment when faced with bone loss. Like other revision procedures, outcomes following revision UCL surgery are inferior to those seen with primary reconstruction. Further research and investigation must be conducted on revision UCL surgery in order to develop evidence-based guidelines and treatment recommendations that will optimize outcomes.

References

1. Feltner ME. Three-dimensional interactions in a two-segment kinetic chain, part II: application to the throwing arm in baseball pitching. Int J Sport Biomech. 1989;5:420–50.
2. Fleisig GS, Andrews JR, Dillman CJ, Escamilla RF. Kinetics of baseball pitching with implications about injury mechanisms. Am J Sports Med. 1995;23:233–9.
3. Cain EL, Andrews JR, Dugas JR, Wilk KE, McMichael CS, Walter JC 2nd, Riley RS, Arthur ST. Outcome of ulnar collateral ligament reconstruction of the elbow in 1281 athletes: results in 743 athletes with minimum 2-year follow-up. Am J Sports Med. 2010;38:2426–34.
4. Mauro CS, Dines JS, ElAttrache NS. Ulnar collateral ligament tears: special considerations. In: Dines JS, Altchek DW, Andrews J, ElAttrach NS, Wilk KE, Yocum LA, editors. Sports medicine of baseball. Philadelphia: Wolters Kluwer Health/Lippincott Williams & Wilkins; 2012. p. 247–8.
5. Regan WD, et al. Biomechanical study of ligaments around the elbow joint. Clin Orthop Relat Res. 1991;271:170–9.
6. Hamner DL, et al. Hamstring tendon grafts for reconstruction of the anterior cruciate ligament: biomechanical evaluation of the use of multiple strands and tensioning techniques. J Bone Joint Surg Am. 1999;81(4):549–57.
7. Petty DH, Andrews JR, Fleisig GS, Cain EL. Ulnar collateral ligament reconstruction in high school baseball players: clinical results and injury risk factors. Am J Sports Med. 2004;32(5):1158–64.
8. Lee GH, Limpisvasti O, Park MC, McGarry MH, Yocum LA, Lee TQ. Revision ulnar collateral ligament reconstruction using a suspension button fixation technique. Am J Sports Med. 2010;38:575–80.
9. Rohrborough JT, Altchek DW, Hyman J, Williams RJ III, Botts JD. Medial collateral ligament reconstruction of the elbow using the docking technique. Am J Sports Med. 2002;30:541–8.
10. Azar FM, Andrews JR, Wilk KE, Groh D. Operative treatment of ulnar collateral ligament injuries of the elbow in athletes. Am J Sports Med. 2000;28:16–23.
11. Conway JE, Jobe FE, Glousman RE, Pink M. Medial instability of the elbow in throwing athletes: treatment by repair or reconstruction of the ulnar collateral ligament. J Bone Joint Surg Am. 1992;74:67–83.
12. Vitale MA, Ahmad CS. The outcome of elbow ulnar collateral ligament reconstruction in overhead athletes. AJSM. 2008;36:1193–205.
13. Dines JS, Fealy S, Strauss EJ, et al. Outcomes analysis of revision total shoulder replacement. J Bone Joint Surg Am. 2006;88:1494–500.
14. Djurasovic M, Marra G, Arroyo JS, Pollock RG, Flatow EL, Bigliani LU. Revision rotator cuff repair: factors influencing results. J Bone Joint Surg Am. 2001;83:1849–55.

15. Dines JS, Yocum LA, Frank JB, ElAttrache NS, Gambardella RA, Jobe FW. Revision surgery for failed elbow medial collateral ligament reconstruction. Am J Sports Med. 2008;36:1061–5.
16. Bruce JR, Andrews JR. Ulnar collateral ligament injuries in the throwing athlete. J Am Acad Orthop Surg. 2014;22(5):315–25.
17. Wear SA, Thornton DD, Schwartz ML, Weissmann RC 3rd, Cain EL, Andrews JR. MRI of the reconstructed ulnar collateral ligament. AJR Am J Roentgenol. 2011;197(5):1198–204.
18. Bucknor MD, Stevens KJ, Steinbach LS. Elbow imaging in sport: sports imaging series. Radiology. 2016;279(1):12–28.
19. Savoie FH, Morgan C, Yaste J, Hurt J, Field L. Medial ulnar collateral ligament reconstruction using hamstring allograft in overhead throwing athletes. J Bone Joint Surg Am. 2013;95(12):1062–6.
20. Conway JE. The DANE TJ procedure for elbow medial ulnar collateral ligament insufficiency. Tech Shoulder Elbow Surg. 2006;7:36–43.
21. Dines JS, ElAttrache NS, Conway JE, Smith W, Ahmad CS. Clinical outcomes of the DANE TJ technique to treat ulnar collateral ligament insufficiency of the elbow. Am J Sports Med. 2007;35:2039–44.
22. Jones KJ, Conte S, Patterson N, ElAttrache NS, Dines JS. Functional outcomes following revision ulnar collateral ligament reconstruction in Major League Baseball pitchers. J Shoulder Elb Surg. 2013;22:642–6.
23. Camp CL, Desai V, Conte S, et al. Revision ulnar collateral ligament reconstruction in professional baseball: current trends, surgical techniques, and outcomes. Orthop J Sports Med. 2019;7(8):2325967119864104.

Medial Ulnar Collateral Ligament Injuries in Baseball Position Players

28

Timothy B. Griffith and Gary M. Lourie

Introduction

Since 1974, when Dr. Frank Jobe first described the medial ulnar collateral ligament reconstruction (UCLR) on Tommy John, a pitcher for the Los Angeles Dodgers, there has been an abundance of orthopedic research published describing medial ulnar collateral ligament (UCL) injuries and UCLR surgery in baseball pitchers. However, despite occurring less frequently than in pitchers, UCL injuries are being increasingly recognized and treated in baseball position players; defined as those playing defensive positions other than pitchers. There is a paucity of research dedicated to describing the epidemiology, treatment, and performance outcomes in this patient population.

Pathoanatomy and Epidemiology

The anterior bundle of the UCL serves as the primary restraint of the throwing athlete's elbow to valgus stress [1, 2]. While the shoulder is maximally externally rotated and the elbow flexed, excessive, repetitive valgus torque is placed on the medial elbow during the late cocking and early acceleration phases of throwing, both in pitchers and position players. Repetitive microtrauma occurs as the torque force generated on the UCL exceeds its capacity for load to failure, leading to UCL insufficiency and rupture. This process results in medial elbow instability, lateral radiocapitellar compression, posterior extension overload, and shear stresses of the medial olecranon tip and fossa [3]. Related pain, instability, and even neurologic symptoms can be devastating to throwing performance and the ability to return to play (RTP) or return to the same level of play (RSL), and was initially considered to be a career-ending injury prior to the advent of UCLR [4–6].

The rate of UCL injuries in professional baseball players has been dramatically increasing [7, 8]. The prevalence of UCLR is high, with 15% of minor league (MiLB) and 25% of major league (MLB) pitchers having surgery during their careers [9]. When UCLR surgery in professional baseball players is necessary, RTP and RSL rates of 80–90% and 70–80%, respectively, have been described [10–12]. The majority of published studies have combined position players with pitchers when evaluating the epidemiology and surgical results of UCLR [13–15]. In 2010, a study of 1210 baseball players described 125 UCL injuries (10.3%) in position players [10]. In 2015, a systematic review of 2019 baseball players requiring UCLR, comprised from 20 separate

T. B. Griffith (✉)
Peachtree Orthopedics, Atlanta Braves, Atlanta, GA, USA
e-mail: tgriffith@pocatlanta.com

G. M. Lourie
The Hand and Upper Extremity Center of Georgia, Atlanta Braves, Atlanta, GA, USA

J. S. Dines et al. (eds.), *Elbow Ulnar Collateral Ligament Injury*,
https://doi.org/10.1007/978-3-030-69567-5_28

studies, found that 14.5% of the combined cohort were position players [11]. Conte, in 2015, in a large survey study of 5088 professional baseball players, questioned 2382 position players during the 2012 season regarding their history of UCLR. 60, or 3%, of position players had previously undergone UCLR during their careers [9]. In an analysis of injury trends in MLB players from 1998 to 2015, published in 2016, the authors found a significant yearly increase in the incidence of UCLRs. 39 of 400 (10%) UCLRs over the 18 year time period were performed on position players [8]. Studies specifically evaluating the outcomes of UCLR in position players have further categorized their cohorts as infielders, outfielders, and catchers, with a fairly equitable distribution of injuries being described. Begly et al., while evaluating the performance outcomes after UCLR of 35 position players from 1984 to 2015, noted a distribution of 10 infielders (28%), 16 outfielders (46%), and 9 catchers (26%) in their cohort [16]. In 2018, Camp et al., in a report on UCLR outcomes on 167 position players, the largest to date, noted a distribution of 62 infielders (37.1%), 58 outfielders (34.7%), and 47 catchers (28.1%) [17]. Throwing injuries dominate as the most common cause of UCL injuries in position players, though a case report of an acute ulnar collateral ligament tear in a third baseman while batting has been reported [18].

Presentation and Evaluation

The initial work-up of a baseball position player with a suspected UCL injury starts with a thorough history. The player's position, level of play (MiLB vs. MLB), and handedness in throwing and batting are noted. The chronicity of the patient's symptoms, whether any inciting traumatic events have occurred, concurrent neurologic, mechanical or "popping" symptoms, and relevant positional symptoms, such as the phase of throwing that causes pain, are further assessed. The occurrence of associated or prior kinetic chain musculoskeletal injuries, especially to the shoulder, cervical spine, core, and hips are important to investigate. Recent changes to training regimens, a prior need for surgery or imaging, prior time on the Injured List (IL), and changes in throwing mechanics are noted. Prior treatments, such as rest, injections, surgery, and the results of these modalities should be assessed.

Physical examination of the athlete's elbow involves inspection, palpation, range of motion evaluation, and stability testing. The exam starts with inspection for elbow swelling and fullness, especially medially. The clinician should then palpate the medial elbow for tenderness, starting at the medial epicondyle and flexor pronator mass. The MUCL, which originates from the anteroinferior surface of the medial epicondyle and inserts at the sublime tubercle at the medial aspect of the coronoid, can be palpated with the elbow flexed at 90 or greater degrees of flexion under the flexor pronator mass [3, 19]. While no physical exam test is definitive, tenderness over the proximal and/or distal MUCL may suggest a ligamentous injury. The radiocapitellar joint, olecranon, and olecranon tip should be palpated as well. The ulnar nerve should be evaluated for stability and with provocative, sensory, and motor testing for signs of ulnar neuritis. Range of motion, including flexion, extension, pronation, and supination, should then be evaluated. Pain and lack of extension may indicate posteromedial olecranon impingement. Finally, stability testing is performed. The manual valgus stress test is performed by creating a valgus stress with the elbow in 30 degrees of flexion and maximal pronation. It is important to note that both elbows should be examined and compared. A positive test involves increased elbow opening or recreation of the patient's pain. The moving valgus stress test is 100% sensitive and 75% specific for MUCL injury. This test involves placing a valgus stress on the athlete's elbow from flexion to extension in an arc of 70–120 degrees of flexion. A positive test is indicated by apprehension, pain, or subjective instability during this maneuver [20]. Evaluation of the ipsilateral shoulder with comparison to the contralateral shoulder is also critical. Evaluation of shoulder range of motion, especially for co-existing glenohumeral internal rotation deficit (GIRD), external rotation, and/or forward flexion limitations is paramount as these deficiencies have been demonstrated as independent risk factors for subsequent elbow injury [21]. Further evaluation for scapular weakness, dyskinesia, and rotator cuff weakness is also necessary. Functional assessment of the lower kinetic chain by means of a deep squat, single leg squat, hop testing, and plank testing is helpful in identifying deficiencies in the lower extremities, core, and lumbar spine.

Pre-operative imaging of the athletic elbow, especially in the case of suspected MUCL injury, involves plain elbow radiographs and magnetic resonance arthrogram imaging (MRA). Anteroposterior, lateral, and oblique radiographic views are obtained to evaluate for osteoarthritis, osteophytes, osteochondral lesions, loose bodies, and malalignment. Olecranon axial views may be obtained to reveal the characteristic posteromedial osteophyte in valgus extension overload. Contralateral comparison radiographs are helpful, especially in the pediatric or adolescent population. Stress radiographs in adults may be helpful but are often deferred in favor of an MRA. MRA, as the primary means of assessing soft tissue and articular cartilage, is helpful to assess for full and partial thickness MUCL tears, osteochondral lesions not detected by plain radiographs, and flexor-pronator mass injury (Fig. 28.1). The above combined pre-operative imaging is important for planning of a successful surgery involving MUCL reconstruction and treatment of associated pathology.

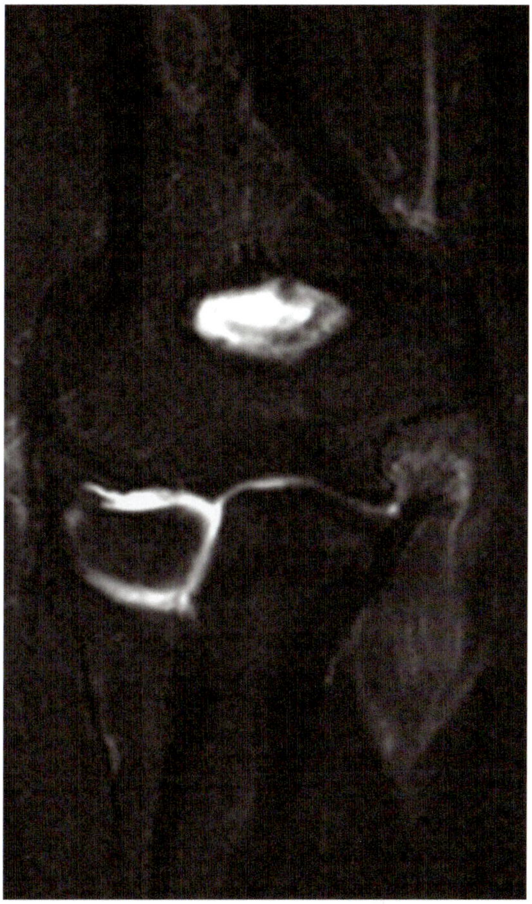

Fig. 28.1 MR arthrogram revealing a complete, proximal UCL tear

Treatment

The treatment of UCL injuries in position players is identical to the treatment in pitchers. Partial tears are typically treated conservatively, including 6 weeks of rest, modalities, strengthening and stretching, adjunctive use of biologics, and a gradual return to throwing. A study assessing the clinical utility of a magnetic resonance imaging (MRI)-based classification system in predicting success for non-operative versus operative treatment in throwers, regardless of position, revealed that distal partial tears and complete tears were more likely to undergo surgical treatment [22, 23]. The non-operative treatment of full thickness UCL tears in throwing athletes frequently leads to a poor return to previous level of competition [6]. Subjective symptoms and the inability to perform in sport due to medial elbow pain in the presence of a full thickness UCL tear, or a partial tear that has failed a conservative treatment regimen, serve as the primary indications for surgery. The current gold standard surgical procedure for the treatment of UCL injuries in position players is UCLR, utilizing autograft tissue to reconstruct the UCL using humeral and ulnar tunnels.

Since the original description of UCLR by Jobe, a variety of technique modifications, methods of securing the graft, and graft types have been described [24]. Most Major League Baseball team physicians utilize either the modified Jobe (figure-of-eight) or docking techniques for UCLR [12]. In order to reduce ulnar neuropraxia and minimize bone removal from the medial epicondyle during traditional figure-of-eight drilling for the modified Jobe technique, the docking technique was developed in 2002 [25]. This technique described a muscle-splitting approach and the use of a single socket in the medial epicondyle. This technique does not require obligatory ulnar nerve transposition and has demonstrated a 92% RTP and 2.8% incidence of ulnar neuropraxia [25, 26]. Both palmaris longus and gracilis autografts have been utilized in UCLR, both with acceptable outcomes. In 2019, in the largest known study evaluating the outcomes of UCLR based on graft type and tunnel configuration in 566 professional pitchers, the authors found no difference in RTP, RSL, time to return, subsequent elbow injuries, or need for subsequent or revision elbow surgery between the modified Jobe and docking techniques, nor between palmaris autograft or gracilis autograft tissue [12]. Therefore, surgeon preference should be employed for selection of the reconstruction technique and graft type for the treatment of UCL tears in position players (Fig. 28.2). Ulnar nerve transpositions are recommended only when preoperative ulnar nerve symptoms are present. UCL repair has demonstrated promising results in the treatment of young baseball players with a partial UCL tear that has failed conservative treatment or for the full thickness tear of the ligament from the proximal or distal attachment without broad ligament damage or tissue deficiency; however, the indications for this procedure continue to evolve [27, 28].

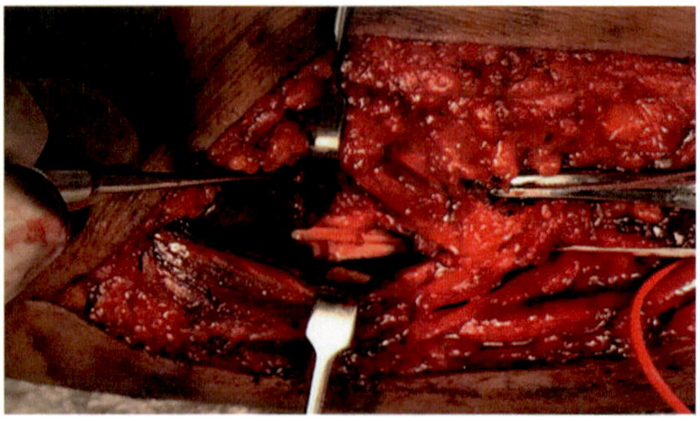

Fig. 28.2 UCLR with palmaris autograft using the Docking technique

Postoperative Rehabilitation Protocol

The operative extremity remains in a plaster splint for 1 week. The elbow is then placed in a hinged brace and motion from 30 to 90 degrees of flexion is initiated. Starting week three, motion is progressed to a range from 15 to 105 degrees of flexion. Removal of the brace and physical therapy, aimed at shoulder and elbow range of motion and scapula and forearm strengthening, occurs at 6 weeks. Plyometric and position-specific training is initiated at weeks 10 through 16. An interval hitting program is started around 12 weeks. Tossing is generally allowed starting at 16 weeks, every other day, at a distance of 45 feet. This distance is increased at regular intervals and decreased if any pain is experienced. Return to play is allowed in position players sooner than in pitchers, but typically occurs 9–12 months after surgery, depending on the player's progression with activity.

Outcomes of UCLR in Position Players

The results of all known published reports on UCLR in position players are summarized in Table 28.1 [8, 10, 16, 17, 29]. Initial studies published on the clinical outcomes of UCLR have combined position players with pitchers when describing their results. In the largest known study of UCL injuries to date, including 1210 baseball players overall, 125 position players were included as part of the analysis over a 19 year period. A RLS rate of 83% with 20% complication rate and average time to RTP of 11.6 months was described; however, the position player cohort was not analyzed separately for position-specific outcomes [10]. Conte et al., in 2016, in a report describing the outcomes of 39 position players at the MLB level that required UCLR over an 18 year time period, described a mean time to RTP of

Table 28.1 Surgical outcomes after ulnar collateral ligament reconstruction in position players

Author	Number of position players	Distribution of cohort by position	Return to play (RTP)/same level (RSL)	Time to RTP	Performance variables	Comparison to controls	Subgroup analysis	Revision rate	Special considerations
Cain et al. [10]	125	Unknown	83% RSL		N/A	N/A	N/A	1%	Position players not analyzed separately
Conte et al. [8]	39	Unknown	Unknown	Average 10.4 months	N/A	RTP 7.4 months faster than pitchers	N/A	Unknown	Noted increased annual incidence of UCLR in MLB players
Begly et al. [16]	26	14 outfielders, 8 infielders, 4 catchers	80% RSL	Unknown	WAR, RBIs, OPS, ISO, batting average, balls on base, HR, double/triple rate	No difference in all variables relative to position-matched cohort	Catchers: RTP 56%, decrease in HR and RBI rates	0%	Switch hitters demonstrated decreased 2 years WAR after UCLR
Camp et al. [17]	167	58 outfielders, 62 infielders, 47 catchers	75.5% RTP in 106 players, 68.8% RSL in 93 players	Average 11 months	N/A	Lower rate of RTP than pitchers, but shorter RTP times	Catchers RTP 58.6%, infielders less time to RTP	4.8%	Noted a significant rise in annual rate of UCLR from 1984 to 2015
Jack et al. [29]	33	14 outfielders, 12 infielders, 7 catchers	84.8% RSL	Average 11.2 months	WAR, Ultimate Zone Rating (UZN)	Catchers had shorter MLB length than controls	No change in UZN, outfielders decrease WAR after UCLR	Unknown	Noted a significant rise in annual rate of UCLR from 1984 to 2015

10.4 months. On average, position players were noted to return 7.4 months faster than pitchers, who returned at 17.8 months [8].

Begly et al., in a report in 2018, described the outcomes of 35 MLB position players after UCLR compared to an age, body mass index (BMI), switch-hitting, position, and plate appearance matched cohort. The distribution of their initial cohort by position included: 16 outfielders (46%), 10 infielders (29%), and 9 catchers (25%). An overall RTP of 80% was noted, but catchers were noted to RTP only 56% of the time. Upon excluding the seven athletes who did not RTP and two additional players who did not achieve 100 plate appearances in either the pre- or post-injury season, a subgroup analysis of performance measures was performed on 26 position players relative to the matched cohort. This group included 14 outfielders (54%), 8 infielders (31%), and 4 catchers (15%). Seven (27%) of these 26 players were switch hitters. The 26 patients who underwent UCLR did not demonstrate statistically significant differences relative to the matched cohort in plate appearances, at bats, or advanced performance statistics such as wins above replacement (WAR), batting average, isolated power (ISO), on-base plus slugging (OPS), runs batted in (RBI), balls on base, and home run (HR), triple, and double rates. When performance measures were compared among positions and pre- versus post-injury performance compared, catchers were found to have statistically greater decreases in their home run rate and lower RBI rates after returning from surgery. The relatively poor performance of catchers was attributed to their more regular and consistent play than pitchers, their significant combined demands of both throwing and batting, and more throws per game than any other position player. Switch hitters after UCLR demonstrated a significant reduction in their two-year WAR relative to switch hitting controls. Defensive metrics in catchers were not analyzed. Also, in this study, specifics on method of UCLR, concomitant elbow disease, rehabilitation specifics, and time required to return to play were not available in the author's analysis [16].

Camp et al., in 2018, published their results in the largest known study describing the outcomes of UCLR in professional baseball position players. Utilizing the MLB Health and Injury Tracking System (HITS) cross-referenced with an online search, all known position players who had ever undergone UCLR were identified. This study overall yielded 167 UCLRs in position players, with a distribution of 62 infielders (37.1%), 58 outfielders (34.7%), and 47 catchers (28.1%), noting a statistically significant rise in the annual rate of UCLRs from 1984 to 2015. When assessed by position, the annual number of UCLR procedures statistically increased for catchers, infielders, and outfielders alike. When evaluated in subgroups, MiLB players were found to experience a near linear increase in their proportion of UCLRs over time, while MLB players sustained a reciprocal decline in their proportion of surgical cases. Of 106 position players who met the inclusion criteria for RTP and 93 players who met inclusion criteria for RSL analysis, 75.5% were able to RTP at an average of 11 months, significantly faster than a UCLR cohort of pitchers. Of those undergoing primary UCLR, 76.2% were able to RTP, while only 69.3% of those undergoing revision UCLR returned. Nearly 68.8% were able to RSL and required an average additional 44 days after their first appearance in a game. Upon subgroup analysis, catchers were able to RTP the least frequently, only 58.6% of the time, relative to 75.6% of infielders and 88.9% of outfielders. Infielders required a statistically significantly less amount of time to RTP, at a mean 294 ± 87 days, relative to 363 ± 122 days and 375 ± 144 days for catchers and outfielders, respectively. The overall revision rate was 4.8%. No statistically significant differences in revision rates were noted based on position or level of play (MLB vs. MiLB). When compared to a known cohort of professional pitchers having undergone UCLR, position players required significantly less time to RTP (342 ± 124 days) than pitchers (435 ± 151 days); however, their ability to RTP (75.5% overall) was lower than that of pitchers (83.7%). The authors theorized that this difference in RTP outcomes may indicate a more severe form of elbow dysfunction or the possession of additional associated factors contributing to elbow injury, such as concurrent shoulder pathology or poor throwing mechanics. The relatively poor outcomes in catchers may be related to throwing volume, both inside and outside of games. Limitations of the study include the data being procured from a database, which lacks detail related to non-operative treatment modality failure, surgical details, and rehabilitation specifics [17].

Jack et al., also in 2018, reported the outcomes of UCLR in 33 MLB position players from 1984 to 2015 in an online search study. The players identified, with a mean age of 30.2 ± 4.2 years and mean MLB experience of 6.3 ± 3.9 years, were compared to a position-matched control group. The study included 7 catchers (21%), 12 infielders (36%), and 14 outfielders (43%). The authors, similar to Camp et al., noted an increase in UCLR in position players over the study period. A RSL rate of 84.8% was noted at a mean 336.9 ± 121.8 days after UCLR. A statistically significant difference in RSL rates of 53.3% and 89.4% was noted when comparing players aged 30 years or older to younger players, respectively. MLB experience did not correlate with outcomes. Relative to position-matched controls at 91.2%, the 1 year MLB career survival rate of position players undergoing UCLR was 73.5%. Catchers in the control group were noted to have significantly longer MLB career survivorship relative to catchers after UCLR, but all other position players after UCLR had similar career lengths and number of games played per season relative to position-matched controls. Twelve players in the study were noted to change positions after surgery, all infielders and outfielders. Outfielders were noted to have a significant decrease in WAR after surgery. No differences in ultimate zone rating was noted for outfielders and infielders post-operatively. Limitations of this study included the use of publicly available data only which may introduce bias, an inability to access surgical details, and limited ability to discern injury severity and rehabilitation specifics [29].

Conclusion

The rate of medial ulnar collateral ligament injuries (UCL) in baseball position players is rising. The treatment of UCL injuries in position players is identical to the treatment in pitchers. Though described less frequently than in pitchers, injuries to the UCL in position players are increasingly necessitating ulnar collateral ligament reconstruction (UCLR). The results of surgery are generally satisfactory, with return to play (RTP) outcomes of 75–80%. Position players typically take less time than pitchers to RTP; however, catchers have been described as having inferior outcomes in performance statistics and ability to RTP. There is a paucity of clinical data in the current literature describing the results of UCLR, epidemiology of UCL injuries, risks of surgery, subsequent injury, performance outcomes, and necessity of revision surgery in position players.

References

1. Morrey BF, An KN. Articular and ligamentous contributions to the stability of the elbow joint. Am J Sports Med. 1983;11(5):315–9.
2. Morrey BF, An KN. Functional anatomy of the ligaments of the elbow. Clin Orthop Relat Res. 1985;201:84–90.
3. Hyman J, Breazeale NM, Altchek DW. Valgus instability of the elbow in athletes. Clin Sports Med. 2001;20(1):25–45. viii
4. Fleisig GS, et al. Kinetics of baseball pitching with implications about injury mechanisms. Am J Sports Med. 1995;23(2):233–9.
5. Loftice J, et al. Biomechanics of the elbow in sports. Clin Sports Med. 2004;23(4):519–30, vii–viii.
6. Rettig AC, et al. Nonoperative treatment of ulnar collateral ligament injuries in throwing athletes. Am J Sports Med. 2001;29(1):15–7.
7. Camp CL, et al. Epidemiology of ulnar collateral ligament reconstruction in major and minor league baseball pitchers: comprehensive report of 1429 cases. J Shoulder Elb Surg. 2018;27(5):871–8.
8. Conte S, Camp CL, Dines JS. Injury trends in major league baseball over 18 seasons: 1998–2015. Am J Orthop (Belle Mead NJ). 2016;45(3):116–23.
9. Conte SA, et al. Prevalence of ulnar collateral ligament surgery in professional baseball players. Am J Sports Med. 2015;43(7):1764–9.
10. Cain EL Jr, et al. Outcome of ulnar collateral ligament reconstruction of the elbow in 1281 athletes: results in 743 athletes with minimum 2-year follow-up. Am J Sports Med. 2010;38(12):2426–34.
11. Erickson BJ, et al. Ulnar collateral ligament reconstruction of the elbow: a systematic review of the literature. Orthop J Sports Med. 2015;3(12):2325967115618914.
12. Griffith TB, et al. Comparison of outcomes based on graft type and tunnel configuration for primary ulnar

collateral ligament reconstruction in professional baseball pitchers. Am J Sports Med. 2019;47(5):1103–10.
13. DeFroda SF, et al. Epidemiology of elbow ulnar collateral ligament injuries among baseball players: National Collegiate Athletic Association Injury Surveillance Program, 2009–2010 through 2013–2014. Am J Sports Med. 2018;46(9):2142–7.
14. Dodson CC, et al. Medial ulnar collateral ligament reconstruction of the elbow in throwing athletes. Am J Sports Med. 2006;34(12):1926–32.
15. Ford GM, et al. Return-to-play outcomes in professional baseball players after medial ulnar collateral ligament injuries: comparison of operative versus nonoperative treatment based on magnetic resonance imaging findings. Am J Sports Med. 2016;44(3):723–8.
16. Begly JP, et al. Performance outcomes after medial ulnar collateral ligament reconstruction in Major League Baseball positional players. J Shoulder Elb Surg. 2018;27(2):282–90.
17. Camp CL, et al. Following ulnar collateral ligament reconstruction, professional baseball position players return to play faster than pitchers, but catchers return less frequently. J Shoulder Elb Surg. 2018;27(6):1078–85.
18. Erickson BJ, et al. An acute ulnar collateral ligament tear in a professional baseball player while batting requiring ulnar collateral ligament reconstruction. J Shoulder Elb Surg. 2018;27(9):e279–82.
19. O'Driscoll SW, et al. Origin of the medial ulnar collateral ligament. J Hand Surg Am. 1992;17(1):164–8.
20. O'Driscoll SW, Lawton RL, Smith AM. The "moving valgus stress test" for medial collateral ligament tears of the elbow. Am J Sports Med. 2005;33(2):231–9.
21. Camp CL, et al. Decreased shoulder external rotation and flexion are greater predictors of injury than internal rotation deficits: analysis of 132 pitcher-seasons in professional baseball. Arthroscopy. 2017;33(9):1629–36.
22. Ramkumar PN, et al. Clinical utility of an MRI-based classification system for operative versus nonoperative management of ulnar collateral ligament tears: a 2-year follow-up study. Orthop J Sports Med. 2019;7(4):2325967119839785.
23. Ramkumar PN, et al. Prognostic utility of an magnetic resonance imaging-based classification for operative versus nonoperative management of ulnar collateral ligament tears: one-year follow-up. J Shoulder Elb Surg. 2019;28(6):1159–65.
24. Jobe FW, Stark H, Lombardo SJ. Reconstruction of the ulnar collateral ligament in athletes. J Bone Joint Surg Am. 1986;68(8):1158–63.
25. Rohrbough JT, et al. Medial collateral ligament reconstruction of the elbow using the docking technique. Am J Sports Med. 2002;30(4):541–8.
26. Camp CL, et al. Ulnar collateral ligament reconstruction of the elbow: the docking technique. Arthrosc Tech. 2016;5(3):e519–23.
27. Dugas JR, et al. Ulnar collateral ligament repair with collagen-dipped FiberTape augmentation in overhead-throwing athletes. Am J Sports Med. 2019;47(5):1096–102.
28. Savoie FH 3rd, et al. Primary repair of ulnar collateral ligament injuries of the elbow in young athletes: a case series of injuries to the proximal and distal ends of the ligament. Am J Sports Med. 2008;36(6):1066–72.
29. Jack RA 2nd, et al. Performance and return to sport after Tommy John surgery among Major League Baseball position players. Am J Sports Med. 2018;46(7):1720–6.

Management of UCL Injuries in Non-throwing Athletes

29

James B. Carr II

Introduction

Injury to the ulnar collateral ligament (UCL) was initially described in javelin throwers by Waris in 1946 [1]. Nearly three decades later, Frank Jobe introduced ulnar collateral ligament reconstruction using a free tendon graft in professional pitcher Tommy John [2]. His subsequent case series of UCL reconstruction in 16 athletes revolutionized the treatment of what was once considered a career ending injury in overhead throwers. The introduction of UCL reconstruction by Jobe sparked a newfound interest in UCL injuries and UCL reconstruction techniques. This led to an abundance of literature focused on UCL injuries, including epidemiology, mechanism of injury, modifications to the UCL reconstruction technique, and outcomes following various treatment strategies.

The overwhelming majority of UCL injuries occur in overhead throwing athletes, especially baseball pitchers, due to the extreme, repetitive valgus force placed on the elbow during the pitching motion. Other overhead throwing athletes, including softball players and javelin throwers, are at a high risk for UCL injury. Furthermore, throwing athletes often require surgical reconstruction in order to return to previous level of competition. As a result, the vast majority of available literature on UCL injuries focuses on results in this specific demographic.

However, UCL injuries are not unique to overhead throwing athletes. A variety of sports other than baseball can place the UCL at risk for injury, either from repetitive valgus stress or more likely from episodic traumatic forces to the elbow. Combat sports (i.e., wrestling, mixed martial arts, jiu-jitsu), contact sports (football, hockey, rugby), and tumbling sports (gymnastics and cheerleading) often expose the elbow to forceful valgus loads and/or frequent weight bearing through the elbow joint, potentially creating a UCL injury.

Given the paucity of literature examining UCL injuries in the non-throwing athlete, management of these types of injuries can present a conundrum for the treating physician. Very few studies include non-throwing athletes in the analysis, and even fewer studies are solely dedicated to UCL injuries in non-throwing athletes. Though supporting literature is scarce, decision making is often based on a variety of factors, including age of the patient, level of competition, sport-specific demands, and timing within the sport season. This chapter presents a summary of the available literature of UCL injuries in non-throwing athletes as well as the author's preferred algorithm for management.

J. B. Carr II (✉)
Sports Medicine Institute, Hospital for Special Surgery, West Palm Beach, FL, USA
e-mail: carrja@hss.edu

J. S. Dines et al. (eds.), *Elbow Ulnar Collateral Ligament Injury*,
https://doi.org/10.1007/978-3-030-69567-5_29

Epidemiology

Like most aspects of UCL injury research, the epidemiology of such injuries is well described in throwing athletes but less so in the non-throwing athlete population [3–7]. This is likely attributable to its presumed lower incidence in non-throwing athletes. One of the first epidemiology studies for UCL injuries in non-throwing professional athletes was performed by Kenter et al. [8] They analyzed acute elbow injuries between 1991 and 1996 in the National Football League (NFL) and found that 19 of 91 (21%) elbow injuries were ulnar collateral ligament tears. The vast majority of these injuries (17 of 19) occurred in players other than quarterback. All players with UCL injuries were treated non-operatively, and all players were able to return to competition with an average time loss of less than one game.

Combat athletes have one of the highest rates of UCL injuries among non-throwing athletes. Frey et al. reviewed injury rates during 21 seasons of judo competitions in France and reported that UCL injuries accounted for 17% of all injuries [9]. Competing at a more elite level was a risk factor for sustaining a UCL injury, likely because of the increased forces transmitted during competition at higher levels of combat. Similarly, another epidemiology study of Brazilian jiu-jitsu athletes found the elbow joint to be the most commonly injured joint with UCL sprains occurring 6 times out of 5022 athlete exposures [10]. Interestingly, the Brazilian jiu-jitsu arm bar was the most commonly implicated mechanism of UCL injury, likely due to the possibility for a forceful valgus load.

One of the most robust epidemiological studies for UCL injuries in non-throwing athletes was performed by Li et al. [11] They analyzed the National Collegiate Athletic Association (NCAA) Injury Surveillance Program for UCL injuries between the academic years of 2009 and 2013 across 25 varsity NCAA sports. During the five seasons surveyed, there were a total of 109 UCL injuries reported, accounting for an overall UCL injury rate of 0.29 per 10,000 athlete exposures. Surprisingly, the majority of UCL injuries (83 out of 109, 76.1%) occurred in non-throwing athletes. The other 26 UCL injuries (23.9%) occurred in a throwing athlete, including baseball, softball, and javelin throwers. Wrestling and football were the most commonly played non-throwing sports for UCL injuries. However, UCL injuries in throwing athletes accounted for more time missed with a greater proportion of athletes missing more than 3 weeks of competition (36.4% vs 9.1% in throwing and non-throwing athletes, respectively). UCL injuries in throwing athletes also more commonly resulted in surgical intervention (11.1%) compared to non-throwing athletes (1.3%).

While data is still limited, a non-throwing, contact trauma to the elbow is the most likely mechanism for a UCL injury in a non-throwing athlete. UCL injuries in non-throwing athletes likely do not garner as much attention as their throwing athlete counterparts due to the less morbidity and decreased incidence of surgery often seen in non-throwing athletes.

Mechanism of Injury

The UCL originates from the humeral medial epicondyle and has a broad insertion onto the sublime tubercle [12]. It is composed of the anterior bundle, the posterior bundle, and the transverse ligament. The UCL is the primary soft tissue restraint to valgus load of the elbow, with the anterior bundle being the most important stabilizer. Therefore, recreation of the anterior bundle is the primary goal of UCL reconstruction surgery.

In the throwing athlete, the UCL is often injured from repetitive valgus stress incurred during the late cocking and early acceleration phases of the throwing motion. This can result in microtrauma to the ligament and eventual attritional failure. In the non-throwing athlete, there are a variety of potential mechanisms of injury to the UCL with acute trauma being the most common denominator. For example, in combat sports, a single, forceful valgus stress can be applied to the arm during a combat maneuver, most frequently an arm bar. A sudden external rotation force during an arm bar can especially result in a large valgus force to the elbow, which can result in a traumatic UCL injury [10]. Bracing the body from a fall can also result in a sudden valgus force that can lead to UCL injury. Similarly, UCL injuries occur in contact sports, such as football or rugby, most commonly from engaging the arm in extension during a block or from a sudden traumatic collision or fall [8].

Gymnastics and cheerleading place unique forces across the athlete's elbow because it becomes a weight bearing joint during many of the tumbling techniques. Koh et al. analyzed the weight bearing forces through the elbow joint in gymnasts performing a back handspring [13]. They found that ground reactive forces at the hand during upper extremity loading created a compressive force on the elbow that averages 2.37 times bodyweight and a valgus force that averages 0.03 × body weight × body height. As a result of frequent upper extremity weight bearing with associated valgus loads, gymnasts can develop both attritional and traumatic injuries to the UCL. Therefore, gymnasts are a unique subset of athletes with specialized demands on the elbow that must be considered when developing a treatment plan.

Understanding the mechanism of UCL injury in a non-throwing athlete is critical for developing a successful treatment plan. Because non-throwing athletes often sustain traumatic UCL injuries without chronic, attritional changes, they may be more amenable to non-operative management than their throwing athlete counterparts. The following section will discuss treatment options with respective results in the non-throwing athlete as well as the author's preferred algorithm.

Treatment Outcomes

Treatment options for a UCL injury include non-operative versus operative management. There are different surgical options, including ligament reconstruction or ligament repair with or without augmentation. Determining the appropriate treatment option depends on a variety of factors, including the type of sport played, level of competition, timing within the season, and shared decision making with the athlete. Unlike throwing athletes, some non-throwing athletes have a better likelihood of succeeding with non-operative management since they do not place repetitive valgus stress on the elbow. Gymnasts are a unique subgroup of non-throwing athletes that do place repetitive valgus stress on the elbow, so decision making can be more difficult in this population.

UCL injuries occur on a spectrum based on degree (partial, complete, or avulsion) and location (proximal, midsubstance, or distal). These factors often have prognostic implications and can influence treatment decisions. While there is extensive literature investigating treatment outcomes in throwing athletes, the available literature for non-throwing athletes is relatively sparse. The current section reviews outcome literature for various treatment options in non-throwing athletes.

Non-operative Management

While non-operative management tends to be unsuccessful in certain patterns of UCL injuries in throwing athletes, it is more successful in non-throwing athletes. Early studies reported poor return to sport rates in throwing athletes following non-operative management. Rettig et al. reported results in 31 overhead throwing athletes with UCL injury treated non-operatively with 2–3 months of bracing and progressive rehabilitation [14]. Only 13 patients (42%) were able to return to sport at an average of 24.5 weeks. Subsequent studies have highlighted the possibility of return to sports following a partial UCL injury, even in throwing athletes depending on tear pattern with partial proximal grade 1 or 2 UCL injuries having the best chance of full recovery [15].

In the non-throwing athletes, there is limited data on return to sport following non-operative management of a UCL injury. Nicolette et al. reported on five collegiate division I female gymnasts who sustained a UCL injury [16]. Every patient experienced a traumatic mechanism with a sudden valgus load applied to the elbow during a back handspring or fall from an elevated competition surface. Each patient had a magnetic resonance imaging (MRI) confirming a high grade partial or complete tear of the UCL without significant ligament attenuation. Following a structured rehabilitation protocol, 4 out of 5 gymnasts returned to sport an average of 3.98 weeks following the injury. Similarly, McCrum et al. presented a case series of 3 professional hockey players who sustained an acute, traumatic UCL injury from a collision or fall onto the ice [17]. MRI evaluation discovered two partial ligament tears and 1 complete proximal avulsion. All athletes returned to competition at an average of 36 days post-operatively following structured rehabilitation and a series of two leukocyte poor platelet rich plasma (PRP) injection (one injection 2 days and 1 week following the injury).

Platelet-rich plasma is an emerging biologic agent for the treatment of partial UCL tears. There are no studies evaluating the use of PRP for partial UCL tears in non-throwing athletes as all studies evaluate PRP in throwing athletes [18–20]. These results have been encouraging with similar return to sport rates as non-operative management of low-grade UCL injuries. However, it should be noted that these studies are often limited by a lack of control group.

Operative Management with UCL Reconstruction

While dedicated case series of UCL injuries in non-throwing athletes are rare, some larger studies have included non-throwing athletes with throwing athletes. These provide the majority of available evidence for the role of UCL reconstruction in the non-throwing athlete. Unfortunately, this does limit the generalizability of these studies to non-throwing athletes since the overall amount of such patients remains limited.

One study reports outcomes of UCL reconstruction specifically in non-throwing athletes. Fuller et al. reported results in 66 United States military members with 86.4% of patients reporting no significant disability in their elbow at final follow-up [21]. A total of 83.3% of patients reported a good or excellent outcome. Interestingly, 47% of patients had a previous history of playing a throwing sport, most commonly being a baseball pitcher.

Multiple studies have reported outcomes following UCL reconstruction with a mixed cohort of throwing and non-throwing athletes. Jones et al. reported 55 adolescent athletes status post UCL reconstruction using the docking technique [22]. There were three gymnasts in the group. While 87% of patients in the overall cohort reported an excellent Conway score, only one out of three had an excellent Conway score at final follow-up with only one patient returning to gymnastics. However, it should be noted that the two gymnasts who did not return to competition had advanced osteochondral capitellar injuries that underwent microfracture at the time of surgery.

Similarly, Erickson et al. reported on 187 patients after UCL reconstruction at a single institution [23]. The cohort was largely baseball players except for two gymnasts and one cheerleader. One gymnast (50%) and the cheerleader were able to return to the previous level of competition.

Operative Management with UCL Repair

UCL repair has historically had poor results with return to sport rates typically around 50–63% in overhead athletes [24, 25]. However, with the knowledge of the spectrum of UCL injuries (i.e., partial vs complete tears and distal vs proximal tears) as well as different athletic demands based on the sport, UCL repair has gained renewed interest. The use of collagen dipped suture augmentation for UCL repair has also contributed to renewed interest as results have been more promising with newer techniques [26–28].

Savoie et al. reported a series of 60 patients with UCL insufficiency treated with primary repair [28]. All patients failed a 3 month trial of rehabilitation and had injury to the UCL at a single site within the ligament. Most patients were overhead athletes, but there were nine non-overhead athletes (two basketball players, two cheerleaders, and five gymnasts). Nearly 93% of patients returned to the same level of sport at mean 6 months postoperatively, including every non-throwing athlete.

Richard et al. analyzed UCL repair following acute traumatic injury [29]. Seven out of ten athletes were non-throwing athletes (football, golf, swimming, wrestling, and volleyball) and underwent repair with non-absorbable suture and a humeral tunnel. Nine out of ten athletes returned to the same level of sport between 4 and 6 months. The only athlete who did not return to sport was a senior football player who did not play professionally.

Preferred Algorithm

Acute traumatic UCL injuries in the non-throwing athlete can often be treated non-operatively due to the different mechanism of injury and different athletic demands compared to UCL insufficiency in the throwing athlete. For throwing athletes, UCL reconstruction remains the gold standard for UCL insufficiency that does not respond to rest and conservative management. Most non-throwing athletes can successfully be treated non-operatively. Collision athletes who do not throw are especially amenable to non-operative management, and this is the preferred first-line treatment for this subset of athletes. For tumbling and gymnastic athletes, treatment varies and is based on individual scenarios and shared decision making. Many gymnasts can be treated non-operatively, but if they do not respond after a 4–6 week trial of conservative management, then operative management should be recommended. When surgery is chosen, then reconstruction remains the gold standard though new techniques with UCL repair are promising, yet with insufficient data to support its regular use currently.

Conclusions

Unlike overhead throwing athletes who often experience attritional breakdown of the UCL, non-throwing athletes often experience UCL insufficiency after a single traumatic episode without chronic, attritional compromise of the ligament. Therefore, the mechanism of injury usually leads to damage at a single location of the ligament that is often amenable to non-operative management. Furthermore, the demands of the medial elbow differ significantly between throwing and non-throwing athletes because non-throwing athletes do not place repetitive valgus stress on the elbow. Therefore, non-operative management of UCL injury in non-throwing athletes can often result in appropriate healing with full return to sport. After failure of conservative management, surgical treatment is a reasonable option with generally good to excellent results. In the setting of a high grade partial or complete tear near one insertion site, UCL repair is a possibility though long-term outcome data is limited.

References

1. Waris W. Elbow injuries of javelin-throwers. Acta Chir Scand. 1946;93(6):563–75.
2. Jobe FW, Stark H, Lombardo SJ. Reconstruction of the ulnar collateral ligament in athletes. J Bone Jt Surg Ser A. 1986;68(8):1158–63.
3. Camp CL, Conte S, D'Angelo J, Fealy SA. Epidemiology of ulnar collateral ligament reconstruction in Major and Minor League Baseball pitchers: comprehensive report of 1429 cases. J Shoulder Elb Surg. 2018;27(5):871–8.
4. Erickson BJ, Nwachukwu BU, Rosas S, Schairer WW, McCormick FM, Bach BR, et al. Trends in medial ulnar collateral ligament reconstruction in the United States: a retrospective review of a large private-payer database from 2007 to 2011. Am J Sports Med. 2015;43:1770–4.
5. Mahure SA, Mollon B, Shamah SD, Kwon YW, Rokito AS. Disproportionate trends in ulnar collateral ligament reconstruction: projections through 2025 and a literature review. J Shoulder Elb Surg. 2016;25(6):1005–12.
6. Erickson BJ, Harris JD, Tetreault M, Bush-Joseph C, Cohen M, Romeo AA. Is Tommy John surgery performed more frequently in major league baseball pitchers from warm weather areas? Orthop J Sport Med. 2014;2(10):1–6.
7. Zaremski JL, Horodyski M, Donlan RM, Brisbane ST, Farmer KW. Does geographic location matter on the prevalence of ulnar collateral ligament reconstruction in collegiate baseball pitchers? Orthop J Sports Med. 2015;3(11):2325967115616582. https://doi.org/10.1177/2325967115616582. PMID: 26740953; PMCID: PMC4687835.

8. Kenter K, Behr CT, Warren RF, O'Brien SJ, Barnes R. Acute elbow injuries in the National Football League. J Shoulder Elb Surg / Am Shoulder Elb Surg [et al]. 2000;9(1):1–5.
9. Frey A, Lambert C, Vesselle B, Rousseau R, Dor F, Marquet LA, Toussaint JF, Crema MD. Epidemiology of judo-related injuries in 21 seasons of competitions in France: A prospective study of relevant traumatic injuries. Orthop J Sports Med. 2019;7(5):2325967119847470. https://doi.org/10.1177/2325967119847470. PMID: 31211149; PMCID: PMC6545656.
10. Scoggin JF 3rd, Brusovanik G, Izuka BH, Zandee van Rilland E, Geling O, Tokumura S. Assessment of injuries during Brazilian Jiu-Jitsu Competition. Orthop J Sports Med. 2014;2(2):2325967114522184. https://doi.org/10.1177/2325967114522184. PMID: 26535299; PMCID: PMC4555620.
11. Li NY, Goodman AD, Lemme NJ, Owens BD. Epidemiology of elbow ulnar collateral ligament injuries in throwing versus contact athletes of the National Collegiate Athletic Association: Analysis of the 2009–2010 to 2013–2014 Seasons. Orthop J Sports Med. 2019;7(4):2325967119836428. https://doi.org/10.1177/2325967119836428. PMID: 31008136; PMCID: PMC6457031.
12. Erickson BJ, Fu M, Meyers K, Camp CL, Altchek DW, Coleman SH, Dines JS. The middle and distal aspects of the ulnar footprint of the medial ulnar collateral ligament of the elbow do not provide significant resistance to Valgus Stress: A Biomechanical Study. Orthop J Sports Med. 2019;7(2):2325967118825294. https://doi.org/10.1177/2325967118825294. PMID: 30800692; PMCID: PMC6378449.
13. Koh TJ, Grabiner MD, Weiker GG. Technique and ground reaction forces in the back handspring. Am J Sports Med. 1992;20(1):61–6.
14. Rettig AC, Sherrill C, Snead DS, Mendler JC, Mieling P. Nonoperative treatment of ulnar collateral ligament injuries in throwing athletes. Am J Sports Med. 2001;29(1):15–7.
15. Frangiamore SJ, Lynch TS, Vaughn MD, Soloff L, Forney M, Styron JF, Schickendantz MS. Magnetic resonance imaging predictors of failure in the nonoperative management of ulnar collateral ligament injuries in professional baseball pitchers. Am J Sports Med. 2017;45(8):1783–9. https://doi.org/10.1177/0363546517699832. Epub 2017 Apr 11. PMID: 28398820.
16. Nicolette GW, Gravlee JR. Ulnar collateral ligament injuries of the elbow in female division I collegiate gymnasts: a report of five cases. Open Access J Sport Med. 2018;9:83–9.
17. McCrum CL, Costello J, Onishi K, Stewart C, Vyas D. Return to play after PRP and Rehabilitation of 3 elite ice hockey players with ulnar collateral ligament injuries of the elbow. Orthop J Sports Med. 2018;6(8):2325967118790760. https://doi.org/10.1177/2325967118790760. PMID: 30148179; PMCID: PMC6100131.
18. Deal JB, Smith E, Heard W, O'Brien MJ, Savoie FH 3rd. Platelet-Rich plasma for primary treatment of partial ulnar collateral ligament tears: MRI correlation with results. Orthop J Sports Med. 2017;5(11):2325967117738238. https://doi.org/10.1177/2325967117738238. PMID: 29164165; PMCID: PMC5686880.
19. Podesta L, Crow SA, Volkmer D, Bert T, Yocum LA. Treatment of partial ulnar collateral ligament tears in the elbow with platelet-rich plasma. Am J Sports Med. 2013;41(7):1689–94.
20. Dines JS, Williams PN, ElAttrache N, Conte S, Tomczyk T, Osbahr DC, et al. Platelet-rich plasma can be used to successfully treat elbow ulnar collateral ligament insufficiency in high-level throwers. Am J Orthop (Belle Mead NJ). 2016;45(5):296–300.
21. Fuller JB, Dunn JC, Kusnezov NA, Nesti LJ, Kilcoyne KG. Outcome measures after medial ulnar collateral ligament reconstructions in a military population. J Shoulder Elb Surg. 2019;28(2):317–23.
22. Jones KJ, Dines JS, Rebolledo BJ, Weeks KD, Williams RJ, Dines DM, Altchek DW. Operative management of ulnar collateral ligament insufficiency in adolescent athletes. Am J Sports Med. 2014;42(1):117–21. https://doi.org/10.1177/0363546513507695. Epub 2013 Oct 21. PMID: 24145949.
23. Jones KJ, Dines JS, Rebolledo BJ, Weeks KD, Williams RJ, Dines DM, Altchek DW. Operative management of ulnar collateral ligament insufficiency in adolescent athletes. Am J Sports Med. 2014;42(1):117-21. https://doi.org/10.1177/0363546513507695. Epub 2013 Oct 21. PMID: 24145949.
24. Azar FM, Andrews JR, Wilk KE, Groh D. Operative treatment of ulnar collateral ligament injuries of the elbow in athletes. Am J Sports Med. 2000;28(1):16–23.
25. Conway JE, Jobe FW, Glousman RE, Pink M. Medial instability of the elbow in throwing athletes. Treatment by repair or reconstruction of the ulnar collateral ligament. J Bone Jt Surg Ser A. 1992;74(1):67–83.
26. Gilliam BD, Douglas L, Fleisig GS, Aune KT, Mason KA, Dugas JR, et al. Return to play and outcomes in baseball players after superior labral anterior-posterior repairs. Am J Sports Med. 2018;46(1):109–15.
27. Jones CM, Beason DP, Dugas JR. Ulnar collateral ligament reconstruction versus repair with internal bracing: Comparison of cyclic fatigue mechanics. Orthop J Sports Med. 2018;6(2):2325967118755991. https://doi.org/10.1177/2325967118755991. PMID: 29479544; PMCID: PMC5818096.
28. Savoie FH, Trenhaile SW, Roberts J, Field LD, Ramsey JR. Primary repair of ulnar collateral ligament injuries of the elbow in young athletes: a case series of injuries to the proximal and distal ends of the ligament. Am J Sports Med. 2008;36(6):1066–72.
29. Richard MJ, Aldridge JM, Wiesler ER, Ruch DS. Traumatic valgus instability of the elbow: Pathoanatomy and results of direct repair. J Bone Jt Surg Ser A. 2008;90(11):2416–22.

Ulnar Collateral Ligament Injury in Female Athletes

30

Elizabeth C. Gardner, Joe Manzi, Kathryn McElheny, and Asheesh Bedi

Introduction

Traditionally, injury to the ulnar collateral ligament (UCL) of the elbow has been associated with the male baseball pitcher. This is emphasized by the fact that the eponym for the classic reconstruction of this ligament is known as "Tommy John" surgery, named for the then Los Angeles Dodgers pitcher who underwent surgery by Dr. Frank Jobe in 1974. However, while less commonly reported, injuries to the UCL have now been described in the female athlete population. Recognition of this injury and knowledge of treatment options in female athletes is vital to achieve optimal results.

Epidemiology and Pathoanatomy

The function of the UCL has been well described in this text and elsewhere. In brief, the anterior bundle of the UCL serves as the primary stabilizer against valgus stress to the elbow within a functional range of motion, from 25° to 125° of flexion. In response to valgus load at the elbow, the UCL helps to provide a stabilizing varus force. No matter the specific sport, recurrent valgus stress at the elbow results in a triad of pathologic lesions: traction to the medial structures, compression of the lateral structures and posteromedially directed shear, and compression of the olecranon.

While the function of the UCL is thought to be similar in both sexes, there have not been any studies comparing the biomechanical properties of female UCL to those of the better studied male UCL. However, as previous study of females' anterior cruciate ligaments has demonstrated significant differences, including a lower percentage of collagen [1], less elasticity, and failure at 30% less load than males' [2], it is reasonable to think that there may be similarly important differences in the UCL. Additionally, certain important anatomic differences in the male and female body do exist. The upper torso and arm of female athletes typically possess less muscle mass and strength than the male athlete, and as such, female athletes generate less muscle torque and power. At the elbow, the carrying angle is greater, and there is often more ligamentous laxity in female athletes. Though defined, Goldfarb et al. believed this carrying angle difference to be of little clinical significance [3]. Even so, it is important to keep these distinctions, known and potential, in mind

E. C. Gardner
Department of Orthopaedic Surgery, Yale University, New Haven, CT, USA

J. Manzi · K. McElheny (✉)
Sports Medicine Institute, Hospital for Special Surgery, New York, NY, USA
e-mail: mcelhenyk@hss.edu

A. Bedi
Department of Orthopaedic Surgery, University of Michigan, Ann Arbor, MI, USA

J. S. Dines et al. (eds.), *Elbow Ulnar Collateral Ligament Injury*,
https://doi.org/10.1007/978-3-030-69567-5_30

when considering risk factors for UCL injury and its treatment.

Injuries to the UCL in female athletes, as in their male counterparts, typically occur through one of two mechanisms. The first is a single extraordinary valgus force to the elbow that causes an acute rupture of the ligament. In these rarer cases of an acute, traumatic rupture, some patients, particularly those of younger age, may experience a bony avulsion of the ligament from the sublime tubercle of the ulna. The more common mechanism is chronic microtrauma, which leads to microtears and eventual ligament attenuation, or complete tearing. With or without partial tearing at the proximal or distal attachments, this may render the ligament nonfunctional.

Biomechanics of UCL Injury in Women

Since 1946, when Waris [4] first described injury to the UCL in a group of 17 elite javelin throwers, many other sports have been implicated (Table 30.1). Female athletes participating in the following sports have been reported to have suffered UCL injuries: softball [5], gymnastics [6, 7], baseball [6], calf roping [5], cheerleading [5], javelin [4, 6], tennis [5, 6], baton twirling [5], judo [6], swimming [6], equestrian [6], alpine skiing [5], and handball [6]. In the largest published study of UCL injuries in female athletes, none of the patients competed professionally [5].

Of all overhead athletic motions, the baseball pitch is considered to be one of the most violent in its effect on the shoulder and elbow. As such, the baseball pitching motion has been extensively studied. It has been repeatedly shown that the greatest varus torque occurs during the late cocking and early acceleration phases of pitching, when varus torque is necessary to prevent valgus extension of the elbow. Werner et al. showed that while the UCL is thought to be the primary contributor to varus torque, contraction of the wrist flexor-pronator group also provides a stabilizing force. In their study, Werner et al. found a maximum varus torque of 120 Nm in their cohort of male baseball pitchers. This high value is thought to exceed the intrinsic strength of the UCL, thus explaining the high incidence of UCL injuries in this population.

Table 30.1 Sports with reported UCL injuries in female athletes

Softball	Gymnastics
Baseball	Calf roping
Cheerleading	Javelin
Tennis	Baton twirling
Judo	Swimming
Equestrian	Alpine skiing
Handball	–

Chu et al. [8] performed a biomechanical comparison of the pitching motions of elite male and female baseball pitchers. They found that female athletes displayed significantly slower ball velocity, which is not surprising considering that the women had a smaller body height and mass than their male counterparts. There were other differences in the kinetics and kinematics of the female baseball pitch, including a maximum elbow varus torque of approximately 75 % of males' values, at 46 Nm. While this value is likely below the load limit of the male UCL, without specific knowledge of the biomechanical properties of the female UCL, it is impossible to know if this can adequately explain the relative paucity of UCL injuries in female athletes. Chu et al. did find that when normalized for body height and weight, the peak varus torque values were very similar between the genders.

Barrentine et al. [9] have described the softball windmill pitch in a way similar to that of the baseball pitch, as is shown in Fig. 30.1. The motion is separated into four phases: wind-up, stride, delivery, and follow through. In their study of eight healthy female softball pitchers, they demonstrated that there is significantly less varus torque produced during windmill pitching than in baseball pitching, and theorized that this is the reason why UCL injuries are rarely seen in these athletes. Their data are presented in Fig. 30.2. In fact, in his report of UCL injuries in women, Argo [5] found that of eight injured softball players, only one was a pitcher.

There have been several studies that have investigated the biomechanics of javelin

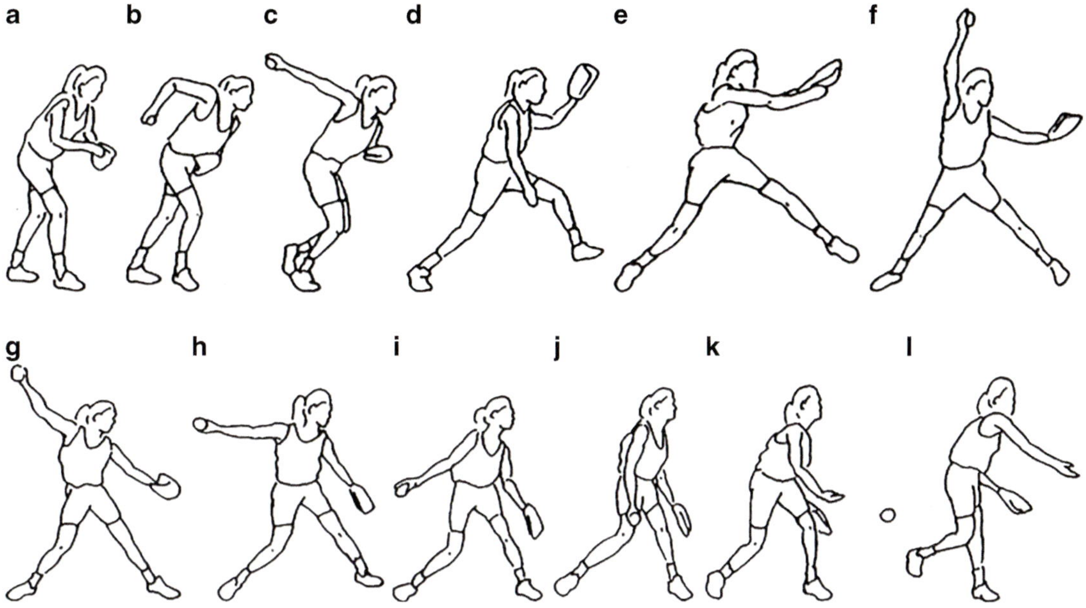

Fig. 30.1 Sequence of motion in windmill pitching. (**a–c**) Wind-up. (**d–f**) Stride. (**g–j**) Delivery. (**k, l**) Follow through

throwing, although they have focused primarily on performance rather than joint stress or load [10, 11]. The elbow is held in extension until the moment of the final foot strike, in order to lengthen the acceleration path of the javelin and thus generate a higher release speed. From the instant of final foot strike to release, called the thrust phase, the elbow flexes rapidly. As much as 70 % of the release speed of the javelin spear is generated in the last 0.1 s, during which the elbow flexion velocity nears 1900°/s [11]. Unfortunately, there has not been specific measurement of the varus torque generated during javelin throwing. In Dines' [12] report of UCL reconstruction in javelin throwers, he offered the similar observation that while the at-risk position during baseball pitching is during the late-cocking and early acceleration phases, in javelin throwers, maximum angular velocities occur during the thrust phase of the throw. There have been no studies specifically examining the biomechanics of female javelin throwers, and thus injury mechanism must be inferred from these male studies.

Tennis remains a very popular overhead sport for both sexes. Elliott et al. [13] investigated the loading of the shoulder and elbow joint during the tennis serve in male and female athletes. Men recorded significantly higher service speeds and had higher peak absolute elbow varus torque (78.3 vs. 58.2 Nm). They also noted that players who flexed the front knee by 7.6° in the backswing phase of the serve, while having a similar serve speed, demonstrated larger normalized varus torque when the arm was in the maximally externally rotated position, when compared with those players who flexed the front knee by 14.7°. The reason why a more effective knee bend decreases elbow varus torque in unclear.

The biomechanics of gymnastics have also been studied to explain the risk for UCL injury in these athletes. Elements such as the back handspring or handstand transform the elbow into a weight-bearing joint. During the performance of these skills, a compressive and valgus load is transmitted through the elbow joint [5]. Nicolette et al. [14] suggest that stress to the UCL is in fact quite frequent. Given the commonness of backhand spring maneuvers, considered a basic transitory step in many gymnast activities often performed hundreds of times a day, continuous valgus force across the UCL is endured. Nicolette states that increased bony stability in extension and increased articular contact during pronation

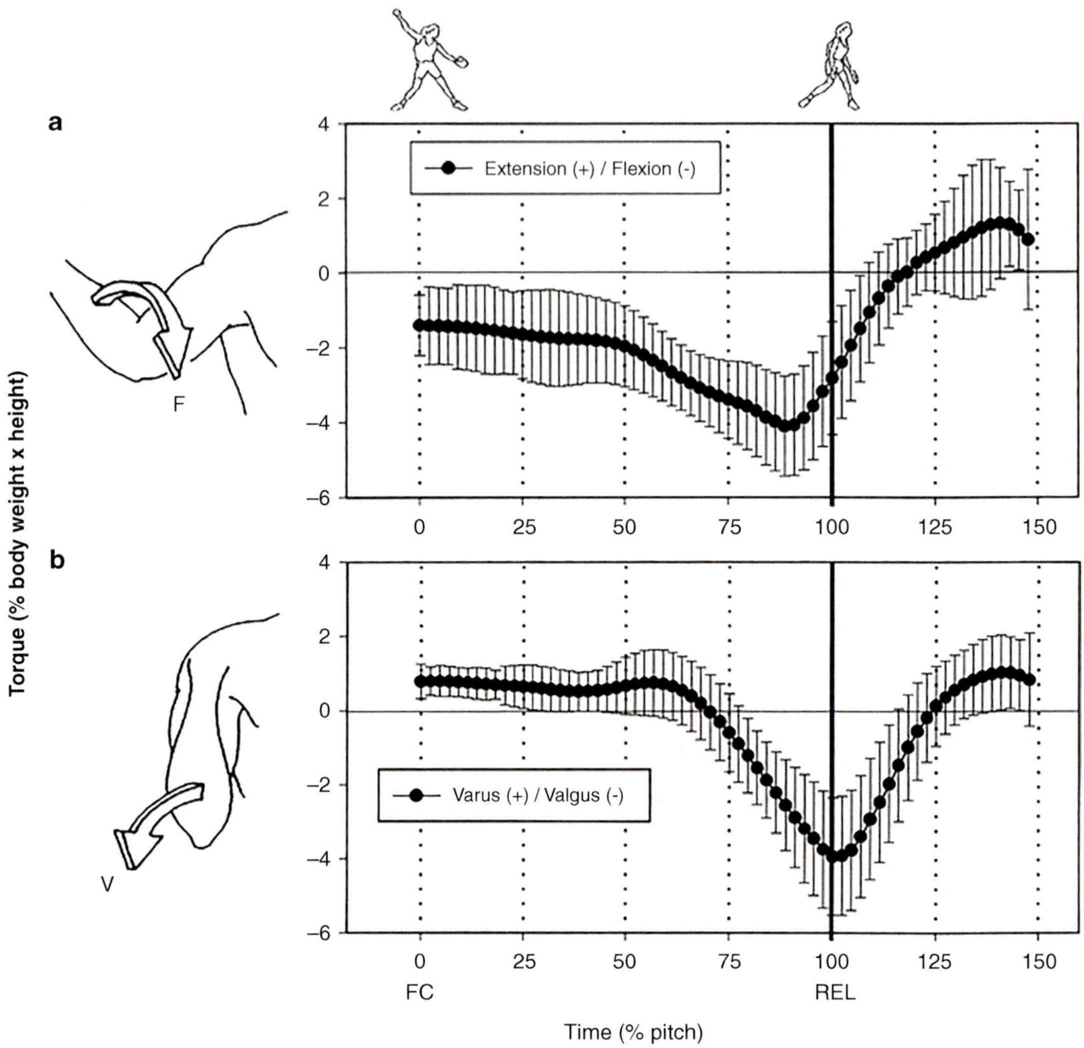

Fig. 30.2 Torque applied to the forearm at the elbow for varus(+)/valgus(−) versus time. (**a, b**), Graphs represent mean and standard deviation data for all subjects. The instances of foot contact (FC) and ball release (REL) are shown

may in fact prevent damage, potentially explaining why UCL injury is relatively rare in these athletes.

Reeser et al. [15] examined the biomechanics of the upper limb during the volleyball spike and serve in an effort to understand this popular women's overhead sport. They found that maximum elbow varus torque was produced near the time of maximum external rotation of the arm, during which arm cocking is decelerated and forward rotation is initiated. Of all skills tested, cross-body spike, straight-ahead spike, roll shot, jump serve, and float serve, the highest elbow varus torque was found to occur during the jump serve (43.3 Nm). This value is lower than the maximum varus torque seen in female baseball pitchers as discussed above and helps to explain why UCL injuries have not been reported to occur in this dynamic overhead sport.

Presentation and Evaluation

As with all patients, initial evaluation of female athletes with a suspected UCL injury starts with a thorough history. This includes the patient's sport and level of participation. The events surrounding the initial onset of symptoms and their chronicity are critical. Patients should be questioned regarding the details of current symptoms, including pain, popping sensation during activity, and paresthesias. Previous treatment, such as rest, injections, and surgery, and its effect should be noted. Also important are details regarding the athlete's performance since the time of injury, such as speed and accuracy of throwing and ability to perform sport-specific skills.

The physical examination of male and female patients with medial elbow pain is similar and should include inspection, palpation, and motion of the bilateral upper extremities and neck. Female patients with UCL injuries commonly have point tenderness just distal to the medial epicondyle. It is important to thoroughly evaluate for the presence of epicondylitis, although UCL injury and medial epicondylitis may be present concurrently. The integrity of the ligament should be carefully evaluated. Typically this occurs with the humerus stabilized while a valgus force is applied to a slightly flexed elbow (30°). The clinician then evaluates for the presence of tenderness overlying the UCL and joint space opening. Other tests, such as the "milking maneuver" and "Moving Valgus Stress Test" may be utilized as well. A neurovascular examination, specifically of the ulnar nerve, is also critical. It is important to note the presence or absence of the palmaris longus tendon, in case it may be needed for reconstruction.

Imaging of the elbow may include plain radiographs with or without valgus stress, dynamic ultrasound, arthrograms, and contrast or noncontrast computed tomography (CT) and magnetic resonance imaging (MRI). X-rays may reveal avulsion fracture, or secondary findings suggestive of chronic instability such as ossification of the ligament, loose bodies, or marginal osteophytes. Instability may be demonstrated on stress radiographs or dynamic ultrasound. It should be noted that it may be necessary to evaluate the uninjured elbow as well, in order to provide a comparison. The use of contrast dye in arthrograms, CT, or MRI may aid in the evaluation of the UCL by highlighting medial capsule rupture or even partial, undersurface tears in the case of CT or MRI.

Indications and Procedures

As with male patients, the initial treatment of all UCL injuries in female athletes is nonoperative. Consisting primarily of overhead activity cessation and a progressive rehabilitation program, this is an imperative part of the treatment algorithm. It is generally recommended that athletes undergo at least 3–6 months of nonoperative treatment. In a report of 31 throwing athletes, Rettig et al. [16] evaluated patients with UCL injuries that were all treated nonoperatively. His protocol involved an initial phase of throwing rest for 2–3 months with anti-inflammatories and therapeutic modalities to treat symptoms. Athletes were also placed into a long-arm splint or brace at 90° at night as needed to control pain. Once the athlete became pain-free, the splint or brace was discontinued. A progressive upper extremity strengthening was initiated with a throwing program instituted at 3 months. In this study, 42% of patients were able to return to their previous level of competition at an average of 24.5 weeks (range 13–54 weeks). There were only three women in this study and the specific results for these patients were not reported. Additionally, there were no predictive findings in either the patient's history or physical exam that was useful in predicting the success of nonoperative treatment.

An alternative nonoperative intervention considered in Podesta et al. [17] is the use of autologous platelet rich plasma (PRP) injections adjacent to and into the damaged UCL. This study protocol included 28 male and 6 female athletes with symptomatic MRI grade 1/2 partial UCL lesions, refractory to nonoperative treatment with attempted return to play. Autologous concentrates of PRP were injected under ultrasound guidance followed by a rehabilitation program of 12–14 weeks with sport specific training to follow. At an average follow-up of 70 weeks, 88% of patients returned to the same level of play with no complaints. Results were not stratified by sex or sport of play; however, the population included a majority of baseball players, as well as softball, tennis, and volleyball. Dines et al. [18] retrospective analysis of PRP injections in 44 baseball players spanning high school to professional showed 34% of patients returning to preinjury level and 39% returning to a lower level of competition.

If symptoms persist despite an adequate course of conservative treatment, then operative intervention may be considered. Understanding the pathoanatomy that underlies these injuries is essential when making treatment decisions. When an avulsion is present, repair through drill holes, or using suture anchors may be possible, as the ligamentous tissue itself is often not extensively injured. However, in cases of ligament attenuation, with or without partial tearing, the condition of the injured ligament must be closely assessed. If the tissue remaining is of good quality, then primary repair, with possible augmentation, may be considered. In their report of 14 direct ligament repairs in college and professional male baseball players, Conway and Jobe [19] found that while ten of 14 players had a good or excellent result, only 50 % were able to return to their previous level of play.

If the tissue has been extensively damaged, or if there is a complete tear of the ligament, then a classic reconstruction with grafting should be performed. There have been multiple surgical techniques described in the literature, which have been detailed elsewhere in this text. It is this author's preference to perform the reconstruction with a palmaris autograft when possible, utilizing a docking technique. And, while it is our practice to perform a nerve transposition only when preoperative ulnar nerve symptoms are present, this issue remains controversial within the orthopedic community. Current literature has not shown a benefit of one reconstruction technique over another in the treatment of female patients with UCL injury, and thus the chosen method should be based on surgeon preference.

Unfortunately, very little has been written about the specific treatment of UCL injuries in women. In the largest single report of the operative treatment of UCL injuries, Cain's [20] cohort of 1281 procedures included only 28 female patients. Similarly, in Vitale's [21] review of 285 patients, 99 % were male. Unfortunately, neither study stratified their results by gender. However, while bearing in mind the gender differences mentioned previously, one may use the male-dominated literature for guidance on treatment and outcomes. Table 30.2 summarizes the find-

Table 30.2 Women included in major studies of the treatment of UCL injuries

Authors	Data collection	Overall number of UCL patients	Number of female patients	Treatment for female patients
Andrews and Timmerman [22]	1986–1990	14	0/14	N/A
Argo et al. [5]	1994–2001	19	19/19	1/19 recon; 18/19 repair +/− augment
Azar et al. [23]	1988–1994	91	0/91	N/A
Cain et al. [20]	1988–2006	1281	28/1281	Not reported
Conway et al. [19]	1974–1987	70	1/70	1/1 recon
Dines et al. [24]	2006–2009	25	Not reported	Not reported
Dodson et al. [25]	2000–2003	100	0/100	N/A
Kodde et al. [6]	2001–2007	20	13/20	13/13 recon
Koh et al. [26]	Not Reported	20	0/20	N/A
Paletta and Wright [27]	1998–2000	25	0/25	N/A
Petty et al. [28]	1995–2000	27	0/27	N/A
Rettig [16]	1994–1997	31	3/31	3/3 non-op
Rohrbough [29]	1995–1999	36	1/36	1/1 recon
Savoie et al. [30]	1994–2001	60	13/60	13/13 recon
Thompson et al. [31]	1992–1996	83	1/83	1/1 recon
Total		1902	79	30 recon; 18 repair +/− augment; 3 non-op

ings of the largest UCL outcomes studies, with special attention paid to any included female patients. In most of the studies, the female patients have been treated according to the algorithm applied to the male patients. With the exception of Argo et al., when surgery was necessary, a reconstruction was performed utilizing the preferred technique of the author.

Argo [5] published the largest study of the treatment of UCL injuries in female patients, reporting on 19 women. They played sports including softball, gymnastics, and tennis. The most common pathology in this group was a distal soft tissue avulsion, occurring in 8 of 19 patients. These were repaired with suture anchors. He also commonly encountered central ligament attenuation, sometimes with partial tearing. He treated these athletes by plication of the ligament, with anchor reinforcement or flexor-pronator mass augmentation as necessary. In only one of 19 cases was a traditional UCL reconstruction performed, in this case using a palmaris autograft; the fixation technique was not described. This tendency toward ligament repair with potential augmentation, and away from reconstruction, is in contrast to treatment that has been described in the male athlete population, and represents a potential key difference in the treatment of male and female patients with UCL injuries.

Rehabilitation

Rehabilitation after UCL reconstruction in a female athlete does not differ from that of the male population, which is discussed extensively elsewhere in this text. Typically patients are placed into a hinged elbow brace for 6–8 weeks postoperatively, allowing progressive increase in the range of motion of the elbow. Strengthening of the wrist and forearm, along with scapular stabilization and shoulder isometric muscle training, begins soon after surgery. Isotonic exercises of the wrist and elbow are begun approximately 1 month after surgery, with eccentrics starting 1 month later. Plyometrics are introduced at 10 weeks postoperatively, and a throwing program is typically delayed until 14 weeks postoperatively.

The benefit of a primary repair, when possible, is that it allows for an accelerated rehabilitation program. In his protocol, Argo's [5] female UCL repair patients were progressed along 4 weeks ahead of those who underwent reconstruction. They were started on a sport-specific program within the brace, including a throwing progression when appropriate, at 4–6 weeks postoperatively. Perhaps as a result of this, he found that his repair patients were able to return to full athletic participation at an average of 2.5 months, whereas in Cain's [20] large report of reconstruction patients, the athletes did not return to full competition for an average of 11.6 months. Argo attributed this quick recovery to the less invasive nature of repair as compared to reconstruction. Additionally, as was discussed earlier in this chapter, due to anatomic gender differences in muscle mass and strength, as well as sport-specific demands, female athletes tend to place less strain on the UCL. This likely allows earlier return to "full function" when compared to their male counterparts.

Conclusion

Though infrequently reported, female athletes do suffer injuries to the UCL of the elbow. These occur during participation in a wide variety of sports, including softball, tennis, javelin, and gymnastics. The mechanism of injury is often chronic microtrauma; however, ligament avulsion is commonly seen as well. Extensive damage to the ligament necessitates reconstruction. To this point, there has not been any research to suggest a different approach to reconstruction in the female athlete, and thus the procedure performed is the same one classically described in the male athlete. However, when the ligament is not as extensively injured, Argo has reported excellent results with primary repair, although his study is limited by a small sample size. For this reason, in contrast to current literature regarding the treatment of male throwers, repair should be considered in these female patients competing at or below the college level. This offers the benefit of a less invasive procedure and potentially an earlier return to sport. However, treatment recommendations for the female athlete with a UCL injury are limited by the paucity of literature regarding both the biomechanics of the female ligament as well as outcome data in this patient population.

References

1. Hashemi J, et al. The human anterior cruciate ligament: sex differences in ultrastructure and correlation with biomechanical properties. J Orthop Res. 2008;26(7):945–50.
2. Chandrashekar N, et al. Sex-based differences in the tensile properties of the human anterior cruciate ligament. J Biomech. 2006;39:2943–50.
3. Goldfarb CA, Patterson JM, Sutter M, Krauss M, Steffen JA, Galatz L. Elbow radiographic anatomy: measurement techniques and normative data. J Shoulder Elbow Surg. 2012;21(9):1236–46.
4. Waris W. Elbow injuries of javelin throwers. Acta Chir Scand. 1946;93:563–75.
5. Argo D, et al. Operative treatment of ulnar collateral ligament insufficiency of the elbow in female athletes. Am J Sports Med. 2006;34(3):431–7.
6. Kodde IF, et al. Long-term results after ulnar collateral ligament reconstruction of the elbow in European athletes with interference screw techniques and triceps fascia autograft. J Shoulder Elbow Surg. 2012;21:1656–63.
7. Grumet RC, et al. Bony avulsion of the medial ulnar collateral ligament in a gymnast: a case report. J Shoulder Elbow Surg. 2010;19(7):e1–6.
8. Chu Y, et al. Biomechanical comparison between elite female and male baseball pitchers. J Appl Biomech. 2009;25:22–31.
9. Barrentine SW, et al. Biomechanics of windmill softball pitching with implications about injury mechanisms at the shoulder and elbow. J Orthop Sports Phys Ther. 1998 Dec;28(6):405–14.
10. Bartlett RM, et al. The biomechanics of javelin throwing. J Sports Sci. 1988;6:1–8.
11. Morris C, et al. Biomechanical factors critical to performance in the men's javelin throwing during the final thrust phases. Sports Med. 1996;21:438–46.
12. Dines JS, et al. Elbow ulnar collateral ligament reconstruction in javelin throwers at a minimum 2-year follow-up. Am J Sports Med. 2012;40(1):148–51.
13. Elliott B, et al. Technique effects on upper limb loading in the tennis serve. J Sci Med Sport. 2003;6(1):76–87.
14. Nicolette GW, Gravlee JR. Ulnar collateral ligament injuries of the elbow in female division i collegiate gymnasts: a report of five cases. Open Access J Sports Med. 2018;9:183–9. https://doi.org/10.2147/oajsm.s159624.
15. Reeser JC, et al. Upper limb biomechanics during the volleyball serve and spike. Sports Health. 2010;2:368–74.
16. Rettig AC, et al. Nonoperative treatment of ulnar collateral ligament injuries in throwing athletes. Am J Sports Med. 2001;29(1):15–7.
17. Podesta L, et al. Treatment of partial ulnar collateral ligament tears in the elbow with platelet-rich plasma. Am J Sports Med. 2013;41(7):1689–94. https://doi.org/10.1177/0363546513487979.
18. Dines JS, Williams PN, ElAttrache N, Conte S, Tomczyk T, Osbahr DC, Dines DM, Bradley J, Ahmad CS. Platelet-rich plasma can be used to successfully treat elbow ulnar collateral ligament insufficiency in high-level throwers. Am J Orthop (Belle Mead, N.J.). 2016;45(5):296–300.
19. Conway JE, et al. Medial instability of the elbow in throwing athletes. J Bone Joint Surg Am. 1992;74(1):67–83.
20. Cain EL Jr, et al. Outcome of ulnar collateral ligament reconstruction of the elbow in 1281 athletes: results in 743 athletes with minimum 2-year follow-up. Am J Sports Med. 2010;38(12):2426–34.
21. Vitale MA, et al. The outcome of elbow ulnar collateral ligament reconstruction in overhead athletes: a systematic review. Am J Sports Med. 2008;36(6):1193–205.
22. Andrews JR, Timmerman LA. Outcome of elbow surgery in professional baseball players. Am J Sports Med. 1995;23(4):407–13.
23. Azar FM, et al. Operative treatment of ulnar collateral ligament injuries of the elbow in athletes. Am J Sports Med. 2000;28(1):16–23.
24. Dines JS, et al. Clinical outcomes of the DANE TJ technique to treat ulnar collateral ligament insufficiency of the elbow. Am J Sports Med. 2007;35(12):2039–44.
25. Dodson CC, et al. Medial ulnar collateral ligament reconstruction of the elbow in throwing athletes. Am J Sports Med. 2006;34(12):1926–32.
26. Koh JL, et al. Ulnar collateral ligament reconstruction in elite throwing athletes. Arthroscopy. 2006;22(11):1187–91.
27. Paletta GA, Wright RW. The modified docking procedure for elbow ulnar collateral ligament reconstruction: 2-year follow-up in elite throwers. Am J Sports Med. 2006;34(10):1594–8.
28. Petty DH, et al. Ulnar collateral ligament reconstruction in high school baseball players. Am J Sports Med. 2004;32(5):1158–64.
29. Rohrbough JT, et al. Medial collateral ligament reconstruction of the elbow using the docking technique. Am J Sports Med. 2002;30(4):541–8.
30. Savoie FH, et al. Primary repair of ulnar collateral ligament injuries of the elbow in young athletes. Am J Sports Med. 2008;36(6):1066–72.
31. Thompson WH, et al. Ulnar collateral ligament reconstruction in athletes: muscle-splitting approach without transposition of the ulnar nerve. J Shoulder Elbow Surg. 2001;10:152–7.

Ulnar Collateral Ligament Injuries in High-School-Aged Athletes

31

Ryan R. Thacher, Alex J. Anatone, Lauren M. Fabian, and Orr Limpisvasti

Background

Medial-sided elbow injuries in young athletes are extremely common, especially in youth and high school baseball players. By high school age, many baseball players have already begun to play for several teams, practice for several hours each day, and play year-round baseball. Shoulder and elbow pain has been reported between 50% and 80% in adolescent baseball players at least some time during the season, more commonly in young pitchers and catchers than position players [1–3]. Radiographic findings consistent with the phenomenon of "Little League Elbow" such as apophyseal widening, fragmentation, and hypertrophy have been noted in 23–90% of both symptomatic and asymptomatic skeletally immature players [1, 4]. As adolescents reach skeletal maturity, however, their injuries tend to affect the ulnar collateral ligament (UCL) rather than the growth plate or osseous structures.

R. R. Thacher (✉)
Department of Orthopedic Surgery, Hospital for Special Surgery, New York, NY, USA
e-mail: thacherr@hss.edu

A. J. Anatone
Hospital for Special Surgery, New York, NY, USA

L. M. Fabian
Orthopaedic Specialty Group, Fairfield, CT, USA

O. Limpisvasti
Kerlan-Jobe Orthopaedic Clinic, Los Angeles, CA, USA

Since Jobe published his report of UCL reconstruction, or "Tommy John" surgery in 1986, the procedure has become more common among professional, college, and high school athletes [5]. Petty and Andrews noted that throughout the 1990s and 2000s, there was an increasing trend in younger players who required surgery to continue playing. At one institution between the years of 1988 and 1994, 85 UCL reconstructions were performed, and 7 (8%) were done on high school players. By contrast, between 1995 and 2003, 609 players underwent UCL reconstruction, and 77 (13%) were high school players. Not only did the overall number of cases increase, but there was also a 50% increase in the proportion of high school players who required surgery [6]. Between the years 2002 and 2011, the rates of UCL reconstructions in some parts of the country nearly doubled and studies suggest that baseball players aged 15–19 are experiencing the fastest growing rates of UCL reconstruction per year of any age group [7, 8].

While an increasing number of young athletes have required UCL reconstruction, a disturbing lack of understanding about the injury is still prevalent in the community among players, coaches, and parents. Ahmad et al. administered a questionnaire to assess players', coaches', and parents' perceptions of Tommy John surgery, and found that 30% of coaches and 51% of high school players believed surgery can be performed on uninjured players to enhance performance.

J. S. Dines et al. (eds.), *Elbow Ulnar Collateral Ligament Injury*,
https://doi.org/10.1007/978-3-030-69567-5_31

Similarly, 28 % of players and 20 % of coaches believed that performance after surgery would be better than pre-injury, and a significant number of those surveyed underestimated both risk factors for injury and the time frame it would take after surgery to return to play [9]. In this age group, the challenge to inform and educate patients and families about risk factors, prevention, and indications for surgery is paramount.

Anatomy and Physiology

For athletes with developing musculoskeletal systems, the physis is generally considered to be the most vulnerable link. High-school-age throwers (aged 14–18) compete during various phases of developing skeletal maturity, strength progression, and increasing physical demands of the sport. Throwing, and especially pitching, requires a complex movement that involves the entire body including the legs, core, and entire upper extremity, including the shoulder and elbow. Soft tissue and bony adaptive changes occur during adolescence if a young athlete competes consistently.

Though there is little literature focused on adaptive changes to the elbow, investigators have shown that significant adaptive changes occur in the shoulder in high-school-age athletes. Even younger little-league-age throwers demonstrate differences in the range of motion of their dominant shoulder compared to their nondominant side as a response to the physiologic stresses of throwing. These include an increase in external rotation, reduced internal rotation, and increased inferior laxity in the dominant arm. These changes become more pronounced as the adolescent gets older, particularly during the early high school years (age 13–14), and tend to stay stable once he has reached skeletal maturity [10, 11]. Because there is an increase in external rotation with a complementary decrease in internal rotation, there may be a side-to-side difference in shoulders, but in asymptomatic players, the total arc of motion is usually within 5°. This phenomenon is seen more frequently in pitchers than position players [12]. These changes in range of motion are not only a soft-tissue response to the stress of throwing, but also represent osseous changes including increased retroversion of both the humerus and glenoid in the throwing shoulder compared to the nondominant side [13–16]. Deficits in shoulder range of motion beyond physiologic changes in young pitchers have been linked to increased stress across the elbow during throwing as well as an increased risk for both shoulder and elbow injury [17, 18].

In the elbow, the primary stress of throwing creates a valgus moment on the medial side. In early adolescence, the apophysis of the skeletally immature elbow is particularly vulnerable to these forces. Hang et al. examined 343 little league players in Taiwan, and found that 100 % of pitchers and catchers, and 90 % of position players demonstrated hypertrophy of the medial apophysis on radiographs. Separation and fragmentation of the medial epicondylar apophysis were also common findings, both in symptomatic and asymptomatic elbows [1]. Before the physis has closed, the UCL is intimately associated with the periosteum, and is less vulnerable to injury than the apophysis. Once the physis has closed, however, the UCL is injured more frequently than the bone [19].

Risk Factors/Prevention

For adolescent and high school athletes, injury prevention is paramount. As these young athletes enter high school, they often compete for multiple teams and for most months out of the year if the climate allows. As they enter puberty, they begin to develop bigger and stronger muscles, and with talent, they throw harder and faster. With these changes, risk factors for UCL injury have been explored.

As throwing and pitching are complex movements involving the entire body, healthy shoulder motion is important to preventing elbow injuries as well. Shanley et al. found that among high school softball and baseball players, those with large mean deficits in internal rotation were at greater risk for shoulder or elbow injury, and that *a* >25° loss of passive internal rotation was predictive of injury. There was a trend towards total range of motion deficit as a risk for injury, though this was not statistically significant [17]. Among 60 high-school- and college-aged patients with diagnosed UCL tears Garrison et al. found that there was no difference in elbow extension, glenohumeral internal rotation deficit, or horizontal abduction, but those pitchers with UCL tears had less shoulder total range of motion than uninjured players [18]. A recent study by Sakata et al. demonstrated that a strength and stretching program designed to improve range of motion of the shoulder and hip and to decrease thoracic kyphosis was an effective approach to preventing medial elbow injuries in young throwing athletes [20].

Proper pitching mechanics are important for preventing pitching injury. Davis et al. analyzed five common pitching parameters among pitchers aged 9–18, including (1) leading with hip, (2) early cocking with hand on top of the ball, (3) elbow higher than the hand, (4) shoulder closed (not "opening up" too early), and (5) leading stride foot centered and pointed towards home plate. They found that young pitchers who performed three or more of the above correctly showed lower humeral torque and valgus loads on the elbow than those who did not. Older pitchers tended to follow parameters more correctly than younger ones [21]. Even those children with proper pitching mechanics cannot generate as large torques as adults, and therefore, these must come from increased strength and musculature [22] (Figs. 31.1, 31.2, 31.3, and 31.4).

Pitch type and pitch counts are also important in assessing the risk to a young pitcher. Lyman et al. examined 476 pitchers aged 9–14, and

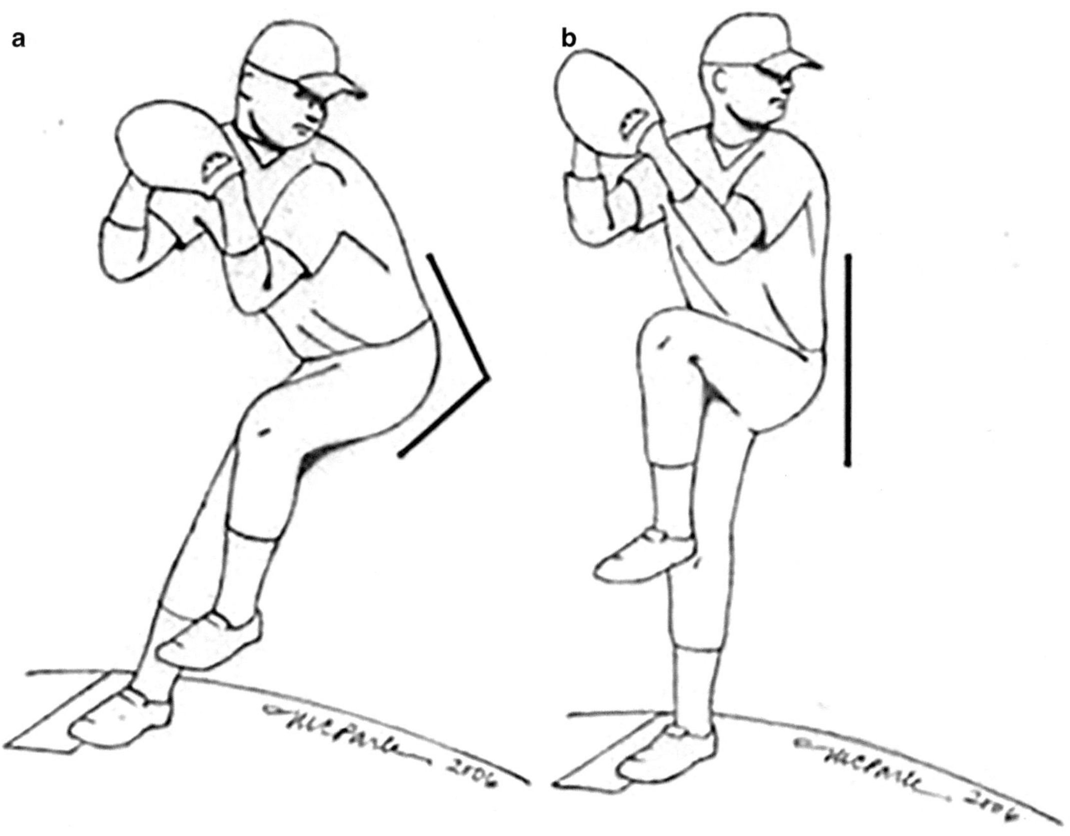

Fig. 31.1 Parameter 1: leading towards home plate with the hips. (**a**) Correct position defined by the pelvis leading the trunk towards home plate during the early cocking phase. (**b**) The incorrect position with a vertical torso in the early cocking phase, not leading with the hips [21]

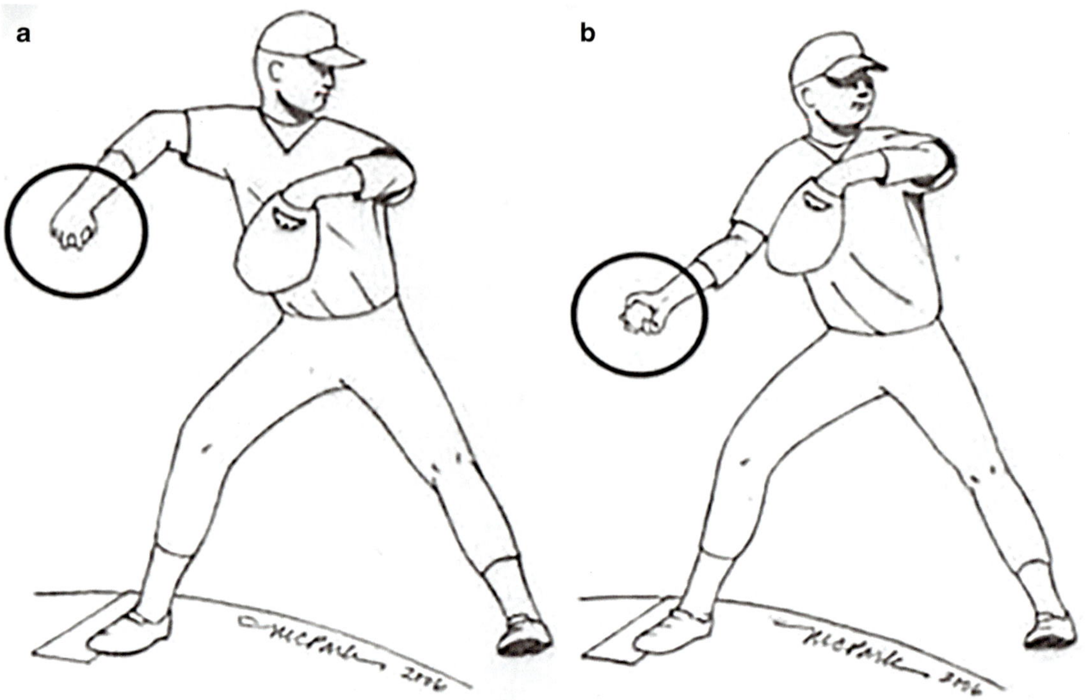

Fig. 31.2 Parameter 2: hand on top position. (**a**) Correct position defined by the throwing hand on top of the ball with the forearm in pronation as it comes out of the glove. (**b**) The incorrect position with the hand under the ball with the forearm in supination as it comes out of the glove [21]

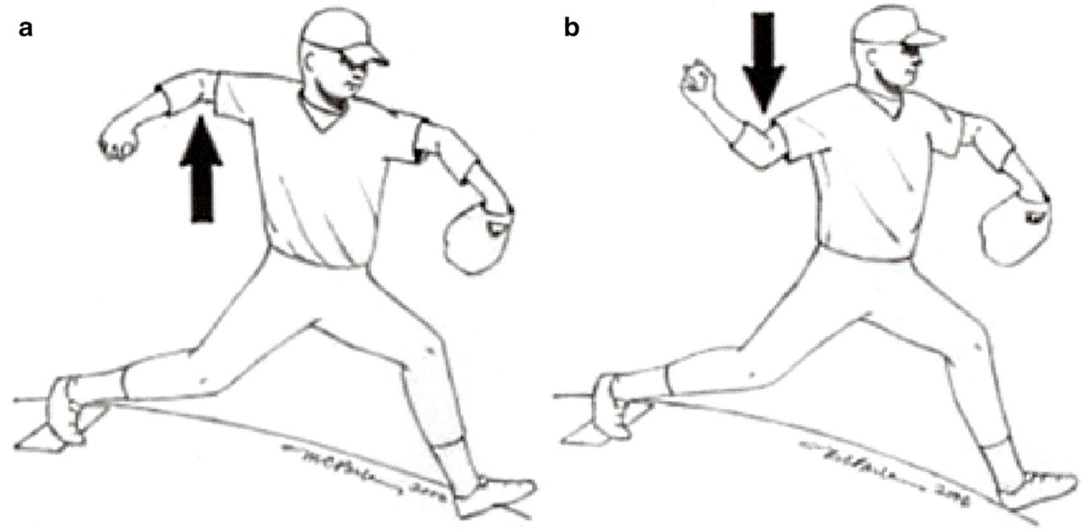

Fig. 31.3 Parameter 3: arm in throwing position. (**a**) Correct position defined by the elbow reaching maximum height by stride foot contact. (**b**) Incorrect performance with the elbow below the hand as with stride foot contact [21]

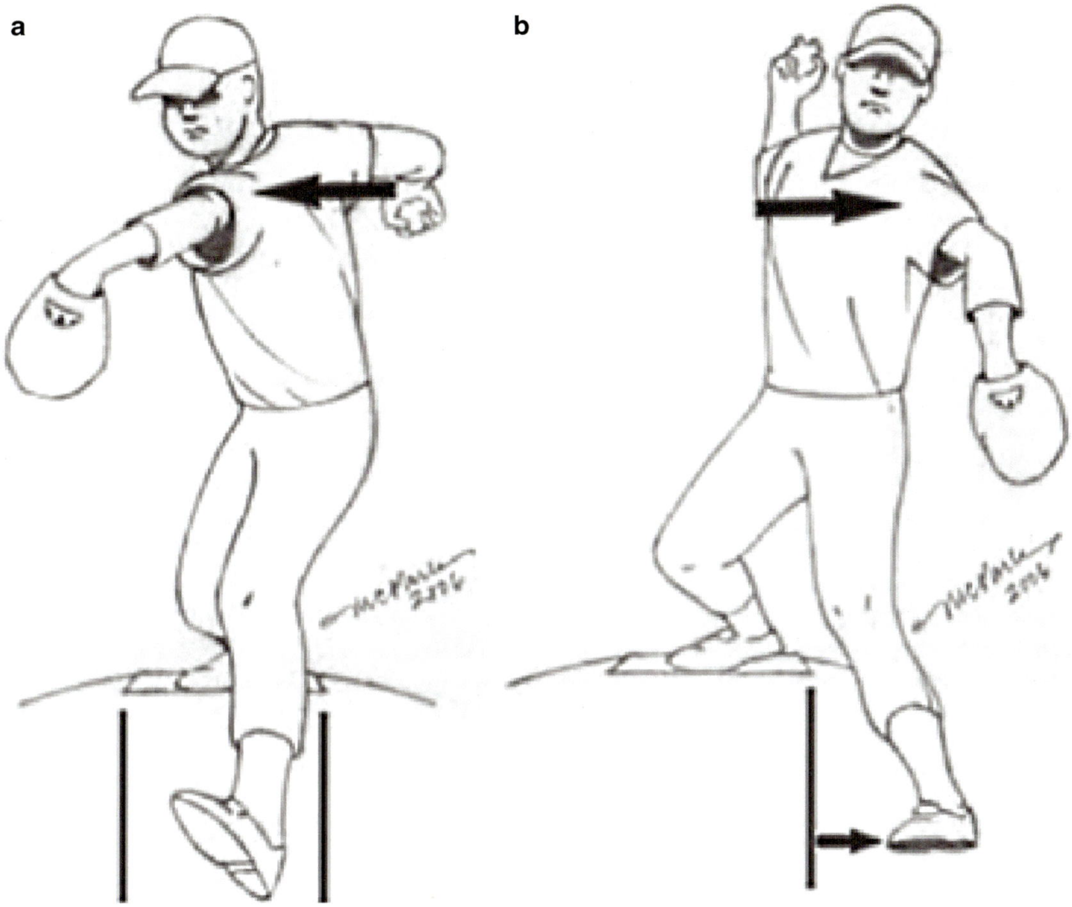

Fig. 31.4 Parameter 4: closed-shoulder position. (**a**) Correct position defined by the lead shoulder pointing towards home plate at stride foot contact. (**b**) Incorrect position with the torso facing forward with stride foot contact (opening up too early). Parameter 5: stride foot towards home plate. (**a**) Correct position defined by the stride foot pointing towards home plate at contact. (**b**) Incorrect position with the foot not pointed towards home plate [21]

found that the curveball was associated with 52 % chance of shoulder pain and the slider with an 86 % risk of elbow pain especially in the 13- to 14-year-old age group [2]. The curveball has been shown to correlate with the highest valgus stress over the elbow with increasing age and strength [22, 23]. Multiple studies have shown a significant correlation between the pitch count and the rate of elbow injuries [2, 24]. Olsen et al. have shown that increased number of months pitching and increased pitch counts per game and per year were all associated with higher risks of injury. Furthermore, those patients who had more frequent starts, participated in showcases, and used more nonsteroidal anti-inflammatory drugs (NSAIDs) during the season had a higher rate of injury. Interestingly, there was no difference in self-rating, stretching, pitch type, or age of the injured players [24]. A recent magnetic resonance imaging (MRI) study examining the progression of elbow pain and UCL injuries in youth baseball players identified year-round play as a risk factor for injury [25]. Norton et al. identified age, height, playing for multiple teams, and subjective arm fatigue as risk factors for shoulder and elbow pain in high school aged baseball players, but did not identify pitch type or innings pitched as risk factors [26].

Pitch velocity has been shown to correlate with stress on the UCL injury. Hurd et al. used high-speed video studies with 3D motion analysis and have shown that the internal elbow adduction moment increases with the increasing pitch velocity in high-school-aged pitchers. Players who are taller and heavier than their age-matched counterparts have a higher rate of injury, suggesting that youth pitchers who are strong and talented enough to pitch with high velocity may be at increased risk for elbow injuries [24, 27]. Furthermore, Fleisig et al. analyzed the pitching kinematics of youth through professional pitching levels, and found that the greatest elbow torques were in the late cocking and acceleration phase of the pitch, and increased with increasing pitcher level [22]. Studies have also identified working with a private coach as an independent risk factor for elbow pain, perhaps due to increased throwing reps and a bias toward higher level players who throw harder. Our understanding of the risk factors associated with UCL injury in high-school baseball players continues to evolve [28]. Nonetheless, many authors have put together safety recommendations for adolescent baseball pitchers [6, 24, 29] (Tables 31.1, 31.2, and 31.3).

Table 31.1 Recommended maximum number of pitches by age group

Age (years)	Maximum pitches/games	Maximum games/week
8–10	50	2
11–12	65	2
13–14	75	2
15–16	90	2
17–18	105	2

Recommendations were modified with permission from the USA Baseball Medical & Safety Advisory Committee [29]

Table 31.2 Recommended minimum rest after pitching

	Number of pitches			
Age (years)	1 day of rest	2 days of rest	3 days of rest	4 days of rest
8–10	20	35	45	50
11–12	25	35	55	60
13–14	30	35	55	70
15–16	30	40	60	80
17–18	30	40	60	90

Recommendations were modified with permission from the USA Baseball Medical & Safety Advisory Committee [29]

Table 31.3 Age recommended for learning various pitches

Pitch	Age (years)
Fastball	8
Change-up	10
Curveball	14
Knuckleball	15
Slider	16
Forkball	16
Splitter	16
Screwball	17

Recommendations were modified with permission from the USA Baseball Medical & Safety Advisory Committee [29]

Evaluation

History

When a high school athlete seeks medical attention for elbow pain, it is usually due to an inability to perform at their prior level. The player will most commonly report a discrete incident in which he felt a pop on the medial side of the elbow, or an episode of "giving way." Symptoms of ulnar nerve irritation may also be present, including an electrical sensation down the arm radiating to the ring and small fingers. This may be the product of hematoma or a subluxing ulnar nerve. Other players may report a more insidious or chronic pain that usually occurs during the late cocking and acceleration phase, and the player may notice that he has lost velocity or accuracy when he throws or pitches.

Physical Examination

The thrower with an acute UCL injury may have swelling and ecchymoses along the medial side of the elbow and forearm. There may be a flexion contracture of the elbow, though this is common with both injured and uninjured throwers and may not be correlated to UCL injury [1]. Tenderness to palpation directly over the UCL distal to the medial epicondyle is the most common finding. The expected amount of elbow laxity even with a complete UCL disruption is only a few millimeters at most, and is thus a very subtle finding.

The most common provocative maneuvers used to evaluate the UCL are the valgus stress test, the milking maneuver, and the moving valgus stress test [30]. In the classic valgus stress test, the examiner stabilizes the humerus and applies a valgus force to the elbow at 30° of flexion. This level of flexion minimizes the bony contribution to stability of the ulnohumeral joint. The milking maneuver may be performed entirely by the patient, in which he supinates the forearm, and bends the elbow past 90°. Using the other hand, he grabs the thumb and pulls downward, producing a valgus force on the elbow. The examiner may then palpate the UCL for instability and pain. The modified milking maneuver is performed by the examiner, in which the examiner pulls the thumb down with the patient's elbow in 70° of flexion, producing a valgus force. This position has shown the greatest valgus laxity in a cadaveric model when the UCL is sectioned [30]. With the other hand, the examiner can palpate the medial elbow for subtle laxity. O'Driscoll and associates described the moving valgus stress test, in which the examiner holds the patient's forearm with one hand and the humerus with the other, applying a steady valgus force while flexing and extending the elbow [31]. The athlete will experience pain in the arc from 70° to 120°, with a maximum pain at 90° of flexion, if there is a UCL injury. Advantages of this technique include that it closely mimics the throwing motion, it eliminates shoulder rotation which may confound other exam maneuvers, and pain in the arc of motion is common.

In addition to examining the integrity of the UCL, care must be taken to evaluate the ulnar nerve. Attempting to elicit a Tinel sign along the cubital tunnel, and evaluating the nerve for subluxation during range of motion with gentle palpation will help guide treatment of the nerve. Care must be taken to rule out other injuries, such as flexor-pronator avulsions, medial epicondyle fractures, and loose bodies in the elbow.

Imaging

With plain radiographs, high school athletes in variable phases of skeletal maturity may show variable findings. These may include widening or separation of the medial epicondylar physis, fragmentation of the epicondylar ossification center, or calcification in the substance of the UCL [1]. Occasionally, one may find a sublime tubercle fracture. Though stress radiographs of bilateral elbows may be diagnostic, medial widening tends to be very subtle (only 2–3 mm), and is operator dependent. A recent study of over 270 baseball players with UCL injuries identified 0.4 mm of medial widening on stress radiographs as suggestive of UCL injury, and 0.6 mm or greater of widening consistent with full thickness UCL tear [32]. However, even in uninjured players, a side-to-side difference in elbow laxity has also been reported, so stress radiographs may be of limited value [33].

Magnetic resonance imaging (MRI) is helpful in diagnosing both UCL injuries as well as injuries to other structures, including findings that may be missed on X-ray [34]. With current high-quality MRI, the UCL may be well visualized in the absence of intraarticular contrast. Sugimoto and Ohsawa compared MRIs of the UCL in symptomatic and normal elbows in both skeletally immature and skeletally mature patients [19]. They found that in normal immature elbows, the periosteum was an extension of the UCL, and that the UCL has a different signal from the mature ligaments. In skeletally immature symptomatic elbows, there was segmentation of subchondral bone and resorption of the ossification center, either with or without tear of the UCL, suggesting apophyseal pathology. In mature elbows, a tear in the UCL was seen more often (Figs. 31.5 and 31.6).

One should treat MRI findings with caution, as even in asymptomatic high school pitchers will show some subtle changes on MRI. Wei et al. examined nine skeletally immature players, and found that though MRI was more sensitive than radiographs for abnormalities about the elbow, there were no significant differences

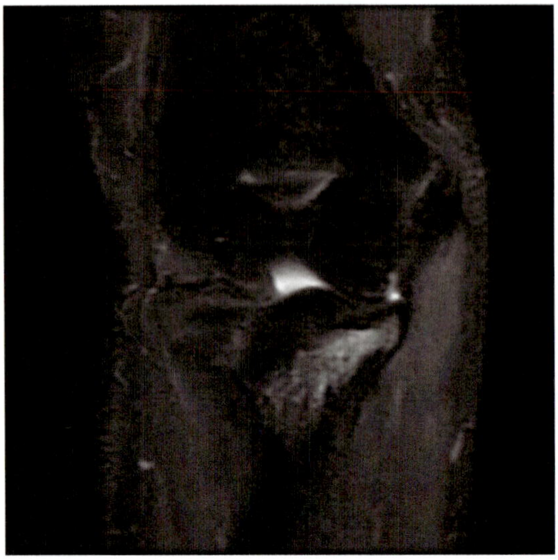

Fig. 31.5 Proton-density sequence MRI of a 15-year-old pitcher and catcher with medial elbow pain. Note that the ulnar collateral ligament is intact, but there is significant bony edema and separation at the medial epicondylar apophysis

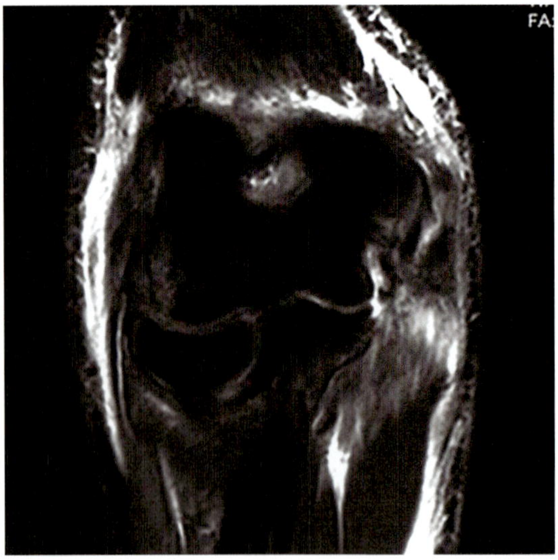

Fig. 31.6 Proton-density sequence MRI of an 18-year-old pitcher with medial elbow pain. Note that the ulnar collateral ligament is completely avulsed from the ulnar attachment (positive "T-sign")

between the dominant and nondominant sides [34]. Hurd et al. examined bilateral elbow MRIs of 23 high school pitchers, and found that only 13 % of the players had normal findings, whereas most players had asymmetrical thickening of the anterior band of the UCL, posteromedial subchondral sclerosis, a posteromedial osteophyte, or chondromalacia, and 43 % of the players had multiple of these findings [35]. Therefore, it is important to correlate MRI findings with the physical exam prior to initiating a treatment plan.

More recently, dynamic ultrasound has been utilized to identify UCL injuries and medial elbow pathology in throwing athletes. Studies have demonstrated the ability to identify increased ligament thickness, ulnohumeral joint space gapping, hypoechoic foci, and increased calcifications in injured throwers [36, 37]. These studies, which have focused primarily on professional athletes, suggest that ultrasound may be an efficient and cost effective modality for assessing medial elbow injuries. However, further studies, particularly with a younger, high-school aged population are needed to fully assess the value of this diagnostic tool.

Treatment

Conservative Management

Conservative management of UCL injuries to the elbow consists of several phases, including rest, modalities, strengthening and stretching, and a gradual return to sport-specific activities such as throwing.

A number of rehabilitation programs have been described for overhead throwing athletes, but they all share several common concepts [38–40]. The first phase of rehabilitation aims to improve pain, normalize range of motion and muscle balance, and improve proprioception. This phase involves cessation or modification of throwing in addition to anti-inflammatory medications and therapeutic modalities such as ultrasound, electric stimulation, and ice. Intermediate phases involve progressive strengthening and dynamic stability of the flexors and pronators of the forearm to enhance neuromuscular control, and improve power and endurance for return to sport. Focus should be paid to strengthening the flexor-pronator mass, and particularly the flexor carpi ulnaris and flexor digitorum superficialis, which provide dynamic valgus stability to the throwing elbow [41]. Range of motion, strength, and stability of both the shoulder and elbow joint are essential before returning to the throwing motion. The final phases of rehabilitation return the player to a slow progressive throwing program and return to competitive throwing while continuing maintenance strength and flexibility drills.

Rettig et al. examined 31 throwing athletes with UCL tears initially treated with conservative management. After a period of 3 months rest and rehabilitation, 42 % of athletes were able to return to their preinjury level of competition. These athletes took an average of 24.5 weeks to return to play, with a range of 13–54 weeks. Unfortunately, no risk factors were able to be identified for patients who failed conservative management, including age, acute versus insidious onset, or length of symptoms prior to treatment [38].

Research into the use of minimally invasive treatment options for the management of UCL injuries, including platelet rich plasma (PRP) and other biologics, is ongoing. In a retrospective review of 44 baseball players (mean age 17.3, range 16–28 years) treated with PRP for UCL insufficiency, Dines et al. demonstrated good to excellent results in 32/44 (73%) with early return to play [42]. A separate study by Podesta et al. of 34 patients (age range 12–33) with partial UCL tears who failed nonop management demonstrated 88% return to play without complaints at an average of 70 months of follow up following PRP injection [43]. Studies suggest that upward of a third of orthopedic surgeons utilize PRP in their practices for management of UCL injuries [44]. Nonetheless, at this stage our best support for PRP remains in small, uncontrolled case series in athletes predominantly at the high school level, which may not be applicable beyond that population. Further research is warranted to further explore the efficacy of PRP as it pertains to a broader patient population and to identify ideal therapeutic parameters, including PRP concentration and injection timing. Other biologic therapy, including the use of stem cells, has been suggested as possible treatment adjuncts for UCL injuries; however, these remain theoretical at this stage.

Operative Intervention

When conservative management has failed, many young players will elect surgical treatment as an option to help them return to play. In the high school age group, several options are available for surgical management. The gold standard for surgical management of UCL tears in the high-school athlete is ligament reconstruction. Petty et al. retrospectively evaluated outcomes of 27 high school athletes who had undergone reconstruction of the UCL during high school, and found that 74 % were able to return to their previous level of play at 11 months, though only 37 % of the athletes went on to play in college. Those who stopped playing baseball did so either because of continual pain and dysfunction (7 %), or they abandoned baseball for other interests (15 %) [6].

Savoie et al. reported a series of 60 young patients with symptomatic UCL tears treated with a primary direct repair of the ligament, either through drill holes or suture anchors. In patients with an average age of 17.2, 93 % reported excellent results, and 58 out of 60 athletes were able to return to their previous level of play within 6 months [45]. The authors advocate this alternative approach to reconstruction for young athletes whose ligament tissue quality is excellent, and those who have not experienced the attritional changes from chronic injury.

An alternative technique for ligament repair, which bolsters the repair with an internal brace, or graft augment, has gained popularity in recent years. This technique, which uses a collagen-coated tape to support and reinforce the ligament repair, has demonstrated similar strength to gold-standard UCL reconstruction in biomechanical studies with increased resistance to gapping at low cyclic loads. Supporters of this approach also hail its ability to decrease soft tissue damage and limit bone loss during surgery [46–48]. Limited clinical data on the outcomes of patients treated with this surgical technique exists at this time, however.

Failure of the ligament repair or reconstruction in this population has been reported from 7% to 26 %, either early or after return to unrestricted play. Other complications, such as transient ulnar neuropathy, are seen in 5–7% of patients either with or without ulnar nerve transposition at the time of surgery.

Rehabilitation

After surgical repair or reconstruction, the elbow should be immobilized for 1 week to allow for soft tissue healing. Active wrist, elbow, and shoulder range of motion should be initialized immediately after removal of the splint. Full range of motion and strengthening exercises may begin at 4–6 weeks, but patients should be cautioned against progressing too quickly, and should avoid valgus stress. After 8–10 weeks, more progressive strengthening may continue, with initiation of plyometric exercises, and continued strengthening of the flexor-pronator mass. A throwing program may begin at 4 months postoperatively, with gradual progression of distance, velocity, and intensity. Shoulder strength, motion, and proper throwing mechanics should be emphasized at this time to prevent reinjury. If there is any return of symptoms, a period of rest and modification of activities is essential, and throwing should not resume until the athlete is pain-free. Strength and flexibility maintenance should continue throughout, and return to competition may resume in 1 year. Depending on the level of competition, however, some players may take 18 months or more to return to their previous level of play. Young athletes and families must be informed and agreeable to a significant rehabilitation effort prior to return to play.

Summary

In recent years, an increasing number of high-school-aged athletes suffer from elbow UCL injuries. Though conservative management and surgical interventions such as ligament repair or reconstruction may be variably successful in helping young athletes return to play, all require significant time off [6, 38, 42]. In a population of young athletes that may finish their careers at the high school or college level, it is important to counsel patients and families, who may misunderstand the implications of UCL tears [9]. Prevention of injuries to both the shoulder and elbow is paramount in the adolescent and high-school-aged population. Focus should be placed on proper throwing technique and minimizing risk factors such as overuse during the season, year-round throwing, and pitches such as the fast ball and curve ball [2, 6, 21, 22, 24].

References

1. Hang DW, Chao CM, Hang YS. A clinical and roentgenographic study of Little League elbow. Am J Sports Med. 2004;32(1):79–84. (PubMed PMID: 14754727).
2. Lyman S, Fleisig GS, Andrews JR, Osinski ED. Effect of pitch type, pitch count, and pitching mechanics on risk of elbow and shoulder pain in youth baseball pitchers. Am J Sports Med. 2002;30(4):463–8. (PubMed PMID: 12130397).
3. Makhni EC, Morrow ZS, Luchetti TJ, Mishra-Kalyani PS, Gualtieri AP, Lee RW, Ahmad CS. Arm Pain in youth baseball players: a survey of healthy players. Am J Sports Med. 2015;43(1):41–6. (PubMed PMID: 25367016).
4. Benjamin HJ, Briner WW Jr. Little league elbow. Clin J Sport Med. 2005;15(1):37–40. (PubMed PMID: 15654190).
5. Jobe FW, Stark H, Lombardo SJ. Reconstruction of the ulnar collateral ligament in athletes. J Bone Joint Surg Am. 1986;68(8):1158–63. (PubMed PMID: 3771597).
6. Petty DH, Andrews JR, Fleisig GS, Cain EL. Ulnar collateral ligament reconstruction in high school baseball players: clinical results and injury risk factors. Am J Sports Med. 2004;32(5):1158–64. (PubMed PMID: 15262637).
7. Hodgins JL, Vitale M, Arons RR, Ahmad CS. Epidemiology of medial ulnar collateral ligament reconstruction: a 10-year study in New York State. Am J Sports Med. 2016;44(3):729–34. (PubMed PMID: 26797699).
8. Erickson BJ, Nwachukwu BU, Rosas S, Schairer WW, McCormick FM, Bach BR, Rush-Joseph CA, Romeo AA. Trends in medial ulnar collateral ligament reconstruction in the United States: A retrospective review of a large private-payer database from 2007-2011. Am J Sports Med. 2015;43(7):1770–4. (PubMed PMID: 26129959)
9. Ahmad CS, Grantham WJ, Greiwe RM. Public perceptions of Tommy John surgery. Phys Sportsmed. 2012;40(2):64–72. (PubMed PMID: 22759607).
10. Meister K, Day T, Horodyski M, Kaminski TW, Wasik MP, Tillman S. Rotational motion changes in

the glenohumeral joint of the adolescent/Little League baseball player. Am J Sports Med. 2005;33(5):693–8. (PubMed PMID: 15722284).
11. Levine WN, Brandon ML, Stein BS, Gardner TR, Bigliani LU, Ahmad CS. Shoulder adaptive changes in youth baseball players. J Shoulder Elbow Surg. 2006;15(5):562–6. (PubMed PMID: 16920368).
12. Sethi PM. Quantitative assessment of glenohumeral translation in baseball players: a comparison of pitchers versus nonpitching athletes. Am J Sports Med. 2004;32(7):1711–5. (PubMed PMID: 15494337).
13. Crockett HC, Gross LB, Wilk KE, Schwartz ML, Reed J, O'Mara J, et al. Osseous adaptation and range of motion at the glenohumeral joint in professional baseball pitchers. Am J Sports Med. 2002;30(1):20–6. (PubMed PMID: 11798991).
14. Reagan KM, Meister K, Horodyski MB, Werner DW, Carruthers C, Wilk K. Humeral retroversion and its relationship to glenohumeral rotation in the shoulder of college baseball players. Am J Sports Med. 2002;30(3):354–60. (PubMed PMID: 12016075).
15. Osbahr DC, Cannon DL, Speer KP. Retroversion of the humerus in the throwing shoulder of college baseball pitchers. Am J Sports Med. 2002;30(3):347–53. (PubMed PMID: 12016074).
16. Mair SD, Uhl TL, Robbe RG, Brindle KA. Physeal changes and range-of-motion differences in the dominant shoulders of skeletally immature baseball players. J Shoulder Elbow Surg. 2004;13(5):487–91. (PubMed 15383802).
17. Shanley E, Rauh MJ, Michener LA, Ellenbecker TS, Garrison JC, Thigpen CA. Shoulder range of motion measures as risk factors for shoulder and elbow injuries in high school softball and baseball players. Am J Sports Med. 2011;39(9):1997–2006. (PubMed PMID: 21685316).
18. Garrison JC, Cole MA, Conway JE, Macko MJ, Thigpen C, Shanley E. Shoulder range of motion deficits in baseball players with an ulnar collateral ligament tear. Am J Sports Med. 2012;40(11):2597–603. (PubMed PMID: 23019251).
19. Sugimoto H, Ohsawa T. Ulnar collateral ligament in the growing elbow: MR imaging of normal development and throwing injuries. Radiology. 1994;192(2):417–22. (PubMed PMID: 8029407).
20. Sakata J, Nakamura E, Suzuki T, Suzukawa M, Akaike A, Shimizu K, Hirose N. Efficacy of a prevention program for medial elbow injuries in youth baseball players. Am J Sports Med. 2018;46(2):460–9. (PubMed PMID: 29095655).
21. Davis JT, Limpisvasti O, Fluhme D, Mohr KJ, Yocum LA, Elattrache NS, et al. The effect of pitching biomechanics on the upper extremity in youth and adolescent baseball pitchers. Am J Sports Med. 2009;37(8):1484–91. (PubMed PMID: 19633301).
22. Fleisig GS, Barrentine SW, Zheng N, Escamilla RF, Andrews JR. Kinematic and kinetic comparison of baseball pitching among various levels of development. J Biomech. 1999;32(12):1371–5. (PubMed PMID: 10569718).
23. Dun S, Loftice J, Fleisig GS, Kingsley D, Andrews JR. A biomechanical comparison of youth baseball pitches: is the curveball potentially harmful? Am J Sports Med. 2008;36(4):686–92. (PubMed PMID: 18055920).
24. Olsen SJ 2nd, Fleisig GS, Dun S, Loftice J, Andrews JR. Risk factors for shoulder and elbow injuries in adolescent baseball pitchers. Am J Sports Med. 2006;34(6):905–12. (PubMed PMID: 16452269).
25. Holt JB, Pedowitz JM, Stearns PH, Bastrom TP, Dennis MM, Dwek JR, Pennock AT. Progressive elbow magnetic resonance imaging abnormalities in Little League baseball players are common: A 3-year longitudinal evaluation. Am J Sports Med. 2019;4:363546519888647. (PubMed PMID: 31801034).
26. Norton R, Honstad C, Joshi R, Silvis M, Chinchilli V, Dhawan A. Risk factors for elbow and shoulder injuries in adolescent baseball players: A systematic review. Am J Sports Med. 2019;47(4):982–90. (PubMed PMID: 29630388).
27. Hurd WJ, Jazayeri R, Mohr K, Limpisvasti O, Elattrache NS, Kaufman KR. Pitch velocity is a predictor of medial elbow distraction forces in the uninjured high school-aged baseball pitcher. Sports Health. 2012;4(5):415–8. (PubMed PMID: 23016114. Pubmed Central PMCID: 3435942).
28. Pennock AT, Pytiak A, Stearns P, Roocroft JH, Dwek J, Kruk P, Bastrom TP. Preseason assessment of radiographic abnormalities in elbows of little league baseball players. J Bone Joint Surg Am. 2016;98(9):761–7. (PubMed PMID: 27147689).
29. Andrews JR, Fleisig GS. USA Baseball News Medical & Safety Advisory Committee special report: how many pitches should I allow my child to throw? USA Baseball News. 1996;1996:1.
30. Safran M, Ahmad CS, Elattrache NS. Ulnar collateral ligament of the elbow. Arthroscopy. 2005;21(11):1381–95. (PubMed PMID: 16325092).
31. O'Driscoll SWM. The "moving valgus stress test" for medial collateral ligament tears of the elbow. Am J Sports Med. 2005;33(2):231–9. (PubMed PMID: 15701609).
32. Bruce JR, Hess R, Joyner P, Andrews JR. How much valgus instability can be expected with ulnar collateral ligament (UCL) injuries? A review of 273 baseball players with UCL injuries. J Shoulder Elbow Surg. 2014;23(10):1521–6. (PubMed PMID: 25220199).
33. Ellenbecker TS, Mattalino AJ, Elam EA, Caplinger RA. Medial elbow joint laxity in professional baseball pitchers. A bilateral comparison using stress radiography. Am J Sports Med. 1998;26(3):420–4. (PubMed PMID: 9617406).
34. Wei AS, Khana S, Limpisvasti O, Crues J, Podesta L, Yocum LA. Clinical and magnetic resonance imaging findings associated with Little League elbow. J Pediatr Orthop. 2010;30(7):715–9. (PubMed PMID: 20864859).
35. Hurd WJ, Eby S, Kaufman KR, Murthy NS. Magnetic resonance imaging of the throwing elbow in the unin-

jured, high school-aged baseball pitcher. Am J Sports Med. 2011;39(4):722–8. (PubMed PMID: 21228309).

36. Atanda AJ, Buckley PS, Hammoud S, Cohen SB, Nazarian LN, Ciccotti MG. Early anatomic changes of the ulnar collateral ligament identified by stress ultrasound of the elbow in young professional baseball pitchers. Am J Sports Med. 2015;43(12):2943–9. (PubMed PMID: 26403208).
37. Ciccotti MG, Atanda A, Nazarian LN, Dodson CC, Holmes L, Cohen SB. Stress sonography of the ulnar collateral ligament of the elbow in professional baseball pitchers: a 10-year study. Am J Sports Med. 2014;42(3):544–51. (PubMed PMID: 24473498).
38. Rettig AC, Sherrill C, Snead DS, Mendler JC, Mieling P. Nonoperative treatment of ulnar collateral ligament injuries in throwing athletes. Am J Sports Med. 2001;29(1):15–7. (PubMed PMID: 11206249).
39. McFarland EG, Ireland ML. Rehabilitation programs and prevention strategies in adolescent throwing athletes. Instr Course Lect. 2003;52:37–42. (PubMed PMID: 12690839).
40. Wilk KE, Meister K, Andrews JR. Current concepts in the rehabilitation of the overhead throwing athlete. Am J Sports Med. 2002;30(1):136–51. (PubMed PMID: 11799012).
41. Park MC, Ahmad CS. Dynamic contributions of the flexor-pronator mass to elbow valgus stability. J Bone Joint Surg Am. 2004;86-A(10):2268–74. (PubMed PMID: 15466738).
42. Dines JS, Williams PN, ElAttrache N, Conte S, Tomczyk T, Osbahr DC, Dines DM, Bradley J, Ahmad CS. Platelet-rich plasma can be used to successfully treat elbow ulnar collateral ligament insufficiency in high-level throwers. Am J Orthop (Belle Mead NJ). 2016;45(5):296–300. (PubMed PMID: 27552453).
43. Podesta L, Crow SA, Volkmer D, Bert T, Yocum LA. Treatment of partial ulnar collateral ligament tears in the elbow with platelet-rich plasma. Am J Sports Med. 2013;41(7):1689–94. (PubMed PMID: 23666850).
44. Hurwit DJ, Garcia GH, Liu J, Altchek DW, Romeo A, Dines J. Management of ulnar collateral ligament injury in throwing athletes: a survey of the American Shoulder and Elbow Surgeons. J Shoulder Elbow Surg. 2017;26(11):2023–8. (PubMed PMID: 28941974).
45. Savoie FH 3rd, Trenhaile SW, Roberts J, Field LD, Ramsey JR. Primary repair of ulnar collateral ligament injuries of the elbow in young athletes: a case series of injuries to the proximal and distal ends of the ligament. Am J Sports Med. 2008;36(6):1066–72. (PubMed PMID: 18443280).
46. Dugas JR. Ulnar collateral ligament repair: An old idea with a new wrinkle. Am J Orthop (Belle Meade NJ). 2016;45(3):124–7. (PubMed PMID: 26991563).
47. Dugas JR, Walters BL, Beason DP, Fleisig GS, Chronister JE. Biomechanical comparison of ulnar collateral ligament repair with internal bracing versus modified Jobe reconstruction. Am J Sports Med. 2016;44(3):735–41. (PubMed PMID: 26717972).
48. Jones CM, Beason DP, Dugas JR. Ulnar collateral ligament reconstruction versus repair with internal bracing: Comparison of cyclic fatigue mechanics. Orthop J Sports Med. 2018;6(2):2325967118755991. (PubMed PMID: 29479544).

Medial Apophysitis in Adolescent Throwers

32

Peter N. Chalmers and Garrett V. Christensen

Introduction

UCL injuries occur in older adolescents and adults but are quite uncommon in young throwers. In contrast, skeletally immature athletes are much more likely to suffer from a spectrum of medial epicondyle pathologies such as medial epicondyle apophysitis, medial epicondyle avulsion fractures, posteromedial elbow impingement, or capitellar osteochondritis dissecans [1, 2]. The increased likelihood of physeal rather than ligamentous damage is due to the relative strength of the adolescent ligamentous structures in comparison to the relatively weaker physis.

In contrast to skeletally mature adults, children and adolescents have *apophyses*. Apophyses are bony outgrowths that serve as insertion sites of ligaments and tendons, which are then separated from the main body of the larger bone by growth plates. Examples of apophyses include the tibial tubercle of the lower extremity and medial humeral epicondyle of the upper extremities [3]. The medial epicondyle physis is the single weakest medial elbow structure in youth before skeletal maturity—and is considered the origin of most elbow pathologies in young throwers [4–6]. Though the term "Little Leaguer's Elbow" is very loosely used to describe nearly any progressive, atraumatic elbow pain in a young thrower, the phrase most precisely describes medial epicondyle apophysitis. Medial epicondyle apophysitis is most likely to occur in younger children—especially those under ten years [4–6].

The medial elbow apophyseal pain can be severe and may affect a thrower's velocity, accuracy, and may lead to long-term deformity. Some experts believe that medial elbow injuries in adolescent throwers can be prevented with proper throwing mechanics and limited pitch counts in youth sports [7, 8]. However, in high-velocity throwers growing quickly, this condition may occur even with perfect mechanics. Interestingly, it is reported that catchers have a higher incidence of medial epicondyle apophysitis than even pitchers. This has been hypothesized to be the result of throwing from the squatting position, as it may increase the stress placed on the elbow [6]. It may also be due to the high number of throws typically thrown by catchers.

Unfortunately, elbow pain is common in adolescent throwers. Studies show that approximately 25% of pitchers aged 9–12 report elbow pain during a season. Larson et al. assessed over 100 Little League pitchers aged 11 and 12 years. Elbow pain was present in 21%, and radiographs of 29% showed changes such as fragmentation, physeal

P. N. Chalmers (✉) · G. V. Christensen
Department of Orthopaedic Surgery, University of Utah, Salt Lake City, UT, USA

J. S. Dines et al. (eds.), *Elbow Ulnar Collateral Ligament Injury*,
https://doi.org/10.1007/978-3-030-69567-5_32

widening, or irregularity of the medial epicondyle [9]. Another study by Hang et al. evaluated over 300 Little League players. They found that all pitchers and catchers, and 90% of fielders had radiographic changes of the medial epicondyle [6].

Pathogenesis

The pathogenesis of medial epicondyle apophysitis is rooted in the fact that the medial epicondyle is the last ossification center of the elbow to fuse to the humerus—often not coalescing until 15 years of age or later [10]. Thus, when throwing athletes repeatedly place excessive valgus tension forces on the immature, unfused medial epicondylarphysis, irritation of the physis is common [5, 11, 12]. Medial epicondyle apophysitis is more likely during an athlete's growth spurt, as faster growth correlates with a widening of the physis. Widening likely weakens the physis, increasing the risk of both chronic overuse and acute injury [13–15].

The pitching motion is divided into six distinct phases. As a pitcher progresses through each phase, he or she converts energy that is largely generated through the lower-extremity and core musculature, into kinetic energy. This energy is then transferred through the shoulder and elbow into the hand and ball, generating acceleration, then ultimately trajectory velocity.

The six phases of the pitch include (1) wind-up, (2) stride, (3) cocking, (4) acceleration, (5) deceleration, and (6) follow-through. Each phase has a specific purpose—allowing energy transfer. The wind-up is preparatory and puts the body in a position to generate force. The stride phase begins the process of velocity generation and positions the arm in the cocking position. This phase is completed after the leading foot strikes the ground, and the pelvis rotates to face the direction of the throw [16].

The next two phases—cocking and acceleration—are the most significant in regards to elbow pathology. These phases put an incredible amount of tension on the medial elbow structures and cause an immense force requiring correction by these structures. The cocking phase permits the transfer of energy from the legs and core into potential energy stored in the shoulder capsule [16].

It begins as the hands separate, and the stride foot strikes the ground. The shoulder becomes maximally externally rotated, up to 180°. The shoulder abducts to 90° [17–20]. The elbow is variably flexed—usually just under 90°. The late cocking phase is the critical moment of peak valgus torque about the elbow leading to most injuries. As the arm continues externally rotating backward, a varus force is required to prevent valgus hyperextension of the elbow. Tensile forces on the medial elbow structures are tremendous. The UCL provides its contribution; however, it is not strong enough to withstand the stress alone [21]. The UCL provides approximately 55% of the overall valgus stability [20, 22].

The flexor-pronator mass also fires. Its contraction creates additional counter-force against valgus hyperextension. During this period, the triceps and anconeus fire as well—likely stabilizing the elbow joint by compression. This bony stabilization decreases the total stress assigned to the UCL [20]. In a skeletally immature thrower, this considerable force repetitively pulling distally on the medial epicondyle apophysis can lead to microtrauma of the relatively fragile physis. This microtrauma is the origin of medial epicondyle apophysitis.

Next, the pitcher's torso rapidly turns 90° toward home plate, transferring energy from the pelvis through the torso [23]. This is the end of the cocking phase. The acceleration phase then begins. The energy stored in the torso and shoulder capsule is transmitted into the baseball through the elbow joint. The shoulder begins explosively internally rotating. The torque placed on the UCL and medial epicondyle remains elevated. The elbow extends. The wrist flexes. The phase is over when the ball is released [17–20].

The deceleration phase begins with ball release and is characterized by internal rotation of the shoulder. Several muscle groups, including the rotator cuff, are critical in countering the distractive momentum of the arm. The follow-through phase then allows the pitcher's body to get into fielding position, and the pitch is complete.

Presentation

The typical presentation is progressive medial elbow pain in a young throwing athlete, which is generally focal and localized to the medial epicondyle. It is most likely to occur in pitchers and catchers, though positional players are certainly at-risk and develop these injuries, though less frequently [6]. It can also occur in other athletes that subject the elbow to abnormal valgus loads, such as gymnasts, volleyball players, and javelin throwers. Pitchers often have decreased throwing velocity compared to their baseline and may lose control or command [24].

The pain generally does not radiate and is worse with throwing or any activity that requires the common flexor-pronator mass of the forearm to contract. Most patients report that this pain is relatively mild, if present at all, at rest. Usually, there are no associated ulnar nerve symptoms, although ulnar traction neuropathy can occur in overhead throwers and can be concomitant in rare cases.

An examiner should perform a very detailed history and physical exam. Relevant history includes player age, height, and weight, as some studies show increased risk with taller athletes [25]. A detailed history of injury should be obtained. This should include the timing of the pain, the factors that worsen the pain, and any previous treatment trials [2]. The number of games played per week, the number of months played per year, and the number of teams played should be ascertained.

A detailed history of injury should be obtained including timing of onset, provocative factors, and any previous treatment trials. The quality and location of pain are critical to investigate. Another vital piece of information to gather is *when* during the throwing motion the pain is worst. This information should be gathered because medal elbow pathology tends to worsen during the late cocking and acceleration phases of throwing, as described above [2, 26].

Physical exam should follow. The inspection of the affected extremity in comparison to the unaffected side gives valuable information. Any gross misalignment, joint swelling, abrasions, atrophy, or hypertrophy should be noted. Swelling is infrequent and should increase the examiner's suspicion for more sinister pathologies like medial epicondyle avulsion fractures or lateral elbow pathologies [7].

The location of tenderness is important in relation to the bony landmarks of the elbow. Several landmarks should be palpated for pathology: the common flexor-pronator mass should be evaluated for pain, which could suggest tendon damage or medial epicondyle avulsion fracture. The soft spot of the elbow, as well as the posteromedial and posterolateral ulnotrochlear joint lines, should be evaluated for synovitis [2]. Next, the examiner should palpate the medial epicondyle, medial collateral ligament, as well as the sublime tubercle of the ulna. The radiocapitellar joint, olecranon, and olecranon physis should be palpated.

Range-of-motion, as well as strength of the elbow and surrounding musculature, should be assessed. Active and passive elbow flexion, extension, pronation, and supination should be examined for pain. In some cases of apophysitis, full elbow extension can be rather painful, and an examiner may note a flexion contracture in a minority of patients [5, 26].

The strength of the wrist flexors, interosseous muscles of the hand, as well as elbow flexors should be tested. Some patients with medial apophysitis can have pain at full extension, as this increases tension on the flexor-pronator mass and subsequently, the medial epicondyle. They may also have symptoms of traction ulnar neuropathy, which may weaken wrist flexion.

To evaluate elbow stability, one should perform the moving valgus stress test as well as the milking maneuver [5, 27, 28]. The moving valgus stress test is performed by applying a valgus stress to the elbow throughout the elbow's flexion-extension arc. The milking maneuver is done by applying valgus stress on the elbow while the elbow is flexed to 90°, and the forearm is supinated [2]. Apprehension, instability, or severe pain with these two maneuvers should make an examiner suspicious of UCL injuries or medial epicondyle avulsion fractures rather than apophysitis. Valgus instability in medial epicondyle apophysitis is uncommon.

The ulnar nerve should also be assessed as it traverses the cubital tunnel. An examiner should perform the Tinel test over the cubital tunnel by tapping the ulnar nerve just proximal to the cubital tunnel with fingers or a reflex hammer. Next, the elbow should be held in a flexed position for >60 seconds. If either of these tests produces distal pain, tingling, or numbness that is similar to their presenting pain, the test is considered positive.

Diagnosis

Diagnosis of medial epicondyleapophysitis is mainly clinical and based on the presentation, as described above. However, avulsion fractures and other osseous medial elbow pathologies are possible. Thus, anteroposterior, oblique, and lateral elbow radiographs should always be obtained and carefully evaluated. These radiographs are often normal but can show sclerosis of the apophysis or widening of the physis [29] (Fig. 32.1). Fragmentation of the apophysis, though uncommon, can also occur [6]. Distal avulsion fractures of the UCL from the sublime tubercle can also occur.

It is essential to compare radiographs to the contralateral extremity since physeal findings are usually quite subtle. Though not routinely necessary for diagnosis, magnetic resonance imaging (MRI) is more sensitive and can be helpful to confirm physeal widening, apophyseal sclerosis, and bone marrow edema [28] (Fig. 32.2). These changes are generally localized to the medial epicondyle, but in more severe cases can cause inflammation that extends to the adjacent medial humeral metaphysis. MRI can also be helpful to evaluate for tears of the UCL and flexor-pronator. Clinicians must be thoughtful and skeptical with the interpretation of radiologic studies, though, as up to 85% of symptomatic throwers will have no plain radiograph or MRI findings. In addition, almost 50% asymptomatic elbows may demonstrate radiographic abnormalities [6, 28, 30]. Thus, clinicians must treat the patient, not the radiographs.

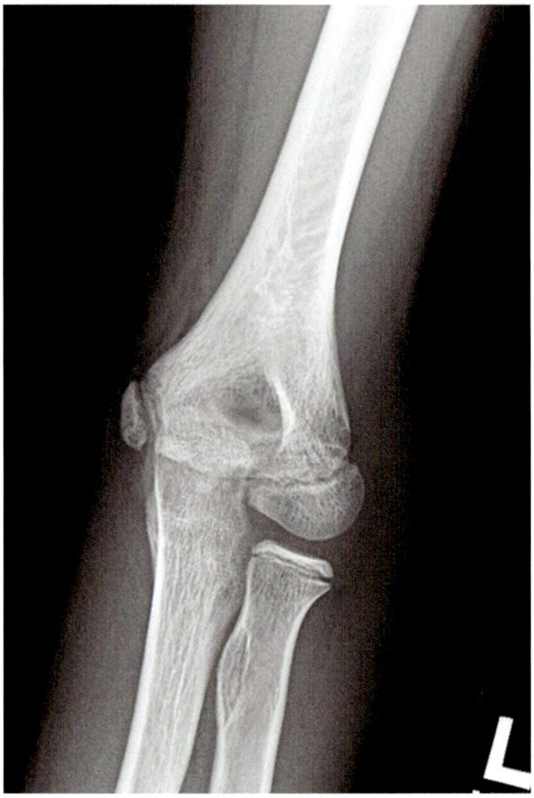

Fig. 32.1 Radiographic appearance of medial epicondyle apophyseal widening with cortical irregularity of the apophysis in a 13-year-old male baseball player

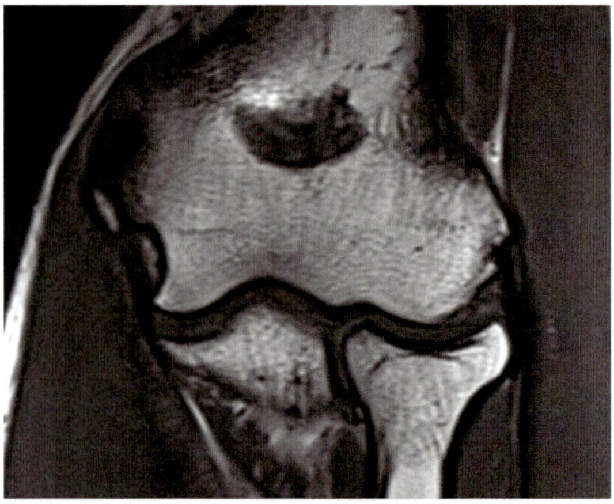

Fig. 32.2 Magnetic resonance imaging appearance of the long-term effects of medial epicondyle apophysitis in an adult baseball pitcher

Prevention

Before the treatment of medial epicondyle apophysitis is reviewed, it is crucial to keep in mind that many of these injuries are avoidable. Most throwing pathologies in adolescents occur due to *overuse* rather than acute injuries. Overuse injuries are an ever-increasing dilemma, as participation in organized sports is increasing, and more athletes are participating in only one sport [31, 32]. This early specialization allows athletes more time to throw, putting their young arms at risk of injury [33, 34]. Overuse injuries have become problematic enough that the American Academy of Pediatrics recommends no athlete specialize in a single sport before puberty [35].

Aside from overspecialization at a young age, several other risk factors increase the likelihood of a thrower becoming injured. These risk factors have been evaluated extensively, and accepted injury-prevention guidelines should always be followed. First and foremost, avoidance of pitching while fatigued is critical. Throwing while fatigued can result in altered throwing mechanics and susceptibility to injury [24]. In one retrospective study comparing pitchers who required elbow surgery vs. healthy controls, pitchers who threw while they were fatigued increased their risk of severe injury by a staggering 36 times [36].

Pitch counts are extremely important. To be specific, pitchers should adhere to recommended pitch counts as well as rest periods. The USA Baseball Pitch Smart program has age-specific guidelines that are widely accepted by the Little League Baseball Organization [37] (Table 32.1). As stated above, most adolescent throwing pathologies are due to overuse. This is supported by several studies that have shown 2–5 times increased risk of injury with pitching over 600 pitches in one season, pitching greater than eight months of the year, or pitching greater than 100 innings per year [36, 38]. Older adolescents are more likely to violate pitch count recommendations [39]. Unfortunately, pitch counts are not often understood or respected by coaches. Fazarale et al. showed that under 50% of youth baseball coaches surveyed could answer questions about pitch counts and rest periods correctly [40]. In another study of youth baseball coaches, Knapik et al. showed that only 56% of coaches "always" tracked pitch counts [41].

Other, less quantifiable recommendations should also be followed. For example, pitchers should not also play catcher for their team, as this vastly increases the number of total throws in the long term. Abstinence of all overhead throwing activities for a minimum of 2–4 months each year is advised as this gives the arm time to heal without exposure to tension forces. Throwers should always properly warm up before pitching. It is also recommended that adolescents avoid pitches other than fastballs and change-ups.

Playing for multiple teams at the same time has been shown to increase risk of injury by up to 22%, and pitching multiple games on the same day is not recommended [25]. Once removed from the mound, a pitcher should not return to pitch, nor should an adolescent pitch for three consecutive days regardless of pitch count. Lastly, and very importantly, if a thrower complains of pain, he or she must not throw until they are appropriately evaluated [31].

Table 32.1 Pitch smart – pitching guidelines. https://www.mlb.com/pitch-smart/pitching-guidelines

Age	Daily max (pitches in game)	Rest for 0 day	Rest for 1 day	Rest for 2 days	Rest for 3 days	Rest for 4 days	Rest for 5 days
7-8	50	1-20	21-35	36-50	N/A	N/A	N/A
9-10	75	1-20	21-35	36-50	51-65	66+	N/A
11-12	85	1-20	21-35	36-50	51-65	66+	N/A
13-14	95	1-20	21-35	36-50	51-65	66+	N/A
15-16	95	1-30	31-45	46-60	61-75	76+	N/A
17-18	105	1-30	31-45	46-60	61-80	81+	N/A
19-22	120	1-30	31-45	46-60	61-80	81-105	106+

Treatment

Medial epicondyle apophysitis is primarily treated nonoperatively. The critical component of treatment is the cessation of throwing as well as any other aggravating factors—generally for 6–12 weeks. Athletes are discouraged, though, from discontinuing training altogether. This period of upper extremity rest is an ideal time for throwers to train their lower extremities and core, which are the first muscle groups to fatigue while pitching [24]. Throwers should also continue to develop proper mechanics, which may prevent injury in the future [42]. During this period, pitchers and their parents and coaches will often bend the rules to negotiate more activity, i.e., by weight lifting, continuing to hit, or by having the pitcher play in the infield. Generally, if any of these activities cause pain, they should be discouraged, and pitchers should be warned that any activity can prolong the condition and prevent the physis from healing. The quickest recovery is with complete rest. Historically casting was even recommended. In cases where compliance will be questionable, this can be considered, although the authors prefer a removable brace for hygiene and to allow frequent motion exercises to prevent stiffness.

In addition to discontinuation of throwing, symptomatic management of medial elbow pain may be augmented with ice and non-steroidal anti-inflammatory analgesics. A structured physical therapy regimen should also be recommended at the physician's discretion to aid young athletes with core and peri-scapular muscle strengthening and to improve shoulder and elbow range of motion [43].

After the 6–12-week period of upper-extremity rest has been completed, athletes should begin a 6-week graduated throwing and strengthening program, which should integrate into the athlete's physical therapy regimen. This time is critical and should be used to improve throwing mechanics and continue strengthening both upper and lower extremities as well as core musculature. The thrower may return to sport once the 6-week throwing program is completed if he or she is entirely symptom-free [2, 7].

Occasionally, symptoms persist despite standard-of-care management, and in this case, advanced imaging should be considered to ensure that there is no occult pathology. If athletes are still endorsing pain after more than six weeks of rest, they should take the remainder of the season off, and a short period of splinting or cast immobilization may be considered [44, 45]. Thankfully, once skeletal maturity is reached, this problem typically wholly resolves.

Further along the spectrum of medial epicondyle injury lie displaced medial epicondyle avulsion fractures. These fractures usually present with acute medial elbow pain immediately after a throwing event rather than chronic overuse injuries. Avulsion fractures of the medial epicondyle account for about 12% of all pediatric elbow fractures and usually present in children aged 9–14 [46, 47].

Osbahr et al. presented a case series of eight adolescent throwers with acute avulsion fractures of the medial epicondyle. None of these patients had preexisting elbow pain. According to published treatment algorithms, those with a displacement of less than 5 mm were treated nonoperatively while those with greater than 5 mm displacement were treated with open reduction and internal fixation. Both groups had excellent outcomes, and return to play was just under eight months on average [48].

Lawrence et al. also show excellent results with both operative and nonoperative treatment of avulsion fractures following the published algorithm. All throwers returned to play at the appropriate level, and none of the pitchers felt their performance was limited after treatment [49]. More robust research needs to be undertaken in this space, though, as there is disagreement when defining thresholds of displacement requiring operative fixation and the relative indications for surgery [50, 51].

Throwers are a unique population, and though some have proposed 5 mm of displacement as the operative threshold, the senior author typically treats any amount of displacement operatively, as even minimal displacement can result in laxity of the UCL—possibly decreasing performance long term. Surgical fixation is generally done with 1–2 screws or Kirschner wires utilizing the tension-band technique.

References

1. Magra M, Caine D, Maffulli N. A review of epidemiology of paediatric elbow injuries in sports. Sports Med. 2007;37(8):717.
2. Saltzman BM, Chalmers PN, Mascarenhas R, Cole BJ, Romeo AA. Upper extremity physeal injury in young baseball pitchers. Phys Sportsmed. 2014;42(3):100–11.
3. Adirim TA, Barouh A. Common orthopaedic injuries in young athletes. Curr Paediatr. 2006;16(3):205–10.
4. Otoshi K, Kikuchi S, Kato K, Sato R, Igari T, Kaga T, et al. Age-specific prevalence and clinical characteristics of humeral medial epicondyle apophysitis and osteochondritis dissecans: ultrasonographic assessment of 4249 players. Orthop J Sport Med. 2017;5(5):2325967117707703.
5. Klingele KE, Kocher MS. Little league elbow: Valgus overload injury in the paediatric athlete. Sports Med. 2002;32(15):1005–15.
6. Hang DW, Chao CM, Hang YS. A clinical and roentgenographic study of Little League elbow. Am J Sports Med. 2004;32(1):79–84.
7. Mautner K, Blazuk J. Overuse throwing injuries in skeletally immature athletes – diagnosis, treatment, and prevention. Curr Sports Med Rep. 2015;14(3):209–14.
8. Toritsuka Y, Nakagawa S, Koyanagi M, et al. Shoulder and elbow evaluation of pitchers in National High School Baseball Invitational Tournaments and National High School Baseball Championships from 1993 to 2016 in Japan. J Orthop Sci. 2019;S0949-2658(19):30189–7.
9. Larson RL, Singer KM, Bergstrom R, Thomas S. Little league survey: the Eugene study. Am J Sports Med. 1976;4(5):201–9.
10. Kocher MS, Waters PM, Micheli LJ. Upper extremity injuries in the paediatric athlete. Sports Med. 2000;30(2):117–35.
11. Maffulli N, Longo UG, Spiezia F, et al. Sports injuries in young athletes: long-term outcome and prevention strategies. Phys Sportsmed. 2010;38:29–34.
12. Maffulli N, Longo UG, Spiezia F, et al. Aetiology and prevention of injuries in elite young athletes. Med Sport Sci. 2011;56:187–200.
13. Wik EH, Martínez-Silván D, Farooq A, Cardinale M, Johnson A, Bahr R. Skeletal maturation and growth rates are related to bone and growth plate injuries in adolescent athletics [published online ahead of print, 2020 Feb 8]. Scand J Med Sci Sports. 2020. 10.1111/sms.13635.
14. Digby KH. The measurement of diaphyseal growth in proximal and distal directions. J Anat Physiol. 1916;50:187–8.
15. Bright RW, Burstein AH, Elmore SM. Epiphyseal-plate cartilage: a biomechanical and histological analysis of failure modes. J Bone Joint Surg Am. 1974;56:688–703.
16. Chalmers PN, Wimmer MA, Verma NN, et al. The relationship between pitching mechanics and Injury: a review of current concepts. Sports Health. 2017;9(3):216–21.
17. Dillman CJ, Fleisig GS, Andrews JR. Biomechanics of pitching with emphasis upon shoulder kinematics. J Orthop Sports Phys Ther. 1993;18(2):402–8.
18. Fleisig GS, Barrentine SW, Escamilla RF, Andrews JR. Biomechanics of overhand throwing with implications for injuries. Sports Med. 1996;21(6):421–37.
19. Fleisig G, Chu Y, Weber A, Andrews J. Variability in baseball pitching biomechanics among various levels of competition. Sports Biomech. 2009;8(1):10–21.
20. Werner SL, Fleisig GS, Dillman CJ, Andrews JR. Biomechanics of the elbow during baseball pitching. J Orthop Sports Phys Ther. 1993;17(6):274–8.
21. Paulino FE, Villacis DC, Ahmad CS. Valgus extension overload in baseball players. Am J Orthop (Belle Mead NJ). 2016;45(3):144–51.
22. Bryce CD, Armstrong AD. Anatomy and biomechanics of the elbow. Orthop Clin North Am. 2008;39(2):141–v.
23. Pappas AM, Zawacki RM, Sullivan TJ. Biomechanics of baseball pitching. A preliminary report. Am J Sports Med. 1985;13(4):216–22.
24. Erickson BJ, Sgori T, Chalmers PN, et al. The impact of fatigue on baseball pitching mechanics in adolescent male pitchers. Arthroscopy. 2016;32(5):762–71.
25. Chalmers PN, Sgroi T, Riff AJ, et al. Correlates with history of injury in youth and adolescent pitchers. Arthroscopy. 2015;31:1349–57.
26. Tisano BK, Estes AR. Overuse injuries of the pediatric and adolescent throwing athlete. Med Sci Sports Exerc. 2016;48(10):1898–905.
27. Brogdon BS, Crow MD. Little Leaguer's elbow. Am J Roentgenol. 1960;83:671–5.
28. Wei AS, Khana S, Limpisvasti O, Crues J, Podesta L, Yocum LA. Clinical and magnetic resonance imaging findings associated with Little League elbow. J Pediatr Orthop. 2010;30(7):715–9.
29. Wong TT, Dana JL, Ayyala RS, Kazam JK. Elbow injuries in pediatric overhead athletes. Am J Roentgenol. 2017;209(4):849–59.
30. Kijowski R, Tuite MJ. Pediatric throwing injuries of the elbow. Semin Musculoskelet Radiol. 2010;14(4):419–29.
31. Fleisig GS, Andrews JR. Prevention of elbow injuries in youth baseball pitchers. Sports Health. 2012;4(5):419–24.

32. Malina RM. Early sport specialization: roots, effectiveness, risks. Curr Sports Med Rep. 2010;9(6):364–71.
33. Myer GD, Jayanthi N, Difiori JP, Faigenbaum AD, Kiefer AW, Logerstedt D, et al. Sport specialization, Part I: does early sports specialization increase negative outcomes and reduce the opportunity for success in young athletes? Sports Health. 2015;7(5):437–42.
34. Myer GD, Jayanthi N, DiFiori JP, Faigenbaum AD, Kiefer AW, Logerstedt D, et al. Sports specialization, Part II: alternative solutions to early sport specialization in youth athletes. Sports Health. 2016;8(1):65–73.
35. Brenner JS. Sports specialization and intensive training in young athletes. Pediatrics. 2016;138(3):e20162148.
36. Olsen SJ, Fleisig GS, Dun S, Loftice J, Andrews JR. Risk factors for shoulder and elbow injuries in adolescent baseball pitchers. Am J Sports Med. 2006;34(6):905–12.
37. USA Baseball. Pitch smart – pitching guidelines [Internet]. MLB Advanced Media 2020. Retrieved 19 Feb 2020, from https://www.mlb.com/pitch-smart/pitching-guidelines.
38. Lyman S, Fleisig GS, Waterbor JW, Funkhouser EM, Pulley L, Andrews JR, et al. Longitudinal study of elbow and shoulder pain in youth baseball pitchers. Med Sci Sports Exerc. 2001;33(11):1803–10.
39. Riff AJ, Chalmers PN, Sgroi T, et al. Epidemiologic comparison of pitching mechanics, pitch type, and pitch counts among healthy pitchers at various levels of youth competition. Arthroscopy. 2016;32(8):1559–68.
40. Fazarale JJ, Magnussen RA, Pedroza AD, Kaeding CC, Best TM, Classie J. Knowledge of and compliance with pitch count recommendations: a survey of youth baseball coaches [published correction appears in Sports Health. 2013; 5(6):569. Best, Thomas M [added]; Classie, Justin [added]]. Sports Health 2012;4(3):202–204.
41. Knapik DM, Continenza SM, Hoffman K, Gilmore A. Youth baseball coach awareness of pitch count guidelines and overuse throwing injuries remains deficient. J Pediatr Orthop. 2018;38(10):e623–8.
42. Leahy I, Schorpion M, Ganley T. Common medial elbow injuries in the adolescent athlete. J Hand Ther. 2015;28(2):201–11.
43. Pearce McCarty L 3rd. Approach to medial elbow pain in the throwing athlete. Curr Rev Musculoskelet Med. 2019;12(1):30–40.
44. Chen FS, Diaz VA, Loebenberg M, Rosen JE. Shoulder and elbow injuries in the skeletally immature athlete. J Am Acad Orthop Surg. 2005;13(3):172–85.
45. Difelice GS, Meunier MJ, Paletta GA. Elbow injury in the adolescent athlete. In: Altchek DW, Andrews JR, editors. The Athlete's Elbow. New York, NY: Lippincott, Williams &Wilkins; 2001. p. 231–48.
46. Pace GI, Hennrikus WL. Fixation of displaced medial epicondyle fractures in adolescents. J Pediatr Orthop. 2017;37(2):e80–2.
47. Wilkins KE. Fractures involving the medial epicondylarapophysis. In: Rockwood Jr CA, Wilkins KE, King RE, editors. Fractures in children, vol. 3. Philadelphia: JB Lippincott; 1991.
48. Osbahr DC, Chalmers PN, Frank JS, Williams RJ 3rd, Widmann RF, Green DW. Acute, avulsion fractures of the medial epicondyle while throwing in youth baseball players: a variant of Little League elbow. J Shoulder Elbow Surg. 2010;19(7):951–7.
49. Lawrence JTR, Patel NM, Macknin J, Flynn JM, Cameron D, Wolfgruber HC, et al. Return to competitive sports after medial epicondyle fractures in adolescent athletes. Am J Sports Med. 2013;41(5):1152–7.
50. Gottschalk HP, Eisner E, Hosalkar HS. Medial epicondyle fractures in the pediatric population. J Am Acad Orthop Surg. 2012;20(4):223–32.
51. Griffith TB, Kercher J, Clifton Willimon S, Perkins C, Duralde XA. Elbow injuries in the adolescent thrower. Curr Rev Musculoskelet Med. 2018;11(1):35–47.

Complications of Ulnar Collateral Ligament Reconstruction

33

Travis G. Maak, Peter N. Chalmers, Brandon J. Erickson, and Robert Z. Tashjian

Introduction

Injury to the ulnar collateral ligament (UCL) commonly occurs when a valgus load is placed on the elbow, which results in distraction of the medial side and compression of the lateral aspect of the elbow. Osseous restraints of the elbow account for approximately 50% of elbow stability, while the other 50% is provided by various soft tissue restraints [1, 2]. Hence, this distraction force places significant tensile stress on the UCL and may lead to partial or complete rupture. A complete rupture often results in significant valgus instability, particularly in overhead athletes such as javelin throwers, pitchers, quarterbacks, and volleyball players, among others. Complete, symptomatic tears of the UCL often require repair or reconstruction in overhead athletes due to the required continued valgus forces during athletic participation. Pitchers often lose accuracy and velocity, and are unable to return to sport (RTS) without surgical intervention. Several techniques have been developed to optimize RTS rates and performance upon RTS in these athletes. While in most circumstances UCL reconstruction (UCLR), also known as "Tommy John surgery," has led to encouraging results and has allowed many athletes to continue participation at high levels [3, 4], complications have occurred.

Analysis of prior complications following UCLR provides crucial information that can be used to improve upon the current reconstructive techniques and avoid intraoperative and postoperative pitfalls. Various complications have been previously documented including transient and permanent neuropathies involving the ulnar, saphenous, and median nerves, neuroma formation, hematoma, infection, donor site harvest tenderness, postoperative stiffness, retear of flexor-pronator muscle, stress fracture of the ulnar bone bridge, and fracture of the medial epicondyle.

Complications Related to Surgical Variables

Vitale et al. performed a systematic review of UCL reconstruction including an analysis of surgical variables that impacted outcomes and complications [5]. The authors found a lower overall complication rate following UCLR in which the flexor-pronator mass was split rather than detached (muscle-splitting approach). Only eight

T. G. Maak · P. N. Chalmers · R. Z. Tashjian (✉)
Department of Orthopaedic Surgery, University of Utah, Salt Lake City, UT, USA
e-mail: Robert.tashjian@hsc.utah.edu

B. J. Erickson
Department of Sports Medicine, Rothman Orthopaedic Institute, New York, NY, USA

J. S. Dines et al. (eds.), *Elbow Ulnar Collateral Ligament Injury*,
https://doi.org/10.1007/978-3-030-69567-5_33

of 91 patients (9%) had complications when a muscle-splitting approach was utilized, as compared to 15 of 65 (23%) in which detachment of the flexor-pronator mass was used. Following this systematic review, Cain et al. published the largest retrospective review of 1281 patients, with 743 athletes available for a minimum of 2-year follow-up [6]. These authors documented a 20% (148/743) complication rate, with 16% (121/743) of these being minor postoperative ulnar nerve neuropraxias. Reoperation occurred 62 times in 55 patients, with arthroscopic osteophyte debridement as the most common surgery performed (53/62) followed by revision UCL reconstruction (9/62). Other complications included medial epicondyle avulsion fracture and graft harvest site superficial infection. A more recent systematic review of UCLR by Erickson et al. that included 20 studies and 2019 patients found an overall complication rate of 10.4% [7]. Transient ulnar neuritis was the most frequent complication (159, 75.4% of complications) followed by donor site issues including pain, wound dehiscence, weakness, and paresthesia (27, 12.8% of complications), need for revision UCLR (14, 6.6%), stiffness (6, 2.8%), reactive synovitis (3, 1.4%), postoperative hematoma (2, 0.9%), and ulnar tunnel fracture (2, 0.9%).

Nerve Injury

Ulnar nerve injury deserves specific evaluation regarding complications that occur as a result of UCLR. Particular attention and study have been paid to management of the ulnar nerve during UCL reconstruction due to the high prevalence and sequelae of this complication. Prior studies have found no difference in performance or RTS rate among professional baseball pitchers who underwent UCLR with or without subsequent ulnar nerve transposition, indicating a reflexive transposition of the nerve at the time of UCLR may be unnecessary [8]. Some authors have advocated for routine ulnar nerve transposition, while others only transpose the nerve if the patient is symptomatic preoperatively [9–12]. Submuscular transposition has resulted in transient ulnar nerve symptoms in 8.5% of patients with 12.7% of those requiring reoperation [13]. Prior data have also demonstrated that ulnar neuropathy can occur in up to 2% of patients following UCLR with no preoperative symptoms [10]. Cain et al. documented a 16% prevalence of postoperative ulnar nerve paresthesias following routine ulnar nerve transposition in UCLR, and attributed this high rate to the routine relatively complete dissection and exposure of the ulnar nerve from the cubital tunnel. Some have suggested that performing a UCLR without ulnar nerve dissection or transposition in cases in which no preoperative ulnar nerve symptoms exist may reduce this high level of ulnar neuropathy. The authors do not routinely transpose the ulnar nerve. Rather, when patients preset with preoperative paresthesias or motor weakness, a concomitant anterior subcutaneous ulnar nerve transposition is performed at the time of UCLR. Regardless of how the nerve is dealt with, in every case careful attention must be paid to the management of the ulnar nerve intraoperatively especially when drilling the posterior aspect of the ulnar tunnel and the posterior exit hole in the medial epicondyle.

Careful evaluation and follow-up of ulnar nerve injury following UCLR has demonstrated that the majority of these are isolated to sensory paresthesias of the ring and small fingers that resolve within the first 6 postoperative weeks [6]. Motor involvement was identified in a single case, which required reoperation and neurolysis. In this case, motor function fully returned at 10 months and sensory paresthesias resolved by 48 months. Interestingly, postoperative ulnar nerve dysfunction has not been shown to affect outcome. Cain et al. documented an 85 and 83% return to play in athletes with and without postoperative ulnar nerve symptoms, respectively [6].

Infection

Postoperative infection represents a devastating complication of any surgical procedure. Fortunately, previously documented infection rates following UCLR have been extremely low.

Azar et al. documented an 8.8% (8/91) complication rate, of which two were superficial infections at the palmaris site, and one was a superficial infection at the elbow [9]. All of these infections were superficial surgical site infections and were managed accordingly. The systematic review performed by Vitale et al. evaluated eight studies of UCLR including the study by Azar et al. [5, 9] This was the only case series in which infection was documented as a complication resulting in a total infection prevalence of three in 410 cases or 0.73% [5]. This systematic review did not document any cases of reoperation for postoperative infection. These data suggest that postoperative infection following UCLR occurs infrequently and rarely involves more than a superficial site infection.

Motion Loss and Arthrofibrosis

Periarticular ligamentous reconstruction can result in postoperative decreased range of motion due to anisometric ligament attachment, over constraint of the joint, and arthrofibrosis. Prior studies have reported decreased range of motion following UCLR ranging from an average loss of extension of 3–17° and an average loss of flexion from 3 to 5°. However, loss of extension in professional baseball pitchers is not uncommon, and often is present preoperatively. Conway et al. [6] evaluated 71 patients following UCLR and documented an average extension loss of 17° (range 2–25°). Extension loss, however, was not categorized as a postoperative complication in this article due to the fact that many overhead athletes lack full extension in their dominant throwing arm at baseline. Paletta et al. evaluated 25 patients following UCLR for an average 2.5-year follow-up and documented an average extension loss of 3° and average flexion loss of 5° [11]. These decreased ranges of motion did not require further operative intervention. Two studies each documented a single case (1%) of postoperative stiffness requiring reoperation, although postoperative ranges of motion were not documented in either study [9, 10].

The aforementioned data suggest that UCLR may result in reduced postoperative range of motion in many cases. The absolute reduction in motion is minimal, and in most cases is 5 ° or less for both flexion and extension. In only a single documented case was reoperation necessary for postoperative stiffness [9]. Even in elite baseball pitchers, this reduced motion remained asymptomatic, did not impact return to play, and did not require reoperation [11]. Nevertheless, care must be taken to identify the center of the medial epicondyle and the sublime tubercle to ensure anatomic, isometric UCLR. Early range of motion should be considered following a 6-week period of splint immobilization to improve postoperative motion and reduce the risk of arthrofibrosis.

Reconstruction Construct Failure

Multiple theoretical mechanisms for construct failure exist including graft tunnel fracture, graft rupture, recurrent instability due to loosening, or continued surgical site pain. As the number of UCLR procedures have increased, so has the number of revision UCLR. Liu et al. reported that of the 235 MLB pitchers who had undergone UCLR from 1999 to 2015, 31 pitchers (13.2%) underwent revision UCLR. Interestingly, aside from graft rupture, the multiple other potential modes of failure have been rarely documented as complications following UCLR. In fact, only one documented case of postoperative stress fracture of the ulnar bridge was reported among the 410 cases that were included in a recent systematic review [5]. This case occurred in the case series that employed the docking technique, but did not require operative intervention and resolved with observation alone [11]. Cain et al. documented a 1% (9/743) rate of UCL revision due to reconstruction construct failure [6]. Five of these cases were due to avulsion fractures of the medial epicondyle at the tunnel site. Four of these cases required ORIF, and one case was managed with isolated immobilization . Other authors have employed the docking technique in an effort to minimize this risk [11, 12]. It is somewhat difficult to report the exact revision rate following UCLR as there is a subset of patients who may forgo revision UCLR despite a graft rupture and simply stop playing their overhead sport.

Complications Related to Graft Harvest Site

Many different types of grafts were used in the published cases to date. These types include palmaris longus, Achilles tendon, gracilis, semitendinosus, and extensor tendon of the fourth toe. Azar et al. documented a 4% (4/91) complication rate at the graft harvest site including two cases of superficial infection and two cases of stiffness or tenderness [9]. None of these complications required reoperation. Notably all four of these cases occurred following the use of palmaris longus despite the use of two other graft types. However, interpretation of these data must be made cautiously, as 63/78 of the reconstructions were performed using palmaris longus in this study. Some authors have avoided the use of ipsilateral plamaris longus due to the concern for scar formation at the wrist flexion crease of the throwing arm and concern regarding the possible role of the palmaris longus in dynamic stabilization of the elbow during varus stress [14]. This philosophy, however, has not been universally adopted or substantiated clinically, and as such, ipsilateral palmari longus autograft is the most common graft used in UCLR [6]. Cain et al. also documented a 4% (27/743) graft harvest site complication rate with the majority of these cases relating to superficial site infections that were treated with oral antibiotics [6]. A potential way to avoid this complication is by using an allograft. One study demonstrated equivalent outcomes between allograft and autograft for UCL reconstruction [15]. One possible complication of UCLR is future injury risk. While future lower extremity injury risk did not differ based on the side of hamstring harvest in UCLR, when comparing future injury risk between players who underwent UCLR with hamstring vs. palmaris autograft, evidence has shown a higher future injury risk to the lower extremity in players that underwent UCLR with hamstring autograft and a slightly higher upper extremity injury risk for those who underwent UCLR with palmaris autograft [16, 17].

Complications Related to Posteromedial Impingement

Many case series have documented arthroscopic posteromedial osteophyte excision with concomitant UCLR. Continued pain related to an inadequate posteromedial olecranon osteophyte excision necessitating reoperation is rare, and was documented in a single case in a systematic review [9]. The low prevalence of this complication is notable given the combined high prevalence (19% or 71/378) of this concomitant procedure. Cain et al. documented persistent pain from olecranon osteophytes as the most common reason for reoperation in their series [6]. Of the 62 subsequent reoperations that were performed in this study, 85% (53/62) involved arthroscopic debridement of an olecranon osteophyte. Notably, 19% (10/53) of the patients that required reoperation for an olecranon osteophyte had an excision of the olecranon osteophyte at the index UCLR. These data suggest that care must be given to completely addressing this concomitant pathology in these valgus extension overload patients. Interestingly, no cases of postoperative UCLR failure were documented due to iatrogenic overresection of the posteromedial osteophyte despite this inherent possibility.

Medial Epicondyle Fractures

One of the more rare complications following UCLR is an avulsion fracture of the medial epicondyle secondary to the tunnel within the medial epicondyle. This complication most likely occurs because the tunnel within the medial epicondyle is either made too large, or is placed too medial (closer to the medial cortex of the bone) and weakens the area. Andrews et al. initially reported this rare complication in seven patients [18]. All but one of these fractures occurred as a result of throwing, and six of the seven were treated with open reduction internal fixation (ORIF) of the fracture. A recent study reported the results following ORIF of all medial epicondyle fractures sustained following UCLR in professional baseball players [19]. A total of 15 pitchers underwent ORIF of medial epicondyle fractures between 2010 and 2016, the majority of which were treated with screw fixation. Overall 73.3% were able to RTS while 55% RTS at the same level or higher. No significant differences existed in performance metrics from pre- to post-surgery, and when these players were compared to a group of controls who did not sustain a medial epicondyle fracture, players in the ORIF group pitched fewer innings than controls after surgery but had no other significant differences in performance metrics.

Other Complications

While the majority of complications fall into the aforementioned complication categories, some other complications have been reported in small frequencies. These complications include retear of flexor-pronator muscle and wound hematoma. The retear of the flexor-pronator muscle and wound hematoma each occurred in 1% (1/83) of cases in a series that employed a muscle-splitting approach through the flexor-pronator muscle [20].

Summary

UCLR has demonstrated reproducibly excellent results with a very low rate of serious complications. The most common complications include ulnar neuropathy, infection, and construct failure. Transient ulnar neuropathy represents the most common postoperative complication and completely resolves with observation by 6 weeks in most cases. Subcutaneous transposition of the ulnar nerve has demonstrated a low rate of reoperation due to ulnar nerve symptoms, while submuscular transposition has required a much higher reoperation rate. Postoperative infection most commonly involves the graft harvest site and often can be adequately treated with oral antibiotics. Careful attention to ulnar nerve management, tunnel placement, and close follow-up can minimize complications and optimize postoperative outcomes following UCLR.

References

1. Erickson BJ, Gupta AK, Harris JD, Bush-Joseph C, Bach BR, Abrams GD, et al. Rate of return to pitching and performance after Tommy John Surgery in Major League Baseball Pitchers. Am J Sports Med. 2014;42(3):536–43. https://doi.org/10.1177/0363546513510890. Epub 2013 Dec 18. PMID: 24352622.
2. Erickson BJ, Bach BR Jr, Cohen MS, Bush-Joseph CA, Cole BJ, Verma NN, et al. Ulnar collateral ligament reconstruction: the rush experience. Orthop J Sports Med. 2016;4(1):2325967115626876.
3. Erickson BJ, Chalmers PN, Bush-Joseph CA, Verma NN, Romeo AA. Ulnar collateral ligament reconstruction of the elbow: a systematic review of the literature. Orthop J Sports Med. 2015;3(12):2325967115618914.
4. Lin F, Kohli N, Perlmutter S, Lim D, Nuber GW, Makhsous M. Muscle contribution to elbow joint valgus stability. J Shoulder Elbow Surg/Am Shoulder Elbow Surg. 2007;16(6):795–802.
5. Morrey BF. Applied anatomy and biomechanics of the elbow joint. Instr Course Lect. 1986;35:59–68.
6. Vitale MA, Ahmad CS. The outcome of elbow ulnar collateral ligament reconstruction in overhead athletes: a systematic review. Am J Sports Med. 2008;36(6):1193–205.
7. Cain EL Jr, Andrews JR, Dugas JR, Wilk KE, McMichael CS, Walter JC 2nd, et al. Outcome of ulnar collateral ligament reconstruction of the elbow in 1281 athletes: results in 743 athletes with minimum 2-year follow-up. Am J Sports Med. 2010;38(12):2426–34.
8. Erickson BJ, Chalmers PN, D'Angelo J, Ma K, Romeo AA. Performance and return to sport after ulnar nerve decompression/transposition among professional baseball players. Am J Sports Med. 2019;47:363546519829159.
9. Azar FM, Andrews JR, Wilk KE, Groh D. Operative treatment of ulnar collateral ligament injuries of the elbow in athletes. Am J Sports Med. 2000;28(1):16–23.
10. Dodson CC, Thomas A, Dines JS, Nho SJ, Williams RJ 3rd, Altchek DW. Medial ulnar collateral ligament reconstruction of the elbow in throwing athletes. Am J Sports Med. 2006;34(12):1926–32.
11. Paletta GA Jr, Wright RW. The modified docking procedure for elbow ulnar collateral ligament reconstruction: 2-year follow-up in elite throwers. Am J Sports Med. 2006;34(10):1594–8.

12. Rohrbough JT, Altchek DW, Hyman J, Williams RJ 3rd, Botts JD. Medial collateral ligament reconstruction of the elbow using the docking technique. Am J Sports Med. 2002;30(4):541–8.
13. Conway JE, Jobe FW, Glousman RE, Pink M. Medial instability of the elbow in throwing athletes. Treatment by repair or reconstruction of the ulnar collateral ligament. J Bone Joint Surg Am Vol. 1992;74(1):67–83.
14. Koh JL, Schafer MF, Keuter G, Hsu JE. Ulnar collateral ligament reconstruction in elite throwing athletes. Arthroscopy. 2006;22(11):1187–91.
15. Savoie FH 3rd, Morgan C, Yaste J, Hurt J, Field L. Medial ulnar collateral ligament reconstruction using hamstring allograft in overhead throwing athletes. J Bone Joint Surg Am Vol. 2013;95(12):1062–6.
16. Erickson BJ, Chalmers PN, D'Angelo J, Ma K, Ahmad CS, Dines JS, et al. Side of hamstring harvest does not affect performance, return-to-sport rate, or future hamstring injuries after ulnar collateral ligament reconstruction among professional baseball pitchers. Am J Sports Med. 2019;47(5):1111–6.
17. Erickson BJ, Chalmers PN, D'Angelo J, Ma K, Dines JS, Romeo AA. Do outcomes or subsequent injuries differ after ulnar collateral ligament reconstruction with palmaris versus hamstring autograft? Am J Sports Med. 2019;47(6):1473–9.
18. Schwartz ML, Thornton DD, Larrison MC, Cain EL, Aaron DG, Wilk KE, et al. Avulsion of the medial epicondyle after ulnar collateral ligament reconstruction: imaging of a rare throwing injury. AJR Am J Roentgenol. 2008;190(3):595–8.
19. Erickson BJ, Chalmers PN, D'Angelo J, Ma K, Romeo AA. Open reduction internal fixation of medial epicondyle fractures after ulnar collateral ligament reconstruction in professional baseball pitchers. Orthop J Sports Med. 2019;7(6):2325967119852896.
20. Thompson WH, Jobe FW, Yocum LA, Pink MM. Ulnar collateral ligament reconstruction in athletes: muscle-splitting approach without transposition of the ulnar nerve. J Shoulder Elbow Surg/Am Shoulder Elbow Surg. 2001;10(2):152–7.

34 Sport-Specific Outcomes for Ulnar Collateral Ligament Reconstruction

Thomas O'Hagan, Charlton Stucken, Alex E. White, and Christopher C. Dodson

Introduction

Injury to the ulnar collateral ligament (UCL) most commonly occurs in overhead throwing athletes, particularly baseball pitchers, but is also seen in other specific subsets of athletes [1–10]. Prior to the first UCL reconstruction performed by Jobe in 1974, the UCL rupture was a catastrophic event in professional baseball pitchers [7]. Improvements in diagnosis, surgical technique, and rehabilitation programs have significantly improved outcomes for athletes.

The subsets of athletes most commonly associated with UCL injuries are baseball players, javelin throwers, softball players, tennis players, gymnasts, wrestlers, and football players [11–15]. Injury to the UCL in these athletes causes pain and valgus instability, which can adversely affect athletic performance in various ways depending on the sport. Therefore, surgical treatment is often necessitated in order to return both recreational and high-level athletes back to their respective sports. In this chapter, we look to explore outcomes specific to various sports in order to guide treatment and set expectations for return to sport.

T. O'Hagan · C. Stucken · C. C. Dodson
Rothman Institute, Philadelphia, PA, USA

A. E. White (✉)
Department of Orthopedic Surgery, Hospital for Special Surgery, New York, NY, USA
e-mail: whitea@hss.edu

Baseball

The first description of injury to the UCL was in 1946 and involved a review of javelin throwers [10]. It was not until 1974 that Dr. Jobe performed the first successful UCL reconstruction on Los Angeles Dodger pitcher Tommy John, which eventually allowed him to return to professional baseball in 1976 [7]. Over the last half century, the injury has become well recognized in overhead throwing athletes with baseball pitchers at the highest risk [1].

Overhead throwing places high valgus stress and extension forces on the elbow, which place the UCL at risk. Baseball pitchers are at a unique risk due to the sheer number of pitches thrown over the course of a season. During late cocking and early acceleration of each pitch, enormous valgus loads are placed on the elbow, which have been estimated to approach the tensile strength of the UCL [16–18].

Initial management of UCL tears in the baseball player consists of a period of rest followed by return to sport with a structured throwing program. However, in the professional athlete as well as many college and even high school baseball players, prolonged attempts at rest or activity

J. S. Dines et al. (eds.), *Elbow Ulnar Collateral Ligament Injury*,
https://doi.org/10.1007/978-3-030-69567-5_34

modification are often not well tolerated by the athlete. Furthermore, various studies have demonstrated poor results in symptomatic throwers with nonoperative treatment alone. An older study by Barnes and Tullos reported only 50% of symptomatic throwing athletes returned to play out of 100 subjects when treated nonoperatively [19]. A 2016 study by Ford et al., however, showed nonoperative treatment in the form of rehabilitation to be successful in throwers with incomplete UCL injuries (grades I, IIA, and IIB), with 93% returning to sport at or above their previous level [20].

Various surgical techniques have been utilized to address a ruptured UCL in baseball players, with the two major divisions being repairs versus reconstruction [6, 9, 12, 15, 21, 22]. Historically, direct repair has been considered less reliable for returning patients to their previous level of sport when compared to reconstruction. In 2010, Cain and Andrews reviewed the outcomes of 743 athletes and found 83% returned to the same level of sport after reconstruction while only 70% returned after repair [1]. Newer UCL repair techniques utilizing internal bracing, however, have demonstrated promising clinical and biomechanical results when compared to UCL reconstruction [22–24]. Dugas et al. reported the results of their modified UCL repair technique with collagen-coated FiberTape (Arthrex) in overhead throwers with complete or partial avulsion of the UCL from either the sublime tubercle or medial epicondyle. They showed that 92% of patients returned to the same or higher level of competition at a mean time of 6.7 months. Eighty-one percent of their patients were baseball pitchers and 11% were baseball non-pitchers [22].

A number of biomechanical studies have likewise shown encouraging results for UCL repair techniques that use internal bracing [25]. A biomechanical study by Dugas et al. comparing UCL repair with internal bracing to the modified Jobe reconstruction showed greater resistance to gapping in the repair group [25]. Similarly, Bodendorfer et al. showed the UCL repair with internal bracing construct to have a similar biomechanical profile when compared to the docking technique for UCL reconstruction [23].

Numerous studies report outcomes of operative reconstruction or repair of the UCL; however, not all specify outcome by individual sport (Table 34.1). Conway et al. looked at throwing athletes undergoing UCL reconstruction between 1974 and 1987 with minimum 2-year follow-up [13]. Of the 56 patients who underwent reconstruction, 52 were baseball players. Of these 52 baseball players, 35 (67%) had an excellent result, defined as the ability to return to the same sport at the same or higher level for at least 12 months. Outcomes were worse for pitchers of which 62% had excellent results as compared to position players of which 85% had excellent results although these differences were not statistically different in this study.

Andrews and Timmerman reviewed 72 professional baseball players undergoing elbow surgery between 1986 and 1990, 14 of whom underwent UCL reconstruction [11]. Twelve of the 14 (86%) were able to return to play at the same level. Later, Azar and Andrews reported on 59 throwing athletes undergoing UCL reconstruction between 1988 and 1994 [12]. While the authors do not differentiate results by sport, they do specify results on 37 professional baseball players in the group with 73% returning to their previous level of play or higher. This includes 11 of 15 (73%) major league players, 4 of 6 (67%) triple-A players, 4 of 5 (80%) double-A players, and 8 of 11 (73%) single-A players returning to their previous level of play or higher. The average time to return to competitive throwing in the baseball players in this study averaged approximately 1 year.

Petty and Andrews reported on 27 high school baseball players who underwent UCL reconstruction between 1995 and 2000 [26]. They found that 20 out of 27 (74%) baseball players returned to competition at or above their previous level. The average time to return was 11 months. Eleven percent (3/27) were catchers, while the remaining 24/27 athletes were pitchers; however, no distinction among outcomes were reported between the pitchers and catchers with respect to return to previous level of play.

Paletta and Wright retrospectively reviewed 25 professional and scholarship collegiate base-

Table 34.1 UCL reconstruction and repair outcomes in baseball players

Authors	Data collection period	Number of baseball players in study	Type of procedure	Number of pitchers	Level of play	Percentage returning to play (RTP)
Conway et al. [13]	1974–1987	52	Reconstruction	45	20 majors 18 minors 10 college 4 high school	35/56 (67%) RTP at previous level or higher
Andrews and Timmerman [11]	1986–1990	14	Reconstruction	Not reported	14 professional	12/14 (86%)[a] RTP at previous level or higher
Azar et al. [12]	1988–1994	37	Reconstruction	Not reported	15 majors 6 triple-A 5 double-A 11 single-A	27/37 (73%) RTP at previous level or higher
Petty et al. [26]	1992–1996	27	Reconstruction	24	27 high school	20/27 (74%) RTP at previous level or higher
Paletta and Wright [8]	1995–2000	25	Reconstruction	25	1 majors 3 triple-A 6 double-A 7 single-A 3 independent minors 5 college	23/25 (92%) RTP at previous level or higher
Dodson et al. [14]	2000–2003	96	Reconstruction	91	17 professional 63 college 16 high school	90/100 (90%)[b] RTP at previous level or higher
Cain and Andrews [1]	1998–2006	710	Reconstruction	Not reported	45 majors 188 minors 346 college 131 high school	584/710(82%)[c] RTP at previous level or higher
Dugas et al. [22]	2013—2019	102	Repair with internal bracing	90	1 professional 31 college 74 high school 1 middle school 4 recreational	102/111(92%)[d] RTP at previous level or higher
Camp et al. [27]	2005—2014	106	Reconstruction	0, all position players	Minor League and Major League[e]	75.5% RTP at any level 68.8% RTP at previous level or higher 58.6% Catchers RTP at any level 75.6% Infielders RTP at any level 88.9% Outfielders RTP at any level
Griffith et al. [28]	2010—2014	566	Reconstruction	566	134 majors 432 minors	79.9% RTP at any level 71.2% RTP at same or greater level

(continued)

Table 34.1 (continued)

Authors	Data collection period	Number of baseball players in study	Type of procedure	Number of pitchers	Level of play	Percentage returning to play (RTP)
Marshall et al. [29]	2002—2016	54	Primary and Revision Reconstruction	54	54 major	94% RTP at any level (primary reconstruction: 96% RTP) 80% RTP at MLB level
Jack et al. [30]	1984—2015	34	Reconstruction	0, all position players	34 major	84.8% RTP at LMB level 53.3% RTP at MLB level if age ≥30 years 89.4% RTP at MLB level in age < 30 years

UCL ulnar collateral ligament

[a]Authors do not specify at what level players returned

[b]Authors' results include four non-baseball athletes

[c]The study included ten athletes who underwent direct repair and some of these may be included in the overall baseball player results

[d]Authors' results include nine non-baseball athletes

[e]Exact distribution of minor league versus major league not reported

ball pitchers undergoing UCL reconstruction [8]. This study was unique at the time in that all subjects were baseball pitchers. Twenty-three of the 25 pitchers (92%) returned to the same level or higher with a mean time to return to competitive throwing of 11.5 months. There was no difference between professional and collegiate players.

Dodson et al. reported on 100 consecutive overhead-throwing athletes treated with UCL reconstruction between 2000 and 2003 [14]. They found that 90% of 100 throwing athletes were able to return to the same level or higher after reconstruction. While the investigators did not stratify outcomes by individual sport, the results are relevant in a discussion of sports specific outcomes of baseball players due to the high percentage of baseball players in their study. Ninety-six of the 100 athletes were baseball players, with 91 being pitchers and five positions players. Among the baseball players, 16 played professionally, 60 played at the collegiate level, and 15 were high school pitchers.

The largest study of UCL reconstruction to date was performed by Cain and Andrews in which they reported on 743 patients undergoing surgical intervention for UCL tears [1]. Of these, 733 underwent reconstruction and 10 underwent repair of the ligament between 1998 and 2006. Overall results demonstrated 610 of 733 (83%) athletes undergoing reconstruction and 7 of 10 (70%) athletes undergoing repair returned to their previous level of play or higher. Among these athletes, 710 were baseball players: 45 major league players, 188 minor league players, 346 collegiate players, and 131 high school and recreational baseball players.

In that same study, Cain and Andrews looked closely at results of baseball players stratifying outcomes by level of play [1]. In their review, 34 of 45 (75.5%) major league players returned to same level with seven returning to the minor leagues and four not returning to sport. Looking at minor league players, 138 of 188 (73%) returned to the same level or higher. An additional 24 of the 188 minor league players (13%) returned to the minor leagues, however, at a lower level (i.e., triple-A to double-A). Among college players, 304 of 346 (88%) returned to the same level or higher. This included five college players eventually advancing to major league baseball, and 66 eventually advancing to minor league baseball. Among the high school athletes, 108 of 131 (83%) returned to the same level of play or higher. Overall, the average time to initiation of throwing was 4.4 months and average time to full competition was 11.6 months after reconstruction.

Camp et al. studied a mixed cohort of Major League and Minor League Baseball position players who underwent UCL reconstruction between the years 2005 and 2014. They determined that 75.5% of position players returned to play at any level at an average of 342 days from surgery. They also showed that of all position players, catchers returned to play at the lowest rate at just 58.6%, followed by infielders at 75.6%, and outfielders at 88.9%. On the whole, however, they compared return to play rates of these position players to an established cohort of pitchers and showed an inferior rate of return for position players (75.5% for position players vs. 83.7% for pitchers) [27].

A large study of UCL reconstruction outcomes in Minor League and Major League Baseball pitchers was performed by Griffith et al. between the years 2010 and 2014 [28]. This study showed no difference in rates of return to play or return to play at the same level or higher based on the type of graft or reconstruction technique. The return to play rate for the group of 566 pitchers was 79.9%, with 71.2% returning to the same level or higher. On average, it took 518.2 days for players to return to their prior level of competition or higher.

Marshall et al. reported the results of 54 UCL reconstructions at a single institution in Major League Baseball pitchers between the years 2002 and 2016 [29]. Their cohort of patients included 46 primary and eight revision reconstructions with an overall return to play rate at 94%, with 80% returning to pitch at the Major League Baseball level. The rates were even higher in primary reconstructions—96% return to play and 82% return to Major League Baseball. This group also showed improvements in earned run average (ERA), walks plus hits per inning pitched (WHIP), and fastball velocity at least by the second year after surgery.

A study by Jack II et al. identified return to play differences based on age in Major League Baseball position players [30]. They included 33 players between the years 1984 and 2015 and showed that overall 84.8% were able to return to play at their previous level at a mean 336.9 days postoperatively. However, they demonstrated that position players who were ≥30 years of age returned to play at a meager 53.3%, while those players <30 years of age returned at a rate of 89.4%. Finally, Jack II and colleagues revealed that the overall 1-year Major League Baseball career survival rate was only 73.5% in players who underwent UCL reconstruction compared to 91.2% in a control group.

As is evident from the above findings, outcomes for return of baseball players after UCL reconstruction has improved over the last 40-plus years. This trend is likely a result of improved clinical diagnosis, advancements in surgical techniques, and more structured rehabilitation throwing programs [6, 9, 12, 15, 21, 31]. Certainly, the overwhelming majority of athletes sustaining these injuries are baseball players as is evident by the high percentage of these athletes in the aforementioned studies.

Important to consider when reviewing the literature on sports specific outcomes after UCL reconstruction are the numerous variables with respect to each athlete's history and treatment method. Specific surgical techniques can potentially affect outcomes and current published data describes flexor pronator mass detachment, retraction, as well as muscle-splitting techniques [9]. However, a large study recently showed no significant difference in outcomes based on tunnel configuration, ulnar nerve transposing technique, or graft choice in professional baseball pitchers [28]. Also important is the presence of previous operations on the same elbow, as it has been shown that a history of prior procedures on the ipsilateral elbow yield poorer outcomes [13]. Another consideration is additional procedures performed at the time of reconstruction, which can also affect outcomes [9]. All of these factors must be taken into account when evaluating outcomes in baseball players or other athletes.

Baseball and specifically pitching represents a unique activity in sports that places a huge amount of force on the elbow in a repetitive manner placing the UCL at risk. It is for this reason that evaluating UCL reconstruction outcomes specifically for baseball players is important. The average starting major league pitcher throws over 3000 live game pitches per year, and as youth baseball becomes a year round sport, younger baseball players throw more and more. Studies have shown the valgus force reaches 290 N, resulting in angular velocity in excess of 2400–3000°/s [17, 32]. Taking these factors into consideration, it is not difficult to see why sport-specific outcomes, specifically with respect to pitching, are important to consider when looking at results of ulnar ligament reconstruction.

Author's preferred treatment: It is our experience that expectations for baseball players to return to the previous level are similar to the current literature, and thus we provide expectations that 85–90% of baseball players will return to their previous level of play after UCL reconstruction. Reconstruction involves a muscle-splitting technique utilizing a docking or figure-eight technique. Players may begin throwing at 4 months at which time a structured throwing program is implemented. Return to full competitive throwing takes place at approximately 1 year after UCL reconstruction. Similarly to the current literature, our indications for UCL repair with internal bracing include partial tears with at least one bony attachment (either proximal or distal) intact. Even with these indications, however, reconstruction using a docking technique is preferred, unless the patient has short term goals for return to play or less consideration for career longevity.

Additional Sports

Most of the attention regarding injuries to the UCL has been placed on baseball players, specifically pitchers. However, it has also been reported in other overhead athletes, including javelin throwers, quarterbacks, softball pitchers, and tennis players. Each sport requires different throwing mechanics, and with each change in motion, there are different stresses imparted to the elbow. The common denominator in these sporting activities is a repetitive valgus stress to the elbow. The role of surgical reconstruction of the UCL in the elbow is sport specific and must be individualized to the patient (Table 34.2).

Javelin Throwers

Although baseball pitchers garner most of the attention regarding UCL injuries, the first reported diagnosis of a UCL tear was made in 1946 in a javelin thrower [10]. Numerous studies have analyzed the biomechanics of the javelin throw [33–35]. The javelin event involves throwing a 2.6 m spear weighing at least 800 g. The generation of a large release of speed is the major contributing factor in a long distance throw, and throwers lengthen the path of acceleration of the javelin by maintaining an extended elbow for as long as possible until foot strike [36]. The throwing motion is broken down into four phases:

Table 34.2 Outcomes of non-baseball UCL injuries

Study	Sport	Number of patients	Treatment	Outcomes
Dines et al. [3]	Javelin	10 (2 partial, 8 complete)	Reconstruction	9 excellent, 1 fair
Conway et al. [13]	Javelin	3 (of 71)	Reconstruction	3 excellent
Kodde et al. [38]	Javelin	6 (of 20)	Reconstruction	6 return to play
Cain et al. [1]	Javelin	15 (of 1281)	Reconstruction	Overall 83% return to play
Dodson et al. [4]	Football	10 (4 grade I, 3 grade II, 3 grade III)	9 Non-OP, 1 repair	10 return to play
Kenter et al. [41]	Football	2 (both grade I)	2 Non-OP	2 return to play
Dodson et al. [14]	Football	2 (of 100)	Reconstruction	Overall 90% return to play
Argo et al. [44]	Softball	8 (of 19)	Repair	Overall 94% return to play

approach run, cross steps, delivery stride, and thrust phase. The time between final foot contact and release is called the thrust phase. During this thrust phase, the elbow flexes through a range of 40–60°, which is comparable to baseball pitchers [34]. As contrasted with baseball pitchers who undergo rapid *extension*, javelin throwers undergo rapid *flexion*. During this rapid flexion, the flexion angular velocity approaches 1900°/s (compared with 2400°/s in baseball pitchers), imparting a large valgus force on the medial side of the elbow [3, 36]. For these throwers, as much as 70% of the release speed of the javelin is developed in the last second [35].

There is no literature describing nonoperative outcomes of UCL injuries in javelin throwers. The sole article in the English language on nonoperative treatment of UCL injuries in throwing athletes does include two javelin throwers [37]. However, the results of these two javelin throwers were not separated from the 29 baseball players; overall 42% of athletes returned to previous level of competition at an average of 24.5 months after rest and rehabilitation exercises.

Besides several series of outcomes after UCL reconstruction that include a few javelin throwers, there is only one report that focuses specifically on reconstruction in this group of athletes [3]. Dines et al. evaluated ten javelin throwers who underwent UCL reconstruction after failing a course of nonoperative management that included rest, physical therapy, and a structured attempt to return to throwing [3]. All patients had positive physical examination findings and magnetic resonance imaging (MRI) showed partial tears in two and complete tears in eight. These patients all underwent UCL reconstruction with docking technique, and at the 2-year follow-up, nine had excellent outcomes, and one had a fair outcome. The average time to start throwing was 8 months, and the average time to return to the previous level of competition was 15 months. All ten patients were subjectively satisfied with their clinical outcome.

Other reports only include a few javelin throwers among their other reconstructions, which are mostly baseball players [1, 13, 38]. Conway et al. included three (of 71 patients) javelin throwers, and all three had excellent results; however, they do not describe changes to postoperative protocol nor specifically address these athletes' results [13]. Kodde et al. included six javelin throwers (of 20 patients) who underwent reconstruction; all six returned to play at their preinjury level of sports [38]. The largest series of UCL reconstruction included 15 javelin throwers (of 1281 patients), yet no sport-specific outcomes were included; 83% of all patients included in the study returned to previous level of competition [1].

No consensus postoperative protocol and throwing program exists for javelin throwers in the literature. Dines et al. modified their baseball interval throwing program to account for the specialized movements of the javelin throwing motion [3]. As the javelin is much heavier than a baseball (1.76 vs. 0.32 pounds), they waited 8 months from surgery (as compared to four in baseball players) to begin an interval throwing program. They also focused more on lower extremity and core strengthening to account for the increased weight of the javelin.

Author's preferred treatment: Javelin throwers, like other overhead athletes with UCL insufficiency, can expect to return to their previous level of play after surgical reconstruction or repair with internal bracing. They should be counseled that due to their unique throwing motion and increased weight of the javelin, their return to play will be longer than in baseball players. A postoperative protocol focusing on core and lower extremity strengthening then progressing to a throwing program at 8 months should allow them to return to play at around 15 months.

Football Quarterbacks

The motion of throwing a football is similar to throwing a baseball pitch; however, kinematic and biomechanic distinctions between the two result in a very different injury profile. The lower incidence of elbow injuries in football quarterbacks may be attributed to lower forces and torques throughout the throwing motion [36, 39, 40]. During arm acceleration, the elbow reaches a maximum elbow extension velocity of 1760°/s, as compared with 2400°/s in pitchers [17]. The increased weight of a football (0.9 pounds) as compared with a baseball (0.32 pounds) appears to affect shoulder position and stresses throughout the throwing motion. The follow-through phase used to decelerate the arm is abbreviated in football as the quarterback must be prepared for the impact from an opposing player, possibly lowering forces and torques produced during this phase. Quarterbacks are at risk of elbow injuries from both the chronic throwing motion and acute contact injury.

The largest series of UCL injuries in football players includes ten quarterbacks [4]. Dodson et al. reported on ten national football league (NFL) quarterbacks with UCL injuries; seven occurred as a result of contact injury. Four of the UCL injuries were grade I ligamentous injuries, three were graded as grade II, and three were graded as grade III. Nine of the ten quarterbacks were treated without surgery, while the other one quarterback underwent surgery (grade II injury with return to play in 17 days, implying simple ligamentous repair). Nonoperative treatment consisted of rest, anti-inflammatories, and other forms of local modalities. The average time after nonoperative treatment was 27.4 days (7.8 days for grade I, 7 days for grade II, and 67.3 days for grade III). These results suggest that even a complete tear of the UCL in a quarterback can be managed nonoperatively.

Another study of acute elbow injuries in all NFL players from 1991 to 1996 included 19 acute UCL injuries, including two quarterbacks [41]. Both injuries were acute, grade I injuries and both players were able to return to the same level of play without surgical repair or reconstruction of the UCL. There are also previous reports that included quarterbacks under a broader heading of overhead athletes. In 2006, Dodson et al. reported on the results of 100 overhead athletes undergoing ligament reconstruction, of which two were quarterbacks [14]. The specifics of these two patients are unavailable; however, 90% of these patients were able to compete at the same or higher level. Thompson et al. reported on reconstruction in 83 overhead athletes, including one quarterback, and all patients were able to return to their sport; no information regarding mechanism of injury or rehabilitation was described. Studies by Cain et al. and Dines et al. also reported on 1 and 13 football players, respectively, who underwent ligament reconstruction, but again, specifics are unavailable with overall outcomes of 83% and 86% return to play, respectively [1, 42, 43].

Author's preferred treatment: While successful outcomes have been reported after surgical reconstruction in quarterbacks, the available literature suggests that these players can be successfully treated nonoperatively and return to competitive play.

Softball Pitchers

Softball pitchers present as a unique subset of throwers as their primary motion is underhand. Also, as compared to the overhead throwers in baseball and football, softball pitchers are primarily female. As with overhead throwers, underhand throwers are subject to high forces and torques on the upper extremities, but this force is less than that of baseball pitchers [36, 43]. The maximum stress is imparted upon the elbow just before the ball release when an elbow extension velocity of 570°/s is produced, and at this moment elbow extension is terminated and elbow flexion is terminated. So, while the overhead thrower is extending at ball release, the underhand softball pitcher is flexing the elbow.

In 2006, Argo et al. reported the largest series of UCL insufficiency in female patients, including eight softball players (of 19 patients) [44]. Only one of these players was a pitcher. All patients underwent surgery, yet the majority (18 of 19) underwent repair instead of reconstruction. Of the 18 patients who participated in athletics, 17 (94%) were able to return to their sport at a mean of 2.5 months postoperatively. In terms of rehabilitation, patients were allowed to start throwing in a brace at 6 weeks postoperatively. They attribute this rapid return to activity to less invasive surgery combined with aggressive sport-specific rehabilitation in a brace and a lower functional demand population. Although reasons are unclear, the female athlete, especially the underhand softball pitcher, imparts less stress to the elbow, making injury more amenable to repair. Other reports have included softball players among their UCL reconstructions with favorable results, yet none of these studies include sport-specific outcomes [1]. A recent study highlighted the epidemiology of UCL injuries in the National Collegiate Athletic Association (NCAA) between 2009 and 2014 noting three softball injuries resulting from a throwing mechanism [45]. All three injuries were treated nonoperatively. Outcomes were not reported, but one of the three subjects was restricted from sport participation for less than 21 days, while the remaining two were held out for greater than 21 days [45].

Author's preferred treatment: The focus on the female thrower, with specific attention to softball players, lacks the data and support afforded to the elite, male, overhead thrower. While there is evidence to suggest positive outcomes in ligament reconstruction for these athletes, the only study with a specific focus on the female thrower has shown favorable results with ligament repair. Further research into female throwing injuries is necessary, but the current literature suggests that both operative and nonoperative treatments can be considered in this population.

Other Sports

UCL injuries have also been reported in tennis, gymnastics, and wrestling [1, 38]. Each of these sports places stresses across the medial elbow, but not to the degree of baseball pitcher, thus, the lower frequency of injury. During the tennis serve, the angular velocity of elbow extension was found to reach 982°/s, much less than the 2300°/s in baseball pitchers [46]. While several large series of UCL reconstructions include these athletes, there is no discrete data on treatment algorithms or rehabilitation protocols [1, 3, 44]. Further research is needed to investigate sport-specific protocols and treatment outcomes for athletes who play sports that place the UCL at risk.

Conclusion

Overhead throwing athletes place considerable stresses on the UCL. While our techniques have continued to evolve over time, we should not place our technical advances above the sport-specific needs and demands of our athletes. The role of ligamentous reconstruction in baseball players is well described and widely accepted; however, there is an emerging role for direct ligamentous repair with internal bracing in the appropriate patient. The treatment of throwers outside of baseball still lacks conclusive data and should be researched further. The specific demands, chronicity of injury, and integrity of the ligament should all be taken into consideration when treating javelin throwers, quarterbacks, softball players, and other overhead athletes.

References

1. Cain EL, Andrews JR, Dugas JR, Wilk KE, McMichael CS, Walter JC, Riley RS, Arthur ST. Outcome of ulnar collateral ligament reconstruction of the elbow in 1281 athletes. Am J Sports Med. 2010;38:2426–34.
2. Ciccotti MG, Siegler S, Kuri JAII, Thinnes JH, Murphy DJIV. Comparison of the biomechanical profile of the intact ulnar collateral ligament with the modified Jobe and the Docking reconstructed elbow. Am J Sports Med. 2009;37(5):974–81.
3. Dines JS, Jones KJ, Kahlenberg C, Rosenbaum A, Osbahr DC, Altchek DW. Elbow ulnar collateral ligament reconstruction in javelin throwers at a minimum 2-year follow-up. Am J Sports Med. 2012;40:148–51.
4. Dodson CC, Slenker NS, Cohen SB, Ciccotti MG, DeLuca P. Ulnar collateral ligament injuries of the elbow in professional football quarterbacks. J Shoulder Elbow Surg. 2010;19:1276–80.
5. Gibson BW, Webner D, Huffman GR, Sennett BJ. Ulnar collateral ligament reconstruction in major league baseball pitchers. Am J Sports Med. 2007;35:575–81.
6. Hechtman KS, Zvijac JE, Wells ME, Bemden AB. Long-term results of ulnar collateral ligament reconstruction in throwing athletes based on a hybrid technique. Am J Sports Med. 2011;39:342–7.
7. Jobe FW, Stark H, Lombardo SJ. Reconstruction of the ulnar collateral ligament in athletes. J Bone Joint Surg Am. 1986;68:1158–63.
8. Paletta GA Jr, Wright RW. The modified docking procedure for elbow ulnar collateral ligament reconstruction: 2-year follow-up in elite throwers. Am J Sports Med. 2006;34:1594–8.

9. Vitale MA, Ahmad CS. The outcome of elbow ulnar collateral ligament reconstruction in overhead athletes: a systematic review. Am J Sports Med. 2008;36:1193–205.
10. Waris W. Elbow injuries of javelin throwers. Acta Chir Scand. 1946;93(6):563–75.
11. Andrews JR, Timmerman LA. Outcome of elbow surgery in professional baseball players. Am J Sports Med. 2003;31:332–7.
12. Azar FM, Andrews JR, Wilk KE, Groh D. Operative treatment of ulnar collateral ligament injuries of the elbow in athletes. Am J Sports Med. 2000;28:16–23.
13. Conway JE, Jobe FW, Glousman RE, Pink M. Medial instability of the elbow in throwing athletes: treatment by repair or reconstruction of the ulnar collateral ligament. J Bone Joint Surg Am. 1992;74(1):67–83.
14. Dodson CC, Thomas A, Dines JS, Nho SJ, Williams RJIII, Altchek DW. Medial ulnar collateral ligament reconstruction of the elbow in throwing athletes. Am J Sports Med. 2006;34:1926–32.
15. Thompson WH, Jobe FW, Yocum LA, Pink MM. Ulnar collateral ligament reconstruction in athletes: muscle-splitting approach without transposition of the ulnar nerve. J Shoulder Elbow Surg. 2001;10:152–7.
16. Dillman C, Smutz P, Werner S, et al. Valgus extension overload in baseball pitching. Med Sci Sports Exerc. 1991;23:S135.
17. Fleisig GS, Barrentine SW, Escamilla RF, Andrews JR. Biomechanics of overhand throwing with implications for injuries. Sports Med. 1996;21:421–37.
18. Werner SL, Fleisig GS, Dillman CJ, Andrews JR. Biomechanics of the elbow during baseball pitching. J Orthop Sports Phys Ther. 1993;17:274–8.
19. Barnes DA, Tullos HS. An analysis of 100 symptomatic baseball players. Am J Sports Med. 1978;6:62–7.
20. Ford GM, Genuario J, Kinkartz J, Githens T, Noonan T. Return-to-play outcomes in professional baseball players after medial ulnar collateral ligament injuries. Am J Sports Med. 2016;44(3):723–8.
21. Rohrbough JT, Altchek DW, Hyman J, Williams RJ, Botts JD. Medial collateral ligament reconstruction of the elbow using the docking techniques. Am J Sports Med. 2002;30:541–8.
22. Dugas JR, Looze CA, Capogna B, Walters BL, Jones CM, Rothermich MA, Fleisig GS, Aune KT, Drogosz M, Wilk KE, Emblom BA, Cain EL Jr. Ulnar collateral ligament repair with collagen-dipped FiberTape augmentation in overhead-throwing athletes. Am J Sports Med. 2019;47(5):1096–102.
23. Bodendorfer BM, Looney AM, Lipkin SL, Nolton EC, Li J, Najarian RG, Chang ES. Biomechanical comparison of ulnar collateral ligament reconstruction with the docking technique versus repair with internal bracing. Am J Sports Med. 2018;46(14):3495–501.
24. Moore AR, Fleisig GS, Dugas JR. Ulnar collateral ligament repair. Orthop Clin N Am. 2019;50:383–9.
25. Dugas JR, Walters BL, Beason DP, Fleisig GS, Chronister JE. Biomechanical comparison of ulnar collateral ligament repair with internal bracing versus modified Jobe reconstruction. Am J Sports Med. 2015;44(3):735–41.
26. Petty DH, Andrews JR, Fleisig GS, Cain EL. Ulnar collateral ligament reconstruction in high school baseball players: clinical results and injury risk factors. Am J Sports Med. 2004;32:1158–64.
27. Camp CL, Conte S, D'Angelo J, Fealy SA. Following ulnar collateral ligament reconstruction, professional baseball position players return to play faster than pitchers, but catchers return less frequently. J Shoulder Elbow Surg. 2018;27:1078–85.
28. Griffith TB, Ahmad CS, Gorroochurn P, D'Angelo J, Ciccotti MG, Dines JS, Altchek DW, Camp CL. Comparison of outcomes based on graft type and tunnel configuration for primary ulnar collateral ligament reconstruction in professional baseball pitchers. Am J Sports Med. 2019;47(5):1103–10.
29. Marshall NE, Keller RA, Limpisvasti O, ElAttrache NS. Pitching Performance after ulnar collateral ligament reconstruction at a single institution in Major League Baseball pitchers. Am J Sports Med. 2018;46(3):3245–53.
30. Jack RA, Burn MB, Sochacki KR, McCulloch PC, Lintner DM, Harris JD. Performance and return to sport after Tommy John surgery among Major League Baseball position players. Am J Sports Med. 2018;46(7):1720–6.
31. Leland DP, Conte S, Flynn N, Conte N, Crenshaw K, Wilk KE, Camp CL. Prevalence of medical ulnar collateral ligament surgery in 6135 current professional baseball players. Orthop J Sports Med. 2019;7(9):1–7.
32. Feltner ME. Three-dimensional interactions in a two-segment kinetic chain, part II: application to the throwing arm in baseball pitching. Int J Sport Biomech. 1998;5:420–50.
33. Bartlett RM, Rent RJ. The biomechanics of javelin throwing. J Sports Sci. 1988;6:1–38.
34. Mero A, Komi PV, Korjus T, Navarro E, Gregor R. Body segment contributions to javelin throwing during final thrust phases. J Appl Biomech. 1994;10:166–77.
35. Morris C, Bartlett RM. Biomechanical factors critical for performance in the men's javelin throw. Sports Med. 1996;21:438–46.
36. Loftice J, Fleisig GS, Zheng N, Andrew JR. Biomechanics of the elbow in sports. Clin Sports Med. 2004;23:519–30.
37. Rettig AC, Sherrill C, Snead DS, Mendler JC, Mieling P. Nonoperative treatment of ulnar collateral ligament injuries in throwing athletes. Am J Sports Med. 2001;29:15–7.
38. Kodde IF, Rahusen FT, Eygendaal D. Long-term results after ulnar collateral ligament reconstruction of the elbow in European athletes with interference screw technique and triceps fascia autograft. J Shoulder Elbow Surg. 2012;21:1656–63.
39. Kelly BT, Bachus SI, Williams RJ. Elextromyographic analysis and phase definition of the overhead football throw. Am J Sports Med. 2002;30:837–44.

40. Wick H, Dillman CJ, Werner S. A kinematic comparison between baseball pitching and football passing. Sports Med Update. 1991;6:13–6.
41. Kenter K, Behr CT, Warren RF, O'Brien SJ, Barnes R. Acute elbow injuries in the National Football League. J Shoulder Elbow Surg. 2000;9:1–5.
42. Dines JS, ElAttrache NS, Conway JE, Smith W, Ahmad CS. Clinical outcomes of the DANE TJ technique to treat ulnar collateral ligament insufficiency of the elbow. Am J Sports Med. 2007;35:2039–44.
43. Barrentine SW, Fleisig GS, Whiteside JA, Escamilla RF, Andrews JR. Biomechanics of windmill softball pitching with implications about injury mechanisms. J Orthop Sports Phys Ther. 1998;28:405–15.
44. Argo D, Trenhaile SW, Savoie FHIII, Field LD. Operative treatment of ulnar collateral ligament insufficiency of the elbow in female athletes. Am J Sports Med. 2006;34:431–7.
45. Li NY, Goodman AD, Lemme NJ, Owens BD. Epidemiology of elbow ulnar collateral ligament injuries in throwing versus contact athletes of the National Collegiate Athletic Association. Orthop J Sports Med. 2019;7(4):1–6.
46. Kibler WB. Clinical biomechanics of the elbow in tennis: implications for evaluation and diagnosis. Med Sci Sports Exerc. 1994;26:1203–6.

Rehabilitation of the Overhead Athlete's Elbow

35

Kevin E. Wilk, Todd S. Ellenbecker, and Leonard C. Macrina

Introduction

As has been discussed at length previously, the repetitive overhead-throwing motion of baseball players is responsible for unique and sport-specific patterns of injuries to the elbow. Other athletes can also sustain an elbow injury due to repetitive elbow stresses during javelin throwing, tennis, football throwing, or volleyball. Collision athletes can sustain a traumatic elbow injury too.

The purpose of this chapter is to provide an overview of general rehabilitation principles for the overhead athlete's elbow. Furthermore, specific nonoperative and postoperative treatment guidelines for the thrower's elbow is also discussed.

General Rehabilitation Guidelines

Rehabilitation following elbow injury or elbow surgery follows a sequential and progressive multiphased approach. The ultimate goal of elbow rehabilitation is to return the athlete to their previous functional level as quickly and safely as possible. The following section provides an overview of the rehabilitation process following elbow injury (Table 35.1) and surgery (Table 35.2); rehabilitation protocols for specific pathologies follows.

Phase I: Immediate Motion Phase

The first phase of elbow rehabilitation is the immediate motion phase. The goals of this phase are to minimize the effects of immobilization, reestablish nonpainful range of motion, decrease pain and inflammation, and retard muscular atrophy.

Early range of motion (ROM) activities are performed to nourish the articular cartilage and assist in the synthesis, alignment, and organization of collagen tissue [1–7]. ROM activities are performed for all planes of elbow and wrist motions to prevent the formation of scar tissue and adhesions. Active-assisted and passive ranges of motion exercises are performed at the humero-ulnar joint to restore flexion/extension as well at both the humero-radial and radial-ulnar joints for supination/pronation. Reestablishing full elbow extension, typically defined as preinjury motion, is the primary goal of early ROM activities to minimize the occurrence of elbow flexion contractures [8–10]. The preoperative elbow motion

K. E. Wilk
Physiotherapy Associates, Birmingham, AL, USA

T. S. Ellenbecker (✉)
Medical Services ATP Tour, Rehab Plus Sports Therapy Scottsdale, Scottsdale, AZ, USA
e-mail: todd.ellenbecker@atptour.com

L. C. Macrina
Champion Physical Therapy, Waltham, MA, USA

J. S. Dines et al. (eds.), *Elbow Ulnar Collateral Ligament Injury*,
https://doi.org/10.1007/978-3-030-69567-5_35

Table 35.1 Nonoperative rehabilitation program for elbow injuries

I. Acute phase (week 1)
Goals: improve motion
Diminish pain and inflammation
Retard muscle atrophy
Exercises
1. Stretching for wrist and elbow joint, stretches for shoulder joint
2. Strengthening exercises isometrics for wrist elbow, and shoulder musculature
3. Pain and inflammation control cryotherapy, High voltage stimulation (HVS), ultrasound, and whirlpool

II. Subacute phase (weeks 2–4)
Goals: normalize motion
Improve muscular strength, power, and endurance
Week 2
1. Initiate isotonic strengthening for wrist and elbow muscles
2. Initiate exercise tubing exercises for shoulder
3. Continue use of cryotherapy, etc.

Week 3
1. Initiate rhythmic stabilization drills for elbow and shoulder joint
2. Progress isotonic strengthening for entire upper extremity
3. Initiate isokinetic strengthening exercises for elbow flexion/extension

Week 4
1. Initiate Throwers' Ten Program
2. Emphasize eccentric biceps work, concentric triceps, and wrist flexor work
3. Program endurance training
4. Initiate light plyometric drills
5. Initiate swinging drills

III. Advanced phase (week 1)
Goals: preparation of athlete for return to functional activities
Criteria to progress to advanced phase
1. Full nonpainful ROM
2. No pain or tenderness
3. Satisfactory isokinetic test
4. Satisfactory clinical exam

Weeks 4–5
1. Continue strengthening exercises, endurance drills, and flexibility exercises daily
2. Thrower's Ten Program
3. Progress plyometric drills
4. Emphasize maintenance program based on pathology
5. Progress swinging drills (i.e., hitting)

Weeks 6–8
1. Initiate interval sport program once determined by the physician

Phase I program

Table 35.1 (continued)

IV. Return to activity phase (weeks 6–9)
Weeks 6–9: when you return to play depending on your condition and progress, your physician will determine when it is safe.
1. Continue strengthening Thrower's Ten Program
2. Continue flexibility program
3. Progress functional drills to unrestricted play

Table 35.2 Postoperative rehabilitative protocol for elbow arthroscopy

I. Initial phase (week 1)
Goal: full wrist and elbow ROM, decrease swelling, decrease pain, retardation, or muscle atrophy
A. Day of surgery
Begin gently moving elbow in bulky dressing
B. Post-op day 1 and 2
1. Remove bulky dressing and replace with elastic bandages
2. Immediate post-op hand, wrist, and elbow exercises
   (a) Putty/grip strengthening
   (b) Wrist flexor stretching
   (c) Wrist extensor stretching
   (d) Wrist curls
   (e) Reverse wrist curls
   (f) Neutral wrist curls

C. Post-op day 3–7
1. PROM elbow ext./flexion (motion to tolerance)
2. Begin Progressive Resistive Exercises (PRE) with 1 lb weight
   (a) Wrist curls
   (b) Reverse wrist curls
   (c) Neutral wrist curls
   (d) Pronation/supination
   (e) Broomstick roll-up

II. Intermediate phase (weeks 2–4)
Goal: improve muscular strength and endurance; normalize joint arthrokinematics
A. Week 2 ROM exercises (overpressure into extension)
1. Addition of active range of motion (AROM) elbow flexion and light triceps extension
2. Continue to progress PRE weight and repetitions as tolerable

B. Week 3
1. Initiate biceps and biceps eccentric exercise program
2. Initiate rotator-cuff exercises program
   (a) External rotators
   (b) Internal rotators
   (c) Deltoid
   (d) Supraspinatus
   (e) Scapulothoracic strengthening

Table 35.2 (continued)

III. Advanced phase (weeks 4–8)
Goals: preparation of athlete for return to functional activities
Criteria to progress to advanced phase
1. Full nonpainful ROM
2. No pain or tenderness
3. Isokinetic test that fulfills criteria to throw
4. Satisfactory clinical exam
A. Weeks 4–6
1. Continue maintenance program, emphasizing muscular strength, endurance, and flexibility
2. Initiate interval throwing program phase

must be carefully assessed and recorded. Postoperatively, if the patient was not seen prior to injury or surgery, the athlete should be asked how much elbow extension had been present in the past 2–3 years. Attempting to compare elbow ROM to the contralateral side may not be adequate when restoring back to baseline. The elbow is predisposed to flexion contractures due to the intimate congruency of the joint articulations, the tightness of the joint capsule, and the tendency of the anterior capsule to develop adhesions following injury [7]. The brachialis muscle also attaches to the capsule and crosses the elbow joint before becoming a tendinous structure. Injury to the elbow may cause excessive scar tissue formation of the brachialis muscle, as well as functional splinting of the elbow [7]. Wright et al. [11] reported on 33 professional baseball players prior to the competitive season. The average loss of elbow extension was 7°, and the average loss of flexion was 5.5° compared to the opposite elbow joint. It is critical that postoperative ROM match preoperative motion, especially in the case of ulnar collateral ligament (UCL) reconstruction. This loss of extension ROM can be a deleterious side effect for the overhead athlete.

Another goal of this phase is to decrease the patient's pain and inflammation. Cryotherapy and high-voltage stimulation may be performed as needed to further assist in reducing pain and inflammation. The authors of this chapter have utilized laser therapy extensively in the first phase of the rehabilitation phase with significant benefits. Once the acute inflammatory response has subsided, moist heat, warm whirlpool, and ultrasound may be used at the onset of treatment to prepare the tissue for stretching and improve the extensibility of the capsule and musculotendinous structures. Grade I and II mobilization techniques may also be utilized in the early phases to neuromodulate pain by stimulating type I and type II articular receptors [12, 13].

In addition to the ROM exercises, joint mobilizations may be performed as tolerated to minimize the occurrence of joint contractures. Grade I and II mobilizations are initially used to help decrease pain and inflammation, and later progressed to more aggressive grade III and IV mobilization techniques at end ROM with the intended goal of improving ROM during later stages of rehabilitation when symptoms have subsided. Joint mobilization must include the radio-capitellar and radioulnar joints as well to maintain supination and pronation ROM. Posterior glides of the humero-ulnar joint with oscillations are performed at end ROM to assist in regaining full elbow extension.

If the patient continues to have difficulty achieving full extension using ROM and mobilization techniques, a low-load, long-duration (LLLD) stretch may be performed to produce a deformation (creep) of the collagen tissue, resulting in tissue elongation [14–17]. Anecdotally, this technique seems to be extremely beneficial for regaining full elbow extension. The patient lies supine with a towel roll or a foam pad placed under the distal brachium to act as a cushion and fulcrum. Light resistance exercise tubing is applied to the wrist of the patient and secured to the table or a dumbbell on the ground (Fig. 35.1). The patient is instructed to relax as much as possible for 15 min per treatment. The amount of resistance applied should be of enough magnitude to enable the patient to perform the stretch for the entire duration without pain or muscle spasm. This technique is intended to impart a low load but a long-duration stretch. Patients are instructed to perform LLLD stretches several times per day, totaling at least 60 min of total end-range time (TERT). We typically recommend a 15 min stretch, four times per day. This type of program has been referred to as the TERT program [18] and has been extremely beneficial for patients with a stiff elbow. However, in some patients that are not responding well to the above-mentioned treatment, it may be more beneficial to utilize splinting and bracing to create this LLLD stretch. This would require the patient to wear a splint or brace during the day and at night for several hours while sleeping to improve elbow extension (Fig. 35.2).

The aggressiveness of stretching and mobilization techniques is dictated based on healing constraints of involved tissues, as well as specific pathology/surgery and the amount of motion and end feel. For example, if the patient presents with a decrease in motion and hard end feel without pain, more aggressive stretching and mobilization techniques may be used. Conversely, a patient exhibiting pain before resistance or an empty end feel will be progressed slowly with gentle stretching. In addition, it is beneficial to incorporate interventions to maintain proper glenohumeral (GH) joint ROM as indicated with each individual patient, including stretching and GH joint mobilizations.

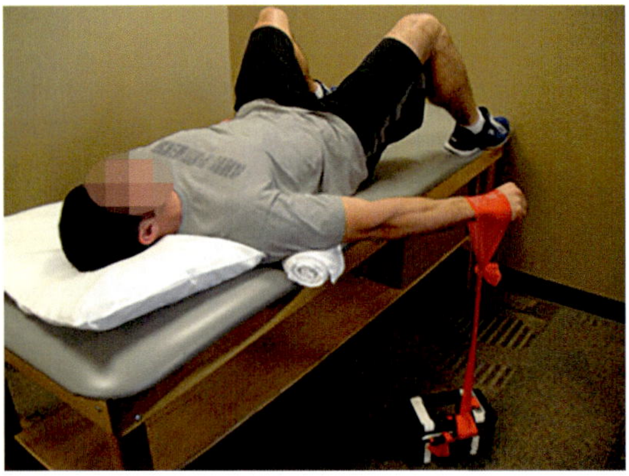

Fig. 35.1 A low-load, long duration stretch into elbow extension is performed using light resistance. The shoulder is internally rotated while the forearm is pronated to best isolate and maximize the stretch on the elbow joint

The early phases of rehabilitation also focus on voluntary activation of muscle and retarding muscular atrophy. Subpainful and submaximal isometrics are performed initially for the elbow flexor and extensor, as well as the wrist flexor, extensor, pronator, and supinator muscle groups. Shoulder isometrics may also be performed during this phase with caution against internal and external rotation exercises if painful as the elbow joint becomes a fulcrum for shoulder isometrics. Alternating rhythmic stabilization drills for shoulder flexion/extension/horizontal abduction/adduction, shoulder internal/external rotation, and elbow flexion/extension/supination/pronation are performed to begin reestablishing pro-

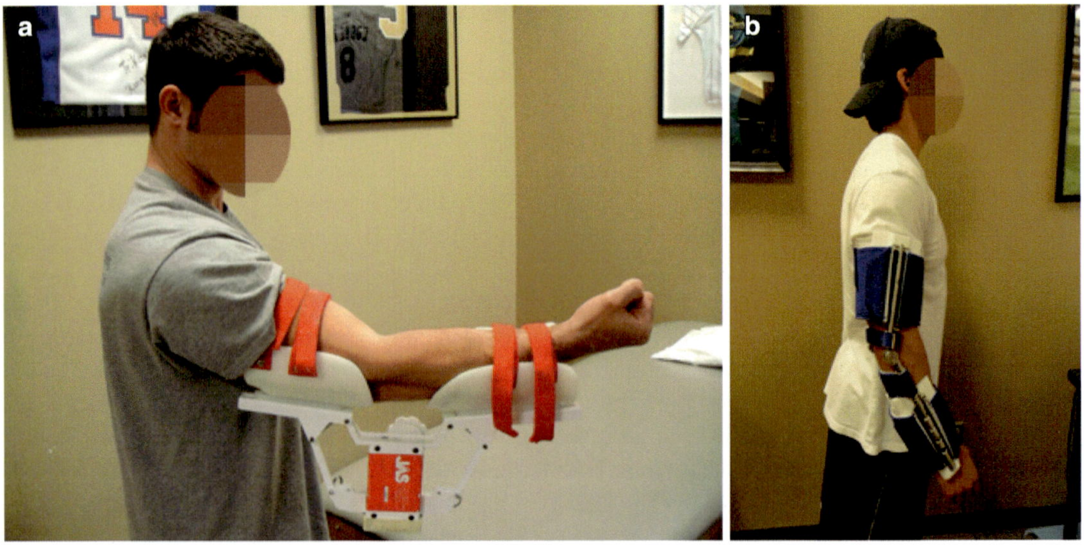

Fig. 35.2 Joint Active System (JAS, Effingham, IL) (**a**), and Dynasplint (Severna Park, MD) (**b**) are two commercial devices commonly used by patients at home to work on elbow extension ROM

prioception and neuromuscular control of the upper extremity. Scapular strengthening and activation exercises are also initiated immediately following surgery.

Phase II: Intermediate Phase

Phase II, the intermediate phase, is initiated when the patient exhibits full throwing ROM as it was prior to the injury, minimal pain, and tenderness, and a good (≥4/5) manual muscle test of the elbow flexor and extensor musculature. The emphasis of this phase includes maintaining and enhancing elbow and upper extremity mobility, improving muscular strength and endurance, and reestablishing neuromuscular control of the elbow complex.

Stretching exercises are continued to maintain full elbow and wrist range of motion. Mobilization techniques may be progressed to more aggressive grade III and IV techniques as needed to apply a stretch to the capsular tissue at end range. Flexibility is progressed during this phase to focus on wrist flexion, extension, pronation, and supination. Elbow extension and forearm pronation flexibility are of particular emphasis in throwing athletes in order to perform efficiently. Shoulder flexibility is also maintained in athletes with emphasis on external and internal rotation at 90° of abduction, flexion, and horizontal adduction (or cross-body stretch). In particular, shoulder external rotation at 90° abduction is emphasized; loss of external rotation may result in increased strain on the medial elbow structures during the overhead-throwing motion [19]. Additionally, internal rotation motion is also diligently performed as internal rotation (IR) ROM of the shoulder may create a protective varus force at the elbow. The rehabilitation program for shoulder joint ROM should consider the total ROM (TROM) and appropriate treatments should be employed to restore equal motion bilaterally [20].

Strengthening exercises are progressed during this phase to include isotonic contractions, beginning with concentric and progressing to include eccentric contractions. Emphasis is placed on elbow flexion and extension, wrist flexion and extension, and forearm pronation and supination. The glenohumeral and scapulothoracic muscles are also placed on a progressive resistance program as long as there is no elbow pain. Emphasis is placed on strengthening the shoulder external rotators and periscapular muscles. A complete upper extremity strengthening program, such as the Thrower's Ten Program [21] may be performed (Appendix A). This program has been designed based on electromyographic studies to illicit activity of the muscles most needed to provide dynamic stability [22, 23]. Strengthening exercises are advanced to include external and internal rotation with exercise tubing at 0° of abduction and active ROM exercises against gravity. These exercises initially include standing scaption in external rotation (full can) [22–24], standing abduction, side-lying external rotation, and prone rowing. As strength returns, the program may be advanced to a program that includes full upper-extremity strengthening with emphasis on posterior rotator-cuff muscles and scapular strengthening.

Neuromuscular control exercises are initiated in this phase to enhance the muscles' ability to control the elbow joint during athletic activities. A decrease in neuromuscular control has also been associated with muscular fatigue. Carpenter et al. [25] observed the ability to detect passive motion of shoulders positioned in 90° of abduction and 90° of external rotation. Results indicate a decrease in the detection of both internal and external rotation movement following an isokinetic fatigue protocol. Voight et al. [26] examined joint angle replication following an isokinetic fatigue protocol. A significant decrease in accuracy was reported following muscle fatigue when comparing both active and passive joint reproduction. Also, Myers et al. [27, 28] studied the effects of fatigue on active angle reproduction at both mid- and end range of internal and external rotation. The authors report that fatigue of the shoulder rotators resulted in decreased accuracy at mid- and end range of motion. These exercises include proprioceptive neuromuscular facilitation exercises with rhythmic stabilizations and manual resistance elbow/wrist flexion drills (Fig. 35.3).

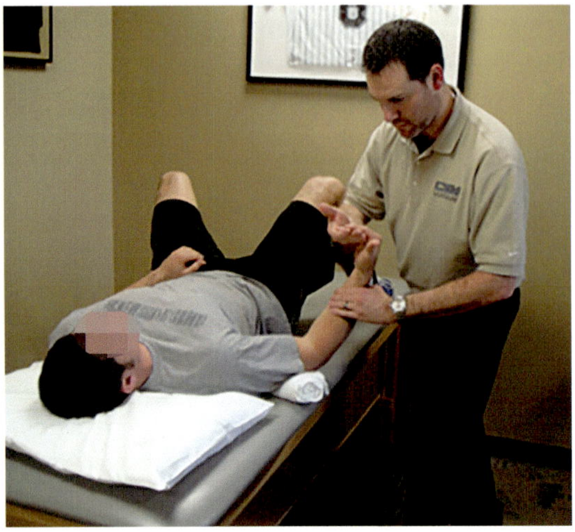

Fig. 35.3 Manual concentric and eccentric resistance exercises for the elbow flexors and wrist flexor pronators

Phase III: Advanced Strengthening Phase

The third phase involves a progression of activities to prepare the athlete for sport participation. The goals of this phase are to gradually increase strength, power, endurance, and neuromuscular control to prepare for a gradual return to sport. Specific criteria that must be met before entering this phase include full nonpainful external rotation (ER) and IR TROM, no pain or tenderness, and strength that is 70% of the contralateral extremity.

Advanced strengthening activities during this phase include a gradual progression to more aggressive strengthening exercises emphasizing higher resistance, functional movements, eccentric contraction, and plyometric activities. Elbow flexion exercises are progressed to emphasize eccentric control. The biceps muscle is an important stabilizer during the follow through phase of overhead throwing to eccentrically control the deceleration of the elbow, preventing pathological abutting of the olecranon within the fossa [29, 30]. Elbow flexion can be performed with elastic tubing to emphasize slow and fast concentric and eccentric contractions. Furthermore, manual resistance may be applied for concentric and eccentric contractions of the elbow flexors. Aggressive strengthening exercises with weight machines are also incorporated during this phase when the athlete demonstrates the ability to safely use these machines with an appropriate amount of weight. These most commonly begin with bench press, seated rowing, and front latissimus dorsi pulldowns. The triceps are primarily exercised with a concentric contraction due to the muscle-shortening activity during the acceleration phase of throwing. During this phase, the overhead athlete may be placed on the advanced Thrower's Ten Program ([31]; Appendix B). This program incorporates exercises and movement patterns specific to the throwing motion, performed in a discrete series, utilizing principles of coactivation, high-level neuromuscular control, dynamic stabilization, muscular facilitation, endurance, and coordination, which serve to restore muscle balance and symmetry in the throwing athlete [31]. Examples include the full can raise with sustained holds while seated on a stability ball (Fig. 35.4) or prone horizontal abduction on a stability ball while performing sustained holds (Fig. 35.5).

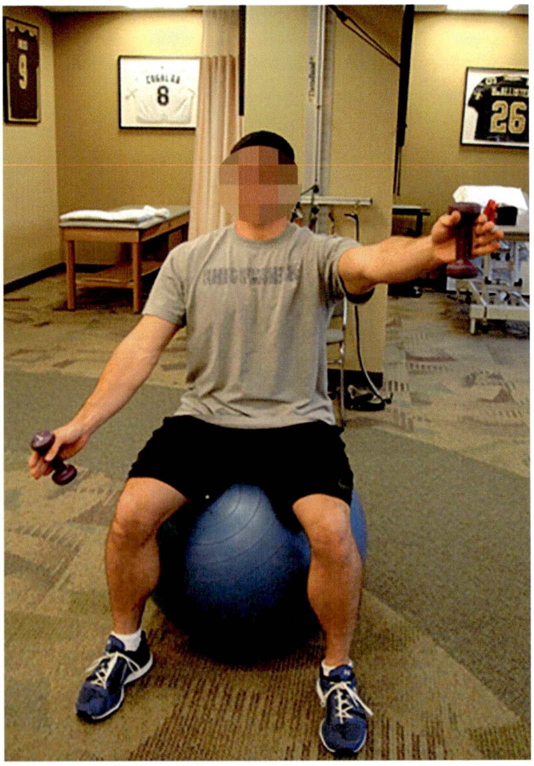

Fig. 35.4 Advanced Thrower's Ten: full can raises with sustained holds while seated on a stability ball

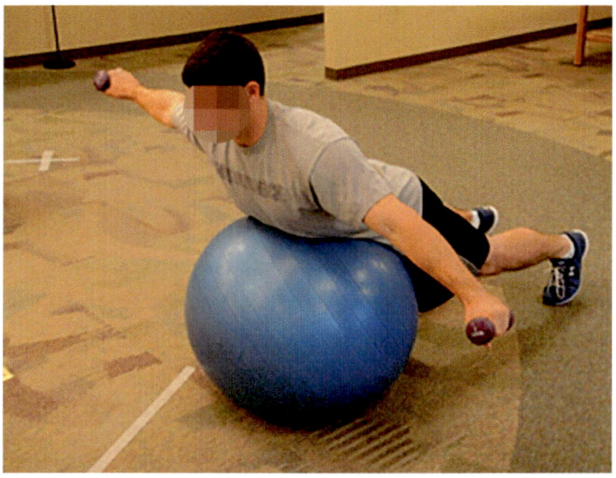

Fig. 35.5 Advanced Thrower's Ten: prone horizontal abduction on a stability ball while performing sustained holds

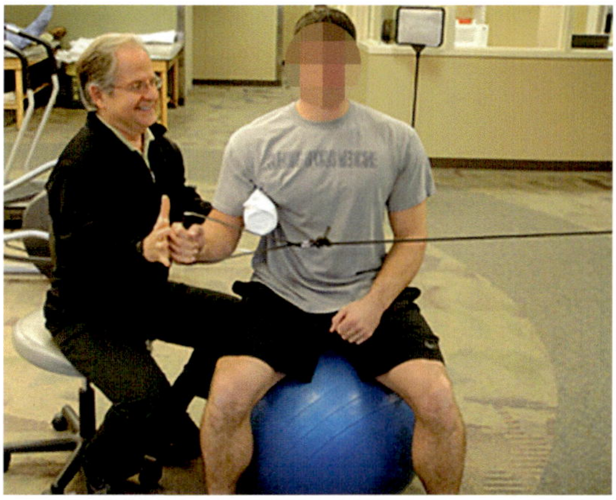

Fig. 35.6 External rotation at 0° abduction with exercise tubing, manual resistance, and rhythmic stabilizations, while the athlete is seated on a stability ball

Neuromuscular control exercises are progressed to include side-lying external rotation with manual resistance. Concentric and eccentric external rotation is performed against the clinician's resistance with the addition of rhythmic stabilizations at end range. This manual resistance exercise may be progressed to standing external rotation with exercise tubing at 0° (Fig. 35.6) and finally at 90°.

Plyometric drills can be an extremely beneficial form of functional exercise for training the elbow in overhead athletes [32, 33]. Plyometric exercises are performed using a weighted medicine ball during the later stages of this phase to train the shoulder and elbow to develop and withstand high levels of stress. Plyometric exercises are initially performed with two hands performing a chest pass, side-to-side throw, and overhead soccer throw. These may be progressed to include one-handed activities such as 90/90 throws with rhythmic stabilization at end range (Fig. 35.7), external and internal rotation throws at 0° of abduction into a trampoline and wall dribbles to improve shoulder musculature endurance. Specific plyometric drills for the forearm musculature include wrist flexion flips (Fig. 35.8) and extension grips. The latter two plyometric drills are an important component to an elbow rehabilitation program, emphasizing the forearm and hand musculature.

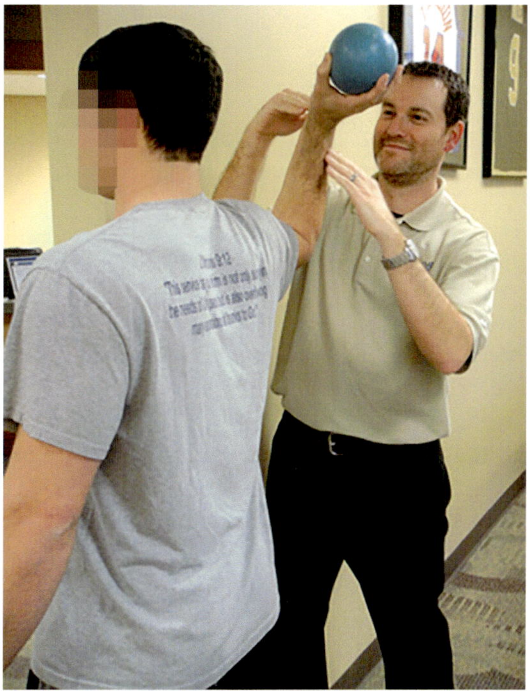

Fig. 35.7 Plyometric wall throws with a 2-pound ball while the rehabilitation specialist performs a rhythmic stabilization at end range

Phase IV: Return to Activity Phase

The final phase of elbow rehabilitation, the return to activity phase, allows the athlete to progressively return to full competition using an

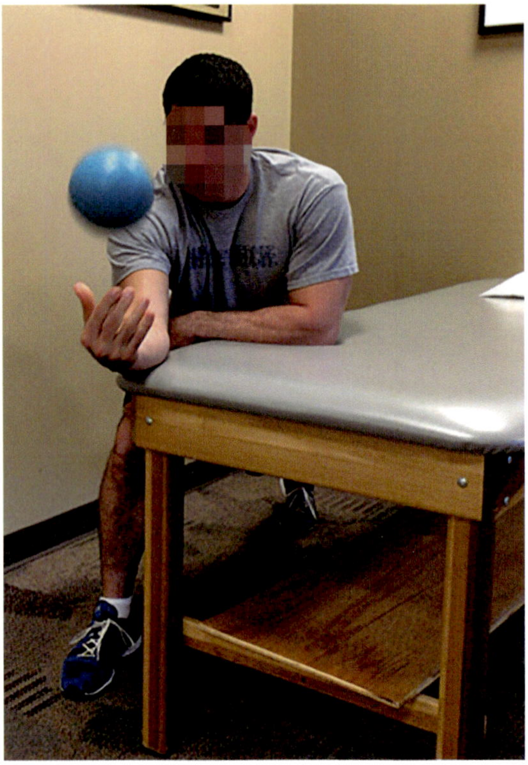

Fig. 35.8 Plyometric wrist flips using a 2-pound medicine ball to strengthen the wrist flexors

interval return to throwing program. Other interval programs are used for the tennis player or golfer [34].

Before an athlete is allowed to begin the return to activity phase of rehabilitation, the athlete must exhibit full pain-free throwing ROM, no pain or tenderness, a satisfactory isokinetic test, and medical clearance through medical doctor (MD) clinical examination. Isokinetic testing is commonly utilized to determine the readiness of the athlete to begin an interval sport program [34]. Athletes are routinely tested at 180 and 300°/s. Our data indicate the bilateral comparison at 180°/s for the throwing arm's elbow flexion to be 10–20% stronger and the dominant extensors are typically 5–15% stronger than the nonthrowing arm [35–37]. Furthermore, we prefer the patient to complete a thorough two and one hand plyometric program prior to the initiation of the interval throwing program.

Upon achieving the previous criteria, we begin a formal interval sport program as described by Reinold et al. [34]. For patients returning to sports that involve the upper extremity such as golf, tennis, baseball, and softball, these patients are placed on an interval sport program. For the overhead thrower, we initiate a long-toss interval throwing program beginning at 45 ft. and gradually progressing to 120 or 180 ft. (player and position dependent, Tables 35.3 and 35.4). Throwing should be performed without pain or significant increase in symptoms. During the long-toss program, as intensity and distance increase, the stresses increase on the patient's medial elbow and anterior shoulder joint. Fleisig et al. [38] reported that the longer throwing distances significantly increased these forces. This is an important component to consider; if a patient with a UCL reconstruction is having pain while long tossing, an appropriate treatment would be to reduce the distance and intensity of the throws before stopping the interval throwing program (ITP). We believe it is important for the overhead athlete to perform dynamic stretching and an abbreviated strengthening program prior to and after performing the interval sport program. Typically, our overhead throwers warm up, stretch, and perform one set of their exercise program before throwing, followed by two additional sets of exercises proceeding throwing. This provides an adequate warm-up but also ensures maintenance of necessary ROM and flexibility of the shoulder joint. The following day, the thrower will exercise their scapular muscles, external rotators, and perform a core stabilization program [34].

Following the completion of a long-toss program, the pitchers will progress to phase II of the throwing program, throwing off a mound (Table 35.5; [34]). In phase II, the number of throws, intensity, and type of pitch are progressed to gradually increase stress on the elbow and shoulder joints. Generally, the pitcher begins at 50% intensity and gradually progressed to 75, 90, and 100% over a 4- to 6-week period of time. Breaking balls are initiated once the pitcher can throw 40–50 pitches at a minimum of 80% intensity, without symptoms.

Table 35.3 Interval throwing program for baseball positional players

45′ phase	60′ phase	90′ phase	120′ phase	150′ phase	180′ phase		
Step 1: A) Warm-up throwing	Step 3: A) Warm-up throwing	Step 5: A) Warm-up throwing	Step 7: A) Warm-up throwing	Step 9: A) Warm-up Throwing	Step 11: A) Warm-up throwing	Step 13: A) Warm-up throwing	*All throws should be on an arc with a crow-hop*
B) 45′ (25 throws)	B) 60′(25 throws)	B) 90′ (25 throws)	B) 120′ (25 throws)	B) 150′ (25 throws)	B) 180′ (25 throws)	B) 180′ (25 throws)	*Warm-up throws consist of 10–20 throws at approximately 30 ft.*
C) Rest 5–10 min	C) Rest 5–10 min	C) Rest 5–10 min	C) Rest 5–10 min	C) Rest 3–5 min	C) Rest 3–5 min	C) Rest 3–5 min	*Throwing program should be performed every other day, three times per week unless otherwise specified by your physician or rehabilitation specialist*
D) Warm-up throwing	D) Warm-up throwing	D) Warm-up throwing	D) Warm-up throwing	D) Warm-up throwing	D) Warm-up throwing	D) Warm-up throwing	*Perform each step _____ times before progressing to next step*
E) 45′ (25 throws)	E) 60′ (25 throws)	E) 90′ (25 throws)	E) 120′ (25 throws)	E) 150′ (25 throws)	E) 180′ (25 throws)	E) 180′ (25 throws)	
Step 2: A) Warm-up throwing	Step 4: A) Warm-up throwing	Step 6: A) Warm-up throwing	Step 8: A) Warm-up throwing	Step 10:A) Warm-up throwing	Step 12: A) Warm-up throwing	F) Rest 3–5 min	
B) 45′ (25 throws)	B) 60′ (25 throws)	B) 90′ (25 throws)	B) 120′ (25 throws)	B) 150′ (25 throws)	B) 180′ (25 throws)	G) Warm-up throwing	
C) Rest 5–10 min	C) Rest 5–10 min	C) Rest 5–10 min	C) Rest 5–10 min	C) Rest 3–5 min	C) Rest 3–5 min	H) 180′ (20 throws)	
D) Warm-up throwing	D) Warm-up throwing	D) Warm-up throwing	D) Warm-up throwing	D) Warm-up Throwing	D) Warm-up Throwing	I) Rest 3–5 min	
E) 45′ (25 throws)	E) 60′ (25 throws)	E) 90′ (25 throws)	E) 120′ (25 throws)	E) 150′ (25 Throws)	E) 180′ (25 Throws)	J) Warm-up Throwing	
F) Rest 5–10 min G) Warm-up throwing	F) Rest 5–10 min G) Warm-up throwing	F) Rest 5–10 min G) Warm-up throwing	F) Rest 5–10 min G) Warm-up throwing	F) Rest 3–5 min. G) Warm-up Throwing	F) Rest 3–5 min G) Warm-up Throwing progressing from	K) 15 throws	
H) 45′ (25 throws)	H) 60′ (25 throws)	H) 90′ (25 throws)	H) 120′ (25 throws)	H) 150′ (25 Throws)	H) 180′ (25 Throws)		
					120 → 90′ Step 14: Return to respective position or progress to step 14 below.		

45 ft. = 13.7 m
60 ft. = 18.3 m
90 ft. = 27.4 m
120 ft. = 36.6 m
150 ft. = 45.7 m
180 ft. = 54.8 m

Table 35.4 Interval throwing program for Baseball pitchers: phase I

45′ Phase	60′ Phase	90′ Phase	120′ Phase
Step 1: A) Warm-up throwing	Step 3: A) Warm-up throwing	Step 5: A) 60′ (10 throws)	Step 7: A) 60′ (5–7 throws)
B) 45′ (25 throws)	B) 60′ (25 throws)	B) 90′ (20 throws)	B) 90′ (5–7 throws)
C) Rest 3–5 min.	C) Rest 3–5 min.	C) Rest 3–5 min.	C) 120′ (15 throws)
D) Warm-up throwing	D) Warm-up throwing	D) 60′ (10 throws)	D) Rest 3–5 min
E) 45′ (25 throws)	E) 60′ (25 throws)	E) 90′ (20 throws)	E) 60′ (5–7 throws)
			F) 90′ (5–7 throws)
			G) 120′ (15 throws)
Step 2: A) Warm-up throwing	Step 4: A) Warm-up throwing	Step 6: A) 60′ (7 throws)	Step 8: A) 60′ (5 throws)
B) 45′ (25 throws)	B) 60′ (25 throws)	B) 90′ (18 throws)	B) 90′ (10 throws)
C) Rest 3–5 min	C) Rest 3–5 min	C) Rest 3–5 min	C) 120′ (15 throws)
D) Warm-up Throwing	D) Warm-up Throwing	D) 60′ (7 throws)	D) Rest 3–5 min
E) 45′ (25 Throws)	E) 60′ (25 Throws)	E) 90′ (18 Throws)	E) 60′ (5 throws)
F) Rest 3–5 min	F) Rest 3–5 min	F) Rest 3–5 min	F) 90′ (10 throws)
G) Warm-up throwing	G) Warm-up throwing	G) 60′ (7 throws)	G) 120′ (15 throws)
H) 45′ (25 throws)	H) 60′ (25 throws)	H) 90′ (18 throws)	H) Rest 3–5 min
			I) 60′ (5 throws)
			J) 90′ (10 throws)
			K) 120′ (15 throws)
Step 9: *Flat throwing*		Step 10:	
A) Throw 60 ft. (10–15 throws)		A) Throw 60 ft. (10–15 throws)	
B) Throw 90 ft. (10 throws)		B) Throw 90 ft. (10 throws)	
C) Throw 120 ft. (10 throws)		C) Throw 120 ft. (10 throws)	
D) Throw 60 ft. (flat ground) using pitching mechanics (20–30 throws)		D) Throw 60 ft. (flat ground) using pitching mechanics (20–30 throws)	
		E) Rest 3–5 min	
		F) Throw 60–90 ft. (10–15 throws)	
		G) Throw 60 ft. (flat ground) using pitching mechanics (20 throws)	

Throwing program should be performed every other day, with one day of rest between steps, unless otherwise specified by your physician

Perform each step 2 times before progressing to the next step

Table 35.5 Interval throwing program: phase II—throwing off the mound

STAGE ONE: FASTBALLS ONLY		ALL THROWING OFF THE MOUND SHOULD BE DONE IN THE PRESENCE OF YOUR PITCHING COACH OR SPORT BIOMECHANIST TO STRESS PROPER THROWING MECHANICS
Step 1:	Interval Throwing	
	15 Throws off mound 50%[a]	
Step 2:	Interval throwing	(Use radar gun to aid in effort control)
	30 Throws off mound 50%	
Step 3:	Interval throwing	
	45 Throws off mound 50%	*Use interval throwing 120 ft (36.6 m) phase as warm-up*
Step 4:	Interval throwing	
	60 Throws off mound 50%	
Step 5:	Interval throwing	
	70 Throws off mound 50%	
Step 6:	45 Throws off mound 50%	
	30 Throws off mound 75%	
Step 7:	30 Throws off mound 50%	
	45 Throws off mound 75%	
Step 8:	10 Throws off mound 50%	
	65 Throws off mound 75%	
STAGE TWO: FASTBALLS ONLY		
Step 9:	60 Throws off mound 75%	
	15 Throws in batting practice	
Step 10:	50–60 Throws off mound 75%	
	30 Throws in batting practice	
Step 11:	45–50 Throws off mound 75%	
	45 Throws in batting practice	
STAGE THREE		
Step 12:	30 Throws off mound 75% warm-up	
	15 Throws off mound 50% BEGIN BREAKING BALLS	
	45–60 Throws in batting practice (fastball only)	
Step 13:	30 Throws off mound 75%	
	30 Breaking balls 75%	
	30 Throws in batting practice	
Step 14:	30 Throws off mound 75%	
	60–90 Throws in batting practice (gradually increase breaking balls)	
Step 15:	SIMULATED GAME: PROGRESSING BY 15 THROWS PER WORKOUT (Pitch Count)	

[a]Percentage effort

Specific Nonoperative Rehabilitation Guidelines

Ulnar Collateral Ligament Injury

Injuries to the UCL are becoming increasingly more common in overhead-throwing athletes, although the higher incidence of injury may be due to our increased ability to diagnose these injuries. The elbow experiences a tremendous amount of valgus stress during overhead throwing [39, 40]. The repetitive nature of overhead-throwing activities such as baseball pitching, javelin throwing, and football passing further increases the susceptibility of UCL injury by exposing the ligament to repetitive microtraumatic forces.

Conservative treatment is attempted with partial tears and sprains of the UCL, although surgical reconstruction may be warranted for complete tears or if nonoperative treatment is unsuccessful. Our nonoperative rehabilitation program is outlined in Table 35.6. ROM is initially permitted in a nonpainful arc of motion, usually from 10 to 100°, to allow for a decrease in inflammation and the proper alignment of collagen tissue. A brace may be used to restrict motion, as well as prevent valgus loading. Furthermore, it may be beneficial to rest the UCL immediately following the initial painful episode of throwing to prevent additionally deleterious stresses on the ligament. Isometric exercises are performed for the shoulder, elbow, and wrist to prevent muscular atrophy. Ice and anti-inflammatory medications are prescribed to control pain and inflammation.

ROM of both flexion and extension is gradually increased by 5–10° per week during the second phase of treatment or as tolerated. Full pain-free ROM should be achieved by at least 3–4 weeks. Elbow flexion/extension motion is encouraged to promote collagen formation and alignment. We attempt to control valgus loading onto the elbow joint to minimize stress on the UCL. Rhythmic stabilization exercises are initiated to develop dynamic stabilization and neuromuscular control of the upper extremity. As dynamic stability is advanced, isotonic exercises are incorporated for the entire upper extremity.

The advanced strengthening phase is usually initiated at 6–7 weeks postinjury. During this phase, the athlete is progressed to the Thrower's Ten (Appendix A) isotonic strengthening program and plyometric exercises are slowly initiated. An interval return to throwing program is initiated once the athlete regains full motion, adequate shoulder and elbow strength (5/5 manual muscle test (MMT)), and dynamic stability of the elbow. The athlete is allowed to return to competition following the asymptomatic completion of the interval sport program. If symptoms reoccur during the interval throwing program, it is usually at longer distances, greater intensities, or with off-the-mound throwing. If symptoms persist, the athlete is reassessed and possible surgical intervention is considered.

Table 35.6 Conservative treatment following ulnar collateral sprains of the Elbow

2. *I. Immediate motion phase (weeks 0 through 2)*
Goals: increase range of motion
Promote healing of ulnar collateral ligament
Retard muscular atrophy
Decrease pain and inflammation
1. ROM:
Brace (optional) nonpainful ROM (20–90°)
AAROM, PROM elbow and wrist (nonpainful range)
2. Exercises:
Isometrics—wrist and elbow musculature
Shoulder strengthening (no ext rotation strengthening)
3. Ice and compression
II. Intermediate phase (*weeks 3 through 6*)
Goals: increase range of motion
Improve strength/endurance
Decrease pain and inflammation
Promote stability
1. ROM:
Gradually increase motion 00–135" (increase 10° per week)
2. Exercises:
Initiate isotonic exercises wrist curls wrist extensions pronation/supination biceps/triceps dumbbells: external rotation, deltoid, supraspinatus, rhomboids, internal rotation
3. Ice and compression
III. Advanced phase (*weeks 6 and 7 through 12 and 14*)
Criteria to progress
1. Full range of motion
2. No pain or tenderness
3. No increase in laxity
4. Strength 4/5 of elbow flexor/extensor
Goals: Increase strength, power and endurance
Improve neuromuscular control
Initiate high speed exercise drills
1. Exercises:
Initiate exercise tubing, shoulder program: Throwers ten program Biceps/triceps program Supination/ pronation Wrist extension/flexion Plyometrics throwing drills
IV. Return to activity phase (*week 12 through 14*)
Criteria to progress to return to throwing:
1. Full nonpainful ROM
2. No increase in laxity
3. Isokinetic test fulfills criteria
4. Satisfactory clinical exam
1. Exercises:
Initiate interval throwing
Continue throwers ten program
Continue plyometrics

Medial Epicondylitis and Flexor-Pronator Tendinitis

Medial epicondylitis occurs due to changes within the flexor-pronator musculotendinous unit. Associated ulnar neuropathy has been reported in 25–60% of patients with medial epicondylitis [41–43]. The underlying pathology is a microscopic or macroscopic tear within the flexor carpi radialis or pronator teres near the origin on the medial epicondyle. Overhead throwers who exhibit flexor-pronator tendinitis may have an associated UCL injury. The tendinitis may develop as a secondary pathology due to the underlying increased laxity. Thus, before initiating a rehabilitation program, it is important for the clinician to accurately examine the UCL for any lesion or pathology. Furthermore, it may be beneficial to determine the number of episodes and chronicity of medial epicondylar complaints. Patients with long histories of medial epicondylitis may exhibit a chronic degeneration known as tendinosis or tendinopathy, not true tendonitis. Conversely, patients with first-time episodes probably exhibit paratendonitis, or tendinitis. The treatment is significantly different for both. Nirschl et al. [44] reported four stages of epicondylitis, beginning with an early inflammatory reaction followed by angiofibroblastic degeneration, leading to structural failure and ultimately fibrosis or calcification. It is critical to identify the condition of the tendon as the stage of the injury will dictate the treatment.

The treatment of tendinopathy is based on a careful examination to determine the exact pathology present. Often patients are diagnosed with "tendonitis" only later to discover that the tendon had undergone a degenerative process referred to tendonosis [42, 45, 46]. The differential diagnosis of tendonosis may be made through magnetic resonance imaging (MRI), ultrasound examination, or tissue biopsy.

The treatment for tendonitis is typically targeted at reducing inflammation and pain. This is accomplished through reducing activities, steroid injections, anti-inflammatory medications, cryotherapy, iontophoresis, light exercise, and stretching.

Conversely, the treatment for tendonosis focuses on increasing circulation to promote collagen synthesis and collagen organization. The treatment would include heat, stretching, slow resistance eccentrics, laser therapy, transverse massage, and soft tissue mobilization. All of this is performed to increase circulation and promote tissue healing. Some authors have advocated dry needling for the pathology or other techniques to promote tendon healing [47, 48].

Several different strategies may be utilized in an attempt to improve collagen regeneration and alignment. Modalities to promote a heating affect and improve the blood flow such as laser, hot packs, and transverse friction massage are often employed. Tendon loading by eccentric exercise and strength training has been shown to improve results in this patient population by increasing collagen synthesis [49] and realigning fiber orientation [50–52]. Other modalities such as laser therapy [53–56] and extracorporeal shockwave therapy [57–59] have shown promising results as well.

Other emerging treatments have shown some promise in treating chronic tendinopathy. The goal of these treatments is to stimulate a regenerative response that has otherwise been difficult thus far. Platelet-rich plasma (PRP) is a promising intervention, in which a small sample of the patient's own blood is separated out, and the platelet-rich layer is injected into the sight of injury. The proposed mechanism delivers humoral mediators and growth factors locally to induce a healing response. Other advantages of PRP are (1) minimally invasive, (2) local response only, and (3) avoids an inflammatory response. Some disadvantages may include the cost of treatment, lack of supporting evidence, and staffing time required to withdraw the blood, spin it down and reinject it into the site of pathology.

Early research on the clinical application of PRP to promote healing and adaptive responses is promising [44, 60–68]. Mishra et al. [66] showed significant benefits to PRP in patients with chronic lateral epicondylitis. Thanasas et al. [69] showed improved visual analog scale visual analog scale (VAS) scores in ultrasound-guided PRP injections versus a single injection of autologous blood in patients with chronic lateral epicondylitis. In a randomized controlled, double-blinded study, Gosens et al. [70] showed improved VAS scores and disabilities of the arm, shoulder and hand (DASH) scores in the PRP group compared to a corticosteroid group even at a 2-year follow-up in patients with chronic lateral epicondylitis. Basic science and controlled studies have yet to truly surmise the efficacy of such a treatment.

The use of pain stimulation or noxious stimulation is gaining popularity as a treatment prior to strength training for the degenerative tissue. The primary goal of this modality is to produce pain at the site of the degenerative tissue. By producing pain, the body will respond by releasing endorphins, which will block any pain response felt by the involved tissue. Once the pain has been reduced, the patient will perform specific exercises designed to progressively load the tendon through eccentric loading to produce collagen synthesis and collagen alignment. The authors of this chapter have found the pain stimulation to be extremely successful in the treatment of patellar and Achilles tendinopathies. However, use of this treatment may be limited for the elbow because of the surrounding contractile tissues of the flexors and extensors that would become activated when the electrical stimulation intensity is increased.

The nonoperative approach for treatment of epicondylitis (i.e., tendinitis and/or paratendonitis) (Table 35.7) focuses on diminishing the pain and inflammation associated with tendinitis and then gradually improving muscular strength. The primary goals of rehabilitation are to control the applied loads and create an environment for healing. The initial treatment consists of iontophoresis, stretching exercises, and light strengthening exercises to stimulate a repair response. Rehabilitation specialists often utilize therapeutic modalities to decrease inflammation and promote tissue healing. There is very limited evidence to support the use of

Table 35.7 Epicondylitis rehabilitation protocol

Phase I acute phase
Goals: decrease inflammation
Promote tissue healing
Retard muscular atrophy
Cryotherapy
Whirlpool
Stretching to increase flexibility wrist extension/flexion elbow extension/flexion forearm supination/pronation
Isometrics wrist extension/flexion elbow extension/flexion forearm supination/pronation
HVGS
Phonophoresis
Friction massage
Lontophoresis (with anti-inflammatory, i.e., dexamethasone)
Avoid painful movements (i.e., gripping, etc.)
Phase II subacute phase
Goals: Improve flexibility
Increase muscular strength/endurance
Increase functional activities/return to function
Exercises:
Emphasize concentric/eccentric strengthening
Concentration on involved muscle group
Wrist extension/flexion
Forearm pronation/supination
Elbow flexion/extension
Initiate shoulder strengthening (if deficiencies are noted)
Continue flexibility exercises
May use counterforce brace
Continue use of cryotherapy after exercise/function
Gradual return to stressful activities
Gradually re-initiate once pain-free movements
Phase III chronic phase
Goals: Improve muscular strength and endurance
Maintain/enhance flexibility
Gradual return to sport/high level activities
Exercises:
Continue strengthening exercises (emphasize eccentric/concentric)
Continue to emphasize deficiencies in shoulder and elbow strength
Continue flexibility exercises
Gradually decrease use of counterforce Brace
Use of cryotherapy as needed
Gradual return to sport activity
Equipment Modification (grip size, string tension, playing surface)
Emphasize maintenance program

these modalities in isolation. Common modalities may include massage, cold laser therapy, iontophoresis, ultrasound, nitric oxide, and extra corporeal shockwave therapy. However, when these modalities are used in combination with exercise or with other modalities, studies have shown improved tissue quality and outcomes [53–59, 71, 72, 73–81].

Recently, the authors have utilized the disposable iontophoresis patch (Hybresis DJO Globa, Vista, CA) for tendinitis. The patch is worn for 2 h with dexamethasone applied. We have observed excellent results clinically. Glass et al. [82] reported the depth of penetration of dexamethasone with iontophoresis to be 13–18 mm in the hip region. Gangarosa et al. [83] reported a 1–3 cm depth of penetration of lidocaine. A recent study performed by Anderson et al. [84] showed the depth of penetration of dexamethasone using iontophoresis is 12 mm following administration of a standard dosage. A high-voltage stimulation and cryotherapy are used following treatment to decrease pain and postexercise inflammation. The athlete should be cautioned against excessive gripping activities. Conversely, patients with tendinosis are treated with transverse friction massage, forceful stretching, and a focus on eccentric strengthening with gradually progressing loads, and warm modalities to promote tendon regeneration.

Once the patient's symptoms have subsided, an aggressive stretching and (high load low repetitions) strengthening program with emphasis on eccentric contractions are initiated. Wrist flexion and extension activities should be performed initially with the elbow flexed 30–45° to decrease stress on the medial elbow structures. A gradual progression through plyometric and throwing activities precedes the initiation of the interval throwing program. Because poor mechanics are often a cause of this condition, an analysis of sport mechanics and proper supervision through the interval throwing program are critical. If nonoperative treatment fails, then the physician may perform a surgical debridement of the necrotic tissue.

Ulnar Neuropathy

There are numerous theories regarding the cause of ulnar neuropathy in throwing athletes. Ulnar nerve changes can result from tensile forces, compressive forces, or nerve instability. Any one or combination of these mechanisms may be responsible for ulnar nerve symptoms. Unless there is gross instability of the ulnar nerve requiring a transposition, a conservative treatment is employed to improve medial elbow dynamic stability during a period of active rest for the athlete.

A leading mechanism for tensile force on the ulnar nerve is valgus stress. This may be coupled with an external rotation-supination stress overload mechanism. The traction forces are further magnified when underlying valgus instability from UCL injuries is present. Ulnar neuropathy is often a secondary pathology of UCL insufficiency.

Compression of the ulnar nerve is often due to hypertrophy of the surrounding soft tissues or the presence of scar tissue. The nerve may also be trapped between the two heads of the flexor carpi ulnaris. Repetitive flexion and extension of the elbow with an unstable nerve can irritate or inflame the nerve. The nerve may sublux or rest on the medial epicondyle, rendering it vulnerable to direct trauma.

There are three stages of ulnar neuropathy [85]. The first stage includes an acute onset of radicular symptoms that are transient in nature. The second stage is manifested by a recurrence of symptoms as the athlete attempts to return to competition. The third stage is associated with persistent motor weakness and sensory changes. Once the athlete presents in the third stage of injury, conservative management may not be effective.

The nonoperative treatment of ulnar neuropathy focuses on diminishing ulnar nerve irritation, enhancing dynamic medial joint stability, and gradually returning the athlete to competition. Often nonsteroidal anti-inflammatory drugs (NSAIDs) are prescribed and rehabilitation includes iontophoresis disposable patch and cryotherapy. Following the diagnosis of ulnar neuropathy, throwing athletes are instructed to discontinue throwing activities for at least 4 weeks, depending on the severity and chronicity of symptoms. The use of a night splint with the elbow flexed to 45° may be beneficial to rest and calm the nerve down. The athlete progresses through the immediate motion and intermediate phases over the course of 4–6 weeks with emphasis placed on eccentric and dynamic stabilization drills while carefully monitoring for onset of ulnar nerve symptoms. Plyometric exercises are utilized to facilitate further dynamic stabilization of the medial elbow. The athlete is allowed to begin an interval throwing program when full pain-free ROM and muscle performance is exhibited without neurological symptoms. The athlete may gradually return to play if progression through the interval throwing program [34] does not reveal neurological symptoms.

Valgus Extension Overload

Valgus extension overload occurs in sporting activities requiring repetitive, forceful extension, such as during the acceleration or deceleration phases of throwing as the olecranon wedges up against the medial olecranon fossa during elbow extension [86]. This mechanism may result in osteophyte formation and potentially loose bodies. Repetitive extension stress from the triceps may further contribute to this injury. There is often a certain degree of underlying valgus laxity of the elbow in these athletes, further facilitating osteophyte formation through compression of the radio-capitellar joint and the posteromedial elbow [87, 88]. Overhead athletes typically present with pain at the posteromedial aspect of the elbow that is exacerbated with forced extension and valgus stress.

A conservative treatment approach is often attempted before considering surgical intervention. Initial treatment involves relieving the posterior elbow of pain and inflammation. The authors recommend the use of ice, laser, and iontophoresis to control inflammation. As symptoms subside and ROM normalizes, dynamic stabilization and strengthening exercises are initiated. Emphasis is placed on improving eccentric strength of the elbow flexors in an attempt to control the rapid extension that occurs at the elbow during athletics. Manual resistance exercises of concentric and eccentric elbow flexion are performed, as well as elbow flexion with exercise tubing. The athlete's throwing mechanics should be carefully assessed to determine if mechanical faults are causing the valgus extension overload (VEO) symptoms or if a UCL injury is present.

Osteochondritis Dissecans

Osteochondritis dissecans of the elbow may develop due to the valgus strain on the elbow joint, which produces not only medial tension but also a lateral compressive force [89]. This is observed as the capitellum of the humerus compresses with the radial head. Patients often complain of lateral elbow pain upon palpation and valgus stress. Morrey [90] described a three-stage classification of pathological progression. Stage one describes patients without evidence of subchondral displacement or fracture, whereas stage two referred to lesions showing evidence of subchondral detachment or articular cartilage fracture. Stage three lesions involve detached osteochondral fragments, resulting in intra-articular loose bodies. Nonsurgical treatment is attempted for stage one patients only and consists of relative rest and immobilization until elbow symptoms have resolved.

Nonoperative treatment includes 3–6 weeks of immobilization at 90° of elbow flexion. However, ROM activities for the shoulder, elbow, and wrist are performed 3–4 times a day. As symptoms resolve, a strengthening program is initiated with isometric exercises. Isotonic exercises are included after approximately 1 week of isometric exercise. Aggressive high-speed, eccentric, and plyometric exercises are progressively included to prepare the athlete for the start of an interval throwing program.

If nonoperative treatment fails or evidence of loose bodies exists, surgical intervention including arthroscopic abrading and drilling of the lesion with fixation or removal of the loose body, is indicated [91–93]. Long-term follow-up studies regarding the outcome of patients undergoing surgery to drill or reattach the lesions have not produced favorable results, suggesting that prevention and early detection of symptoms may be the best form of treatment [91].

Little League Elbow

Little league elbow is a spectrum of medial epicondylar apophyseal injury that ranges from microtrauma to the physis to fracture and displacement of the medial epicondyle through the apophysis. Pain of the medial elbow is common in adolescent throwers. The medial epicondyle physis is subject to repetitive tensile and valgus forces during the arm-cocking and acceleration phases of throwing. These forces may result in microtraumatic injury to the physis with potential fragmentation, hypertrophy, separation of the epiphysis, or avulsion of the medial epicondyle. Treatment varies based on the extent of injury.

In the absence of an avulsion, a rehabilitation program similar to that of the nonoperative UCL program is initiated. Emphasis is placed initially on the reduction of pain and inflammation, and the restoration of motion and strength. Strengthening exercises are performed in a gradual fashion. First isometrics are performed prior to initiating light isotonic strengthening exercises. In young throwing athletes, we emphasize core, legs, and shoulder strengthening. Often these individuals exhibit poor core and scapula control along with weakness of the shoulder musculature. In addition, stretching exercises are performed to normalize shoulder ROM, especially into IR and horizontal adduction. No heavy lifting is permitted for 12–14 weeks. An interval throwing program is initiated as tolerated when symptoms subside, typically after an 8–12-week rest period.

In the presence of a nondisplaced or minimally displaced avulsion, a brief period of immobilization for approximately 7 days is encouraged, followed by a gradual progression of range of motion, flexibility, and strength. An interval throwing program is usually allowed at weeks 6–8. If the avulsion is displaced, an open reduction, internal fixation procedure may be required.

Prevention of Elbow Injuries in Youth Baseball Players

Fleisig et al. [94] have reported approximately 5% of all youth baseball pitchers will suffer a serious elbow or shoulder injury requiring surgery or retirement from pitching within 10 years. The risk factors with the strongest correlation to injury is the amount of pitching, specifically increased pitches per game, innings pitched per season, and months pitched per year. Pitching while fatigued and pitching for concurrent teams and in multiple leagues are also associated with increased risk. Pitchers who also play catcher have increased risk factor. Another risk factor is poor biomechanics. Improper biomechanics increases the torque and force produced about the elbow and shoulder joint during each pitch. Hurd et al. [95] reported pitch velocity in high school pitchers may be a predictor of increased medial elbow distraction forces; thus, the higher the velocity the more the force.

Lastly, recent research from Japan by Kurakowa et al. [96] studied 256 young throwing athletes with a mean age of 11 years regarding medial elbow pain and medial epicondyle abnormality. Medial epiconylar abnormality was observed with ultrasound in 51% of the young throwers. Abnormality of the medical epicondyle was related to pitch velocity and the number of practice days in a week. Based on the findings of this study, an increase in pitch velocity of 10 km/h increased the risk of medial epicondyle abnormality and medial elbow pain by 3 times. These studies show the important role of overuse, overload, and use of proper biomechanics to decrease the risk of medial elbow pain in young throwers.

Specific Postoperative Rehabilitation Guidelines

Ulnar Collateral Ligament Reconstruction

Surgical reconstruction of the UCL attempts to restore the stabilizing functions of the anterior bundle of the UCL [97]. Several surgical procedures exist including the Jobe procedure [98], the docking procedure [99–101], and the DANE procedure [88, 102, 103]. At our center, the procedure that has been used is the modified Jobe procedure in which the palmaris longus or gracilus graft source is taken and passed in a figure-8 pattern through drill holes in the sublime tubercle of the ulna and the medial epicondyle [82]. A subcutaneous ulnar nerve transposition is performed at the time of reconstruction.

A more recent procedure applied particularly for the management of incomplete UCL tears in the overhead athlete is the UCL repair with internal brace technique. This newly developed surgical technique allows for faster postoperative rehabilitation and a quicker return to sports and other functional activities. The faster postoperative rehabilitation is allowed because the collagen-treated internal brace is implanted inside the partially torn UCL ligament to augment the ligament while its healing takes place. There are no bone tunnels, grafts to heal and mature, and no need to prolong recovery time [104].

UCL repair with internal brace technique is reserved for specific types of UCL injury [105]. These include partial or complete tears at the origin or insertion of the UCL with good ligament tissue and low-grade mid-substance partial UCL tears. Within these parameters, surgical repair of the UCL with internal brace can be performed in the presence of open physes. In patients with chronic, attritional damage to the UCL and associated loss of elbow joint stability, reconstruction remains the most appropriate surgical intervention [88, 106]. Therefore, injured athletes with good joint stability and high-quality native ligament tissue are the ideal candidates for UCL repair with internal brace.

The rehabilitation program following the surgical management of UCL injury is based on the specific surgical procedure utilized by the surgeon. We will describe both UCL reconstruction protocols and the protocol for UCL repair with internal brace for the purposes of this chapter.

The rehabilitation program we currently use following UCL reconstruction is outlined in Tables 35.8 and 35.9, and is based on the Fig. 35.8 surgical procedure. One protocol is utilized for accelerated ROM progression (Table 35.8) and the protocol (Table 35.9) is a slightly slower ROM progression. The surgeon determines which protocol is being utilized at the time of the surgery. The athlete is placed in a posterior splint with the elbow immobilized at 90° of flexion for the first 7 days postoperatively. This allows early healing of the UCL graft and fascial slings involved in the nerve transposition. The patient is allowed to perform wrist ROM and gripping and submaximal isometrics for the wrist and elbow. The patient is progressed from the posterior splint to a hinged elbow ROM brace (Fig. 35.9) to protect the healing tissues from valgus stresses that may be detrimental. The brace is discontinued at the beginning of week 5.

Passive ROM activities are initiated immediately to decrease pain and slowly stress the healing tissues. Initially, the focus of the rehabilitation is obtaining full elbow extension while gradually progressing the flexion. Elbow extension is encouraged early on to at least 15°, but if the patient can comfortably obtain full extension, then it is allowed as long as there is no discomfort. A recent study by Bernas et al. [107] produced 3% or less strain in both bands of the reconstructed ligament and approximately 1% strain for the anterior band of the UCL during passive range of motion (PROM) of the elbow joint. The authors determined that in the immediate postoperative period, full elbow extension is safe and does not place excessive stress on the healing graft. Conversely, an elbow flexion to 100° is allowed and should be brought along at about 10° per week until full ROM is achieved by 4–6 weeks postoperatively.

Isometric exercises are progressed to include light resistance isotonic exercises at weeks 3–4,

Table 35.8 Postoperative rehabilitation protocol following ulnar collateral ligament reconstruction using autogenous palmaris longus graft (accelerated ROM)

I. Immediate postoperative phase (0–3 weeks)
Goals: protect healing tissue
Decrease pain/inflammation
Retard muscular atrophy
Protect graft site—allow healing
A. Postoperative week 1
Brace: posterior splint at 90° elbow flexion
Range of motion: wrist AROM ext/flexion immediately postoperative
Elbow postoperative compression dressing (5–7 days)
Wrist (graft site) compression dressing 7–10 days as needed
Exercises: gripping exercises
Wrist ROM
Shoulder isometrics (no shoulder ER)
Biceps isometrics
Cryotherapy: to elbow joint and to graft site at wrist
B. Postoperative week 2
Brace: elbow ROM 15–105° or tolerance
Motion to tolerance
Exercises: continue all exercises listed above
Elbow ROM in brace (30–105°)
Initiate elbow extension isometrics
Continue wrist ROM exercises
Initiate light scar mobilization over distal incision (graft)
Cryotherapy: continue ice to elbow and graft site
C. Postoperative week 3
Brace: Elbow ROM 5/10°–115/120°
Motion to tolerance
Exercises: continue all exercises listed above
Elbow ROM in brace
Initiate active ROM wrist and elbow (no resistance)
Initiate light wrist flexion stretching
Initiate active ROM shoulder
Full can
Lateral raises
ER/IR tubing
Elbow flex/extension
Initiate light scapular strengthening exercises
May incorporate bicycle for lower extremity strength and endurance
II. Intermediate phase (weeks 4–7)
Goals: gradual increase to full ROM
Promote healing of repaired tissue
Regain and improve muscular strength
Restore full function of graft site
A. Week 4
Brace: elbow ROM 0–135°
Motion to tolerance
Exercises: begin light resistance exercises for arm (1 lb)
Wrist curls, extensions, pronation, supination
Elbow extension/flexion
Progress shoulder program emphasize rotator cuff and scapular strengthening
Initiate shoulder strengthening with light dumbbells
B. Week 5
ROM: elbow ROM 0–135°
Discontinue brace
Maintain full ROM
Continue all exercises: progress all shoulder and upper extremity (UE) exercises (progress weight 1 lb.)
Week 6
AROM: 0–145° without brace or full ROM
Exercises: Initiate Thrower's Ten Program
Progress elbow strengthening exercises
Initiate shoulder external rotation strengthening without limits
Progress shoulder program
Week 7
Progress Thrower's Ten Program (progress weights)
Initiate proprioceptive neuromuscular facilitation (PNF) diagonal patterns (light)
III. Advanced strengthening phase (weeks 8–14)
Goals: increase strength, power, endurance
Maintain full elbow ROM
Gradually initiate sporting activities
A. Week 8
Exercises: initiate eccentric elbow flexion/extension
Continue isotonic program: forearm and wrist
Continue shoulder program—Thrower's Ten Program
Manual resistance diagonal patterns
Initiate plyometric exercise program (two-hand plyos close to body only)
Chest pass
Side throw close to body
Continue stretching calf and hamstrings
B. Week 10
Exercises: continue all exercises listed above
Program plyometrics to two-hand drills away from body
Side to side throws
Soccer throws
Side throws
C. Week 12–14
Continue all exercises
Initiate isotonic machines strengthening exercises (if desired)
Bench press (seated)
Lat pulldown

(continued)

Table 35.8 (continued)

Initiate golf, swimming
Initiate interval hitting program
Iv. Return to activity phase (weeks 14–32)
Goals: continue to increase strength, power, and endurance of upper extremity musculature
Gradual return to sport activities
A. Week 14
Exercises: continue strengthening program
Emphasis on elbow and wrist strengthening and flexibility exercises
Maintain full elbow ROM
Initiate one hand plyometric throwing (stationary throws)
Initiate one hand wall dribble
Initiate one hand baseball throws into wall
B. Week 16
Exercises: initiate interval throwing program (phase I, long toss program)
Continue Thrower's Ten Program and plyos
Continue to stretch before and after throwing
C. Weeks 22–24
Exercises: progress to phase II throwing (once successfully completed phase I)
D. Weeks 30–32
Exercises: gradually progress to competitive throwing/sports

Table 35.9 Rehabilitation following UCL reconstruction utilizing palmaris longus graft (regular rehabilitation approach)

I. Immediate postoperative phase (0–3 weeks)
Goals: protect healing tissue
Decrease pain/inflammation
Retard muscular atrophy
Protect graft site—allow healing
A. Postoperative week 1
Brace: posterior splint at 90° elbow flexion
ROM: wrist AROM ext/flexion immediately postoperative
Elbow postoperative compression dressing (5–7 days)
Wrist (graft site) compression dressing 7–10 days as needed
Exercises: gripping exercises
Wrist ROM
Shoulder isometrics (no shoulder ER)
Biceps isometrics
Cryotherapy: to elbow joint and to graft site at wrist
B. Postoperative week 2
Brace: elbow ROM 25–100° (Gradually increase ROM—5° ext./10° of flex per week)
Exercises: continue all exercises listed above
Elbow ROM in brace (30–105°)
Initiate elbow extension isometrics

Table 35.9 (continued)

Continue wrist ROM exercises
Scapular strengthening program (manual resistance)
Initiate light scar mobilization over distal incision (graft)
Cryotherapy: continue ice to elbow and graft site
C. Postoperative week 3
Brace: elbow ROM 15–115°
Exercises: continue all exercises listed above
Elbow ROM in brace
Initiate active ROM wrist and elbow (no resistance)
Initiate light wrist flexion stretching
Initiate active ROM shoulder
Full can
Lateral raises
ER/IR tubing
Elbow flex/extension
Initiate light scapular strengthening exercises
May incorporate bicycle for lower extremity strength and endurance
II. Intermediate phase (weeks 4–7)
Goals: gradual increase to full ROM
Promote healing of repaired tissue
Regain and improve muscular strength
Restore full function of graft site
A. Week 4
Brace: elbow ROM 0–125°
Exercises: begin light resistance exercises for arm (1 lb)
Wrist curls, extensions, pronation, supination
Elbow extension/flexion
Progress shoulder program emphasize rotator cuff and scapular strengthening
Initiate shoulder strengthening with light dumbbells
Initiate Thrower's Ten Program without dumbbells
B. Week 5
ROM: elbow ROM 0–135°
Discontinue brace
Continue all exercises: progress all shoulder and UE exercises (progress weight 1 lb.)
Week 6
AROM: 0–145° without brace or full ROM
Exercises: initiate Thrower's Ten Program with isotonics
Progress elbow strengthening exercises
Initiate shoulder external rotation strengthening
Progress shoulder program
Week 7
Progress Thrower's Ten Program (progress weights)
Initiate PNF diagonal patterns (light)
III. Advanced strengthening phase (weeks 8–14)
Goals: increase strength, power, endurance
Maintain full elbow ROM
Gradually initiate sporting activities
A. Week 8

Table 35.9 (continued)

Exercises: initiate eccentric elbow flexion/extension
Continue isotonic program: forearm and wrist
Continue shoulder program—Thrower's Ten Program
Manual resistance diagonal patterns
Initiate plyometric exercise program (two-hand plyos close to body only)
Chest pass
Side throw close to body
Continue stretching calf and hamstrings
B. Week 10
Exercises: continue all exercises listed above
Program plyometrics to two-hand drills away from body
Side to side throws
Soccer throws
Side throws
C. Weeks 12–14
Initiate advanced Thrower's Ten Program at week 12
Continue all exercises
Initiate isotonic machines strengthening exercises (if desired)
Bench press (seated)
Lat pulldown
Initiate golf, swimming
Initiate interval hitting program (see program) week 12
IV. Return to activity phase (weeks 14–32)
Goals: continue to increase strength, power, and endurance of upper extremity musculature
Gradual return to sport activities
A. Week 14
Exercises: continue strengthening program
Emphasis on elbow and wrist strengthening and flexibility exercises
Maintain full elbow ROM
Initiate one hand plyometric throwing (stationary throws)
Initiate one hand wall dribble
Initiate one hand baseball throws into wall
B. Week 16
Exercises: initiate interval throwing program (phase I) [long toss program]
Continue advanced Thrower's Ten Program and plyometrics
Continue to stretch before and after throwing
C. Weeks 22–24
Exercises: progress to phase II throwing (once successfully completed phase I)
D. Weeks 30–32
Exercises: once return to sports utilize Thrower's Ten Program
Continue shoulder and elbow ROM and stretching program
Gradually progress to competitive throwing/sports
Most pitchers return to competitive game pitching at 8–9 months

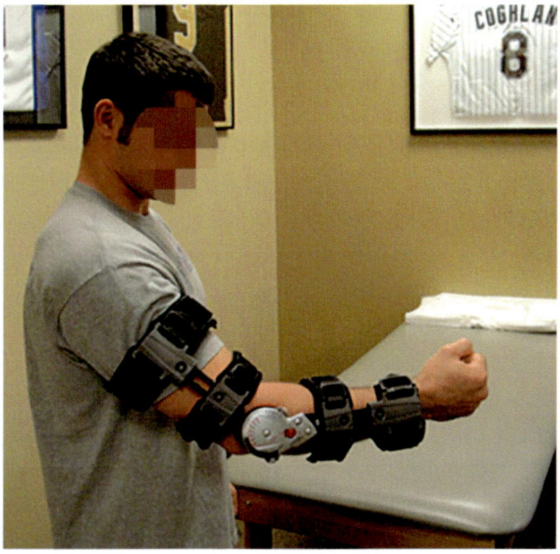

Fig. 35.9 Hinged elbow brace utilized postoperatively to protect the graft from deleterious valgus stresses

while the Thrower's Ten Program (Appendix A) is initiated by week 6. Progressive resistance exercises are incorporated at weeks 8–9. Focus is again placed on developing dynamic stabilization of the medial elbow. Due to the anatomical orientation of the flexor carpi ulnaris and flexor digitorum superficialis overlaying the UCL, isotonic, and stabilization activities for these muscles may assist the UCL in stabilizing valgus stress at the medial elbow [108]. Thus, concentric and eccentric strengthening of these muscles is performed.

Aggressive exercises involving eccentric and plyometric contractions are included in the advanced phase, usually weeks 12–16. The advanced Thrower's Ten Program is initiated at week 12 after surgery. Two-hand plyometric drills are performed at week 12, one-hand drills at week 14. An interval throwing program (Tables 35.3, 35.4, and 35.5) is allowed at week 16 postoperatively. In most cases, throwing from a mound is progressed at 6–8 weeks following the initiation of an interval throwing program and a return to competitive throwing, and off-the-mound throwing is initiated at approximately 24 weeks postoperative. A return to competitive throwing usually occurs at approximately 9–12 months following surgery.

Cain et al. [106] reported on the outcome of UCL reconstruction of the elbow in 743 athletes during a 2-year minimum follow-up. The authors went on to report that UCL reconstruction with subcutaneous ulnar nerve transposition was found to be effective in correcting valgus elbow instability in the overhead athlete and allowed most athletes (83%) to return to previous or higher level of competition in less than 1 year. Major complications were noted in only 4% of the subjects, and most of the complications resolving by 6 months postoperatively. Our most recent follow-up study looking at patients undergoing UCL reconstruction at a mean of 10 years postoperatively has revealed 93% of the patients were satisfied and 90% of the pitchers were able to return to pitching at the same or next level. Only 3% of the patients expressed persistent elbow pain (Osbahr AAOSM Meeting 2013) [109].

The rehabilitation program following UCL reconstruction utilizing the docking procedure is slightly different. Dodson et al. [100] and recently Dr. Altchek (personal communications) have advocated an elbow brace with ROM from 30 to 60° for the first 3 weeks, then 15–90° at week 4 postoperatively. The athlete should obtain full ROM by 6 weeks after the surgery. The surgeons prefer active ROM and no passive ROM for the first 12 weeks. Isotonic strengthening exercises are also initiated at week 8 to improve glenohumeral and scapulothoracic strength. Plyometric activities may be performed at approximately 12 weeks after the surgery to further stress the healing tissues in preparation for the interval throwing program. The athlete may also incorporate heavier strengthening exercise utilizing machine weights at this time. A positional player may begin a hitting program at 5 months postoperatively, which includes first hitting off of a tee, progressing to soft-toss throws, and finally formal batting practice. The interval throwing program is permitted at 4 months postoperatively and formal pitching is typically accomplished at 9–12 months after the surgery. Please refer to Table 35.10 for the entire Dr. Altchek UCL Docking Procedure Rehabilitation Program.

Table 35.10 Rehabilitation following UCL reconstruction utilizing the docking procedure (Altchek protocol)

Postoperative phase I (weeks 1–4)
Goals:
Promote healing: reduce pain, inflammation and swelling
Begin to restore ROM to 15–90°
Promote independence in home therapeutic exercise program
Precautions:
No PROM of the elbow
Brace should be worn at all times
Treatment Recommendations:
Follow brace instructions as per prescription: post-op week 1: splint at 50–60° flexion; post-op weeks 1–3: brace open from 30 to 60° flexion; post-op week 4: brace open from 15 to 90° flexion; elbow AROM in brace; wrist AROM; scapular isometrics; gripping exercises; emphasize patient compliance to home exercise program (HEP) and brace precautions
Minimum criteria for advancement to next phase:
Elbow ROM 15–90° of flexion
Minimal pain or swelling
Postoperative phase II (weeks 4–6)
Goals:
ROM 15–115°
Minimal pain and swelling
Precautions:
Continue to wear brace at all times
Avoid PROM
Avoid valgus stress
Treatment recommendations:
Continue AROM in brace: Remove brace 5 weeks post-op; begin AROM without the brace; begin pain-free isometrics in brace (shoulder FF/ext., elbow flex/ext.); manual scapula stabilization exercises with proximal resistance; modalities as needed; progress/advance patients home exercise program (evaluation based)
Minimum criteria for advancement:
ROM 15° → 115°
Minimal pain and swelling
Postoperative phase III (weeks 6–12)
Goals:
Restore full ROM
All UE strength 5/5
Begin to restore UE endurance
Precautions:
Minimize valgus stress
Avoid PROM by the clinician
Avoid pain with therapeutic exercise
No isolated forearm exercises for 1 year
Treatment recommendations:

Table 35.10 (continued)

Continue AROM; low intensity/long duration stretch for extension; isotonics for scapula, shoulder, elbow; begin IR/ER strengthening at 8 weeks; upper body ergometer (if adequate ROM); neuromuscular drills; PNF patterns when strength is adequate; incorporate eccentric training when strength is adequate; modalities as needed; emphasize patient compliance with home exercise program
Minimum criteria for advancement:
Pain-free
Full elbow ROM
All UE strength 5/5
Postoperative phase IV (weeks 12–16)
Goals:
Restore full strength and flexibility
Restore normal neuromuscular function
Prepare for return to activity
Precautions:
Avoid pain with plyometrics
Treatment recommendations:
Advance IR/ER to 90/90 position; full upper extremity flexibility program; neuromuscular drills; plyometrics program; continued endurance training; address trunk and lower extremities; advance home exercise program
Criteria for advancement:
Complete plyometrics program without symptoms
Normal upper extremity flexibility
Postoperative phase V
Return to sport (months 4–9)
Goals:
Return to activity
Prevent reinjury
Precautions:
Significant pain with throwing or hitting
Avoid loss of strength or flexibility
Treatment recommendations:
Begin interval throwing program at 4 months
Begin hitting program at 5 months
Continue flexibility exercises
Continue strengthening program (incorporate training principles)
Criteria for discharge:
Pain-free
Independence with home therapeutic exercise program
Independent throwing/hitting program

Rehabilitation of the patient following UCL repair with internal brace follows many of the same interventions; however, the sequence and timing of the interventions is accelerated compared to traditional UCL reconstruction [104]. Table 35.11

Table 35.11 Postoperative Rehabilitation for Ulnar Collateral Ligament Repair with Internal Brace

Phase I: Immediate Postoperative Phase (Week 1)
Goals: Protect healing tissue; reduce pain and inflammation; retard muscle atrophy; full wrist range of motion (ROM)
Day of Surgery:
1. Elbow brace locked at 90° for 7 days
2. Passive ROM (PROM) of wrist and hand in locked brace
Post-op Day 1 and 2: Add (all performed in locked elbow brace)
1. Shoulder PROM: flexion, external rotation (ER), and internal rotation (IR) to tolerance
2. Shoulder pendulum exercises
3. Wrist flexors/extensors stretching
4. Putty/griping exercises
Post-op Day 3 through 7: (all exercises performed in locked elbow brace)
1. Continue previous exercises advancing PROM as tolerated
2. Add the following exercises:
(a) Shoulder isometrics: ER, IR, abduction, flexion, and extension performed pain-free, sub-maximal
(b) Scapular strengthening: seated neuromuscular control drills with manual resistance
Progression to next phase is purely time based
Phase II: Controlled Mobility Phase (Weeks 2–5)
Goals: Gradually restore elbow ROM; improve muscular strength and endurance; normalize joint arthrokinematics
Beginning Week 2 (Day 8)
1. Set elbow ROM brace to 30–110°
2. Begin elbow PROM and AAROM 30–110°
3. Initiate elbow AROM for flexion
4. Initiate shoulder AROM in elbow brace
5. Progress scapular strengthening exercises
Seated manual resistance: protraction/retraction; elevation/depression; diagonal patterns
1. Progress to light isotonic strengthening exercises for wrist, elbow, and shoulder at day 10
Beginning Week 3:
1. Progress elbow ROM to 10–125°
2. Initiate Thrower's Ten exercise program
Beginning Week 4:
1. Progress elbow ROM to 0–145°
2. Progress elbow and wrist strengthening exercises
3. Initiate wrist flexion and elbow flexion movements against manual resistance
Criteria for progression to next phase:
Elbow PROM of 10–125°; Minimal pain and tenderness; Good manual muscle testing of key muscles/movements (elbow flexion/extension, wrist flexion, shoulder IR, ER, and scapular abduction)
Phase III: Intermediate Phase (Weeks 6–8)

(continued)

Table 35.11 (continued)

Goals: Restore full elbow ROM; progress upper extremity strength; continue with functional progression
Beginning Week 6:
1. Discontinue elbow brace at week 6
2. Initiate advanced Thrower's Ten program
3. Initiate 2 hand plyometrics: chest pass, side-to-side throw, and overhead pass
4. Initiate prone plank exercise
Beginning Week 8:
1. Progress to 1 hand plyometrics: 90°/90° ball throw, 0° ball throw
2. Continue with Advanced Thrower's Ten program
3. Initiate side plank with shoulder ER strengthening exercise
Criteria for progression to next phase:
Full nonpainful elbow AROM and PROM; no pain or tenderness; appropriate strength of …shoulder and elbow… (70% minimum compared to opposite side); satisfactory clinical exam; completion of current rehabilitation phase without difficulty
Phase IV: Advanced Phase (Weeks 9–14)
Goals: Advanced strengthening exercises; initiate interval throwing program; gradual return to throwing
Beginning Week 9:
1. Continue all strengthening exercises, including advanced Thrower's Ten program and 1 and 2 hand plyometrics program
Beginning Week 10: Initiate
1. Seated chest press machine
2. Seated row machine
3. Biceps/Triceps machine or cable strengthening
4. Interval hitting program
Week 12: Initiate Interval Throwing Program (Phase I)
Criteria to enter next phase:
Full elbow, wrist, and shoulder ROM; no pain or tenderness;
functional or isokinetic test that fulfills criteria for desired activity; satisfactory clinical examination
Phase V: Return to Activity/Play Phase (weeks 14+):
Goals: Gradual return to competitive throwing; continue all exercises and stretches
Week 14–16:
1. Continue all exercises as in weeks 9–12
2. Continue Interval Throwing Program (ITP) Phase 1- Long Toss (week 12)
(a) Each athlete may progress through ITP at different rates/pace
(b) Expected to complete 0–90 ft throws within 3 weeks of starting ITP and 120 ft within 8 weeks
Week 16–20:
1. Continue ROM and stretching programs
2. Continue Advanced Thrower's Ten program
3. Continue Plyometrics
4. Initiate ITP Phase 2 (off the mound) when Phase 1 is complete, and athlete is ready
Week 20+
1. Initiate gradual return to competitive throwing
2. Perform dynamic warm-ups and stretches
3. Continue Advanced Thrower's Ten program
4. Return to competition when athlete is ready (physician decision & rehabilitation team)

contains the authors' protocol for rehabilitation following UCL repair with internal brace.

Rehabilitation Comparison Between UCL Repair with Internal Brace and UCL Reconstruction

Since so many rehabilitation interventions are similar between the internal brace technique and UCL reconstruction, for the purposes of this chapter, we elect to summarize here some of the most significant differences that will guide the clinician along with the detailed protocol in Table 35.11 for clinical application.

For both the UCL reconstruction and UCL repair with internal brace, elbow motion is restricted and held in 90° of flexion for 7 days following the surgery. Surgery to protect the fascial slings used in the concomitant ulnar nerve transposition. Following this first week, elbow motion is generally progressed faster after UCL repair with internal brace with extension allowed to tolerance and full ROM expected by the beginning of week 4. This is in contrast to full elbow ROM, which is expected by the end of week 6 after UCL reconstruction. The Thrower's Ten exercise program is initiated 3 weeks following surgery and the Advanced Thrower's Ten program 4–5 weeks post-surgery in the UCL repair with internal brace program. This is in contrast to week 6, and weeks 8–9 for these exercise applications respectively, for the traditional UCL reconstruction rehabilitation program.

Compared to UCL reconstruction, following UCL repair with internal brace, 2-handed plyometric drills are started 2 weeks sooner (6 weeks post-surgery) and 1-handed drills 8 weeks sooner (8 weeks post-surgery). Isotonic machine resistance exercises are begun at 10 weeks, 2–4 weeks earlier than when they are initiated following UCL reconstruction.

A significant difference between the rehabilitation programs after UCL repair with internal brace compared to UCL reconstruction is the much earlier initiation of interval training programs and return to competitive throwing. With UCL repair with internal brace, interval hitting and golf can be incorporated 10 weeks post-surgery, which is 2–4 weeks sooner than following UCL reconstruction. Long toss (interval throwing phase I) begins at 12 weeks (compared to 16 weeks) post-surgery and throwing off the mound (interval throwing phase II) is initiated 16–20 weeks (compared to 22–24 weeks) post-surgery. A gradual return to competitive throwing begins 5 months following UCL repair with internal brace in contrast to 9–12 months following UCL reconstruction [110].

Ulnar Nerve Transposition

At our center, an ulnar nerve transposition is performed in a subcutaneous fashion using fascial slings. Caution is taken to not overstress the soft tissue structures involved with relocating the nerve while healing occurs [7]. The rehabilitation following an ulnar nerve transposition is outlined in Table 35.12. A posterior splint at 90° of elbow flexion is used for the first week postoperatively to prevent excessive flexion ROM and tension on the nerve. The splint is discharged at the beginning of week 2 and light ROM activities are initiated. Full ROM is usually restored by weeks 3–4. Gentle isotonic strengthening is begun during weeks 3–4 and progressed to the full Thrower's Ten Program by 4–6 weeks following surgery. Aggressive strengthening including eccentric, Advanced Thrower's Ten, and plyometric training is incorporated at week 8 and an interval throwing program at weeks 10–12, if all previously outlined criteria are met, similar to the advanced phase of the UCL protocol. A return to competition usually occurs at week 16 postoperatively.

Table 35.12 Postoperative rehabilitation following ulnar nerve transposition

Phase I: immediate postoperative phase (*weeks 0–1*)
Goals: Allow soft tissue healing of relocated nerve
Decrease pain and inflammation
Retard muscular atrophy
A. Week 1
1. Posterior splint at 90° elbow flexion with wrist free for motion (sling for comfort)
2. Compression dressing
3. Exercises such as gripping exercises, wrist ROM, shoulder isometrics
B. Week 2
1. Remove posterior splint for exercise and bathing
2. Progress elbow ROM (PROM 15–120°)
3. Initiate elbow and wrist isometrics
4. Continue shoulder isometrics
Phase II: intermediate phase (*weeks 3–7*)
Goals: Restore full pain free range of motion
Improve strength, power, and endurance of upper extremity musculature
Gradually increase functional demands
A. Week 3
1. Discontinue posterior splint
2. Progress elbow ROM, emphasize full extension
3. Initiate flexibility exercise for wrist extension/flexion, forearm supination/pronation, and elbow extension/flexion
4. Initiate strengthening exercises for wrist extension/flexion, forearm supination/pronation, elbow extensors/flexors, and a shoulder program
B. Week 6
1. Continue all exercises listed above
2. Initiate Thrower's Ten Program
Phase III: advanced strengthening phase (*weeks 8–12*)
Goals: Increase strength, power, endurance
Gradually initiate sporting activities
A. Week 8
1. Initiate eccentric exercise program
2. Initiate plyometric exercise drills
3. Continue shoulder and elbow strengthening and flexibility exercises
4. Initiate interval throwing program
Phase IV: return to activity phase (*weeks 12–16*)
Goals: gradually return to sporting activities
A. Week 12
1. Return to competitive throwing
2. Continue Thrower's Ten Exercise Program

Posterior Olecranon Osteophyte Excision

Surgical excision of posterior olecranon osteophytes is performed arthroscopically using an osteotome or motorized burr. Approximately 5–10 mm of the olecranon tip is removed concomitantly, and a motorized burr is used to contour the coronoid, olecranon tip, and fossa to prevent further impingement with extreme flexion and extension [111]. Caution is exercised not to remove too much bone and destabilize the elbow, resulting in increased loads on the UCL during forceful throwing [112].

The rehabilitation program following arthroscopic posterior olecranon osteophyte excision is slightly more conservative in restoring full elbow extension secondary to postsurgical pain. ROM is progressed within the patient's tolerance; by 10 days postoperative, the patient should exhibit at least 15–105/110° of ROM, and 5–10 to 115° by day 14. Full ROM (0–145°) is typically restored by day 20–25 post-surgery. The rate of ROM progression is most often limited by osseous pain and synovial joint inflammation, usually located at the tip of the olecranon.

The strengthening program is similar to the previously discussed progression. Isometrics are performed for the first 10–14 days and isotonic strengthening from weeks 2–6. Initially, especially during the first 2 weeks, forceful triceps contractions may produce posterior elbow pain. If this is present, the clinician should either avoid or reduce the force produced by the triceps muscle. The full Thrower's Ten Program is initiated by week 6. An interval throwing program is included by weeks 10–12. The rehabilitation focus is similar to the nonoperative treatment of the valgus extension overload. Emphasis is placed on eccentric control of the elbow flexors and dynamic stabilization of the medial elbow.

Andrews and Timmerman [102] reported on the outcome of elbow surgery in 72 professional baseball players. Sixty-five percent of these athletes exhibited a posterior olecranon osteophyte and 25% of the athletes who underwent an isolated olecranon excision later required an UCL reconstruction [102]. This may suggest that subtle medial instability may accelerate osteophyte formation .

Conclusion

The elbow joint is a common site of injury in athletes, especially in the overhead athlete. In the overhead-throwing athlete, the injury is usually due to the repetitive microtraumatic injuries observed during the act of throwing. In other athletes, such as in collision sports like football, wrestling, soccer, and gymnastics, often the elbow injury is due to macrotraumatic forces to the elbow, as seen in fractures, dislocations, and ligamentous injuries. Rehabilitation of the elbow, whether postinjury or postsurgical, must follow a progressive and sequential order to ensure that healing tissues are not overstressed but also provide appropriate stress at appropriate times to promote proper collagen alignment to withstand forces. The rehabilitation program should limit immobilization and achieve full ROM early, especially elbow extension. Furthermore, it is essential that the rehabilitation program progressively restore strength and neuromuscular control while gradually incorporating sports-specific activities to successfully return the athlete to their previous level of function as quickly and safely as possible. The rehabilitation of the elbow must include the entire kinetic chain (scapula, shoulder, hand, core/hips, and legs) to ensure the athletes' return to high-level sport participation.

References

1. Coutts RD, Toth C, Kaita JH. The role of continuous passive motion in the rehabilitation of the total knee patient. In: Hungerford DS, Krackow KA, Kenna RV, editors. Total knee arthroplasty: a comprehensive approach. Baltimore: Williams and Wilkins; 1984. p. 126–32.
2. Dehne E, Torp RP. Treatment of joint injuries by immediate mobilization. Based upon the spinal adaptation concept. Clin Orthop Relat Res. 1971;77:218–32.
3. Haggmark T, Eriksson E. Cylinder or mobile cast brace after knee ligament surgery. A clinical analy-

sis and morphologic and enzymatic studies of changes in the quadriceps muscle. Am J Sports Med. 1979;7(1):48–56.
4. Noyes FR, Mangine RE, Barber S. Early knee motion after open and arthroscopic anterior cruciate ligament reconstruction. Am J Sports Med. 1987;15(2):149–60.
5. Perkins G. Rest and movement. J Bone Joint Surg Br. 1953;35-B(4):521–39.
6. Salter RB, Simmonds DF, Malcolm BW, Rumble EJ, MacMichael D, Clements ND. The biological effect of continuous passive motion on the healing of full-thickness defects in articular cartilage. An experimental investigation in the rabbit. J Bone Joint Surg Am. 1980;62(8):1232–51.
7. Wilk KE, Arrigo C, Andrews JR. Rehabilitation of the elbow in the throwing athlete. J Orthop Sports Phys Ther. 1993;17(6):305–17.
8. Akeson WH, Amiel D, Woo SL. Immobility effects on synovial joints the pathomechanics of joint contracture. Biorheology. 1980;17(1–2):95–110.
9. Green DP, McCoy H. Turnbuckle orthotic correction of elbow-flexion contractures after acute injuries. J Bone Joint Surg Am. 1979;61(7):1092–5.
10. Nirschl RP, Morrey BF. Rehabilitation. In: Morrey BF, editor. The elbow and its disorders. Philadelphia: WB Saunders; 1985. p. 147–52.
11. Wright RW, Steger-May K, Wasserlauf BL, O'Neal ME, Weinberg BW, Paletta GA. Elbow range of motion in professional baseball pitchers. Am J Sports Med. 2006;34(2):190–3.
12. Maitland GD. Vertebral manipulation. 4th ed. London: Butterworth; 1977.
13. Wyke BD. The neurology of joints. Ann R Coll Surg. 1966;41:25–9.
14. Kottke FJ, Pauley DL, Ptak RA. The rationale for prolonged stretching for correction of shortening of connective tissue. Arch Phys Med Rehabil. 1966;47(6):345–52.
15. Sapega AA, Quedenfeld TC, Moyer RA, Butler RA. Biophysical factors in range-of-motion exercise. Phys Sports Med. 1981;9(12):57–65.
16. Warren CG, Lehmann JF, Koblanski JN. Elongation of rat tail tendon: effect of load and temperature. Arch Phys Med Rehabil. 1971;52(10):465–74 (passim).
17. Warren CG, Lehmann JF, Koblanski JN. Heat and stretch procedures: an evaluation using rat tail tendon. Arch Phys Med Rehabil. 1976;57(3):122–6.
18. McClure PW, Blackburn LG, Dusold C. The use of splints in the treatment of joint stiffness: biologic rationale and an algorithm for making clinical decisions. Phys Ther. 1994;74(12):1101–7.
19. Fleisig GS, Andrews JR, Dillman CJ, Escamilla RF. Kinetics of baseball pitching with implications about injury mechanisms. Am J Sports Med. 1995;23(2):233–9.
20. Wilk KE, Meister K, Andrews JR. Current concepts in the rehabilitation of the overhead throwing athlete. Am J Sports Med. 2002;30(1):136–51.
21. Wilk KE, Obma P, Simpson CD, Cain EL, Dugas JR, Andrews JR. Shoulder injuries in the overhead athlete. J Orthop Sports Phys Ther. 2009;39(2):38–54.
22. Reinold MM, Macrina LC, Wilk KE, et al. Electromyographic analysis of the supraspinatus and deltoid muscles during 3 common rehabilitation exercises. J Athl Train. 2007;42(4):464–9.
23. Reinold MM, Wilk KE, Fleisig GS, et al. Electromyographic analysis of the rotator cuff and deltoid musculature during common shoulder external rotation exercises. J Orthop Sports Phys Ther. 2004;34(7):385–94.
24. Reinold MM, Escamilla RF, Wilk KE. Current concepts in the scientific and clinical rationale behind exercises for glenohumeral and scapulothoracic musculature. J Orthop Sports Phys Ther. 2009;39(2):105–17.
25. Carpenter JE, Blasier RB, Pellizzon GG. The effects of muscle fatigue on shoulder joint position sense. Am J Sports Med. 1998;26(2):262–5.
26. Voight ML, Hardin JA, Blackburn TA, Tippett S, Canner GC. The effects of muscle fatigue on and the relationship of arm dominance to shoulder proprioception. J Orthop Sports Phys Ther. 1996;23(6):348–52.
27. Myers JB, Guskiewicz KM, Schneider RA, Prentice WE. Proprioception and neuromuscular control of the shoulder after muscle fatigue. J Athl Train. 1999;34(4):362–7.
28. Myers JB, Ju YY, Hwang JH, McMahon PJ, Rodosky MW, Lephart SM. Reflexive muscle activation alterations in shoulders with anterior glenohumeral instability. Am J Sports Med. 2004;32(4):1013–21.
29. Andrews JR, Jobe FW. Valgus extension overload in the pitching elbow. In: Andrews JR, Zarins B, Carson WB, editors. Injuries to the throwing arm. Philadelphia: Saunders; 1985. p. 250–7.
30. Fleisig GS, Escamilla RF. Biomechanics of the elbow in the throwing athlete. Op Tech Sports Med. 1996;4(2):62–8.
31. Wilk KE, Yenchak AJ, Arrigo CA, Andrews JR. The advanced throwers ten exercise program: a new exercise series for enhanced dynamic shoulder control in the overhead throwing athlete. Phys Sportsmed. 2011;39(4):90–7.
32. Schulte-Edelmann JA, Davies GJ, Kernozek TW, Gerberding ED. The effects of plyometric training of the posterior shoulder and elbow. J Strength Cond Res. 2005;19(1):129–34.
33. Wilk KE, Voight ML, Keirns MA, Gambetta V, Andrews JR, Dillman CJ. Stretch-shortening drills for the upper extremities: theory and clinical application. J Orthop Sports Phys Ther. 1993;17(5):225–39.
34. Reinold MM, Wilk KE, Reed J, Crenshaw K, Andrews JR. Interval sport programs: guidelines for baseball, tennis, and golf. J Orthop Sports Phys Ther. 2002;32(6):293–8.
35. Brown LP, Niehues SL, Harrah A, Yavorsky P, Hirshman HP. Upper extremity range of motion and isokinetic strength of the internal and external shoulder rotators in major league baseball players. Am J Sports Med. 1988;16(6):577–85.
36. Greenfield BH, Donatelli R, Wooden MJ, Wilkes J. Isokinetic evaluation of shoulder rotational strength

between the plane of scapula and the frontal plane. Am J Sports Med. 1990;18(2):124–8.
37. Wilk KE, Andrews JR, Arrigo CA, Keirns MA, Erber DJ. The strength characteristics of internal and external rotator muscles in professional baseball pitchers. Am J Sports Med. 1993;21(1):61–6.
38. Fleisig GS, Bolt B, Fortenbaugh D, Wilk KE, Andrews JR. Biomechanical comparison of baseball pitching and long-toss: implications for training and rehabilitation. J Orthop Sports Phys Ther. 2011;41(5):296–303.
39. Fleisig GS, Barrentine SW, Escamilla RF, Andrews JR. Biomechanics of overhand throwing with implications for injuries. Sports Med. 1996;21(6):421–37.
40. Werner SL, Fleisig GS, Dillman CJ, Andrews JR. Biomechanics of the elbow during baseball pitching. J Orthop Sports Phys Ther. 1993;17(6):274–8.
41. Gabel GT, Morrey BF. Operative treatment of medical epicondylitis. Influence of concomitant ulnar neuropathy at the elbow. J Bone Joint Surg Am. 1995;77(7):1065–9.
42. Nirschl RP. Medial tennis elbow: surgical treatment. Orthop Trans. 1983;7:298.
43. Vangsness T. The surgical treatment of medial epicondylitis. Orthop Trans. 1988;7:733.
44. Nirschl RP. Prevention and treatment of elbow and shoulder injuries in the tennis player. Clin Sports Med. 1988;7(2):289–308.
45. Kraushaar BS, Nirschl RP. Tendinosis of the elbow (tennis elbow). Clinical features and findings of histological, immunohistochemical, and electron microscopy studies. J Bone Joint Surg Am. 1999;81(2):259–78.
46. Nirschl RP, Ashman ES. Tennis elbow tendinosis (epicondylitis). Instr Course Lect. 2004;53:587–98.
47. James SL, Ali K, Pocock C, et al. Ultrasound guided dry needling and autologous blood injection for patellar tendinosis. Br J Sports Med. 2007;41(8):518–21 (discussion 522).
48. Suresh SP, Ali KE, Jones H, Connell DA. Medial epicondylitis: is ultrasound guided autologous blood injection an effective treatment? Br J Sports Med. 2006;40(11):935. 9 (discussion 939)
49. Langberg H, Ellingsgaard H, Madsen T, et al. Eccentric rehabilitation exercise increases peritendinous type I collagen synthesis in humans with Achilles tendinosis. Scand J Med Sci Sports. 2007;17(1):61–6.
50. Alfredson H, Pietila T, Jonsson P, Lorentzon R. Heavy-load eccentric calf muscle training for the treatment of chronic Achilles tendinosis. Am J Sports Med. 1998;26(3):360–6.
51. Clement DB, Taunton JE, Smart GW. Achilles tendinitis and peritendinitis: etiology and treatment. Am J Sports Med. 1984;12(3):179–84.
52. Shalabi A, Kristoffersen-Wilberg M, Svensson L, Aspelin P, Movin T. Eccentric training of the gastrocnemius-soleus complex in chronic Achilles tendinopathy results in decreased tendon volume and intratendinous signal as evaluated by MRI. Am J Sports Med. 2004;32(5):1286–96.
53. Bjordal JM, Lopes-Martins RA, Iversen VV. A randomised, placebo controlled trial of low level laser therapy for activated Achilles tendinitis with microdialysis measurement of peritendinous prostaglandin E2 concentrations. Br J Sports Med. 2006;40(1):76–80 (discussion 76–80).
54. England S, Farrell AJ, Coppock JS, Struthers G, Bacon PA. Low power laser therapy of shoulder tendonitis. Scand J Rheumatol. 1989;18(6):427–31.
55. Lam LK, Cheing GL. Effects of 904-nm low-level laser therapy in the management of lateral epicondylitis: a randomized controlled trial. Photomed Laser Surg. 2007;25(2):65–71.
56. Stergioulas A, Stergioula M, Aarskog R, Lopes-Martins RA, Bjordal JM. Effects of low-level laser therapy and eccentric exercises in the treatment of recreational athletes with chronic achilles tendinopathy. Am J Sports Med. 2008;36(5):881–7.
57. Ko JY, Chen HS, Chen LM. Treatment of lateral epicondylitis of the elbow with shock waves. Clin Orthop Relat Res. 2001;387:60–7.
58. Wang CJ, Chen HS. Shock wave therapy for patients with lateral epicondylitis of the elbow: a one- to two-year follow-up study. Am J Sports Med. 2002;30(3):422–5.
59. Wang CJ, Ko JY, Chen HS. Treatment of calcifying tendinitis of the shoulder with shock wave therapy. Clin Orthop Relat Res. 2001;387:83–9.
60. Creaney L, Hamilton B. Growth factor delivery methods in the management of sports injuries: the state of play. Br J Sports Med. 2008;42(5):314–20.
61. de Mos M, Koevoet W, van Schie HT, et al. In vitro model to study chondrogenic differentiation in tendinopathy. Am J Sports Med. 2009;37(6):1214–22.
62. de Mos M, van der Windt AE, Jahr H, et al. Can platelet-rich plasma enhance tendon repair? A cell culture study. Am J Sports Med. 2008;36(6):1171–8.
63. Kajikawa Y, Morihara T, Sakamoto H, et al. Platelet-rich plasma enhances the initial mobilization of circulation-derived cells for tendon healing. J Cell Physiol. 2008;215(3):837–45.
64. Lyras D, Kazakos K, Verettas D, et al. Immunohistochemical study of angiogenesis after local administration of platelet-rich plasma in a patellar tendon defect. Int Orthop. 2010;34:143–8.
65. Lyras D, Kazakos K, Verettas D, et al. The effect of platelet-rich plasma gel in the early phase of patellar tendon healing. Arch Orthop Trauma Surg. 2009;129:1577–82.
66. Mishra A, Pavelko T. Treatment of chronic elbow tendinosis with buffered platelet-rich plasma. Am J Sports Med. 2006;34(11):1774–8.
67. Mishra A, Woodall J Jr, Vieira A. Treatment of tendon and muscle using platelet-rich plasma. Clin Sports Med. 2009;28(1):113–25.
68. Sanchez M, Anitua E, Orive G, Mujika I, Andia I. Platelet-rich therapies in the treatment of orthopaedic sport injuries. Sports Med. 2009;39(5):345–54.
69. Thanasas C, Papadimitriou G, Charalambidis C, Paraskevopoulos I, Papanikolaou A. Platelet-rich

plasma versus autologous whole blood for the treatment of chronic lateral elbow epicondylitis: a randomized controlled clinical trial. Am J Sports Med. 2011;39(10):2130–4.
70. Gosens T, Peerbooms JC, van Laar W, den Oudsten BL. Ongoing positive effect of platelet-rich plasma versus corticosteroid injection in lateral epicondylitis: a double-blind randomized controlled trial with 2-year follow-up. Am J Sports Med. 2011;39(6):1200–8.
71. Alfredson H. Chronic midportion Achilles tendinopathy: an update on research and treatment. Clin Sports Med. 2003;22(4):727–41.
72. Enwemeka CS. The effects of therapeutic ultrasound on tendon healing. A biomechanical study. Am J Phys Med Rehabil. 1989;68(6):283–7.
73. Gum SL, Reddy GK, Stehno-Bittel L, Enwemeka CS. Combined ultrasound, electrical stimulation, and laser promote collagen synthesis with moderate changes in tendon biomechanics. Am J Phys Med Rehabil. 1997;76(4):288–96.
74. Harvey W, Dyson M, Pond JB, Grahame R. The stimulation of protein synthesis in human fibroblasts by therapeutic ultrasound. Rheumatol Rehabil. 1975;14(4):237.
75. Jackson BA, Schwane JA, Starcher BC. Effect of ultrasound therapy on the repair of Achilles tendon injuries in rats. Med Sci Sports Exerc. 1991;23(2):171–6.
76. Murrell GA, Szabo C, Hannafin JA, et al. Modulation of tendon healing by nitric oxide. Inflamm Res. 1997;46(1):19–27.
77. Nowicki KD, Hummer CD 3rd, Heidt RS Jr, Colosimo AJ. Effects of iontophoretic versus injection administration of dexamethasone. Med Sci Sports Exerc. 2002;34(8):1294–301.
78. Paoloni JA, Appleyard RC, Nelson J, Murrell GA. Topical nitric oxide application in the treatment of chronic extensor tendinosis at the elbow: a randomized, double-blinded, placebo-controlled clinical trial. Am J Sports Med. 2003;31(6):915–20.
79. Reddy GK, Gum S, Stehno-Bittel L, Enwemeka CS. Biochemistry and biomechanics of healing tendon: part II. Effects of combined laser therapy and electrical stimulation. Med Sci Sports Exerc. 1998;30(6):794–800.
80. Reddy GK, Stehno-Bittel L, Enwemeka CS. Laser photostimulation of collagen production in healing rabbit Achilles tendons. Lasers Surg Med. 1998;22(5):281–7.
81. Wang L, Qin L, Lu HB, et al. Extracorporeal shock wave therapy in treatment of delayed bone-tendon healing. Am J Sports Med. 2008;36(2):340–7.
82. Glass JM, Stephen RL, Jacobson SC. The quantity and distribution of radiolabeled dexamethasone delivered to tissue by iontophoresis. Int J Dermatol. 1980;19(9):519–25.
83. Gangarosa LP Sr, Ozawa A, Ohkido M, Shimomura Y, Hill JM. Iontophoresis for enhancing penetration of dermatologic and antiviral drugs. J Dermatol. 1995;22(11):865–75.
84. Anderson CR, Morris RL, Boeh SD, Panus PC, Sembrowich WL. Effects of iontophoresis current magnitude and duration on dexamethasone deposition and localized drug retention. Phys Ther. 2003;83(2):161–70.
85. Alley RM, Pappas AM. Acute and performance related injuries of the elbow. In: Pappas AM, editor. Upper extremity injuries in the athlete. New York: Churchill Livingstone; 1995. p. 339–64.
86. Wilson FD, Andrews JR, Blackburn TA, McCluskey G. Valgus extension overload in the pitching elbow. Am J Sports Med. 1983;11(2):83–8.
87. Anderson K. Elbow arthritis and removal of loose bodies and spurs and techniques for restoration of motion. In: Altchek DW, Andrews JR, editors. The athlete's elbow. Philadelphia: Lippincott, Williams & Wilkins; 2001. p. 219–30.
88. Azar FM, Andrews JR, Wilk KE, Groh D. Operative treatment of ulnar collateral ligament injuries of the elbow in athletes. Am J Sports Med. 2000;28(1):16–23.
89. Andrews JR, Whiteside JA. Common elbow problems in the athlete. J Orthop Sports Phys Ther. 1993;17(6):289–95.
90. Morrey BF. Osteochondritis dessicans. In: DeLee JC, Drez D, editors. Orthopedic sports medicine. Philadelphia: Saunders; 1994. p. 908–12.
91. Bauer M, Jonsson K, Josefsson PO, Linden B. Osteochondritis dissecans of the elbow. A long-term follow-up study. Clin Orthop Relat Res. 1992;284:156–60.
92. Roberts N, Hughes R. Osteochondritis dissecans of the elbow joint; a clinical study. J Bone Joint Surg Br. 1950;32-B(3):348–60.
93. Woodward AH, Bianco AJ Jr. Osteochondritis dissecans of the elbow. Clin Orthop Relat Res. 1975;110:35–41.
94. Fleisig GS, Andrews JR. Prevention of elbow injuries in youth baseball pitchers. Sports Health. 2012;4(5):419–24.
95. Hurd WJ, Jazayeri R, Mohr K, Limpisvasti O, Elattrache NS, Kaufman KR. Pitch velocity is a predictor of medial elbow distraction forces in the uninjured high school-aged baseball pitcher. Sports Health. 2012;4(5):415–8.
96. Kurakowa D, Muraki T, Ishikawa H, Shingawa K, Nagamoto H, Takahashi H, Yamamoto N, Tanaka M, Itoi E. The influence of pitch velocity on medial elbow pain and medial epicondyle abnormality among youth baseball players. Am J Sports Med. 2020;48(7):1601–7.
97. Andrews JR, Jelsma RD, Joyse ME, Timmerman LA. Open surgical procedures for injuries of the elbow in throwers. Op Tech Sports Med. 1996;4(2):109–13.
98. Jobe FW, Stark H, Lombardo SJ. Reconstruction of the ulnar collateral ligament in athletes. J Bone Joint Surg Am. 1986;68(8):1158–63.

99. Dodson CC, Altchek DW. Ulnar collateral ligament reconstruction revisited: the procedure I use and why. Sports Health. 2012;4(5):433–7.
100. Dodson CC, Thomas A, Dines JS, Nho SJ, Williams RJ 3rd, Altchek DW. Medial ulnar collateral ligament reconstruction of the elbow in throwing athletes. Am J Sports Med. 2006;34(12):1926–32.
101. Rohrbough JT, Altchek DW, Hyman J, Williams RJ 3rd, Botts JD. Medial collateral ligament reconstruction of the elbow using the docking technique. Am J Sports Med. 2002;30(4):541–8.
102. Andrews JR, Timmerman LA. Outcome of elbow surgery in professional baseball players. Am J Sports Med. 1995;23(4):407–13.
103. Dines JS, ElAttrache NS, Conway JE, Smith W, Ahmad CS. Clinical outcomes of the DANE TJ technique to treat ulnar collateral ligament insufficiency of the elbow. Am J Sports Med. 2007;35(12):2039–44.
104. Wilk KE, Arrigo CA, Bagwell MS, Rothermich MA, Dugas JR. Repair of the ulnar collateral ligament of the elbow: rehabilitation following internal brace surgery. J Orthop Sports Phys Ther. 2019;49(4):253–61.
105. Dugas JR, Walters BL, Beason DP, Fleisig GS, Chronister JE. Biomechanical comparison of ulnar collateral ligament repair with internal bracing versus modified Jobe reconstruction. Am J Sports Med. 2016;44(3):735–41.
106. Cain EL Jr, Andrews JR, Dugas JR, et al. Outcome of ulnar collateral ligament reconstruction of the elbow in 1281 athletes: results in 743 athletes with minimum 2-year follow-up. Am J Sports Med. 2010;38(12):2426–34.
107. Bernas GA, Ruberte Thiele RA, Kinnaman KA, Hughes RE, Miller BS, Carpenter JE. Defining safe rehabilitation for ulnar collateral ligament reconstruction of the elbow: a biomechanical study. Am J Sports Med. 2009;37(12):2392–400.
108. Davidson PA, Pink M, Perry J, Jobe FW. Functional anatomy of the flexor pronator muscle group in relation to the medial collateral ligament of the elbow. Am J Sports Med. 1995;23(2):245–50.
109. Osbahr D, Cain EL, Raines B, Fortenbaugh D, Dugas JR, Andrews JR. Long term outcomes after ulnar collateral ligament reconstruction in competitive baseball players: follow-up with a minimum of 10 years. Paper presented at: American Orthopaedic Society for Sports Medicine (AOSSM); July 10, 2013; Chicago, IL.
110. Erickson BJ, Gupta AK, Harris JD, Bush-Joseph C, Bach BR, Abrams GD, San Juan AM, Cole BJ, Romeo AA. Rate of return to pitching and performance after Tommy John surgery in Major League Baseball pitchers. Am J Sports Med. 2014;42(3):536–43.
111. Martin SD, Baumgarten TE. Elbow injuries in the throwing athlete: diagnosis and arthroscopic treatment. Op Tech Sports Med. 1996;4(2):100–8.
112. Andrews JR, Heggland EJ, Fleisig GS, Zheng N. Relationship of ulnar collateral ligament strain to amount of medial olecranon osteotomy. Am J Sports Med. 2001;29(6):716–21.

Sport-Specific Rehabilitation After Ulnar Collateral Ligament Surgery

36

Todd S. Ellenbecker, Kevin E. Wilk, and Lenny Macrina

Introduction

Injury to the ulnar collateral ligament (UCL) occurs secondary to repetitive and/or forceful valgus stress to the human elbow [1]. Initial reports of UCL rupture were published in 1946 by Waris [2] and mainly dealt with a population of 17 elite-level javelin throwers. In their systematic review, Vitale and Ahmad [1] reported on 405 patients who underwent UCL reconstructions from studies with mean ages between 17.4 and 24.5 years. Ninety-nine percent of these patients were males and the majority of these patients were throwing athletes. Nearly all of the study population reviewed in this paper were baseball players, but some populations did include tennis players, javelin throwers, softball players, as well as more traumatic injuries in wrestling and football. For the purposes of this chapter, we discuss mainly sport-specific rehabilitation concepts for the throwing athlete that form by nearly all accounts the vast majority of cases seen in orthopedic and sports medicine settings [1]. This chapter is also meant to compliment the material we have provided in the preceding chapter with more specific rehabilitation principles for treating the overhead athlete following UCL injury.

Sport-Specific Concept

One of the basic tenets of any sports medicine rehabilitation program involves the concept of sport-specific training. Simply stated, this has typically been referred to the incorporation of specific exercises and movement progressions that closely simulate the stressors and movement patterns that are encountered in the sport at initially controlled and submaximal levels along a progression continuum to allow athletes to return to their sport. Several recent articles have dealt with the concepts of return to sport [3, 4] and highlight and profile the specific steps undertaken during the often overlooked later stages of the rehabilitation program.

Two important factors should be discussed here before progressing into the specific rehabilitation

T. S. Ellenbecker (✉)
Medical Services ATP Tour, Rehab Plus Sports Therapy Scottsdale, Scottsdale, AZ, USA
e-mail: todd.ellenbecker@atptour.com

K. E. Wilk
Associate Clinical Director, Champion Sports Medicine, A Select Medical Facility, Birmingham, AL, USA

Vice President of Clinical Education & Research, Select Medical, Birmingham, AL, USA

Director Rehabilitative Research, American Sports Medicine Institute, Birmingham, AL, USA

L. Macrina
Co-Founder and Director of Physical Therapy, Champion PT & Performance, Waltham, MA, USA

J. S. Dines et al. (eds.), *Elbow Ulnar Collateral Ligament Injury*,
https://doi.org/10.1007/978-3-030-69567-5_36

parameters that will form the later part of this chapter. These are the most commonly considered characteristics/definitions of sport-specific rehabilitation and also the less commonly discussed and possibly most important part of sport-specific rehabilitation [5]. The most commonly considered characteristic is that of sport simulation or preparation of the athlete for their activity by focusing on the specific musculature, joint positions, angular velocities, and ultimately simulation of the loads and forces encountered in their particular sport during the rehabilitation process. An example would be the use of a 90° abducted medicine ball bounce drill that simulates the 90/90 position of arm cocking and early acceleration imparting controlled valgus loads to the medial aspect of the elbow (Fig. 36.1). This exercise specifically mimics the sport activity of throwing as well as replicates to some extent the valgus and extension loads on the elbow. This is a very important part of the process and one that is discussed more in this chapter.

The second and often less commonly discussed part of sport specificity actually focuses not specifically on simulation of the actual movement or skill activity but rather on the musculature and movement patterns that emphasize the stabilizing and controlling aspects that are required for proper deceleration and neuromuscular control of the patient's sport activity. An example of this would entail the use of an eccentric deceleration drill with the arm in the 90/90 position focusing on a catch of the ball thrown from behind the patient that results in an eccentric posterior rotator cuff activation and an actual backward throw after deceleration (i.e., it does not simulate the actual throw used in baseball but rather the opposite of the typical throwing response to improve posterior rotator cuff activation; Fig. 36.2). Through the use of this type of complimentary exercise, the rehabilitation specialist is actually addressing the need for stabilizing and muscular control and also providing in this case increased posterior rotator cuff activation and strengthening to a patient population that characteristically has imbalances in the external and internal shoulder rotation strength ratio [6–8]. Both parts of sport-specific rehabilitation will be discussed and are critically important parts of the comprehensive rehabilitation program following UCL reconstruction as well.

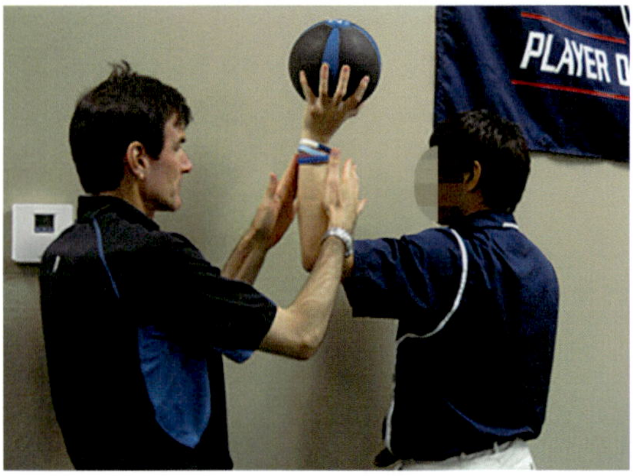

Fig. 36.1 A 90/90 internal rotation plyometric drill with rhythmic stabilization

Kinetic Chain Rehabilitation

Steindler [9] defined the kinetic chain as a "combination of several successively arranged joints constituting a complex motor unit." In rehabilitation, we are completely aware that elbow rehabilitation cannot focus solely on the ulnohumeral articulation but must globally include segments both proximal and distal to the injured elbow [10, 11]. This complementary chapter to the one previous (Wilk et al. Chap. 27) provides greater detail on rehabilitation techniques for the entire upper extremity kinetic chain as well as some core and truly sport-specific exercises that can be included in the rehabilitation process for the patient following UCL reconstruction.

Proximal Upper Extremity Focus

To allow patients to return to full activity following UCL reconstruction requires rehabilitation of the entire upper extremity kinetic chain. Early in the rehabilitation process following UCL reconstruction, a proximal focus can be undertaken to improve scapular stabilization and proximal strength. The challenge for the clinician is to ensure that loads are minimized to protect the healing graft in the medial elbow. Careful attention to eliminate valgus loads to the elbow is followed; however, many proximal exercise progressions can be used to ensure early activation of the scapu-

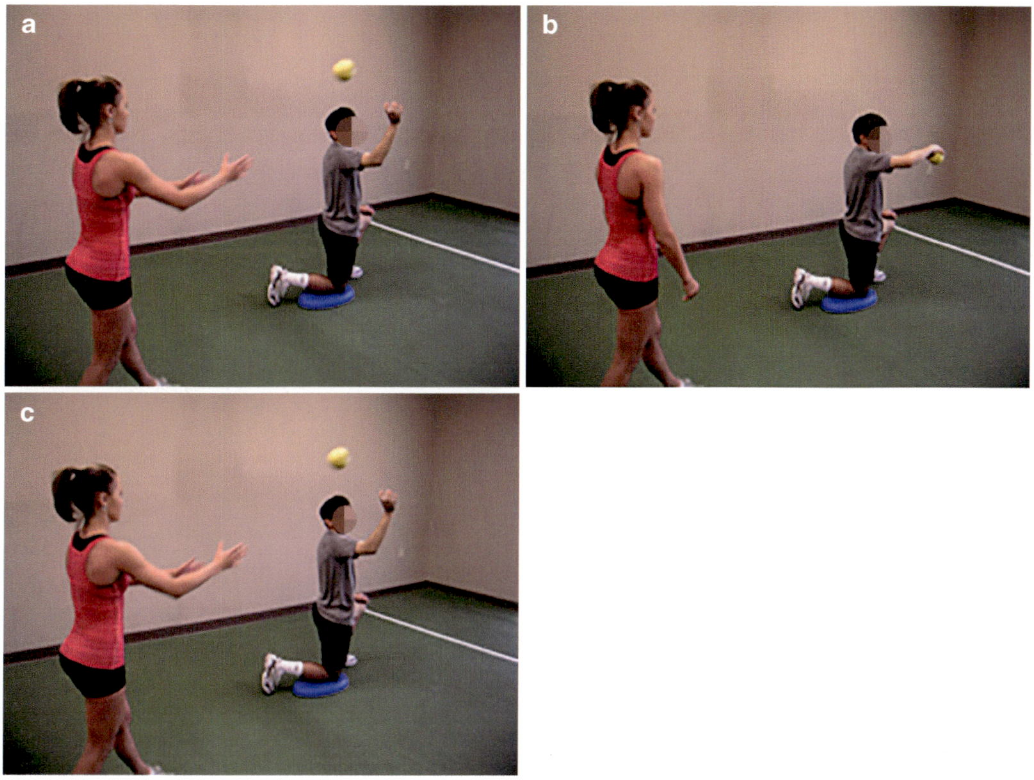

Fig. 36.2 (**a–c**) A 90/90 reverse toss plyometric drill for posterior rotator cuff strengthening

lothoracic and rotator cuff musculature without elbow loading. Exercises such as the dynamic isometric scapular retraction exercise using scapular strap (Fig. 36.3), manual scapular protraction, and retraction resistance provided by the therapist (Fig. 36.4) with direct scapular contacts, which create scapular activation without elbow loading, are recommended. Figure 36.5 shows a serratus punch exercise allowing for serratus anterior activation without elbow loading or movement [12]. Many exercises such as these can be used to facilitate muscular activation of the scapular muscles and can be applied early in the rehabilitation process to address the common finding of scapular dyskinesis in throwing athletes [13, 14]. An extended focus on this region during rehabilitation is an example of sport-specific rehabilitation necessitated by the common finding of scapular dyskinesis in the overhead athlete. Additional exercises outlined by Kibler and colleagues [15] including the robbery, low row, and lawn mower exercise are also important early inclusions in a kinetic chain rehabilitation program.

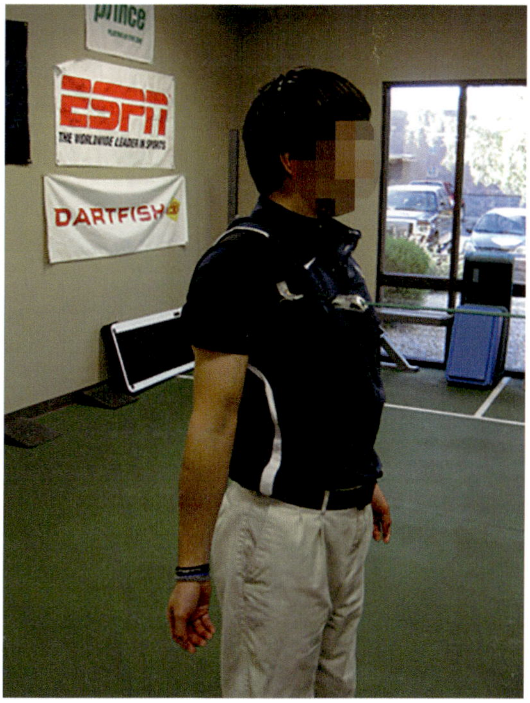

Fig. 36.3 Scapular retraction walk back isometrics with elastic resistance

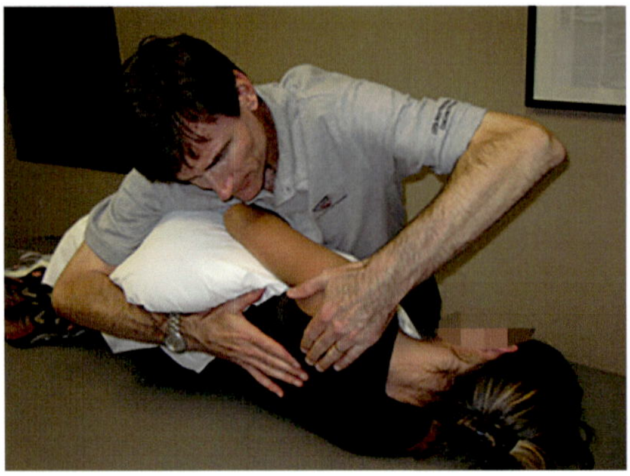

Fig. 36.4 Manual scapular retraction provided by a physical therapist

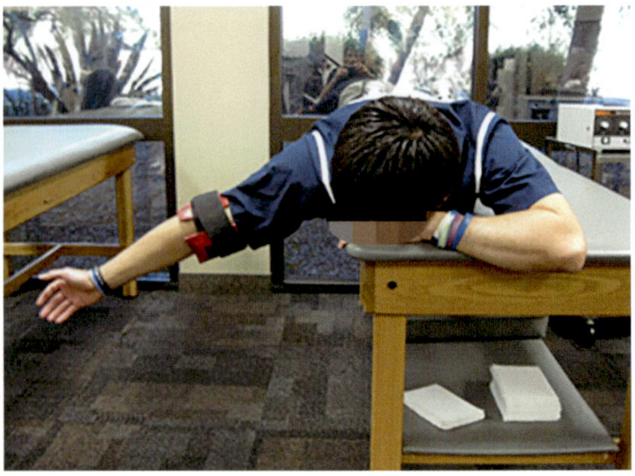

Fig. 36.6 Horizontal abduction for posterior rotator cuff and scapular strengthening with resistance application proximal to the elbow

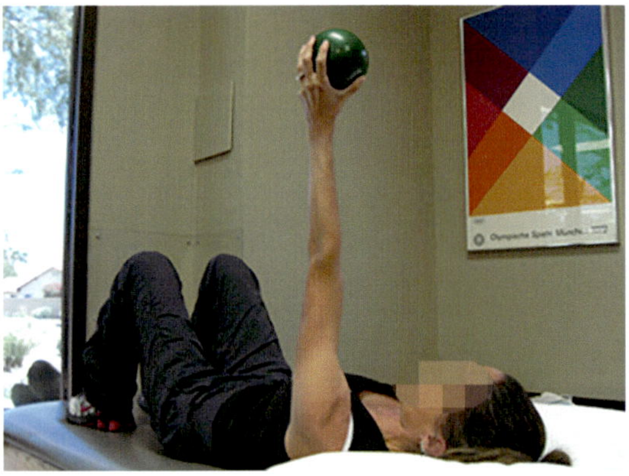

Fig. 36.5 Serratus punch

Exercise for the rotator cuff is also of critical importance. Research has identified modifications and alterations of the normal unilateral external/internal rotation strength ratios with decreased external rotation strength reported in several studies in elite-level throwers [5, 6] and tennis players [16, 17]. Guidelines for inclusion of these exercises include minimization or elimination of elbow loading during early performance through the use of weight application proximal to the ulnohumeral joint. Exercises characterized by high levels of posterior rotator cuff activation including prone horizontal abduction (Fig. 36.6), prone extension [18, 19] in the early phase (weeks 1–6) with the addition of side-lying external rotation, and prone external rotation at 90° abduction are also recommended. Many references exist that cover shoulder rehabilitation with evidence-based exercise progression for the overhead athletes and can serve as a resource for program development following UCL reconstruction [20, 21] .

Sport-specific exercise progressions that can commence in the later stages of rehabilitation (12 weeks) for the overhead athlete following UCL reconstruction with respect to the proximal segments of the upper extremity kinetic chain include isokinetic training of shoulder internal and external rotation (Fig. 36.7) simulating shoulder and elbow positions in the cocking and acceleration phases of the throwing [22] and serving position [23]. Additionally, the shoulder internal rotation portion of this training provided a controlled isokinetically resisted valgus load to the elbow while supported in 90° of elbow flexion in preparation for a return to throwing. To provide greater levels of co-contraction and neuromuscular control, Wilk et al. [24] have recommended advanced throwers ten exercises. One example extremely relevant for the proximal aspect of the upper extremity is the 90/90 external rotation exercise performed with elastic resistance (Fig. 36.8). This is a prime example of the integration of sport-specific positioning and movement patterns coupled with a kinetic chain focus to improve or normalize muscular strength ratios in the shoulder and scapular region of the overhead athlete.

Core and Hip Stabilization of the Overhead Athlete

As mentioned earlier in this chapter, a global, whole body, kinetic chain focus to rehabilitation following UCL reconstruction is recommended [24]. Another key area in addition to early work on the posterior rotator cuff and scapular stabilizers is hip and core strengthening. While it is beyond the scope of this chapter to completely cover these important concepts, it must be emphasized and discussed in any chapter on sport-specific training and rehabilitation for the throwing athlete. The role of the core musculature has been eloquently documented in electromyography (EMG) research showing critically important sequential activation patterns during both the throwing [25] and batting [26] as well as tennis serve [27] functional movement patterns. Early and continual focus on these muscle groups is of paramount importance as an adjunct to the more primary rehabilitation methods utilized during rehab following UCL reconstruction (Chap. 27 , Wilk et al.).

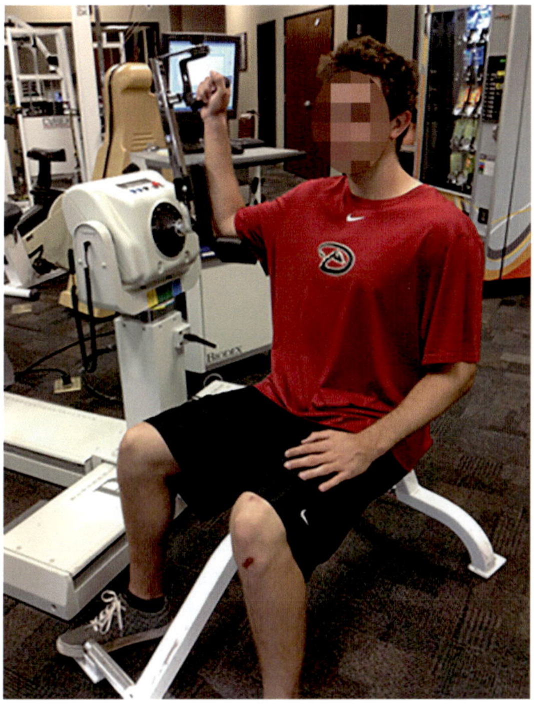

Fig. 36.7 Isokinetic internal/external rotation training in 90° of abduction and 90° of elbow flexion

Many athletes training for sport employ a wide array of sport-specific functional exercises to develop core muscles and enhance core stability. The "core" has been referred to as the lumbopelvic-hip complex, involving the deeper muscles, such as the internal oblique, transversus abdominis, transversospinalis (multifidus, rotatores, semispinalis), quadratus lumborum, and psoas major and minor, and the superficial muscles, such as the rectus abdominis, external oblique, erector spinae (iliocostalis, spinalis, longissimus), latissimus dorsi, gluteus maximus and medius, hamstrings, and rectus femoris [28–30]. We personally consider the core from the supe-

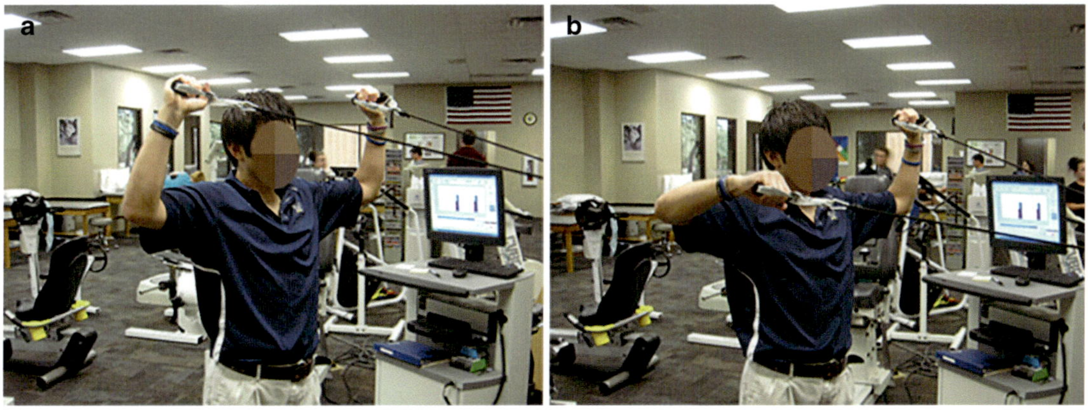

Fig. 36.8 A 90/90 sustained hold external rotation with elastic resistance. (**a**) Start position, bilateral shoulders hold contraction in 90° of external rotation while (**b**) R extremity does dynamic concentric and eccentric contractions of internal and external rotation. Exercise reverses when L shoulder does dynamic movements and R shoulder holds the contraction

rior aspect of the scapula all the way down to pelvis including the proximal hamstrings and quads. This is especially true when training the posterior column of the spine and body. Core muscle development is believed to be important in many functional and athletic activities because core muscle recruitment should enhance core stability and help provide proximal stability to facilitate distal mobility. For optimal core stability, both the smaller deeper core muscles and the larger superficial core muscles must contract in sequence with appropriate timing and tension [31, 32]. Enhanced stability and neuromuscular control of the lumbopelvic-hip complex has been shown to decrease the risk of athletic injuries [33]. Core muscle weakness and deficits in neuromuscular trunk control can increase the injury risk to the trunk and extremities [33]. There are a variety of core exercises employed by athletes to enhance core stability [34–36]. Table 36.1 outlines the characteristic muscle activations during the performance of recommended core exercise progressions followed by a list of basic and core exercises that can be included in any sport-specific rehabilitation program for the throwing athlete. Figures 36.9, 36.10, 36.11, 36.12, and 36.13 display commonly used core exercises that have been studied with EMG demonstrating high activation levels of the core musculature and are recommended for inclusion in the comprehensive rehabilitation programs for overhead athletes following UCL injury. Despite the injured or post-operative segment located in the elbow, these core exercises can form a critically important part of the overall program. Early considerations for these exercises include the use of supine exercise for core activation with no weight bearing or loading of the elbow or upper extremity segments. Progression to exercises with upper extremity weight bearing such as the plank progressions and Swiss ball pikes involves upper extremity loading and can be added in the intermediate and advanced stages of the rehab process to further challenge the core but also place gradually increasing levels of upper extremity loading through the ulnohumeral joint.

The inclusion of these exercises in a UCL rehabilitation program for the injured thrower ensures that attention and focus is generated to the additional segments of the body's kinetic chain.

Glenohumeral Joint Range of Motion

In addition to the attention focused on the elbow, wrist, and forearm for range of motion and mobilization following UCL reconstruction, it is recommended that evaluation and treatment of shoulder range of motion be performed. Use of a technique to measure glenohumeral joint internal and external rotation in the supine position with the scapula stabilized is of critical importance [37, 38] (Fig. 36.14). A "C" shaped stabilization method placing the thumb on the coracoid process and fingers posteriorly along the scapula provides optimal stabilization of the scapula to ensure accurate and reliable measurement of glenohumeral joint internal rotation [37]. Findings of reduced internal rotation range of motion and reduced total rotation range of motion (sum of internal and external rotation) compared to the contralateral uninjured extremity necessitate the use of stretches to improve internal rotation range of motion. Losses of as little as 12° of internal rotation and 5° of total rotation range of motion have been related to shoulder injury in professional baseball pitchers [39]. Additionally, Dines et al. [40] have identified internal rotation deficits in professional baseball pitchers with the UCL injury. This important finding shows the relation between proximal shoulder range of motion and stress to the UCL.

Methods used and recommended to improve internal rotation range of motion include use of the sleeper stretch [41–43] and cross arm stretch [43, 44], as well as clinical methods performed by physical therapists and athletic trainers such as internal rotation positions with scapular stabilization at 90° of glenohumeral joint abduction (Fig. 36.15).

Table 36.1 Relative muscle recruitment of the trunk, upper extremity, and lower extremity musculature in swiss ball exercises versus traditional sit-up and crunch

	Upper and lower rectus abdominal muscles	External and internal oblique muscles	Upper extremity muscles	Low back muscles[a]	Lower extremity muscles
Greatest recruitment (>60% MVIC)	Pike, rollout	Pike, knee-up, skier	Decline push-up, rollout	Pike, hip extension right	Hip extension left
Intermediate recruitment (31–60% MVIC)	Knee-up, skier, hip extension right, hip extension left, decline push-up, crunch, bent knee sit-up	Rollout, hip extension right, hip extension left, decline push-up, crunch, bent knee sit-up	Pike, knee-up, skier, hip extension right, hip extension left	Knee-up, skier, hip extension left, decline push-up, bent knee sit-up, rollout	Sitting march right, skier, knee-up, pike, bent knee sit-up
Least recruitment (0–30% MVIC)	Sitting march right	Sitting march right	Sitting march right, crunch, bent knee sit-up	Sitting march right, crunch	Crunch, rollout, hip extension right, decline push-up
Core training progression: basic to advanced					
I. Basic exercises and drills					
Supine straight leg bridges					
Supine bridge					
Supine abdominal bracing					
Planks (prone on elbows)					
Unilateral dumbbell hold					
Side-lying plank					
II. Intermediate and advanced exercises and drills					
Stability ball rollout on elbows					
Supine bridge into hip abduction					
Russian twists					
Side plank with extremity lift (leg and arm alternating)					
Side plank with shoulder external rotator (ER) with dumbbell					
Unilateral stance on balance pad with elastic-resisted abduction/flexion/extension kicks					

[a]*MVIC* maximum voluntary isometric contraction

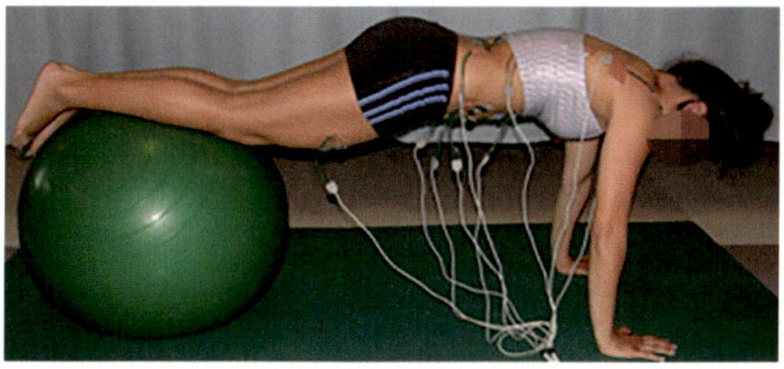

Fig. 36.9 Starting position for the pike, knee-up, skier, decline push-up, hip extension right, and hip extension left

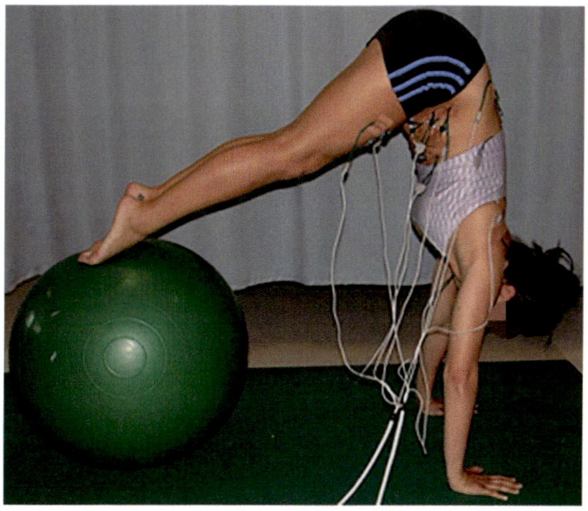

Fig. 36.10 Ending position for the pike

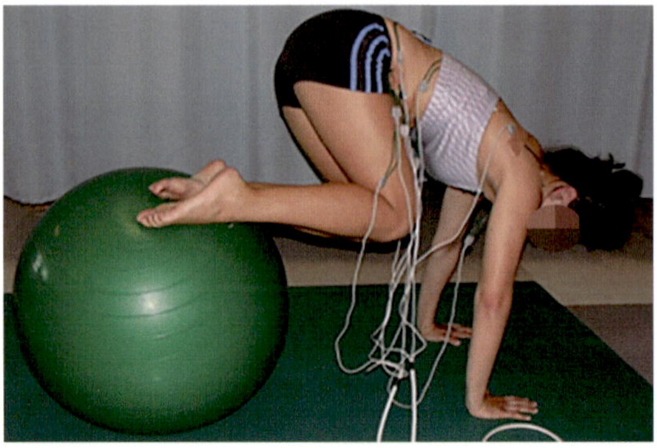

Fig. 36.11 Ending position for the skier

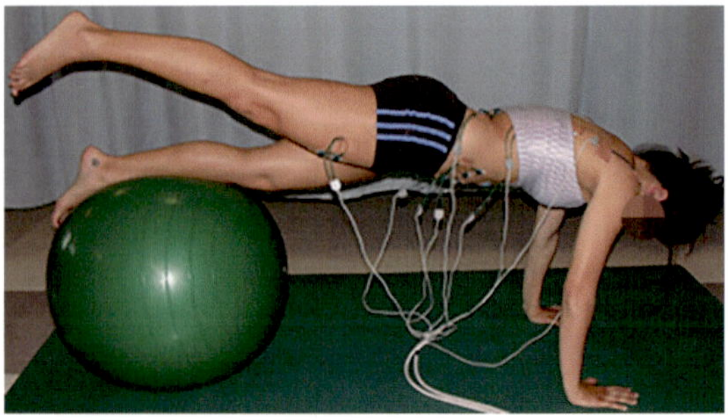

Fig. 36.12 Ending position for the hip extension

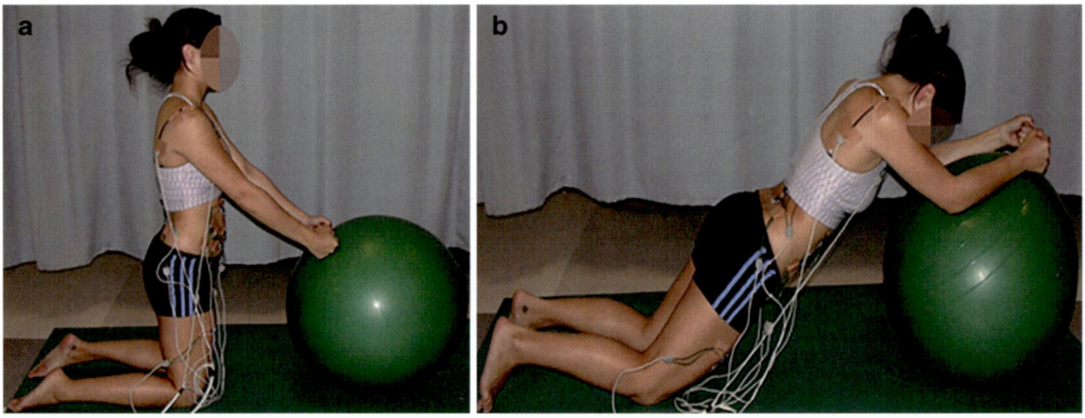

Fig. 36.13 Starting position for the rollout (**a**) and ending position for the rollout (**b**)

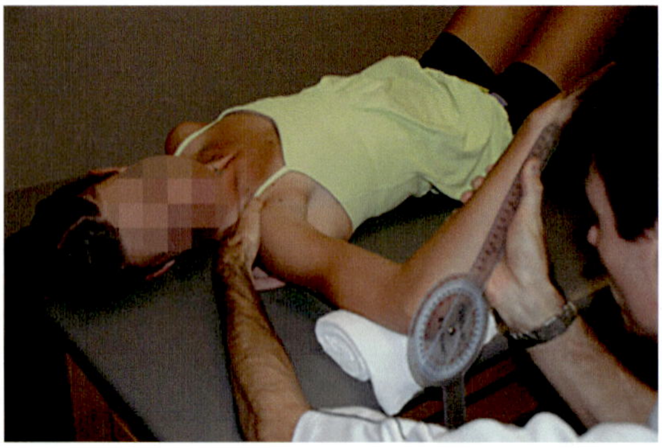

Fig. 36.14 Internal rotation range of motion measurement with scapular stabilization

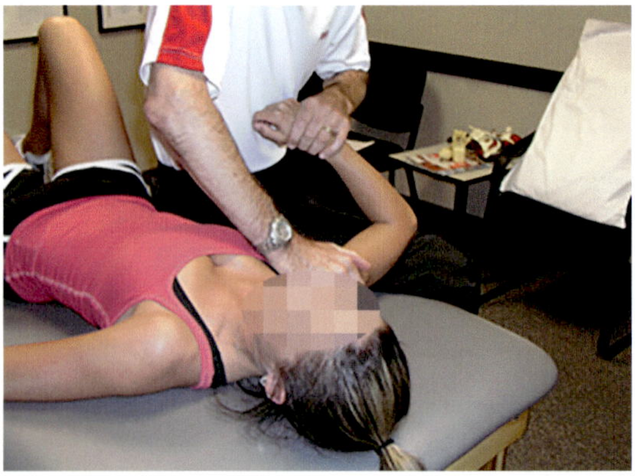

Fig. 36.15 Isolated posterior shoulder stretch with 90° of elevation and scapular stabilization

Functional Activity Progressions (Plyometrics)

One final area of progression to discuss prior to the actual return to sport programs is the use of functional activity progression based on sport-specific rehabilitation training principles. In these exercises, care is taken to simulate and prepare the athlete for the stresses and joint angular velocities that a return to their sport or functional activity will demand. These functional progressions take place after the return of proximal stabilization, and normalized range of motion relationships have been restored. Progression from initially no load (rapid motions) to the use of medicine balls to provide overload is followed.

Throwing Progressions Following UCL Reconstruction

The use of the 90° abducted glenohumeral position is important to simulate the throwing motion. Exercises initially geared at normalizing the external/internal rotator (ER/IR) muscular strength ratio and providing overload to the posterior rotator cuff and scapular musculature are pictured in Figs. 36.2 and 36.16 and form a precursor to the internal-rotation-based exercises with valgus overload in Figs. 36.17 and 36.18. Carter et al. [45] have shown that these posterior rotator cuff exercises when coupled with elastic resistance training can provide improvements in concentric and eccentric internal and external rotation strength in addition to increasing throwing velocity. Additionally, the use of the "towel drill" is recommended to provide simulation of throwing with a small distal load encountered at impact of the towel with the glove of the therapist (Fig. 36.19).

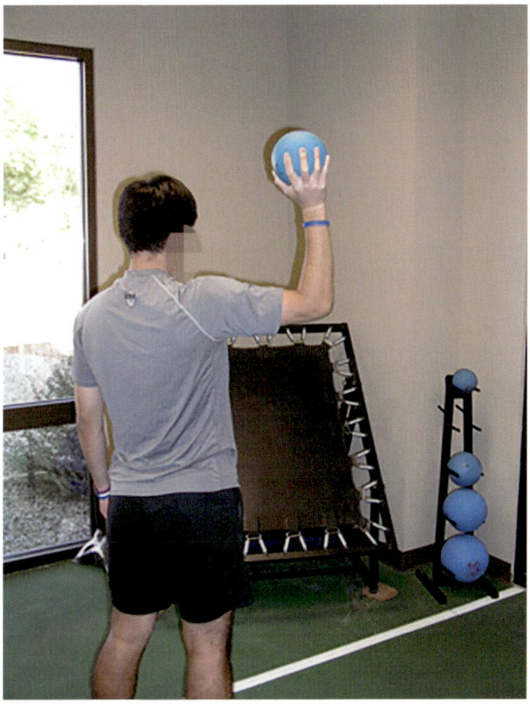

Fig. 36.17 Internal rotation plyo on plyo-back trampoline

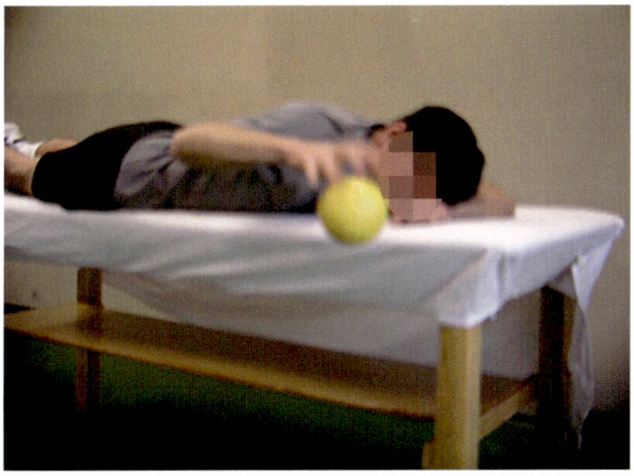

Fig. 36.16 A 90/90 ball drop prone plyometric

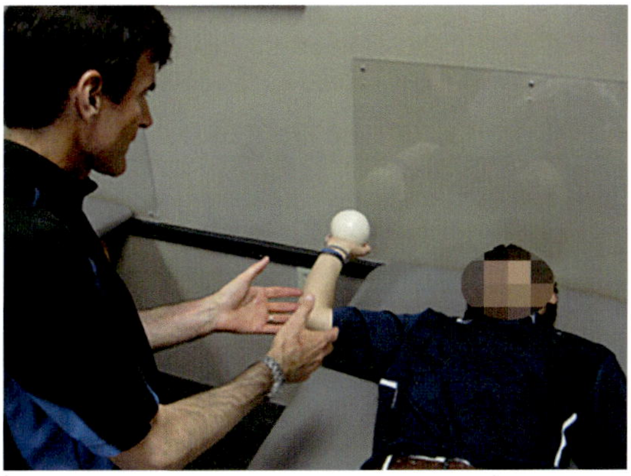

Fig. 36.18 Internal rotation plyo performed in supine position with medicine ball

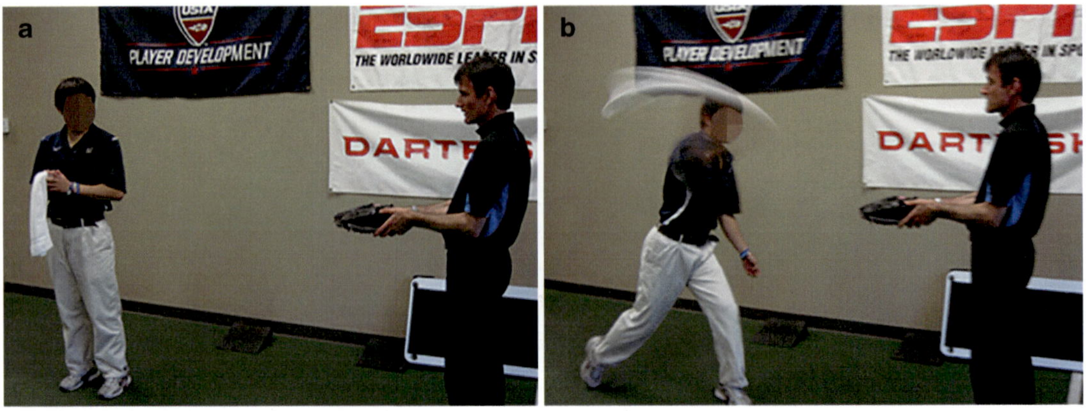

Fig. 36.19 Towel drill: (**a**) start position and (**b**) acceleration with goal of snapping towel against glove held by therapist

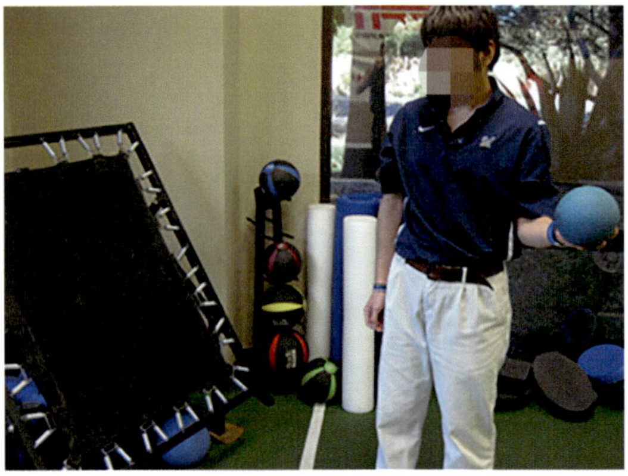

Fig. 36.20 Internal rotation plyometric (arm at side)

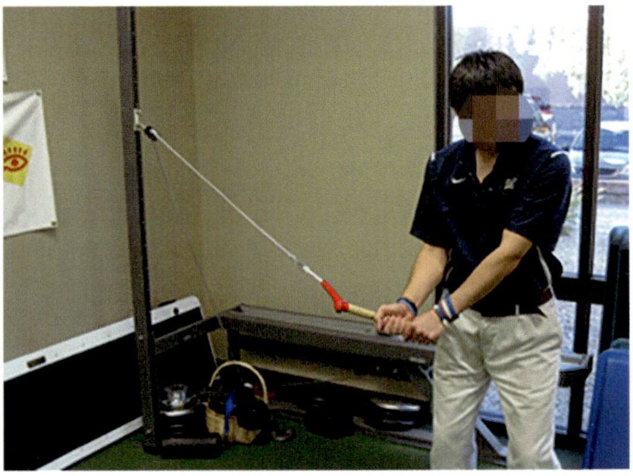

Fig. 36.21 Impulse batting simulation overload drill

Batting Progressions Following UCL Reconstruction

Less attention is often focused on the return to batting following UCL reconstruction. Typically, a progression from swinging without ball contact, to hitting off a tee, followed by soft toss, and then finally facing a live pitcher in batting practice is recommended and followed [46]. Clinically, medicine balls can be used to load trunk rotation off a plyo-back device in addition to simulating valgus loading with the shoulder in more neutral positions of elevation at the side (Fig. 36.20). Additional preparation for batting can be afforded by the use of either elastic or isoinertial devices such as the Impulse (Impulse Inc., Noonan Georgia) where rapid simulation of the batting sequence can be resisted (Fig. 36.21).

Golf Progression Following UCL Reconstruction

Large populations of golfers are not included in many reviews of athletes who suffer UCL injury [1]; however, the trail arm (right arm in a right-handed golfer) can be subjected to medially based loading during the acceleration and contact phases of the golf swing [47]. As such, patients returning to golf would benefit from many of the

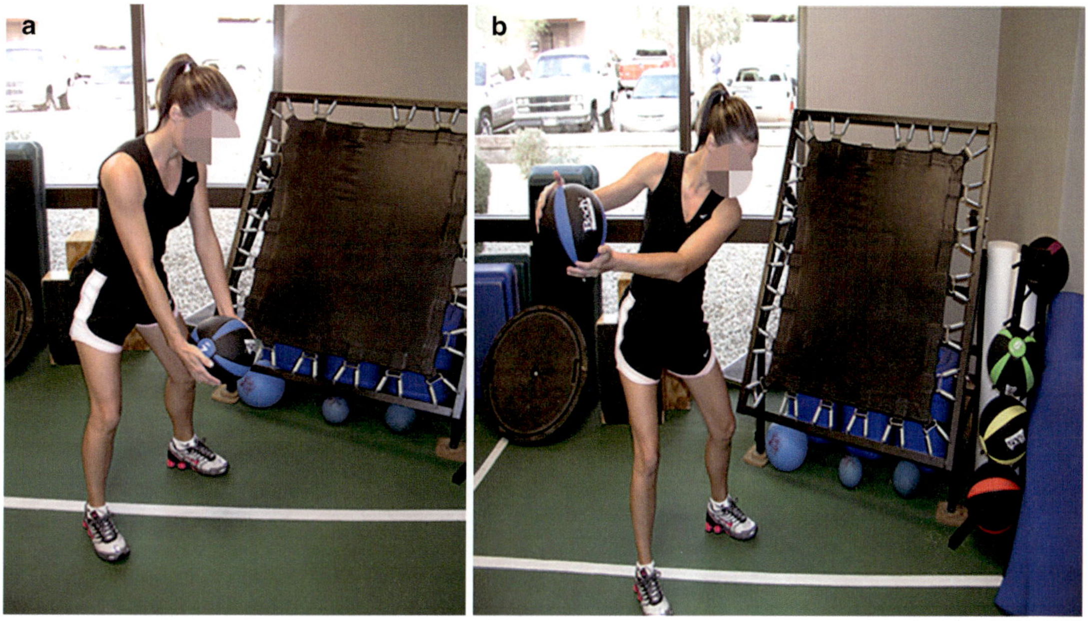

Fig. 36.22 (**a**, **b**) Golf plyo

progressions listed earlier in the batting section. Additionally, the specific characteristics of the golf swing such as a straighter arm at impact compared to batting in baseball, etc., would necessitate the use of more sport-specific applications such as the golf plyometric (Fig. 36.22). Following a return to golf program, such as the one listed in Table 36.2, is recommended to ensure gradual loads are imparted to the medial aspect of the elbow during the return to sport phase of rehabilitation [48].

Tennis Progression Following UCL Reconstruction

UCL injuries are reported in tennis players [1] with both similar valgus loads and elbow flexion positions inherent in the serve and overhand throwing motion [49], as well as unique loading characteristics on the elbow in the forehand and backhand groundstrokes [50]. Similar progressions are followed for serving in tennis players to the material presented in the 90° abducted position with the plyo balls for the throwing athlete. Additionally, to promote coactivation and muscular fatigue both proximally and distally, the statue of liberty exercise (Fig. 36.23) can be used with the oscillation afforded by the flex bar (Thera-band, Performance Health, Akron, OH) with overpressure in both the direction of external rotation (a) and internal rotation (b) to selectively load the medial and lateral aspects of the elbow and provide greater overload for the posterior rotator cuff. Additionally, the use of plyometric groundstroke simulations with alternating patterns of forehand and backhand to challenge foot work and lower extremity movement patterning is highly recommended (Fig. 36.24).

Use of an interval tennis program is also recommended with a more gradual introduction of the forehand groundstroke and greater initial use of the backhand and backhand volley due to smaller medially based loads on the elbow [50] as compared to forehands and forehand volleys. The interval tennis program displayed in Table 36.3 has been modified from other versions previously published [48, 51] for shoulder and nonligamentous injury of the elbow. In addition to the interval tennis program, careful introduction of loading is recommended and can easily be accomplished through the use of foam and low-

Table 36.2 Interval golf program

	Day 1	Day 2	Day 3
Week 1	10 putts	15 putts	20 putts
	10 chips	15 chips	20 chips
	Rest	Rest	Rest
	15 chips	25 chips	20 putts
			20 chips/rest
			10 chips
			10 short irons
Week 2	20 chips	20 chips	15 short irons
	10 short irons	15 short irons	10 medium irons
	Rest	Rest	Rest
	10 short irons	10 short irons	20 short irons
		15 chips	15 chips
Week 3	15 short irons	15 short irons	15 short irons
	10 medium irons/rest	10 medium irons	10 medium irons
	5 long irons	10 long irons/rest	10 long irons/rest
	15 short irons	10 short irons	10 short irons
	Rest	10 medium irons	10 medium irons
	20 chips	5 long irons	10 long irons
		5 woods (off tee)	10 woods (off tee)
Week 4	15 short irons	Play 9 holes	Play 9 holes
	10 medium irons		
	10 long irons		
	10 drives (off tee)		
	Rest/repeat above		
Week 5	Play 9 holes	Play 9 holes	Play 18 holes

Key to golf program: chips = pitching wedge; short irons = W, 9, 8; medium irons = 7, 6, 5; long irons = 4, 3, 2; woods = 3, 5; drives = driver

(1) Always monitor and analyze the mechanics of your golf swing. It may be important to have your swing analyzed by a certified teaching professional to optimize your mechanics and minimize injury risk.

(2) Allow one day of rest after each hitting session to facilitate recovery.

(3) It is important to complete each stage of the program without pain before progressing to the next step.

(4) Minor discomfort is expected with the initiation of the return to golf-interval program; this minor discomfort should be intermittent and golf activity and progression should be stopped, if pain is present during the swing or following any stage of the golf program.

(5) If pain and or swelling persists, discontinue the program until examined by a medical professional. Resume the program at the last step preceding the offending stage.

Adapted from Reinold et al. [46]

compression balls used in junior tennis player development programs (Fig. 36.25).

Emphasis on Proper Mechanics

One final area to discuss of importance in all sport-specific rehabilitation programs is the use of proper sport biomechanics. This most important element is often neglected in many rehabilitation programs and can lead to nonoptimal results and reinjury/reaggravation following an otherwise successful reconstruction of the UCL. To illustrate this concept and show the role of other body segments and their effect on the shoulder and elbow during the tennis serve, the results of research by Elliott et al. will be presented [52]. Elliott et al. measured kinetic and kinematic variables of the serve in professional tennis players and characterized them as having either an effective "leg drive" (front knee flexion angle greater than 14.7°) or an ineffective leg drive (maximal front knee flexion less than 14.7°). Most important from an injury prevention

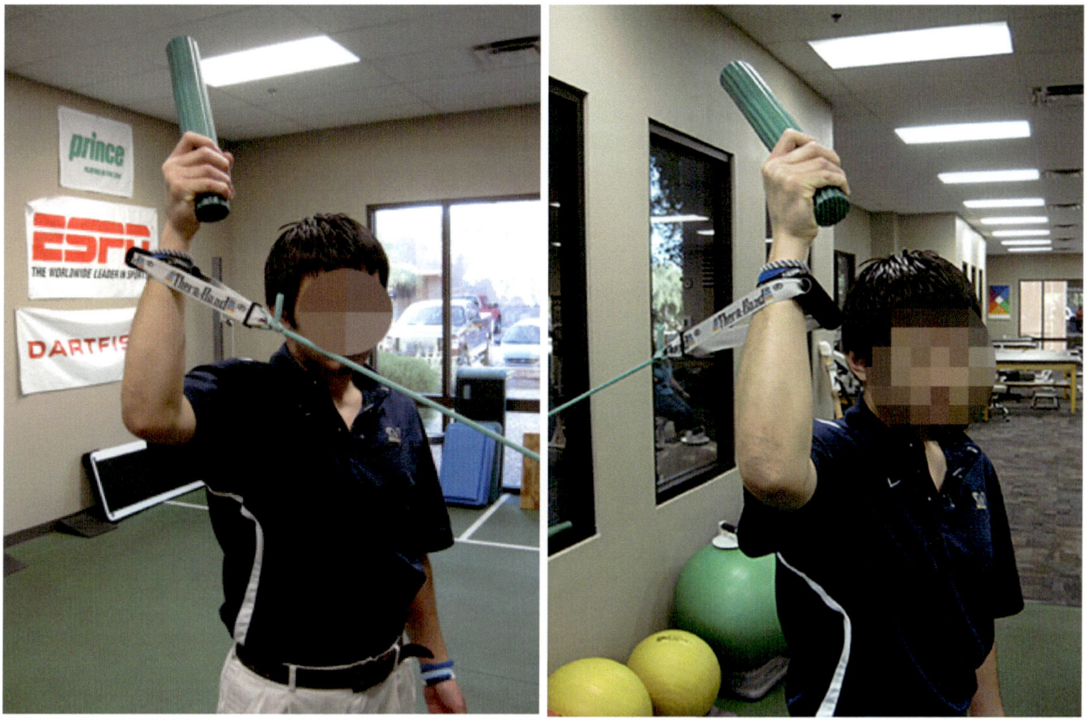

Fig. 36.23 Statue of liberty oscillation exercise: (**a**) external rotation overload and (**b**) internal rotation overload

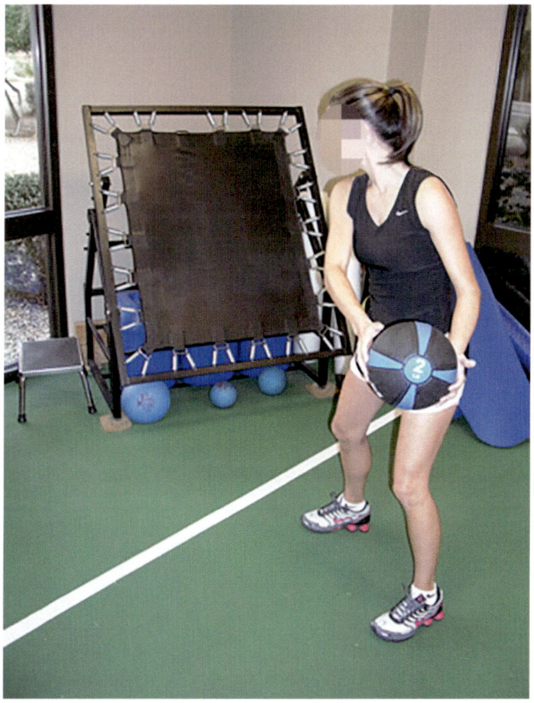

Fig. 36.24 Tennis groundstroke plyometric

risk was the finding in this study of significantly greater medial elbow loading (varus elbow torque 3.9 vs. 5.3%) when comparing the group with greater knee flexion to the group with less knee flexion, respectively [52]. Additionally, the group with a more effective leg drive showed reduced shoulder internal rotation torques when the shoulder was placed in maximal external rotation than the group of elite players who had less leg drive during their serving motion [52]. This study shows the importance of the use of the entire kinetic chain to produce power during the tennis serve and highlights the ramifications of utilizing a pattern of serving biomechanics for the shoulder elbow when the lower extremity and trunk are not optimally integrated.

Additional research was published by Marshall et al. [53] who used a direct linear transformation (DLT) algorithm with eight markers to study the tennis serve of elite players. Using a simulation of delaying internal rotation of the humerus in the mechanical sequence of proximal to distal events, they produced a simulated load

Table 36.3 Modified interval tennis program for patients following UCL reconstruction or medially based elbow injury

Interval tennis program guidelines
Begin at stage indicated by your physical therapist or doctor.
Do not progress or continue program if medial elbow pain is present.
Always stretch your shoulder, elbow, and wrist before and after the interval program, and perform a whole-body dynamic warm-up prior to performing the interval tennis program.
Play on alternate days, giving your body a recovery day between sessions.
Do not use a wallboard or back board as it leads to exaggerated muscle.
Contraction without rest between strokes. Ball feeds or a ball machine are preferred.
Ice your injured arm after each session of the interval tennis program.
It is highly recommended to have your stroke mechanics formally evaluated by a qualified United States Professional Tennis Association (USPTA) tennis teaching professional.
Do not attempt to impart heavy topspin to your groundstrokes until later stages in the interval program.
Contact your therapist or doctor if you have questions or problems with the interval program.
Do not continue to play if you encounter localized medial elbow joint pain.
Interval tennis program:
Perform each stage ________ times before progressing to the next stage. Do not progress to the next stage if you have pain or excessive fatigue on your previous outing; remain at the previous stage until you can perform that part of the program without fatigue or pain.
Stage 1
(a) Have a partner feed 20 backhand groundstrokes to you from the net using a foam tennis ball. (Partner must use a slow, looping feed that results in a waist high ball bounce for player contact.)
(b) Have a partner feed 20 forehand groundstrokes as in stage 1a above with a foam tennis ball.
(c) Rest 5 min.
(d) Repeat 20 backhand feeds as above.
Stage 2
Repeat stage 1 with a low-compression tennis ball (i.e., International Tennis Federation, ITF orange ball). (See Fig. 36.25 for tennis ball varieties used during interval tennis programs.)
Stage 3
Repeat stage 1 with a real (regulation) tennis ball.
Stage 4
(a) Begin as in stage 3 above, with partner feeding 30 backhands and 10 forehands from the net as a warm-up.
(b) Rally with partner from baseline, hitting controlled groundstrokes until you have hit 50–60 strokes. (Alternate between forehands and backhands and allow 20–30 s rest after every 2–3 rallies.) Attempt to hit more backhands than forehands (3:1 ratio on average) to provide a more gradual stress to the medial elbow.
(c) Rest 5 min.
(d) Repeat the rally instructions in "b" above.
Stage 5
(a) Rally groundstrokes (forehands and backhands) from the baseline for 15 min.
(b) Rest 5 min.
(c) Hit 20–25 backhand and 10–15 forehand volleys, emphasizing a contact point in front of your body.
(d) Rally groundstrokes for 15 additional minutes from the baseline.
(e) Hit another 10–15 forehand and backhand volleys as listed above.
Pre-serve interval: (perform prior to stage 6)
(Note. This can be performed off court and is meant solely to determine readiness for progression into stage 6 of the interval tennis program.)
(a) After stretching with racquet in hand, perform serving motion for 10–15 repetitions without a ball or any ball contact.
(b) Using a foam ball, hit 10–15 serves without concern for performance result (only focusing on form, contact point, and the presence or absence of symptoms).
(c) If successful and pain-free, progress to stage 6.
Stage 6
(a) Hit 20–30 min of groundstrokes, mixing in volleys using an 80% groundstroke/20% volley format.
(b) Perform 5–10 simulated serves without a ball.

Table 36.3 (continued)

(c) Perform 5–10 serves using a foam ball.
(d) Perform 10–15 serves using a standard tennis ball at approximately 75% effort. (Note: It is important to hit flat or slice serves not kick serves in the initial phase of the interval tennis program.)
(e) Finish with 10–15 min of groundstrokes.
Stage 7
(a) Hit 30 min of groundstrokes, mixing in volleys using an 80% groundstroke/20% volley format.
(b) Perform 5–10 serves using a foam ball.
(c) Perform 10–15 serves using a standard tennis ball at approximately 75% effort.
(d) Rest 5 min.
(e) Perform 10–15 additional serves as in "d" above.
(f) Finish with 15–20 min of groundstrokes.
Stage 8
(a) Repeat stage 7 listed above increasing the number of serves to 20–25 instead of 10–15.
(b) Before resting between serving sessions, have a partner feed easy short lobs to attempt 4–5 controlled overheads.
Stage 9
Prior to attempting match play, complete steps 1–8 without pain or excess fatigue in the upper extremity. Continue to progress the amount of time rallying with groundstrokes and volleys in addition to increasing the number of serves per workout until 60–80 overall serves can be performed interspersed throughout a workout. Initiate kick serves once the initial stages of the program have been completed. Remember that an average of up to 120 serves can be performed in a singles tennis match; therefore, be prepared to gradually increase the number of serves in the interval program before full competitive play is engaged.

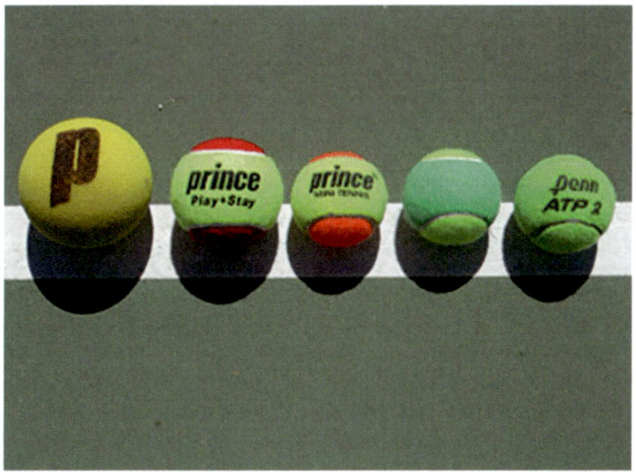

Fig. 36.25 Tennis ball progression (foam, low compression, and regulation)

that was characterized by 53% greater varus torque (valgus load) at the elbow. This simulation was meant to produce a mechanical pattern similar to the one used when the arm lags behind the body similar to hyperangulation and internal rotation of the humerus is delayed in the upper extremity sequence. This rapid humeral internal rotation required to "catch up" resulted in substantially higher medial elbow (valgus loading). These examples are meant to support the need for careful and appropriate biomechanical analysis of the patient's sport performance to ensure proper load sharing by other segments in the kinetic chain as well as proper sequencing and positioning of all segments of the kinetic chain. While the use of high-level biomechanical analysis is optimal, it is not practical in many clinical or nonresearch settings, Davis et al. [54] have shown how visual observation and/or two-dimensional filming can provide meaningful feedback and identification of common flaws in the throwing/pitching motion of young athletes. This important part of the rehabilitation is emphasized and recommended by the authors of this chapter.

Summary

This chapter has provided a review of sport-specific rehabilitation and training principles and contains recommended rehabilitation progressions and kinetic chain interventions for the core, scapula, and glenohumeral regions that are integral parts of a comprehensive rehabilitation program for the patient following UCL reconstructions. Coupled with the protocols, guidelines, and specific rehabilitation interventions in the preceding chapter, these suggested interventions and areas of emphasis can ensure that a comprehensive rehabilitation program is provided for patients following UCL reconstruction.

References

1. Vitale MA, Ahmad CS. The outcome of elbow ulnar collateral ligament reconstruction in overhead athletes. Am J Sports Med. 2008;36(6):1193–205.
2. Waris W. Elbow injuries in javelin throwers. Acta Chir Scand. 1946;93:563–75.
3. Reiman MP, Manske RC. The assessment of function: how is it measured? A clinical perspective. J Man Manip Ther. 2011;19(2):91–9.
4. Verstegen M, Falsone S, Orr R, Smith S. Suggestions from the field for the return to sports participation following anterior cruciate ligament reconstruction: American football. J Orthop Sports Phys Ther. 2012;42(4):337–44.
5. Ellenbecker TS, DeCarlo M, DeRosa C. Effective functional progressions in sport rehabilitation. Champaign: Human Kinetics; 2009.
6. Ellenbecker TS, Mattalino AJ. Concentric isokinetic shoulder internal and external rotation strength in professional baseball pitchers. J Orthop Sports Phys Ther. 1997;25(5):323–8.
7. Wilk KE, Andrews JR, Arrigo CA, Keirns MA, Erber DJ. The strength characteristics of internal and external rotator muscles in professional baseball pitchers. Am J Sports Med. 1993;21:61–6.
8. Byram IR, Bushnell BD, Dugger K, Charron K, Harrell FE, Noonan TJ. Preseason shoulder strength measurements in professional baseball pitchers. Identifying players at risk for injury. Am J Sports Med. 2010;38(7):1375–82.
9. Steindler A. Kinesiology of the human body. Charles C Thomas: Springfield; 1955.
10. Ellenbecker TS, Mattalino AJ. The elbow in sport. Champaign: Human Kinetics; 1997.
11. Ellenbecker TS, Nirschl RP, Renstrom P. Current concepts in examination and treatment of elbow tendon injury. Sports Health. 2013;5(2):186–94.
12. Donatelli RA, Ekstrom RA, Soderberg GL. Surface electromyographic analysis of exercises for the trapezius and serratus anterior muscles. J Orthop Sports Phys Ther. 2003;33(5):247–58.
13. Oyama S, Myers JB, Wassinger CA, Daniel Ricci R, Lephart SM. Asymmetric resting scapular posture in healthy overhead athletes. J Athl Train. 2008;43(6):565–70.
14. Laudner KG, Myers JB, Pasquale MR, Bradley JP, Lephart SM. Scapular dysfunction in throwers with pathologic internal impingement. J Orthop Sports Phys Ther. 2006;36(7):485–94.
15. Kibler WB, Sciascia AD, Uhl TL, Tambay N, Cunningham T. Electromyographic analysis of specific exercises for scapular control in early phases of shoulder rehabilitation. Am J Sports Med. 2008;36:1789–98.
16. Ellenbecker TS, Roetert EP. Age specific isokinetic glenohumeral internal and external rotation strength in elite junior tennis players. J Sci Med Sport. 2003;6(1):63–70.
17. Ellenbecker TS, Davies GJ. The application of isokinetics in testing and rehabilitation of the shoulder complex. J Athl Train. 2000;35(3):338–50.
18. Reinhold MM, Wilk KE, Fleisig GS, et al. Electromyographic analysis of the rotator cuff and deltoid musculature during common shoulder external rotation exercises. J Orthop Sports Phys Ther. 2004;34(7):385–94.
19. Townsend H, Jobe FW, Pink M, Perry J. Electromyographic analysis of the glenohumeral muscles during a baseball rehabilitation program. Am J Sports Med. 1991;19:264–72.
20. Wilk KE, Obma P, Simpson CD, Cain LE, Dugas JR, Andrews JR. Shoulder injuries in the overhead athlete. J Orthop Sports Phys Ther. 2009;39(2):38–54.
21. Ellenbecker TS, Cools A. Rehabilitation of shoulder impingement syndrome and rotator cuff injuries: an evidence based review. Br J Sports Med. 2010;44:319–27.
22. Fleisig GS, Andrews JR, Dillman CJ, et al. Kinetics of baseball pitching with implications about injury mechanisms. Am J Sports Med. 1995;23:233–9.
23. Kovacs M, Ellenbecker TS. An 8-stage model for evaluating the tennis serve. Implications for performance enhancement and injury prevention. Sports Health. 2011;3(6):504–13.
24. Ellenbecker TS, Wilk KE, Altchek DW, Andrews JR. Current concepts in rehabilitation following ulnar collateral ligament reconstruction. Sports Health. 2009;1:301–13.
25. Watkins RG, Dennis S, Dillin WH, Schnebel B, Schneiderman G, Jobe F, Farfan H, Perry J, Pink M. Dynamic EMG analysis of torque transfer in professional baseball pitchers. Spine. 1989;14:404–8.
26. Shaffer B, Jobe FW, Pink M, Perry J. Baseball batting. An electromygraphic study. Clin Orthop Relat Res. 1993;292:285–93.
27. Chow JW, Shim JH, Lim YT. Lower trunk muscle activity during the tennis serve. J Sci Med Sport. 2003;6:512–8.
28. McGill S, Juker D, Kropf P. Appropriately placed surface EMG electrodes reflect deep muscle activity (psoas, quadratus lumborum, abdominal wall) in the lumbar spine. J Biomech. 1996;29:1503–7.
29. McGill SM. Distribution of tissue loads in the low back during a variety of daily and rehabilitation tasks. J Rehabil Res Dev. 1997;34:448–58.
30. Axler CT, McGill SM. Low back loads over a variety of abdominal exercises: searching for the safest abdominal challenge. Med Sci Sports Exerc. 1997;29:804–11.
31. McGill SM. Low back stability: from formal description to issues for performance and rehabilitation. Exerc Sport Sci Rev. 2001;29:26–31.

32. McGill SM, Grenier S, Kavcic N, Cholewicki J. Coordination of muscle activity to assure stability of the lumbar spine. J Electromyogr Kinesiol. 2003;13:353–9.
33. Myer GD, Chu DA, Brent JL, Hewett TE. Trunk and hip control neuromuscular training for the prevention of knee joint injury. Clin Sports Med. 2008;27:425–48.
34. Escamilla RF, Babb E, DeWitt R, Jew P, Kelleher P, Burnham T, Busch J, D'Anna K, Mowbray R, Imamura RT. An electromyographic analysis of traditional and non-traditional abdominal exercises: implications for rehabilitation and training. Phys Ther. 2006a;86(5):656–71.
35. Escamilla RF, McTaggart MSC, Fricklas EJ, DeWitt R, Kelleher P, Taylor MK, Hreljac A, Moorman CT. An electromyographic analysis of commercial and common abdominal exercises: implications for rehabilitation and training. J Orthop Sports Phys Ther. 2006b;36(2):45–57.
36. Escamilla RF, Lewis C, Bell D, Bramblet G, Daffron J, Lambert S, Pecson A, Imamura R, Paulos L, Andrews JR. Core muscle activation in swiss ball exercises compared to traditional abdominal exercises. J Orthop Sports Phys Ther. 2010;40(5):265–76.
37. Wilk KE, Reinold MM, Macrina LC, Porterfield R, Devine KM, Suarez K, Andrews JR. Glenohumeral internal rotation measurements differ depending on stabilization techniques. Sports Health. 2009;1(2):131–6.
38. Ellenbecker TS, Roetert EP, Bailie DS, Davies GJ, Brown SW. Glenohumeral joint total rotation range of motion in elite tennis players and baseball pitchers. Med Sci Sports Exerc. 2002;34(12):2052–6.
39. Wilk KE, Macrina LC, Fleisig GS, Porterfield R, Simpson CD, Harker P, Paparesta N, Andrews JR. Correlation of glenohumeral internal rotation deficit and total rotational motion to shoulder injuries in professional baseball pitchers. Am J Sports Med. 2011;39:329–35.
40. Dines JS, Frank JB, Akerman M, et al. Glenohumeral internal rotation deficits in baseball players with ulnar collateral ligament deficiency. Am J Sports Med. 2009;37(3):566–70.
41. McClure P, Balaicuis J, Heiland D. A randomized controlled comparison of stretching procedures for posterior shoulder tightness. J Orthop Sports Phys Ther. 2007;37:108–14.
42. Laudner KG, Sipes RC, Wilson JT. The acute effects of sleeper stretches on shoulder range of motion. J Athl Train. 2008;43(4):359–63.
43. Manske RC, Meschke M, Porter A, Smith B, Reiman M. A randomized controlled single-blinded comparison of stretching versus stretching and joint mobilization for posterior shoulder tightness measured by internal rotation loss. Sports Health. 2010;2(2):94–100.
44. Moore SD, Laudner KG, McLoda TA, Shaffer MA. The immediate effects of muscle energy technique on posterior shoulder tightness: a randomized controlled trial. J Orthop Sports Phys Ther. 2011;41(6):400–7.
45. Carter AB, Kaminsky TW, Douex AT Jr, Knight CA, Richards JG. Effects of high volume upper extremity plyometric training on throwing velocity and functional strength ratios of the shoulder rotators in collegiate baseball players. J Strength Cond Res. 2007;21(1):208–15.
46. Reinold MM, Wilk KE, Reed J, et al. Interval sport programs: guidelines for baseball, tennis, and golf. J Orthop Sports Phys Ther. 2002;32:293–8.
47. Zheng N, Barrentine SW, Fleisig GS, Andrews JR. Kinematic analysis of swing in pro and amateur golfers. Int J Sports Med. 2008;29(6):487–93.
48. Ellenbecker TS, Wilk KE, Reinold MM, Murphy TF, Paine RM. Use of interval return programs for shoulder rehabilitation. In: Ellenbecker TS, editor. Shoulder rehabilitation: non operative treatment. New York: Theime; 2006.
49. Elliott B, Marsh T, Blanksby B. A three dimensional cinematographic analysis of the tennis serve. Int J Sports Biomech. 1986;2:260–71.
50. Morris M, Jobe FW, Perry J, Pink M, Healy BS. Electromyographic analysis of elbow function in the tennis players. Am J Sports Med. 1989;17:241–7.
51. Ellenbecker TS. Rehabilitation of shoulder and elbow injuries in tennis players. Clin Sports Med. 1995;14(1):87–110.
52. Fleisig G, Nicholls R, Elliott B, Escamilla R. Kinematics used by world class tennis players to produce high-velocity serves. Sports Biomech. 2003;2(1):51–71.
53. Marshall RN, Noffal GJ, Legnani G. Simulation of the tennis serve: factors affecting elbow torques related to medial epicondylitis. Paris: ISB. 1993.
54. Davis JT, Limpisvasti O, Fluhme D, et al. The effect of pitching biomechanics on the upper extremity in youth and adolescent baseball pitchers. Am J Sports Med. 2009;37:1484–91.

Index

J. S. Dines et al. (eds.), *Elbow Ulnar Collateral Ligament Injury*,
https://doi.org/10.1007/978-3-030-69567-5

V

W

Printed by Printforce, the Netherlands